CLINICAL ASTHMA
THEORY AND PRACTICE

Edited by

Jonathan A. Bernstein MD, FAAAAI, FACAAI, FACP, FACCP
Professor of Clinical Medicine, University of Cincinnati College of Medicine
Department of Internal Medicine, Division of Immunology/Allergy Section
Cincinnati, Ohio, USA

Mark L. Levy MBChB (Pret) FRCG
General Practitioner and Senior Research Fellow, Kenton Bridge Medical
Centre London, UK and Edinburgh University, UK

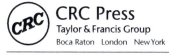
CRC Press
Taylor & Francis Group
Boca Raton   London   New York

CRC Press is an imprint of the
Taylor & Francis Group, an **informa** business

CRC Press
Taylor & Francis Group
6000 Broken Sound Parkway NW, Suite 300
Boca Raton, FL 33487-2742

© 2014 by Taylor & Francis Group, LLC
CRC Press is an imprint of Taylor & Francis Group, an Informa business

No claim to original U.S. Government works

Printed on acid-free paper
Version Date: 20131126

International Standard Book Number-13: 978-1-4665-8561-4 (Hardback)

Visit the Taylor & Francis Web site at
http://www.taylorandfrancis.com

and the CRC Press Web site at
http://www.crcpress.com

CLINICAL ASTHMA

THEORY AND PRACTICE

Dedication

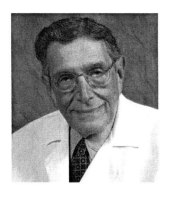

I dedicate this textbook to my father, I. Leonard Bernstein, MD, who was my role model, mentor, and colleague. His thirst for knowledge and devotion to teaching, research, and patient care were the qualities that inspired me to follow him into the field of allergy and clinical immunology. It is especially significant that this textbook focuses on asthma, as this "syndrome" was of particular interest to him, especially as it pertained to the workplace. Through my father, I was able to better appreciate how our understanding of the immunopathogenesis and physiology of asthma leading to improvement in its management and treatment has evolved dramatically over the past 60 years from a condition that was at one time considered to be a psychiatric illness to what is now recognized as a complex inflammatory lung disease influenced by a multitude of environmental and genetic determinants. I. Leonard Bernstein recognized early on that the effective management of asthma required a team approach, reflected in his early work with Dr. Tom Creer who developed the "Living with Asthma" educational model that became the prototypic design for all subsequent behavioral modification education programs. The selection of contributing authors for this book who trained in multiple specialties and disciplines reflects the holistic approach to asthma care advocated by my father. Therefore, it is anticipated that this book, which addresses the spectrum of basic and clinical issues pertaining to asthma, will be appealing to the asthma specialist, the primary care physician, and other ancillary health-care providers that manage asthma patients. Finally, like my father, who would not have been able to devote the amount of time to his profession without the dedicated support of his wife and my mother Miriam, I would be remiss in not expressing my deepest love and gratitude to my wife Lisa, who has been my greatest supporter and partner throughout my career and has given me four fantastic children: Alison, Joshua, Rebecca, and Caren.

Jonathan A. Bernstein

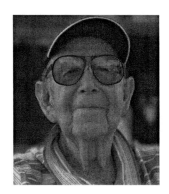

For my father, Hymie Levy.
His unstinting support and the example he set inspired my career.

Mark L. Levy

Contents

SECTION I   The Basics of Asthma

SECTION II   Diagnosis of Asthma

SECTION III   Asthma Triggers

SECTION IV   Asthma Education and Outcomes

SECTION V   Asthma Management and Treatments

SECTION VI   Asthma and Special Populations

SECTION VII   Approach to Asthma Worldwide and in the Primary Care Setting

Foreword

Asthma continues to be a major global problem, which is increasing in prevalence, especially in developing countries. Over 300 million people in the world now suffer from asthma. We have made enormous progress in asthma over the last 50 years with better understanding of its complex pathogenesis and we now have much more effective therapies, so that most patients are now able to lead normal lives. This has been the result of an enormous investment in research, so that the scientific literature is now vast and often difficult to integrate. That is why comprehensive and in-depth books like this are of enormous value in updating readers in a series of chapters written by world experts on this disease. The great strength of this volume is that it adopts a multidisciplinary approach, from basic mechanisms, including genetics, inflammation, immunology, and the identification of different endotypes, through to chapters on the clinical management of patients and how this may be improved. A major strength of the book is in its clinical chapters, which describe diagnosis, triggers, and clinical management in great detail, including the management of asthma in special populations. Of particular importance are the chapters dealing with asthma in the primary care setting, where most asthma is now managed.

Although we understand much more about asthma and have excellent therapies, provided they are used correctly, many unanswered questions remain. We do not know why only some people who are genetically predisposed develop asthma, why asthma appears to improve during adolescence and then often returns at some time in adulthood, or why some patients develop severe asthma—which appears to be a distinct disease. We still do not understand the different phenotypes and endotypes of asthma and how these should be treated differently. Inhaled corticosteroids have revolutionized asthma therapy but are not effective in all patients, and when discontinued, the disease returns. It has been difficult to find new therapies that match existing drugs. Biologics are useful in some patients and selective therapies may only be of value in distinct phenotypes of patients that will need to be identified by further research. We do not have a cure for asthma, or even a treatment that is truly disease modifying. Many of these issues are discussed in the chapters of the book from different perspectives. There is a wealth of information in this book and many people prefer to have a printed book than read different reviews online. The multidisciplinary nature of this book ensures that every aspect of asthma is discussed, providing an outstanding resource for anyone interested in this common disease from general practitioner to basic scientist. I congratulate Jonathan A. Bernstein and Mark L. Levy for bringing together such an excellent group of authors from around the world to give a very comprehensive summary of the state of the art in asthma.

Peter J. Barnes
Imperial College London

It is my distinct pleasure to provide an introduction to this excellent textbook entitled *Clinical Asthma: Theory and Practice*. Indeed, the editors, Drs. Jonathan A. Bernstein and Mark L. Levy, have compiled a set of timely topics and a distinguished panel of world-renowned authors to contribute to this book. The book is dedicated to Dr. Jonathan Bernstein's father, Dr. I. Leonard Bernstein, a leader in the field of allergy and immunology who made many significant contributions to advancing asthma care.

The book is divided into seven sections starting with the basics of asthma and ending with a section on the approach to asthma worldwide and in the primary care setting. The opening section begins with an excellent overview of the epidemiology of asthma and moves its way through the important topics of immunopathogenesis, the rapidly developing topic of genetics and the newly recognized area of endotypes and asthma.

The past 30 years have been marked by the introduction and ongoing revision of asthma guidelines for asthma care. These guidelines, as discussed in individual chapters, must address the individual needs of preschool children, older children, and adults and also allergic diseases, such as rhinitis, that are frequently associated with asthma. To understand the driving forces of asthma, attention is directed to viral infections, pertinent allergens, air pollutants, and exercise-induced asthma. In order to manage these triggers, detailed chapters are provided on the assessment of asthma control and the tools necessary to control the disease, specifically inhaler devices, asthma education, and the importance of assessing medication adherence.

To achieve overall asthma control, it is important to address those special needs of children, adolescents, adults, and the elderly in the principles of management. These topics are covered nicely in individual chapters devoted to these age groups. Separate chapters are also devoted to acute and life-threatening asthma in children and adults. It is not only important to discuss asthma by age, but also to consider associated conditions that can challenge the routine management of asthma, such as obesity, pregnancy, psychological disorders, and the impact of occupational settings. Timely tips on management of these associated conditions are provided.

The approaches to managing asthma can differ significantly across countries in relation to economy, health-care settings and availability of medications. The majority of asthma cases are managed in the primary care setting and we must develop a collaborative relationship among specialists, primary care physicians, and other health-care professionals in order to see a continued reduction in asthma mortality and morbidity. Although much of asthma care is still centered around the relief of symptoms, we are taking major steps in the direction of asthma prevention. This textbook, *Clinical Asthma: Theory and Practice*, highlights the importance of periodically stepping back, reviewing our progress and current knowledge, and projecting ways to further improve asthma management. I would like to thank the editors and authors for sharing their thoughts in moving forward to advance asthma care.

Stanley J. Szefler, MD
National Jewish Health and University of Colorado, Denver

Editors

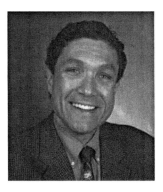

Dr. Jonathan A. Bernstein is professor of clinical medicine in the Department of Internal Medicine, Division of Immunology/Allergy Section at the University of Cincinnati Medical Center and director of clinical research for the Division of Immunology. He received his Bachelor of Arts from Kenyon College in 1981 and his medical degree from the University of Cincinnati College of Medicine in 1985. He completed his residency training in internal medicine at the Cleveland Clinic Hospital from 1985 to 1988 and his allergy/clinical immunology training at Northwestern University from 1988 to 1990. He has been a faculty member of the University of Cincinnati Department of Internal Medicine, Division of Immunology/Allergy Section and a partner of the Bernstein Allergy Group and Clinical Research Center since 1990.

Dr. Bernstein is actively involved in clinical and translational research, in addition to pharmaceutical research, patient care, and teaching. His current research involves a trimellitic anhydride immunosurveillance program, phenotyping chronic rhinitis subtypes, mechanisms of nonallergic rhinitis, seminal plasma hypersensitivity, hereditary and ACE-induced angioedema, chronic urticaria, and environmental interventions in the home and workplace. Dr. Bernstein is the director of clinical research at the University of Cincinnati and is a Drug Information Association (DIA)-certified investigator. He has extensive experience conducting multicenter and physician-initiated clinical therapeutic trials related to asthma, chronic obstructive pulmonary disease, rhinitis, urticaria, hereditary, and angiotensin-converting enzyme-induced angioedema. Dr. Bernstein has published over 165 peer-reviewed articles and clinical reviews, and 35 chapters on a variety of relevant topics in allergy and clinical immunology.

Dr. Bernstein is actively involved in the University of Cincinnati Allergy Fellowship Training Program and in the education of residents and medical students. He is a member of the board of directors for the American Academy of Asthma, Allergy, and Immunology. He is the editor-in-chief of the *Journal of Asthma* and on the editorial board of the *Journal of Allergy and Clinical Immunology*, *Annals of Allergy, Asthma and Immunology*, *Allergy Asthma Proceedings*, and *Journal of Angioedema*. Dr. Bernstein has been voted "best doctor" in Cincinnati from 1999 to 2013 and ranked by U.S. News and World Report as being in the top 1% of doctors in his specialty. He is a member of the University of Cincinnati Alpha Omega Alpha chapter.

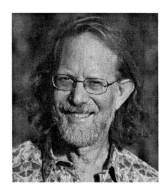

Dr. Mark L. Levy (MBChB [Pret], FRCGP) is a part-time general practitioner (GP) and respiratory lead for Harrow, in London, the United Kingdom, and also a senior clinical research fellow in the Allergy and Respiratory Research Group, Centre for Population Health Sciences: GP Section, University of Edinburgh. During 2011–2014 he was clinical lead for the U.K. National Review of Asthma Deaths (NRAD) being conducted by the Royal College of Physicians on behalf of the U.K. Department of Health.

He completed his medical training in Pretoria, South Africa, in 1974 and worked for two years in academic hospitals, including Chris Hani Baragwanath Academic and J.G. Strijdom Hospitals in Johannesburg. In January 1977, he left South Africa with his wife Celia and has since been actively involved in educational and research activities.

From 1991 to 1995, he chaired the educational committee of the North and West London Faculty of the Royal College of General Practitioners; in this role he was active in the design and implementation of courses for general practitioners and practice nurses. He was medical adviser to Greta Barnes, who started the Asthma Training Centre for nurses (now Education for Health) for a period of 10 years. His interest in respiratory medicine was developed through clinical research and he was one of the first to publish on delayed diagnosis of asthma, in the *BMJ* in 1984. The study demonstrated a 5-year delay and an average of 17 respiratory consultations in diagnosing asthma in children from the first presentation to a doctor. In 1987, he was one of the six founding members and subsequently first chairman and then editor of the Primary Care Respiratory Society U.K. (formerly the General Practitioners in Asthma Group). For 15 years, beginning in 1996, he was editor-in-chief of the *Primary Care Respiratory Journal*, which started as a newsletter and is now the second highest ranked primary care journal worldwide. He is currently one of four expert respiratory advisers for the National Institute for Clinical Excellence (NICE) Quality Outcomes Framework (QoF), which determines outcomes used in the payment process for delivery of primary care services in the U.K.

He has published over 140 papers and editorials in peer-reviewed journals (h-index 20) and co-authored 5 books, one of which, *Asthma at Your Fingertips*, for people with asthma, has been translated into a number of languages; an electronic version is currently being produced.

Together with Professor Onno van Schayck (Maastricht), he formed the Primary Care Scientific Group in the Clinical Assembly of the European Respiratory Society (ERS) and served as secretary and then chairman of this group for a total of 9 years. He has been a member of the U.K. Asthma Guideline development group (acute asthma) since 1992; was recently a member of the NICE Topic Expert Group, which developed and recently published quality outcomes for asthma; and was involved with the development of U.K. guidelines for occupational asthma, oxygen prescribing, and community-acquired pneumonia. He is a member of the Global Initiative for Asthma (GINA) board of directors.

In 2012, he received the Award for Service to Respiratory Medicine from the U.K. Association for Respiratory Technology and Physiology (ARTP), which is the sole professional organization for practitioners working in clinical respiratory physiology and technology within the United Kingdom.

Dr. Mark L. Levy's full curriculum vitae is available at www.consultmarklevy.com, and his wildlife photography is displayed at www.animalswild.com.

Contributors

Neil E. Alexis
Department of Pediatrics
University of North Carolina
Chapel Hill, North Carolina

Kimberly M. Avallone
Department of Psychology
University of Cincinnati
Cincinnati, Ohio

Pedro C. Avila
Division of Allergy-Immunology
Northwestern University
Chicago, Illinois

Leonard B. Bacharier
Department of Pediatrics
Washington University School
   of Medicine
St. Louis, Missouri

Sachin Baxi
Division of Immunology
Harvard Medical School
Boston, Massachusetts

Pallavi Bellamkonda
Department of Internal Medicine
Creighton University Medical Center
Omaha, Nebraska

Rachid Berair
Department of Infection, Immunity
   and Inflammation
University of Leicester
Leicester, United Kingdom

Jonathan A. Bernstein
Department of Internal Medicine
Division of Immunology/Allergy
   Section
University of Cincinnati College of
   Medicine
Cincinnati, Ohio

Eugene R. Bleecker
Center for Genomics and Personalized
   Medicine

Wake Forest University Health Sciences
Winston Salem, North Carolina

Louis-Philippe Boulet
Institute of Cardiology and
   Pneumology Quebec
Laval University
Québec City, Québec, Canada

Jean-Marie Bruzzese
Department of Child and Adolescent
   Psychiatry
New York University School
   of Medicine
New York, New York

Chris Carlsten
Department of Medicine
University of British Columbia
Vancouver, British Columbia

Thomas B. Casale
Department of Medicine
Creighton University
Omaha, Nebraska

Bradley Chipps
Capital Allergy and Respiratory
   Disease Center
Sacramento, California

Chris Cleveland
Division of Allergy-Clinical
   Immunology, National
   Jewish Health
University of Colorado Denver
Denver, Colorado

Chris J. Corrigan
Department of Asthma, Allergy
   and Respiratory Science
King's College London
and
Guy's and St. Thomas' Hospital NHS
   Foundation Trust
and

MRC and Asthma UK Centre in
   Allergic Mechanisms of Asthma
London, United Kingdom

Gina T. Cosia
Morgan Stanley Children's Hospital
   of New York Presbyterian
Columbia University Medical Center
New York, New York

Tolly G. Epstein
Division of Immunology, Allergy,
   and Rheumatology
University of Cincinnati
Cincinnati, Ohio

Claude S. Farah
Woolcock Institute of Medical
   Research
University of Sydney
Glebe, Australia

and

Sydney Medical School
University of Sydney
Camperdown, Australia

and

Department of Respiratory Medicine
Concord Hospital
Concord, Australia

Giovanni A. Fontana
Department of Critical Care Medicine
   and Surgery
University of Florence
Florence, Italy

Erick Forno
Division of Pediatric Pulmonary
   Medicine, Allergy, and Immunology
University of Pittsburgh
Pittsburgh, Pennsylvania

James L. Friedlander
Division of Immunology
Harvard Medical School
Boston, Massachusetts

Peter G. Gibson
School of Medicine and Public Health
University of Newcastle
Newcastle, Australia

and

Department of Respiratory and
    Sleep Medicine
John Hunter Hospital
New Lambton, Australia

and

Woolcock Institute of Medical
    Research
University of Sydney
Sydney, Australia

Paul A. Greenberger
Division of Allergy-Immunology
Department of Medicine
Northwestern University
Chicago, Illinois

Tari Haahtela
Skin and Allergy Hospital
Helsinki University Hospital
Helsinki, Finland

Pranabashis Haldar
Department of Infection, Immunity
    and Inflammation
University of Leicester
Leicester, United Kingdom

Fernando Holguin
Asthma Institute
University of Pittsburgh
Pittsburgh, Pennsylvania

Joy Hsu
Division of Allergy-Immunology
Northwestern University
Chicago, Illinois

Kristen M. Kraemer
Department of Psychology
University of Cincinnati
Cincinnati, Ohio

Federico Lavorini
Department of Internal Medicine
University of Florence
Florence, Italy

Mark L. Levy
Centre for Population Health Sciences
University of Edinburgh
Edinburgh, United Kingdom

Xingnan Li
Center for Genomics and Personalized
    Medicine
Wake Forest University Health
    Sciences
Winston Salem, North Carolina

Vanessa M. McDonald
School of Nursing and Midwifery
and
School of Medicine and Public Health
University of Newcastle
Newcastle, Australia

and

Department of Respiratory and
    Sleep Medicine
John Hunter Hospital
New Lambton, Australia

Alison C. McLeish
Department of Psychology
University of Cincinnati
Cincinnati, Ohio

Deborah A. Meyers
Center for Genomics and Personalized
    Medicine
Wake Forest University Health Sciences
Winston Salem, North Carolina

Paul M. O'Byrne
Department of Medicine
McMaster University
Hamilton, Ontario, Canada

Wanda Phipatanakul
Division of Immunology
Harvard Medical School
Boston, Massachusetts

Annabelle Quizon
Division of Pediatric Pulmonology
University of Miami
Miami, Florida

Christopher Randolph
Center for Allergy, Asthma and
    Immunology
Yale University
Waterbury, Connecticut

Helen K. Reddel
Woolcock Institute of Medical Research
University of Sydney
Glebe, Australia

and

Sydney Medical School
University of Sydney
and
Department of Respiratory Medicine
Royal Prince Alfred Hospital
Camperdown, Australia

Brian H. Rowe
Department of Emergency Medicine
University of Alberta
Edmonton, Alberta, Canada

Glenis K. Scadding
Academic Centre for Medical
    Education
University College London
London, United Kingdom

Guy Scadding
National Heart and Lung Institute
Imperial College London
London, United Kingdom

Beverley J. Sheares
Morgan Stanley Children's Hospital
    of New York Presbyterian
Columbia University
New York, New York

Aziz Sheikh
Allergy and Respiratory Research
    Group
Centre for Population Health Sciences
University of Edinburgh
Edinburgh, United Kingdom

Colin R. Simpson
Allergy and Respiratory Research
    Group
Centre for Population Health Sciences
University of Edinburgh
Edinburgh, United Kingdom

Rebecca E. Slager
Center for Genomics and Personalized
    Medicine
Wake Forest University Health Sciences
Winston Salem, North Carolina

Joseph D. Spahn
Department of Pediatrics
University of Colorado Denver
Denver, Colorado

Lora Stewart
Division of Allergy-Clinical
    Immunology, National Jewish
    Health
University of Colorado Denver
Denver, Colorado

John M. Weiler
Department of Internal Medicine
University of Iowa
Iowa City, Iowa

and

CompleWare Corporation
North Liberty, Iowa

Andrew G. Weinstein
Asthma Management Systems
Department of Pediatrics

Thomas Jefferson Medical University
Philadelphia, Pennsylvania

Barbara P. Yawn
Department of Research
Olmsted Medical Center
Rochester, Minnesota

and

University of Minnesota
Minneapolis, Minnesota

Section I

The Basics of Asthma

1 Epidemiology of Asthma
A Worldwide Perspective

Colin R. Simpson and Aziz Sheikh

CONTENTS

INTRODUCTION

Epidemiology is the study of the causes, distributions, occurrences, and patterns of disease in populations. Epidemiologists are therefore inherently interested in disease definitions (and subtypes) and data sources for estimating both numerators and denominators to establish measures of disease frequency, patterns, and outcomes.[1]

Asthma is now recognized as one of the most important chronic conditions in the world, resulting in considerable morbidity and, in some cases, mortality, and posing a high level of burden on health services and economies worldwide.[2] In the United States, the annual economic cost (direct health care and indirect lost of productivity) is estimated to be $56 billion.[3] While high-income countries are acknowledged to have the highest prevalence, the rate of asthma is also increasing in other countries, possibly as a result of adopting westernized lifestyles.[4] The World Health Organization (WHO) has estimated that 15 million disability-adjusted life years (DALYs) are lost annually due to asthma, representing 1% of the global disease burden.[5] Asthma, the most common chronic childhood disorder, is a common cause of school absence, regular medication use, and hospital admission.[6]

DEFINITIONS OF ASTHMA

Asthma is a disorder that can be defined by its clinical, physiological, and pathological characteristics. A major contribution to understanding asthma in the nineteenth century was made by Henry Hyde Salter (1823–1871), a lecturer in physiology and medicine at Charing Cross Hospital, London, U.K., who surmised that asthma could be caused by extrinsic factors (e.g., animal and vegetable emanations) and inflammation or congestion of mucous surfaces.[7] In the early twentieth century, asthma was widely believed to be a "neurosis" and the pharmacological relief of anxiety became a major therapeutic goal. Francis Rackemann (1887–1973) suggested protein sensitization as a possible cause of asthma, with patients categorized as intrinsic or extrinsic and diagnosed (and treated, often ineffectively) on the basis of skin test findings. Since then, and despite substantial research in the interim years, which has described asthma's pathogenesis, etiology, and epidemiology, an all-encompassing definition of asthma has remained elusive. In fact, it is now known that this condition is complex and manifests as many different clinical phenotypes (discussed later).[8] One of the main issues in diagnosing asthma is its variable and intermittent nature. The heterogeneity of an asthma diagnosis is most apparent in preschool-age children (5 years and younger). A differentiation between viral-associated wheeze and wheezing associated with prematurity or parental smoking is required. A diagnosis of asthma can be considered when wheezing is persistent, it is nocturnally worsened in the absence of a viral infection, and the patient is atopic (in the presence or absence of eczema). A diagnosis in adults can be challenging if hyperventilation, vocal cord dysfunction, or chronic obstructive pulmonary disease (COPD) is present. Occupational asthma may be immunoglobulin E (IgE)- or non-IgE-mediated and is caused by a spectrum of immunological agents or irritants. In the elderly in whom untreated asthma is common, the diagnosis can be confused with left ventricular dysfunction.[9]

The sources of information that clinicians in specialist settings use to diagnose asthma are: a history of the characteristic symptoms such as cough, particularly when awakened at night; wheeze, breathlessness (particularly in young children), and objective evidence of a spontaneously variable or reversible airflow obstruction measured using spirometry; a bronchoconstrictor response to histamine, methacholine, or mannitol; or daily or diurnal variability in peak expiratory flow rates. In primary care, the symptoms of wheeze and cough are often used to determine whether a patient has suspected asthma, and a recording of clinician-diagnosed asthma is made if a patient responds to a bronchodilator (airways reversibility) or an inhaled corticosteroid.[10]

ASTHMA PHENOTYPES

As yet, there is no universally agreed upon asthma phenotype.[9] The currently recognized phenotypes include early-onset, preadolescence asthma, which is mostly allergic in nature and driven by T-helper type 2 (Th2) processes. The later-onset eosinophilic phenotype is more common in women and adults older than 20 years and is pathologically associated with a thickening of the basement membrane zone and characterized by the presence of eosinophilia as determined by sputum, bronchoscopic, or blood analysis. Other phenotypes include: (1) exercise-induced asthma, a non-Th2 asthma where reactive bronchoconstriction occurs in response to sustained exercise, often in individuals with mild asthma; (2) obesity-related asthma; and (3) neutrophilic asthma, in which neutrophils are prominent in airway secretions during acute, severe asthma exacerbations and patients are relatively corticosteroid resistant.[11]

Other asthma phenotypes include aspirin intolerance, asthma related to chronic or persistent respiratory infections,[12] and steroid-resistant asthma, which has several subtypes and is thought to be characterized by the genetic background of the individual.

KEY MEASURES, STUDY DESIGNS EMPLOYED, AND DATA SOURCES AVAILABLE

Several epidemiological study designs and data sources can be used to try and estimate the frequency and patterns of asthma, and to understand the etiology of the disease. The frequency is usually estimated from cross-sectional or cohort studies. The risk factors are determined from cross-sectional, analytical (in particular, cohort and case–control studies), genetic, and experimental studies. The outcomes can be determined using cross-sectional and analytical study designs. Specifically collected or routinely available data can provide the data sources for these studies.

KEY MEASURES OF IMPORTANCE TO EPIDEMIOLOGISTS

The key measures of disease frequency (see Box 1.1) include: (i) the incidence of the disease, which is the rate of

---

BOX 1.1   KEY MEASURES OF DISEASE FREQUENCY

Incidence: The rate of occurrence of new cases in a period of time.

Cumulative incidence: The number of new cases divided by the population at risk.

Person-time incidence: The number of new cases divided by the person-time at risk.

Point prevalence: The proportion of a population with the disease at one point in time.

Period prevalence: The proportion of people with the disease presenting during a period of time, usually 1 year.

Lifetime (ever) prevalence: All people ever diagnosed with the disease in a population.

Case fatality ratio: The proportion of people who die from the disease.

---

occurrence of new cases (which can be expressed as a cumulative or person-time incidence); and (ii) the point, period, or lifetime prevalence. Other indicators of interest to epidemiologists include risk factors, which are any attribute, characteristic, or exposure of an individual that will increase (or reduce) their likelihood of developing a disease.[13] The case fatality ratio refers to the proportion of people who die from the disease.

STUDY DESIGNS

The prospective cohort study design follows groups of individuals who may not have manifested a disease or an outcome at the time of recruitment; it is often used to identify significant host and environmental influences on health and environmental exposures, and their effects on the expression of chronic disease later in life.[14] Large numbers are, however, typically required in order to identify significant differences in the incidence in exposed and nonexposed groups. This requirement for large numbers of cases usually means that cohort studies are expensive to establish and maintain. Genome-wide association studies (GWAS), whereby large cohorts of patients are recruited to detect novel genes and markers associated with disease susceptibility, are a more recently employed study design. GWAS have elicited new lines of enquiry into the etiology and pathogenesis of asthma. Cross-sectional surveys, in which the data and the means of collection are specified in advance and the study population is clearly defined, can be straightforward and inexpensive and are attractive to scientists studying the epidemiology of asthma.[15] Cross-sectional studies also allow exposures and disease status to be assessed simultaneously among individuals in a well-defined population. There can be a specific interval, such as a given calendar year during which a community-wide survey is conducted, or a fixed point in the course of events that varies in real time from person to person.[16]

Case–control studies can be used to explore risk factors by identifying people in a specified population with a disease or any other outcome variable such as asthma or wheezing (cases) and another group of people from the same population who are unaffected by the disease or outcome variable (controls). The occurrence of a possible exposure is then measured in both of these populations. One criterion of the control population is that it should represent people who would have been designated as cases if they had developed the disease. Another criterion of both cases and controls is that the start and the duration of exposure for these two groups be determined. The cases and controls need not be all-inclusive and may represent a subset of a population, for instance, preschool children under 5 years of age. Incidence case–control studies use new asthma presentations as cases and random samples as controls. Prevalence case-control study design uses prevalent cases and controls from non-cases.[17]

DATA SOURCES

Several data sources can be used for studying the epidemiology of asthma. Global population surveys include the International Study of Asthma and Allergies in Childhood (ISAAC) and the European Community Respiratory Health Survey (ECRHS). The ISAAC survey was conducted in 155 participating centers from 56 countries.[18] The survey was a simple one-page questionnaire self-completed by children. For asthma, children were asked whether they had "wheezing or whistling in the chest in the past 12 months." The minimum sample size requirement that was used to estimate the prevalence for each center was 1000 and the 12-month prevalence was calculated by dividing the number of positive responses by the number of completed questionnaires. In the majority of the centers, the response rate was in excess of 80%. The ECRHS was conceived in response to the growing evidence of increasing asthma morbidity and mortality in Europe and elsewhere in the first half of the 1990s.[19] Few studies of asthma prevalence prior to the ECHRS and the ISAAC used standardized definitions or instruments to measure the prevalence of asthma. ECRHS investigators set out to create a standardized questionnaire to estimate asthma prevalence and asthma treatment in young adults aged 20–44 years and, in a subsample, to create a more rigorous examination to determine atopic sensitization, bronchial lability, and suspected risk factors for asthma. Asthma was defined by the ECRHS as having an asthma attack in the last 12 months and/or currently taking asthma medication. The questionnaires were distributed to 140,000 adults in 22 countries and although the primary focus of the ECHRS was to make comparisons between countries in western Europe, other center locations such as Algeria, Australia, Canada, India, New Zealand, and the United States were included.

National health surveys such as those carried out in England and Scotland have also provided a useful source of information with regard to asthma prevalence and have given insights into the health needs of specific populations.[20]

The potential of using information from routine data sources to establish the accurate prevalence of a disease has also emerged.[21] The best routine information available is from developed countries, in particular the United Kingdom and Scandinavia.[22]

FREQUENCY OF ASTHMA

It has been estimated that globally 300 million people have asthma.[13]

FREQUENCY OF ASTHMA BY PLACE

Worldwide comparisons of prevalence rates were determined by the ISAAC cross-sectional survey. The highest prevalence (36.8%) was 20 times higher than the center with the lowest prevalence (1.6%) (Figure 1.1). The highest prevalence was found in English-speaking countries, including the United Kingdom, New Zealand, Australia, and the Republic of Ireland, followed by most centers in the Americas.[23] The lowest prevalence was reported in Indonesia, Greece, China, Taiwan, Uzbekistan, India, and Ethiopia. The ISAAC questionnaire was also used to survey a younger age group of 257,800 children aged 6–7 years and similar patterns of asthma symptoms were found.[18]

The ECRHS found that the incidence rates of childhood asthma (0–15 years) varied from 1.3 in Germany to 6.7 in Australia per 1000 person-years. The incidence of adult-onset asthma was 0.3 in the Netherlands and Belgium, and 2.9 in Australia. The ECRHS also found a sixfold variation in the prevalence of asthma, with high prevalence rates found in the Anglophone countries. A wide range of prevalence rates were observed between countries, with the highest in the Anglophone countries of Australia, the United Kingdom, the United States, and New Zealand, whereas the lowest prevalence rates were in the Mediterranean region and eastern Europe.

FREQUENCY OF ASTHMA BY PEOPLE

The frequency of asthma is highest during childhood and usually peaks in presentation at approximately 5 years of age with a secondary peak during adolescence (Figure 1.2). Women have a higher overall lifetime prevalence of asthma compared to men.[24] However, more male children present with asthma up until 15 years of age, at which time a switch to female preponderance occurs, which is sustained throughout adulthood.[25] The variation among different groups of people of different ethnic backgrounds and countries of birth has also been described; however, the interrelationship between ethnicity and migration is complex, as demonstrated by an analysis of data from the 1% Morbidity Survey in General Practice (MSGP) sample of the U.K. population, which found that all individuals (including whites) born outside the United Kingdom had a consistently lower incidence of asthma than those born within the United Kingdom.[26] Similarly, children born in mainland China who migrated to Hong Kong have

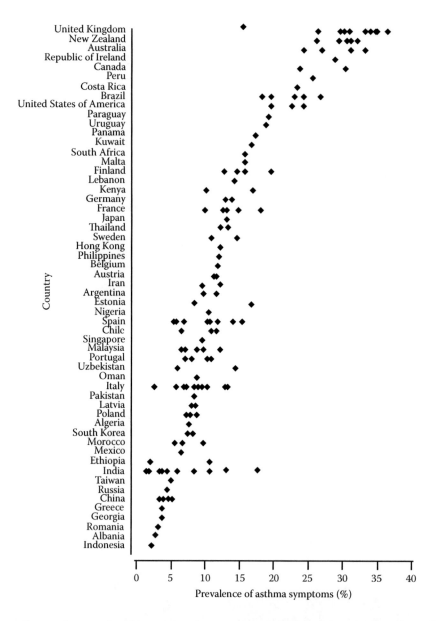

FIGURE 1.1 Twelve-month prevalences of self-reported asthma symptoms from written questionnaires. (Reproduced from The International Study of Asthma and Allergies in Childhood (ISAAC) Steering Committee, *Lancet*, 351, 1225–1232, 1998. With permission.)

been shown to be less likely to wheeze and have atopic disease than indigenous Hong Kong children.[27]

FREQUENCY OF ASTHMA OVER TIME

The observed trends in the rate of a disease are important, as any observed changes in the trajectory of prevalence and incidence can provide a major clue as to its causation, which may help in the strategy for disease prevention. The increasing incidence and prevalence of asthma in the twentieth century have been well documented, although there are still areas where little or no data on asthma trends are available, including parts of Asia, Africa, and South America.[4] Data from Finnish military conscripts, dating back to the 1920s, suggest that the very substantial increases in asthma prevalence began in the 1960s.[28] The ECHRS[29] found that in Spain, the incidence of asthma was

higher in recent birth cohorts than in earlier ones, with subjects born in or later than 1966 having a twofold higher risk of having had asthma attacks than the cohort born between 1946 and 1950. A number of studies in the United Kingdom carried out between the 1960s and the 1990s, in more or less the same population using the same or similar methodologies, have also reported inexorable rises in the prevalence of asthma and atopy.[30] In the MSGP survey of general practices in England and Wales (1991/1992), McCormick et al. found that, in the 10 years between 1981/1982 and 1991/1992, patient consulting rates for asthma increased threefold.[31] Most of these increases in prevalence from the 1980s were driven by the younger age groups. Indeed, during the 1980s, the MSGP4 found that incident rates in young children under 5 years of age in the United Kingdom increased from 192 to 339 per 10,000 people.[31] The increasing rate of new cases continued into the early 1990s,[32]

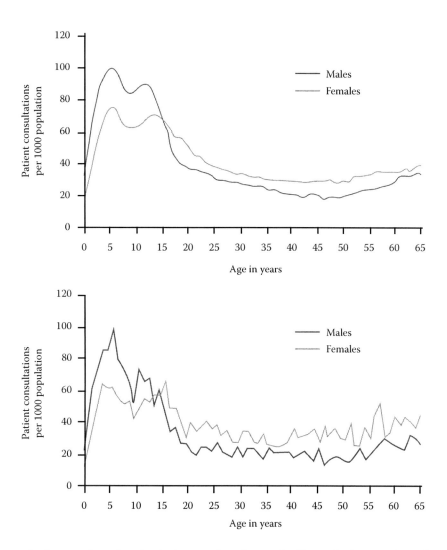

FIGURE 1.2 Patient consultation rates for asthma by single year of age for ages 0–65 years in the general practice research database (*top*) and the continuous morbidity recording database (*bottom*). (Reproduced from Osman, M., Hansell, A.L., Simpson, C.R., et al., *Prim. Care Respir. J.*, 16, 28–35, 2007. With permission.)

but began to plateau by the mid-1990s,[30] and since these studies were carried out, the trend of rising prevalence has either been less dramatic (from 10% in 2001 to 11% in 2005)[6] or it has been reversed to become a decline.[32] Hints that the plateau in prevalence may be real come from the ISAAC phase 3, completed 7 years after phase 1 (1998), which found that although increases in the prevalence of asthma symptoms were common, decreases in the 6–7-year age group did occur in some centers (Figure 1.3).[33] More recent declines in the incidence of asthma in the United Kingdom have also been reported (QRESEARCH database 2001–2005: 1.1%–0.8%).[6] Again, these declines were most marked in the youngest age groups.

There are inherent limitations in using cross-sectional surveys and databases to monitor disease trends with changes in morbidity being difficult to interpret.[34] These changes may reflect a number of varying factors, including changes in incidence, severity, patient expectations, health-care provision, pharmacological management, and changing diagnostic criteria.[35] Whether or not the plateau in asthma incidence and

prevalence merely reflects improvements in the quality of care of asthma or whether the plateau continues especially in the youngest age groups is an important area for further study.

RISK FACTORS FOR ASTHMA

The factors that may influence the development and expression of asthma include host factors, which are related to gene–environment interactions, family history, diet, infections, sex, obesity, and environmental agents including allergens (e.g., house-dust mite allergen), occupational sensitizers, tobacco smoke, outdoor pollution (e.g., car exhaust particulates), and indoor pollution (e.g., fumes from biomass fuels).[9]

The role of genetic variants as risk factors in the population in determining the geographical distribution of asthma prevalence should be noted. Fundamentally, much of asthma is likely to result from the effects of environmental factors on genetically susceptible persons. Allergic IgE-mediated asthma is strongly familial with the heritability of asthma

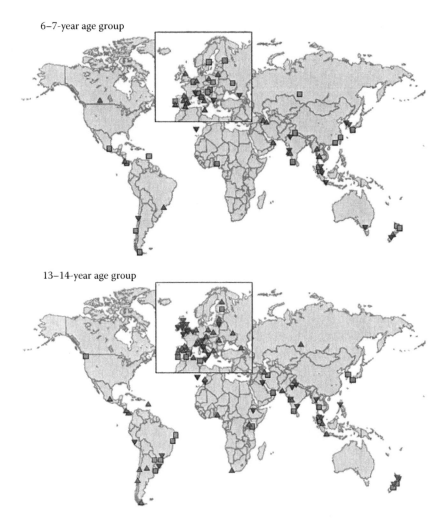

FIGURE 1.3 **(See color insert)** World map showing the direction of change in the prevalence of asthma symptoms for the 6–7-year age group and the 13–14-year age group. Each symbol represents a center. Blue triangle, prevalence reduced by ≥1 SE per year. Green square, little change (<1 SE). Red triangle, prevalence increased by ≥1 SE per year. (Reproduced from Asher, M.I., Montefort, S., Björkstén, B., et al., *Lancet*, 368, 733–743, 2006. With permission.)

being 75%.[36] Studies in identical twins have also demonstrated that 50% of the susceptibility to asthma is due to genetic determinants.[37] GWAS have found genes that may play a role in the development of asthma, for instance, the null allele for the gene encoding filaggrin (*2282del4* and *R501X*).[38] Filaggrin is expressed in the outer epidermis and the oral and nasal mucosa, and helps in the formation of the epithelial barrier, which may impede allergen entry and thereby prevent allergic sensitization. Other GWAS studies have found genes related to asthma, including *ORMDL₃*, which belongs to a family of genes that encode transmembrane proteins anchored in the endoplasmic reticulum.[39] *CCR5Delta32*, which is thought to control pathogen entry into cells, has been found to be associated with asthma in childhood, but not adults.[40] The *ADAM33* gene has a role in the production of ADAM proteins. The ADAM proteins are membrane-anchored metalloproteases with diverse functions, including the shedding of cell-surface proteins such as cytokines and cytokine receptors, which play a role in asthma.[41] It is also possible that variations in asthma may be due to differences in the proportion of individuals in different ethnic groups who carry known or hitherto unknown

genetic polymorphisms[42] and that ethnic variability exists in important gene defects such as filaggrin.[38]

Cross-sectional studies have been used to investigate the effect of risk factors on asthma, in particular, the interaction of dietary factors and asthma. With the westernization of many countries, dietary changes have occurred, including increased use of margarine and vegetable oils. These products contain ω-6 polyunsaturated fatty acids (PUFAs), which are thought to promote an inflammatory environment that favors asthma. Another dietary change that has occurred is a decrease in the consumption of ω-3 PUFAs such as eicosapentaenoic acid present in oily fish, which is thought to have an anti-inflammatory role.[43] Cross-sectional studies have shown beneficial associations between foods containing ω-3 PUFAs and asthma.[44] However, when interventions using dietary supplementation with PUFA were carried out, no clear evidence of any benefits was found.[24] Although no randomized controlled trials have been carried out, evidence from epidemiological studies is supportive with respect to vitamins A, D, and E; zinc; fruits and vegetables; and a Mediterranean diet, for the prevention of asthma.[45] The positive association between diet and asthma may largely reflect, in part, the major limitations of bias and confounding and effect modification. There is difficulty in determining the effect of an exposure (such as diet) within a population on disease occurrence while accounting for factors that correlate with both the exposure and the outcome (confounding) and effect modification, in which the magnitude of the effect on the outcome differs between groups. The recommended adjustments for confounding in studies of diet and asthma include maternal or child characteristics, socioeconomic status, environmental exposures, and other dietary factors. Effect modifiers where interactions should be tested and stratification considered include a family history of disease, season of birth or season of ascertainment of dietary factors, sex, race/ethnicity, place of residence, and breastfeeding.[46]

The exposure to respiratory infections early in life is thought to play a role in asthma. The Oslo Birth Cohort Study recruited 3048 children born in the two main birth clinics in Oslo during a 15-month period beginning in 1992.[47] Questionnaires were allocated to the children's parents at the ages of 6, 12, 18, and 24 months, and at 10 years of age a comprehensive questionnaire was administered to 2540 of 2985 children of the birth cohort. It was found that exposure to lower respiratory tract infections and croup during the first year of life increased the chance of developing asthma by the age of 10 years. Several disadvantages of the cohort methodology were highlighted.[48] One of the major problems of this work was selection bias as a consequence of "dropout" or the failure of subjects to continue in the study (20% of cases had been excluded or had dropped out of this study). However, the authors argued that exclusion and dropout were not related to the determinants of interest and would therefore not be an explanation for the observed relations between infant infection and the risk of asthma.

Significant sex differences in the prevalence of asthma, particularly around adolescence, have led to hypotheses regarding the role of the sex hormones estrogen (which has a proinflammatory effect) and testosterone (which has an antiinflammatory effect).[25] The systemic inflammatory milieu resulting from obesity has also been suggested as a possible risk factor for asthma. This work has been complicated, however, by the physiological alterations in pulmonary physiology caused by obesity, leading to the confusion of asthma with dyspnea and other respiratory symptoms.[49]

It has been widely recognized that air pollutants, which take the form of ambient photochemical oxidants, may exacerbate existing asthma. However, in westernized countries, there was less certainty of a link between pollutants and increases in asthma and atopy.[50] To investigate any link between pollution and allergic disease, Von Mutius and colleagues carried out studies comparing atopy in schoolchildren between Munich (a city in the former West Germany) and Leipzig (a city in East Germany) soon after German reunification. They found that the less polluted and the more westernized lifestyle of Munich had far higher rates of atopy.[51] These findings prompted the study of possible environmental contributors to asthma, in particular for countries in transition from subsistence to affluent consumer economies.[52] It is now largely acknowledged that environmental factors differ between countries, and what may

affect one population may not necessarily influence asthma risk in another; for example, evidence from the ISAAC study suggests that pollution may not be a causal factor for the development of asthma per se (as opposed to asthma exacerbations which may be related), as no correlation between air pollution and asthma prevalence was found.[53]

Another major risk factor for asthma is cigarette smoke. Evidence exists that exposure in utero and in childhood can increase the risk of respiratory symptoms[54] and that, at least in young children, maternal smoking is linked with higher rates of wheezing and recurrent respiratory symptoms.[55] It is acknowledged that smoky environments are unlikely to be the sole cause of the rising asthma prevalence in westernized countries as cigarette smoking has declined dramatically since the early 1970s.[56]

OUTCOMES (MORBIDITY, HEALTH-CARE UTILIZATION, MORTALITY)

Observing the differences and trends in outcomes is important. For clinicians, improving outcomes for patients with asthma is the main goal. Patient outcomes that are more easily quantified at a population level include the number of asthma exacerbations (caused by poor symptom control), primary care consultation frequency, visits to Accident and Emergency Departments, hospitalizations, and deaths. The global rates of mortality are thought to be considerable with 250,000 deaths per year with 1 in every 250 deaths attributable to asthma.[57] Deaths from asthma are most apparent in low- and middle-income countries and in high-income countries where wide socioeconomic disparities and inequitable access to health care exist.[5] Deaths and hospitalizations in these areas are also increasing. For instance, in the United States from 1980 to 1999, the asthma hospitalization and mortality rates grew by 1.4% and 3.4% per year, respectively, with children aged 0–4 years having the largest increase in prevalence and healthcare use, but with adolescents having the highest mortality.[58]

Within-country variations in outcomes by ethnicity are of interest. However, the international data are limited. The best data on ethnic variations come from the United States and the United Kingdom, where studies have, for close to two decades, consistently demonstrated poorer outcomes in black and South Asian ethnic minority groups.[59] In the United States, for instance, the burden of asthma has been found to be disproportionately higher in black children, with large racial disparities for hospitalizations and mortality. When compared with white children, black children were more than three times as likely to be hospitalized and four times as likely to die from asthma.[58] However, the reasons for these poor outcomes remain unclear. A systematic review and a meta-analysis of U.K. data have demonstrated that the differences between ethnic groups within countries—which are substantial—could not be explained by the differences in asthma prevalence, as the prevalence was found to be lower in the ethnic groups in question.[60] Although more robust data from the United Kingdom suggest that the prevalence of multiple wheeze (a proxy for asthma) is high in South Asian children, who are also more likely (than white children) to be hospitalized and, as such, have more persistent and possibly severe asthma.[61] Possible reasons for the increased risk of exacerbations, hospital admissions, and near-fatal episodes in these groups include: (1) an increased genetic risk of severe disease; (2) the impact of migration; (3) an increased risk of exposure to environmental trigger factors; (4) differences in health beliefs and consequently health-seeking behavior; (5) socioeconomic marginalization; (6) poorer quality of asthma care; and (7) differential effectiveness of treatments.[62] Another factor that complicates the use of epidemiological data to understand the reasons for poorer outcomes (and also higher prevalence) includes findings which suggest that many who have migrated from economically developing countries with private health-care systems have only a limited understanding of the notion of prophylactic medication use and are reluctant to use inhaled corticosteroids or other controller treatments when in relatively good health, particularly when coupled with a poor understanding of the disease.[63] Added to this is the persistent problem of institutional deficiencies in care, which disproportionately affect minority ethnic people.[64] The adverse effects of socioeconomic circumstances are also important to consider, as many of those from low-income backgrounds may view their asthma as less of a priority than other day-to-day problems.[64] Low-income families are also less likely to proactively self-manage and are more likely to crisis manage their asthma.[65,66] In such circumstances, individuals may bypass primary care and use the hospital emergency department as their primary place for asthma care.[67]

IMPLICATIONS FOR POLICY, PRACTICE, AND FUTURE RESEARCH

A continuing increase in the number of people with asthma worldwide over the next two decades has been predicted such that it is estimated that there may be an additional 100 million people with asthma by 2025.[5] This will largely result from increases in the proportion of the world's population living in urban areas, in particular in low- to middle-income countries. It is likely, therefore, that without improved access to treatments, hospitalizations and mortality from asthma are likely to increase. As changes in the overall susceptibility of the population to the development of asthma are unlikely to have occurred, the increases in asthma cases are more likely to be due to many different environmental changes, each exerting its own small influences in different people at different ages, living different lifestyles in urban or rural environments.[68] Periodic fluctuations in mortality and the remarkable and still unexplained rise (and peak in high-income countries) in the frequency of asthma across recent decades have been the focus of intensive research, but with mixed and inconclusive findings with regard to asthma etiology. Attention should also be given to identifying the relative importance of risk factors in people living and emigrating from low- to middle-income countries. This lack of understanding may partly be due to a systematic marginalization of many minority ethnic groups from asthma studies,[69] and

it is important that the substantial heterogeneity, which may exist within different ethnic groups with respect to different asthma phenotypes, is investigated.[8]

Unfortunately, due to the complex nature of asthma, purely descriptive studies, even of the magnitude of the ISAAC and the ECHRS, are of relatively limited value when attempting to investigate the frequency and trends and the etiology of a disease (although any new etiological hypothesis will have to fit with what is being shown in these large global surveys).[70] There is, therefore, a need for well-constructed, longitudinal studies that allow the temporal nature of the relationship between exposure and outcome to be studied and firmer conclusions to be drawn. This approach can be both expensive to implement and difficult to ensure adequate follow-up rates over time. In high-income countries, recent advances in physicians' use of electronic patient records[21] and in the linkage between routine data sets[71] may allow a range of factors that are important in relation to allergic disease etiology and outcomes to be assessed and controlled for. Using record linkage of such data (with explicit patient and physician consent), it is also possible to recruit patients into relatively short-term cohort studies and then prospectively collect long-term routine data at relatively little cost. With the prospect of whole population data linkages being made available in the near future, we may not need to wait long for such studies to be initiated.[72] Unlocking whether global differences in asthma prevalence, the increasing rates found in low- to middle-income countries, and poorer outcomes are due to a combination of genetic and early-life environmental factors, or the lack of preventative-related factors are also research priorities that need to be addressed further.

REFERENCES

1. Last JM. *A Dictionary of Epidemiology*. New York: Oxford University Press, 2001.
2. Gupta R, Anderson HR, Strachan DP, et al. International trends in admissions and drug sales for asthma. *Int J Tuberc Lung Dis* 2006;10:138–145.
3. Barnett SB, Nurmagambetov TA. Costs of asthma in the United States: 2002–2007. *J Allergy Clin Immunol* 2011;127:145–152.
4. Anandan C, Nurmatov U, van Schayck OC, et al. Is the prevalence of asthma declining? Systematic review of epidemiological studies. *Allergy* 2010;65:152–167.
5. Masoli M, Fabian D, Holt S, et al. The global burden of asthma: Executive summary of the GINA Dissemination Committee report. *Allergy* 2004;59:469–478.
6. Simpson CR, Sheikh A. Trends in the epidemiology of asthma in England: A national study of 333,294 patients. *J R Soc Med* 2010;103:98–106.
7. McFadden ER. A century of asthma. *Am J Respir Crit Care Med* 2004;170:215–221.
8. Anon. A plea to abandon asthma as a disease concept. *Lancet* 2006;368:705.
9. Global Initiative for Asthma. *Global Strategy for Asthma Management and Prevention*. Available at: http://www.ginasthma.org/uploads/users/files/GINA_Report2011_May4.pdf [Last accessed 25th July 2012].

10. Holgate ST, Frew AJ. Choosing therapy for childhood asthma. *N Engl J Med* 1997;337:1690–1692.

11. Wenzel SE. Asthma phenotypes: The evolution from clinical to molecular approaches. *Nature* 2012;18:716–725.

12. Bel EH. Clinical phenotypes of asthma. *Curr Opin Pulm Med* 2003;10:44–50.

13. World Health Organization. *Health Topics: Risk Factors.* Available at: http://www.who.int/topics/risk_factors/en/ [Last accessed 18/07/2012].

14. Kuh D, Ben-Shlomo Y, Lynch J, et al. Life course epidemiology. *J Epidemiol Commun Health* 2003;57:778–783.

15. Nahhas M, Bhopal R, Anandan C, et al. Prevalence of allergic disorders among primary school-aged children in Madinah, Saudi Arabia: Two-stage cross-sectional survey. *PLoS One* 2012;7:e36848.

16. Hennekens CH, Buring JE. *Epidemiology in Medicine.* Philadelphia: Lippincott Williams & Wilkins, 1987.

17. Pearce N. Classification of epidemiological study designs. *Int J Epidemiol* 2012;41:393–397.

18. Worldwide variations in the prevalence of asthma symptoms: The International Study of Asthma and Allergies in Childhood (ISAAC). *Eur Respir J* 1998;12:315–335.

19. Janson C, Anto J, Burney P, et al. The European Community Respiratory Health Survey: What are the main results so far? European Community Respiratory Health Survey II. *Eur Respir J* 2001;18:598–611.

20. Anandan C, Gupta R, Simpson CR, et al. Epidemiology and disease burden from allergic disease in Scotland: Analyses of national databases. *J R Soc Med* 2009;102:431–442.

21. Anandan C, Simpson CR, Fischbacher C, et al. Exploiting the potential of routine data to better understand the disease burden posed by allergic disorders: Strengths, limitations and future directions in UK datasets. *Clin Exp Allergy* 2006;36:866–871.

22. Punekar YS, Sheikh A. Establishing the incidence and prevalence of clinician-diagnosed allergic conditions in children and adolescents using routinely collected data from general practices. *Clin Exp Allergy* 2009;39:1209–1216.

23. Netuveli G, Hurwitz B, Sheikh A. Lineages of language and the diagnosis of asthma. *J R Soc Med* 2007;100:19–24.

24. Anandan C, Nurmatov U, Sheikh A. Omega 3 and 6 oils for primary prevention of allergic disease: Systematic review and meta-analysis. *Allergy* 2009;64:840–848.

25. Osman M, Hansell A, Simpson CR, et al. Gender specific presentations for asthma, allergic rhinitis and eczema to primary care. *Prim Care Respir J* 2007;16:28–35.

26. Netuveli G, Hurwitz B, Levy M, et al. Ethnic variations in UK asthma frequency, and health service use: A systematic review and meta-analysis. *Lancet* 2005;365:312–317.

27. Wong GWK, Leung TF, Ma Y, et al. Symptoms of asthma and atopic disorders in pre-school children: Prevalence and risk factors. *Clin Exp Allergy* 2007;37:174–179.

28. Haahtela T, Lindholm H, Bjorksten F, et al. Prevalence of asthma in Finnish young men. *BMJ* 1990;301:266–268.

29. Sunyer J, Antó JM, Tobias A, et al. Generational increase of self-reported first attack of asthma in fifteen industrialized countries. European Community Respiratory Health Study (ECRHS). *Eur Respir J* 1999;14:885–891.

30. Anderson HR, Gupta R, Strachan D, et al. 50 years of asthma: UK trends from 1955 to 2004. *Thorax* 2007;62:85–90.

31. McCormick A, Fleming D, Charlton J. *Morbidity Statistics from General Practice. Fourth National Study 1991–1992.* London: HMSO, 1995.

32. Soriano JB, Kiri VA, Maier WC, et al. Increasing prevalence of asthma in UK primary care during the 1990s. *Int J Tuberc Lung Dis* 2003;7:415–421.

33. Asher MI, Montefort S, Björkstén B, et al. Worldwide time trends in the prevalence of symptoms of asthma, allergic rhinoconjunctivitis, and eczema in childhood: ISAAC Phases One and Three repeat multicountry cross-sectional surveys. *Lancet* 2006;368:733–743.

34. Magnus P, Jaakkola JJ. Secular trend in the occurrence of asthma among children and young adults: Critical appraisal of repeated cross sectional surveys. *BMJ* 1997;314:1795–1799.

35. Simpson CR, Helms PJ, Lee AJ, et al. Changing incidence of respiratory presentations in primary care; fact or artefact? *Arch Dis Child* 2005;90:982–983.

36. Cookson W. The alliance of genes and environment in asthma and allergy. *Nature* 1999;402(Suppl):B5–B11.

37. Paitno CM, Martinez FD. Interactions between genes and environment in the development of asthma. *Allergy* 2001;56:279–286.

38. Van den Oord RA, Sheikh A. Filaggrin gene defects and risk of developing allergic sensitisation and allergic disorders: Systematic review and meta-analysis. *BMJ* 2009;339:b2433.

39. Moffatt MF, Kabesch M, Liang L. Genetic variants regulating ORMDL3 expression contribute to the risk of childhood asthma. *Nature* 2007;448:470–473.

40. Srivastava P, Helms PJ, Stewart D, et al. Association of CCR5Delta32 with reduced risk of childhood but not adult asthma. *Thorax* 2003;58:222–226.

41. Van Eerdewegh P, Little RD, Dupuis J, et al. Association of the ADAM33 gene with asthma and bronchial hyperresponsiveness. *Nature* 2002;418:426–430.

42. Hersh CP, Raby BA, Soto-Quiros ME, et al. Comprehensive testing of positionally cloned asthma genes in two populations. *Am J Respir Crit Care Med* 2007;176:849–857.

43. Kim J-H, Ellwood PE, Asher MI. Diet and asthma: Looking back moving forward. *Resp Res* 2009;10:49.

44. Devereux G, Seaton A. Diet as a risk factor for atopy and asthma. *J Allergy Clin Immunol* 2005;115(6):1109–1117.

45. Nurmatov U, Devereux G, Sheikh A. Nutrients and foods for the primary prevention of asthma and allergy: Systematic review and meta-analysis. *J Allergy Clin Immunol* 2011;127:724–733.

46. Nurmatov U, Nwaru BI, Devereux G, et al. Confounding and effect modification in studies of diet and childhood asthma and allergies. *Allergy* 2012;67:1041–1059.

47. Nafstad P, Brunekreef B, Skrondal A, et al. Early infections, asthma, and allergy: 10-year follow-up of the Oslo Birth Cohort. *Pediatrics* 2005;116:255–262.

48. Nafstad P, Magnus P, Jaakkola JJ. Early respiratory infections and childhood asthma. *Pediatrics* 2000;106:E38.

49. Beuther DA, Weiss ST, Sutherland ER. Obesity and asthma. *Am J Respir Crit Care Med* 2006;174:112–119.

50. Britton J. Dietary fish oil and airways obstruction. *Thorax* 1995;50(Suppl 1):S11–S15.

51. Von Mutius E, Fritzsch C, Weiland SK, et al. Prevalence of asthma and allergic disorders among children in united Germany: A descriptive comparison. *BMJ* 1992;305:1395–1399.

52. Hijazi N, Abalkhail B, Seaton A. Diet and childhood asthma in a society in transition: A study in urban and rural Saudi Arabia. *Thorax* 2000;55:775–779.

53. The International Study of Asthma and Allergies in Childhood (ISAAC) Steering Committee. Worldwide variation in prevalence of symptoms of asthma, allergic rhinoconjunctivitis, and atopic eczema: ISAAC. *Lancet* 1998;351:1225–1232.

54. Mannino DM, Moorman JE, Kingsley B, et al. Health effects related to environmental tobacco smoke exposure in children in the United States: Data from the third National Health and Nutrition Examination Survey. *Arch Pediatr Adolesc Med* 2001;155:36–41.

55. Burr ML, Verrall C, Kaur B. Social deprivation and asthma. *Respir Med* 1997;91:603–608.

56. The Scottish Executive. *The Scottish Health Survey 1998.* Edinburgh: The Stationary Office, 2000.

57. World Health Organization. *Global Surveillance, Prevention and Control of Chronic Respiratory Diseases: A Comprehensive Approach, 2007.* Geneva: WHO, 2012.

58. Akinbami LJ, Schoendorf KC. Trends in childhood asthma: Prevalence, health care utilization, and mortality. *Pediatrics* 2002;110:315–322.

59. Simpson CR, Sheikh A. Understanding the reasons for poor asthma outcomes in ethnic minorities: Welcome progress, but important questions remain. *Clin Exp Allergy* 2007;37:1730–1732.

60. Netuveli G, Hurwitz B, Sheikh A. Ethnic variations in incidence of asthma episodes in England & Wales: National study of 502,482 patients in primary care. *Respir Res* 2005;6:120–126.

61. Kuehni CE, Strippoli M-PF, Low N, et al. Wheeze and asthma prevalence and related health-service use in white and south Asian preschool children in the UK. *Clin Exp Allergy* 2007;37:1738–1746.

62. Sheikh A, Griffiths C. Tackling ethnic inequalities in asthma. We now need results. *Respir Med* 2005;99:381–383.

63. Myers P, Ormerod LP. Increased asthma admission rates in Asian patients: Blackburn. *Respir Med* 1992;86:297–300.

64. Zoratti EM, Havstad S, Rpdriguez J, et al. Health service use by African Americans and Caucasians with asthma in a managed care setting. *Am J Respir Crit Care Med* 1998;158:371–377.

65. Moudgil H, Honeybourne D. Differences in asthma management between white European and Indian subcontinent ethnic groups living in socio-economically deprived areas in the Birmingham (UK) conurbation. *Thorax* 1998;53:490–494.

66. Griffiths C, Kaur G, Gantley M, et al. Influences on hospital admission for asthma in south Asian and white adults: Qualitative interview study. *BMJ* 2001;323:962–966.

67. Duran-Tauleria E, Rona RJ. Geographical and socio-economic variations in the prevalence of asthma symptoms in English and Scottish children. *Thorax* 1999;54:476–481.

68. Seaton A, Godden DJ, Brown K. Increase in asthma: A more toxic environment or a more susceptible population? *Thorax* 1994;49:171–174.

69. Sheikh A, Panesar SS, Lasserson T, et al. Recruitment of ethnic minorities to asthma studies. *Thorax* 2004;59:634.

70. Lewis S. ISAAC-a hypothesis generator for asthma? *Lancet* 1998;351:1220–1221.

71. Fischbacher CM, Bhopal R, Povey C, et al. Record linked retrospective cohort study of 4.6 million people exploring ethnic variations in disease: Myocardial infarction in south Asians. *BMC Public Health* 2007;7:142.

72. Scottish Health Informatics Programme. *SHIP Overview.* Available at: http://www.scot-ship.ac.uk/overview [Last accessed 4th July 2012].

2 Immunopathogenesis

Chris J. Corrigan

CONTENTS

CASE PRESENTATION

Jack is a 56-year-old patient who first developed breathlessness and chest tightness at the age of 42. He had no history of childhood asthma or atopic diseases. He had smoked a few cigarettes daily for 2 or 3 years in his youth but did not continue this habit. Spirometry confirmed airway obstruction, which was significantly, but not completely, reversible, consistent with a diagnosis of asthma associated with persistent airway obstruction. There was also a significant degree of gas trapping with elevated residual volume. Jack was treated routinely with inhaled corticosteroids and bronchodilators, which afforded some control of his symptoms, but he remained breathless nearly every day and suffered from two or three admissions to hospital almost every year with presumed infective exacerbations of his disease, which he consistently claimed showed little response to the courses of oral corticosteroid therapy that he was invariably prescribed in these situations. A formal trial of oral corticosteroid therapy for 2 weeks was not associated with a significant (<10%) improvement in his forced expiratory volume in 1 sec (FEV$_1$). A computed tomography (CT) scan of his chest showed generally thickened bronchial walls, consistent with asthma, but no bronchiectasis or interstitial lung disease. Bronchial biopsies taken during a fiber-optic bronchoscopy showed that while there were some infiltrating mucosal eosinophils, neutrophils predominated. Similarly, induced sputum samples showed 6% neutrophils but <2% eosinophils. Jack was treated with a macrolide antibiotic for 3 days each week in addition to his inhaled therapy. This did not convincingly impact his day-to-day symptoms, but it did reduce his acute admissions to hospital.

INTRODUCTION

As a testimony to the inadequacy of current asthma management, nearly 1000 asthmatics still die each year in the United Kingdom. One of the characteristics of patients dying of asthma is the exuberant inflammatory reaction in their airways and the blockage of the airway lumen by thick, inspissated sputum, causing asphyxiation. This has focused attention on the importance of asthma as an inflammatory disease, and the fact that, for a variety of reasons, treatment is still imperfect.

At the same time, the recent availability of biological agents to target very specific pathways thought to be pivotal to the perceived pathophysiological mechanisms of asthma has produced confusing signals in the sense that, in general, they have not been the panacea that was hoped for; if anything, they appear to target a small subset of the asthmatic population, calling into question the validity of these targets and our entire concept of the pathophysiology of asthma.

This chapter contains an account of how the perception of the pathophysiology of asthma has changed in recent decades, the lessons learned from trials of new therapies in real life, and a brief pointer toward future research directions.

CLINICAL PATHOLOGY OF ASTHMA

Asthma may be clinically defined as a syndrome of variable airway obstruction and bronchial hyperresponsiveness. These fundamental abnormalities may result in a variety of symptoms, which vary in prominence between patients. A further variation in the symptomatology of asthma arises from the fact that symptoms are typically diurnally variable according to the endogenous circadian plasma cortisol profile (worse when endogenous production is lowest in the early hours of the morning, or the opposite if the circadian rhythm is reversed), and by the fact that exogenous, environmental trigger factors for the acute exacerbation of airway obstruction and bronchial hyperresponsiveness can be identified in some, but not all patients, and vary between patients. Thus, it is not clear if asthma is driven and triggered exclusively by external environmental stimuli or whether the disease partly reflects inherent disorders of those components of the airways that regulate resistance to airflow, principally the bronchial smooth muscle, but also the epithelial and submucosal linings, which, when edematous, can reduce the internal caliber of the airways. The key clinical features of asthma include:

Variable airway obstruction. Airway obstruction in asthma, as measured by spirometry, may vary spontaneously from none to severe in the course of minutes to hours, and improves after suitable therapy. Breathlessness and impaired exercise tolerance in asthmatics arise from the increased ventilatory effort that is required to move air in and out of abnormally narrow airways and from the obstruction of the small airways, which causes "gas trapping" in the alveoli, which, in turn, results in hyperinflation of the chest and reduced tidal volume. Airway obstruction also results in a feeling of tightness in the chest, which may be perceived as wheeze.

Nonspecific bronchial hyperreactivity. Nonspecific bronchial hyperreactivity refers to the tendency of the smooth muscle cells of asthmatic airways to constrict in response to a very wide variety of nonspecific (i.e., nonimmunological) environmental as well as pharmacological stimuli (including, for example, cold air, smoke, exercise, aerosol sprays, and dust) that do not cause clinically significant bronchoconstriction in nonasthmatics. The mechanism of this remarkable phenomenon remains obscure. It is further exacerbated by excessive mucus production and edema of the airway mucosa, both of which further narrow the internal airway lumen, increasing the degree of obstruction produced by a given degree of smooth muscle constriction. Bronchial hyperreactivity causes excessive cough and contributes to bronchospasm. Again, different stimuli may provoke bronchospasm in different patients.

HISTOPATHOLOGY

Asthma is invariably characterized by inflammatory changes throughout the submucosa of the airways, but not the alveoli or the lung parenchyma. This has naturally led to the assumption that this inflammation is primarily responsible for the clinical features of the disease, although the evidence to support this assertion remains largely circumstantial.[1,2] The first principal characteristic of asthmatic inflammation

is mucosal infiltration with inflammatory cells, particularly mononuclear cells (macrophages and cluster of differentiation 4 [CD4+] T lymphocytes) and granulocytes (eosinophils and neutrophils). Some severe asthmatics appear, in addition, to have elevated numbers of mucosal mast cells,[3] but this is not universal; mast cells are present in all mucosal surfaces even in normal individuals. Although invariably observed in asthma, these changes do not allow a definitive diagnosis of asthma on histopathological grounds, at least when studying bronchial biopsies; for example, there is considerable overlap with chronic obstructive pulmonary disease (COPD). Some chronic, severe asthmatics show a paucity of mucosal eosinophils but a more prominent neutrophil leukocyte infiltrate, and there has been much discussion about whether this can be correlated with the clinical phenotypes of asthma and the response of individual patients to conventional asthma therapy.[4] The problem is that most of these studies are based on "snapshot" samples of the bronchial mucosa at a single point in time; there is little information on how mucosal inflammation in individual asthmatics may vary with time or, for example, during exacerbations of the disease. Claims have also been made, based largely on counting the relative percentages (but not the total numbers) of eosinophils and neutrophils in induced sputum from asthmatics, that it is possible to identify a distinct clinical phenotype of "noneosinophilic asthma."[5] Notwithstanding the validity or the general applicability of these observations, sputum induction is itself a procedure that increases bronchial inflammation and it is not clear whether the relative proportions of granulocytes observed in induced sputum represent those within the bronchial mucosa. Furthermore, the relative percentages of cells do not reflect the actual numbers. Consequently, it seems justified to state that it has so far not been possible to associate etiological and clinical subdivisions of asthma with reproducible and discernible variabilities in the histopathology of asthma.

It has been stated that evidence of these inflammatory changes being responsible, in whole or in part, for the clinical pathology of asthma remains largely circumstantial. The cornerstones of this evidence are that mucosal inflammation in asthma is universal and that anti-inflammatory asthma therapy, such as inhaled corticosteroid therapy, reduces the infiltration of the bronchial mucosa by inflammatory cells (and thereby the production of their inflammatory mediators) in concert with an improvement in the objective markers of asthma severity, such as airway obstruction and bronchial hyperresponsiveness.[6] Nevertheless, it is still not possible to point to a particular cell or mediator and apportion its contribution, if any, to the day-to-day variability of airway obstruction and bronchial hyperresponsiveness in asthmatics. Future clarification of the histopathology of asthma is required to facilitate the discovery of valid and clinically effective new treatments for this disease.

The second principal characteristic of asthmatic airway inflammation is the variable presence of structural changes in the airways, collectively termed *remodeling*.[7] These include hypertrophy and hyperplasia of the airway smooth muscle cells, increased numbers of mucous goblet cells in the airway epithelium, deposition of extracellular matrix proteins (including collagen, fibronectin, and tenascin) beneath the epithelial basement membrane and in the submucosa, and neovascularization resulting in a proliferation of the vascular capillary beds within the submucosa. Some of these changes are not specific for asthma; for example, many chronic inflammatory processes involving the bronchial mucosa (asthma, COPD, bronchiectasis) are associated with mucous hypertrophy. Smooth muscle hypertrophy, hyperplasia and extracellular matrix protein deposited within the mucosa of the airways appear to be more asthma specific. These features have attracted great interest because they have been postulated to contribute to the accelerated decline in lung function and the irreversibility of airway obstruction observed in some, but not all asthmatics. Again, there are interpretational problems with this hypothesis. As already mentioned, some of these changes, such as airway mucosal edema due to neovascularization and blockage because of excessive mucus production, might intuitively be surmised to contribute to variable airway obstruction, while the deposition of extracellular protein might cause irreversible changes in airway function. However, as yet there is little or no direct evidence that they actually do so. Currently, remodeling changes in the asthmatic bronchial mucosa are widely assumed to result from the release of mediators from infiltrating inflammatory cells. While it is true that certain cytokines such as transforming growth factor beta (TGF-β) produced by eosinophils can cause bronchial mucosal fibroblasts to secrete fibrotic proteins such as collagen, while others such as interleukin-25 (IL-25) produced by T lymphocytes and other cells can promote neovascularization,[8] there are still many doubts about the cause and effect relationship between inflammation and remodeling largely because it is so difficult to characterize the natural progression of these two phenomena. Confusingly, of the few studies conducted in children, some have reported that severe asthma is associated with airway remodeling,[9,10] whereas others[11] suggest that remodeling changes predispose to, but predate clinical asthma. Such studies cast doubt on the tenet that remodeling is caused by inflammation and, in turn, contributes to asthma symptoms and physiology. In both children and adults, remodeling changes have been linked to asthma severity but less clearly to disease longevity,[9,10,12] suggesting that they are not necessarily cumulative, and even possibly at least partially reversible over time.

PATHOPHYSIOLOGY OF ASTHMA: ESTABLISHED VIEWS

ROLE OF IMMUNOGLOBULIN E (IgE)-MEDIATED MECHANISMS

IgE-mediated mechanisms, and in particular the IgE-mediated degranulation of mast cells and basophils by cross-linking surface-bound, allergen-specific IgE leading to the release of histamine and other mediators, were traditionally considered the central contributing factor for understanding asthma causation and exacerbation, particularly before the possible importance of chronic airway inflammation was recognized. As late as the 1980s, the pathophysiology of asthma was still viewed by many as a periodic, histamine-induced spasm of the bronchial smooth muscle caused by allergen-induced degranulation of the bronchial mucosal mast cells. This view of asthma pathogenesis was curious in retrospect because it glossed over many obvious, inexplicable inconsistencies, for example, that antihistamine therapy is of little or no clinical benefit in the management of chronic asthma, or that not all atopic persons with the propensity to develop allergen-specific IgE in their airways develop asthma whereas some nonatopic persons, who apparently do not manufacture allergen-specific IgE (at least none that can be detected systemically), do, nonetheless, develop asthma. The understanding of the possible role of IgE antibodies in the pathophysiology of asthma has recently been expanded, firstly by the recognition that IgE may play multiple, additional roles in inflammatory processes; for example, IgE antibodies are of very high avidity and may play a vital role in the capture of antigens by antigen-presenting cells at mucosal surfaces, whether they are allergens or not. Secondly, it has become clear that IgE synthesis may take place de novo in the bronchial mucosa of nonatopic, as well as atopic persons,[13] which raises the intriguing possibility that IgE antibodies against allergens or indeed other antigens could, in theory, be manufactured in the bronchial mucosa of asthmatics regardless of their conventional atopic status and play a role in the disease. Thirdly, and finally, the ability of the nonanaphylactogenic monoclonal anti-IgE antibody omalizumab to reduce exacerbations and, in many cases, the need for systemic corticosteroid therapy in many studies across the world involving both children and adults with severe asthma[14] clearly implicate IgE-mediated mechanisms, at least in some patients, in regulating the stability and arguably also the severity of asthma. This antibody binds to the constant region of the IgE molecule, which is why it does not cross-link adjacent IgE molecules and cause anaphylaxis, and prevents the binding of IgE to both its high- and low-affinity receptors FcεRI and FcεRII (CD23). Thus, omalizumab has the propensity to block the full range of the potential immunological functions of IgE in asthma. To date, clinical studies of its effectiveness have been directed exclusively at atopic asthmatics, since the initial assumption with anti-IgE therapy, based on the time-honored view of the pathophysiology of asthma expounded at the beginning of this section, was that it would ameliorate asthma primarily by inhibiting the allergen-induced release of histamine from sensitized bronchial mucosal mast cells by blocking the binding of their FcεRI receptors to allergen-specific IgE. Interestingly, there are already isolated reports of its efficacy in nonatopic asthma,[15] and further studies will undoubtedly follow. Although the efficacy of omalizumab seems to confirm a role for IgE in the pathophysiology of asthma at least in some patients, it seems unlikely that it acts universally by inhibiting allergen-induced mast cell degranulation. There is currently little understanding of which other IgE-mediated processes might be relevant to the pathophysiology of asthma. It is also salient to note that approximately one-third of apparently eligible atopic asthmatics treated with omalizumab show no significant clinical response[14] and, to date, there is no understanding of what distinguishes a responder from a nonresponder. Whatever the reasons for this variability in response, these observations could be interpreted to suggest that IgE does not necessarily play a pivotal role in the pathophysiology of asthma in every person, even if they are atopic.

T-HELPER TYPE 2 (TH2) T LYMPHOCYTES AND ASSOCIATED INFLAMMATORY PATHWAYS

Since the end of the 1980s, when asthma began to be recognized as a chronic inflammatory disease of the bronchial mucosa, the analysis of the nature of this inflammation through a multitude of observational studies in human asthmatics, allergen challenge of both human subjects and animals, and substantial *in vitro* data[1,2] pointed quite firmly to the involvement of CD4+ Th2 T lymphocytes with their capacity to secrete a wide variety of cytokines and chemokines that are not only able to promulgate the inflammatory granulocyte infiltrate which characterizes asthma, including mast cell, eosinophilic and basophilic inflammation, but also B cell switching to IgE synthesis and a range of asthma-associated remodeling changes in the airway mucosa. Many, but not all of the key cytokines implicated so far in the pathophysiology of asthma include those encoded in the IL-4 cluster on chromosome 5q31: IL-3, IL-4, IL-5, IL-9, IL-13, and granulocyte/macrophage colony-stimulating factor (GM-CSF), and, in addition, chemokines, which are chemoattractive to eosinophils, such as eotaxin, or Th2 T lymphocytes such as the thymus and activation-regulated chemokine (TARC) and the macrophage-derived cytokine (MDC).[16] There is accumulating evidence that the 5q31 cytokines are coregulated.[17]

As with inflammatory cells, however, the evidence for the involvement of these cytokines in the pathophysiology of human asthma, although extensive, has remained (until very recently with the development of biological agents able to inhibit or neutralize particular cytokines or their receptors) largely circumstantial. As knowledge of these mediators has increased, so the chasm of ignorance about what precisely they might do that is relevant to the spectrum and the day-to-day variability of the symptoms and clinical pathophysiology of human asthma has widened. This has resulted in some unpleasant surprises, for example, the Th2 T cell/IL-5/eosinophil axis, considered one of the cornerstones of asthma pathogenesis. Although eosinophil maturation in the bone marrow, recruitment into the airways, and survival in the tissues are potentially influenced by IL-3, IL-5, and GM-CSF, most attention has been focused on IL-5 as many studies have suggested that IL-5 is consistently overexpressed in the asthmatic bronchial mucosa, often to a degree that can be correlated in snapshot studies with the degree of airway obstruction, and that its local production by T cells is reduced in concert with the treatment and amelioration of asthma with corticosteroids.[1,2] Furthermore, IL-5 acts uniquely on eosinophils, which even now are considered a hallmark of the asthma process, with

many studies suggesting that the percentages of eosinophils in asthmatic airways, at least as measured in induced sputum, predict the clinical responsiveness to, or compliance with corticosteroid therapy,[18] even though, as mentioned earlier, it has never been clear precisely how eosinophils might cause the clinical symptoms of asthma. For all these reasons, IL-5 was considered a key molecular target for the treatment of asthma.

With the advent of modern biological agents, it became possible to address the hypothesis that IL-5 is a key molecular target for asthma treatment. A number of humanized, monoclonal anti-IL-5 antibodies have become available, including mepolizumab, reslizuamb, and benralizumab. The treatment of patients with mild/moderate asthma with intravenous mepolizumab did not result in a significant clinical or functional improvement either following acute allergen challenge[19] or in day-to-day asthma symptoms following more prolonged therapy,[20] despite causing substantial reductions in the numbers of eosinophils in the peripheral blood and induced sputum from the airways. These findings surprised the asthma research community. Despite suggestions that the unexpectedly poor efficacy of anti-IL-5 therapy might reflect its inability to remove eosinophils from the airway mucosa completely,[21] the writing on the wall seemed clear: anti-IL-5 therapy was apparently not going to be the panacea for asthma treatment that had been anticipated based on observational studies of its pathophysiology. Two smaller but important subsequent placebo-controlled studies[22,23] of mepolizumab therapy in severe asthmatics with persistently high percentages of eosinophils in their induced sputum despite systemic corticosteroid therapy found that the treatment was associated with a significant reduction in disease exacerbations. Thus, mepolizumab and similar anti-IL-5 strategies may be of therapeutic benefit in a subset of chronic, severe, corticosteroid-dependent asthmatics (possibly those with high percentages of eosinophils in their induced sputum, but since the effects of mepolizumab were not assessed in "low-sputum eosinophil" patients in these studies, this cannot be deduced with certainty). What these findings tell us about the pathophysiology of asthma and the role of IL-5 and eosinophils in the disease is uncertain.

This uncertainty about the role of mediators of Th2-type inflammation in asthma does not seem to have deterred the pharmaceutical industry, which has plunged headlong into identifying new asthma treatments based on their effects in a wide variety of animal "model" experiments typically involving sensitization of the animal to an antigen by vaccination, intraperitoneally or otherwise, followed by an inhalation challenge with the same antigen. These manipulations are designed to recapitulate the Th2 T lymphocyte paradigm in the airways of the animals in the short term, and have facilitated the development of a wide variety of interventional approaches targeted at particular Th2 cytokines or their receptors, including monoclonal antibodies, soluble cytokine receptors, gene fusion proteins, and siRNA technology. Unfortunately, it has proven all too easy using such "models" to show that the blockade of any particular single mediator such as IL-5, IL-4, or IL-13 or, alternatively, overexpression in the airway's through genetic engineering can have profound effects on the airway's inflammatory and remodeling changes. The "real-life" results with anti-IL-5 strategies in human asthmatics, however, seem to advocate a greater degree of caution.

The therapeutic outcomes of targeting other Th2 mediators in human asthma, including IL-4 and IL-13, have so far proven similarly disappointing, although it is, as yet, too early to make firm conclusions.[24] What one might conclude is that future drug development should not rely completely on the outcomes of short-term models in animals involving artificial antigen sensitization, which do not model chronic asthma, obviously in terms of its longevity but also in terms of its complex interactions with environmental influences such as infectious agents, environmental pollutants, and allergens, and endogenous influences such as hormones, drugs, and stress, repeatedly and over a prolonged period of time.[25] Another possible conclusion from the observation that only a subset of patients appears to respond to single biological agents is that asthma may be composed of mechanistic subtypes that have yet to be identified. The identification of biomarkers of responsiveness to particular biologics is the new priority,[26,27] and this will undoubtedly increase our understanding of the contribution of inflammatory mediators to the clinical pathology of asthma. It is not inconceivable that the precise pathophysiology of asthma, taking into account the genetic, environmental, psychosocial, hormonal, pharmacological, and temporal influences on the nature of the disease, differs to a degree in every patient, but hopefully research in the future will delineate major strands.

In addition to cytokines and chemokines, cysteinyl leukotrienes, which are primarily products of activated eosinophils, promote vascular leakage and thus edema of the lining of the airways, and are also the most potent known natural constrictors of the bronchial smooth muscle. They have been implicated in the pathophysiology of asthma in the sense that some, but not all asthmatic patients respond favorably to leukotriene $CysLT_1$ receptor blockers such as montelukast and zafirlukast.[28]

The antigenic drive to Th2 T lymphocyte activation in asthma is unknown. Again, largely as a result of the perceived importance of allergen-induced, IgE-dependent mast cell degranulation as a drive to asthma, there is a widespread tacit assumption that inflammation in asthma is driven largely by T cells that recognize inhaled allergens, some of which may also interact with allergen-specific B lymphocytes resulting in allergen-specific IgE production and the atopic phenotype. Until it is possible routinely to identify the allergen specificity of activated T lymphocytes within the bronchial mucosa, the assertion that a majority of these cells recognize allergen epitopes must remain hypothetical. It is quite possible that other antigens may drive Th2 lymphocyte activation in asthma in particular circumstances. It is also possible to hypothesize that Th2 lymphocyte activation becomes self-propagating with time, similar to what has been observed with autoimmune

disease. This, in turn, may result from a defective inhibition of these cells by T regulatory cells.[29,30]

PATHOPHYSIOLOGY OF ASTHMA: NEW VIEWS

WHY DO SOME PEOPLE DEVELOP ASTHMA BUT NOT OTHERS?

This is, of course, a question applicable to many diseases of uncertain etiology, but it is a very fundamental one since a clear answer to the question of why asthma appears and then remits, at least clinically, in some persons but not others would likely embrace a lot of the fundamental understanding of its pathogenesis. If asthma is indeed driven primarily by Th2 T lymphocyte activation, one might hypothesize that there are differences between individuals in the local environment of the bronchial mucosa yet to be discovered, which result either in the propagation of T lymphocyte activation on the one hand or its suppression on the other. These differences might reside in the structure of the mucosa itself and the results of its interactions with environmental stimuli. The risk of developing asthma tends to run in families. Twin studies estimate the proportion of the asthma risk to be 50%–60% genetically determined, and the remainder is likely accounted for by extensive and complex interactions of gene effects with environmental influences. Genome screens have linked the inheritance of various chromosomal regions with an increased risk of asthma.[31] Some of these regions contain genes encoding cytokines such as IL-4 or IL-13 or their receptors, which have been implicated in asthma pathogenesis, suggesting that genetic variability in the expression or actions of these mediators may contribute to asthma risk. More recent positional cloning strategies[31] have identified new genes, such as *ADAM33*, the products of which do not play a role in known asthma pathways, but are involved in the normal development of the airways during embryogenesis, supporting the possibility that a variability, as yet uncharacterized, in the structure or development of the airways predisposes some individuals to asthma. The implication is that such variability might directly, or indirectly through its interaction with environmental influences, either promote or inhibit the development of clinical asthma by regulating mucosal inflammation or other mechanisms.

ASTHMA AS AN EPITHELIAL DISEASE

There is accumulating evidence that diseases of the atopic march, including asthma, eczema, chronic rhinosinusitis, and food allergies, arise from defects in the epithelial barrier function, which may facilitate, at least in theory, the penetration of environmental factors such as allergens, viruses, and pollutants into the submucosa.[32-35] Abnormalities in the production or function of proteins that maintain the epithelial barrier could constitute one group of potentially heritable factors predisposing individuals to the development of these diseases. Impaired repair and "healing" of the airway epithelium is another well-described feature of asthma histopathology that may have a role in generating remodeling changes. Indeed, the recent fascinating obervation[36] that simple repetitive distortion of the airway wall through bronchoconstriction can cause epithelial growth factor release and remodeling changes raises the possibility that these changes initially arise independently of the asthma process as a "wound healing" response to repetitive epithelial distortion, although they may later become relevant to asthma pathophysiology if, for example, they eventually result in irreversible airway obstruction.

ASTHMA AS A DISEASE OF INNATE IMMUNITY

Asthmatics may exhibit deficiencies in their innate immune responses, which may, in turn, influence the microbiome of the airways[37] and the susceptibility of individuals to respiratory tract infections.[38] Rhinoviral infections are the principal cause of asthma exacerbation[38] and there is some evidence that such infections may program the airway dendritic cells to potentiate Th2-type inflammation.[39,40] Furthermore, asthmatic airway epithelial cells appear to be deficient in their innate response to rhinoviral infection mediated through the Toll-like receptor 3 (TLR3).[41] This observation and the observations[42,43] that the development of asthma and allergies in childhood can be associated with exaggerated bronchiolitic responses to rhinoviral infection together again suggest that one, possibly principal, facet of the pathophysiology of asthma may be epithelial cell abnormality.

ASTHMA AS A DISEASE OF BRONCHIAL SMOOTH MUSCLE

Inappropriate bronchoconstriction and airway hyperresponsiveness to multiple environmental and pharmacological stimuli would appear first and foremost to reflect abnormalities of the airway smooth muscle, so it might be considered somewhat surprising that none of the aforementioned accounts of the pathophysiology of asthma involves the bronchial smooth muscle. The fact is that although hypertrophy and hyperplasia of the smooth muscle cells have been recognized as a feature of asthma pathophysiology for decades, next to nothing is known about what causes these cells to constrict with inappropriate force in response to such a wide range of stimuli in asthmatics. Experiments are very difficult because although it is now possible to routinely culture the human airway smooth muscle cells from bronchial biopsies or resections, it is not so easy to measure the force that they generate in culture, particularly against an appropriate *in vivo* load. The hyperresponsiveness of asthmatic bronchial smooth muscle cells to a wide range of agonists is clearly unlikely to reflect upregulation of the receptors for every one of these agonists or their corresponding signaling pathways. Recently, more sense of this phenomenon has been made from the observation that asthmatic bronchial smooth muscle cells abnormally express proteins that regulate intracellular calcium homoeostasis, and thereby the resting intracellular free calcium concentration and thus the force with which the smooth muscle cell will respond to any stimulus that causes a transient intercellular calcium flux, which,

in turn, triggers contraction. For example, a deficiency of the expression of the SERCA protein[44] has recently been implicated in raising the baseline intercellular calcium in asthmatic smooth muscle cells, increasing their motility and the secretion of remodeling cytokines, and probably also their force of contraction, although this is difficult to measure. Another protein that regulates intracellular calcium in the smooth muscle cells is the calcium-sensing receptor. This is a pleiotropic, G protein-coupled receptor, which plays a fundamental role in mineral ion metabolism.[45] While extracellular calcium ions are the physiological ligand for this receptor, it is also activated by a range of polycations that are elevated in asthma, such as poly-L-arginine, poly-L-lysine, and spermine.[45] Fascinatingly, eosinophil basic proteins such as eosinophil cationic protein are also polycations. If eosinophil basic proteins have the propensity to "reset" resting intracellular calcium in the airway smooth muscle cells in asthmatics, this would provide the first clear link between eosinophilic inflammation in asthma and one of the cardinal facets of its pathophysiology.

CONCLUSIONS

As stated, the traditional pathogenesis of asthma discussed herein does not appear to explain the patient variability of the disease progression, its severity, or the response to different therapies. The complex nature of asthma influenced by a spectrum of environmental and genetic determinants and the redundancy in the pathophysiological effects of mediators, chemokines, and cytokines make it unlikely that treatments designed to target one facet of this disease will be successful. The future development of novel asthma therapies may need to be restricted to a specific patient profile or endotype based on the pathogenic features of the patient's disease.

REFERENCES

1. Corrigan C. T cells and cytokines in asthma and allergic inflammation. In: Kay AB, Kaplan AP, Bousquet J, Holt PG (eds.), *Allergy and Allergic Diseases*, 2nd edn. Oxford: Wiley-Blackwell, 2008.
2. Lemanske RF, Busse WW. Asthma: Clinical expression and molecular mechanisms. *J Allergy Clin Immunol* 2010;125:S95–S102.
3. Balzar S, Fajt ML, Comhair SA, et al. Mast cell phenotype, location and activation in severe asthma. Data from the Severe Asthma Research Program. *Am J Respir Crit Care Med* 2011;183:299–309.
4. Wenzel SE. Asthma phenotypes: The evolution from clinical to molecular approaches. *Nat Med* 2012;18:716–725.
5. Haldar P, Pavord ID. Non-eosinophilic asthma: A distinct clinical and pathologic phenotype. *J Allergy Clin Immunol* 2007;119:1043–1052.
6. Corrigan CJ, Levy ML, Dekhuijzen PR, et al. The ADMIT series—Issues in inhalation therapy. 3. Mild persistent asthma: The case for inhaled corticosteroid therapy. *Prim Care Respir J* 2009;18:148–158.
7. James AL, Wenzel S. Clinical relevance of airway remodeling in airway diseases. *Eur Respir J* 2007;30:134–155.

8. Corrigan CJ, Wang W, Meng Q, et al. T-helper cell type 2 (Th2) memory T cell-potentiating cytokine IL-25 has the potential to promote angiogenesis in asthma. *Proc Natl Acad Sci USA* 2011;108:1579–1584.

9. Payne DNR, Rogers AV, Adelroth E, et al. Early thickening of the reticular basement membrane in children with difficult asthma. *Am J Respir Crit Care Med* 2003;167:78–82.

10. De Blic J, Tillie-Leblond I, Tonnel AB, et al. Difficult asthma in children: An analysis of airway inflammation. *J Allergy Clin Immunol* 2004;113:94–100.

11. Pohunek P, Warner JO, Turzikova J, et al. Markers of eosinophilic inflammation and tissue re-modelling in children before clinically diagnosed bronchial asthma. *Pediatr Allergy Immunol* 2005;16:43–51.

12. Chetta A, Foresi A, Del Donno M, et al. Airways remodelling is a distinctive feature of asthma and is related to severity of disease. *Chest* 1997;111:852–857.

13. Takhar P, Corrigan CJ, Smurthwaite L, et al. Class switch recombination to IgE in the bronchial mucosa of atopic and non-atopic asthmatics. *J Allergy Clin Immunol* 2007;119:213–218.

14. Di Domenico M, Bisogno A, Polverino M, et al. Xolair in asthma therapy: An overview. *Inflamm Allergy Drug Targets* 2011;10:2–12.

15. Menzella F, Piro R, Facciolongo N, et al. Long-term benefits of omalizumab in a patient with severe non-allergic asthma. *Allergy Asthma Clin Immunol* 2011;7:9.

16. Pease JE. Targeting chemokine receptors in allergic disease. *Biochem J* 2011;434:11–24.

17. Strempel JM, Grenningloh R, Ho IC, et al. Phylogenetic and functional analysis identifies Ets-1 as a novel regulator of the Th2 cytokine gene locus. *J Immunol* 2010;184:1309–1316.

18. Hargreave F. Quantitative sputum cell counts as a marker of airway inflammation in clinical practice. *Curr Opin Allergy Clin Immunol* 2007;7:102–106.

19. Leckie MJ, ten Brinke A, Khan J, et al. Effects of an interleukin-5 blocking monoclonal antibody on eosinophils, airways hyperresponsiveness and the late asthmatic response. *Lancet* 2000;356:2144–2148.

20. Flood-Page P, Swenson C, Faiferman I, et al. A study to evaluate safety and efficacy of mepolizumab in patients with moderate persistent asthma. *Am J Respir Crit Care Med* 2007;176:1062–1071.

21. Flood-Page PT, Menzies-Gow AN, Kay AB, et al. Eosinophil's role remains uncertain as anti-interleukin-5 only partially depletes numbers in asthmatic airways. *Am J Respir Crit Care Med* 2003;176:199–204.

22. Nair P, Pizzichini MM, Kjarsgaard M, et al. Mepolizumab for prednisolone-dependent asthma with sputum eosinophilia. *N Engl J Med* 2009;360:985–993.

23. Haldar P, Brightling CE, Hargadon B, et al. Mepolizumab and exacerbations of refractory eosinophilic asthma. *N Engl J Med* 2009;360:973–984.

24. Holgate ST. Pathophysiology of asthma: What has our current understanding taught us about new therapeutic approaches? *J Allergy Clin Immunol* 2011;128:495–505.

25. Holgate ST, Davies DE, Powell RM, et al. Local genetic and environmental factors in asthma disease pathogenesis: Chronicity and persistence mechanisms. *Eur Respir J* 2007;29:793–803.

26. Shirtcliffe P, Weatherall M, Travers J, et al. The multiple dimensions of airways disease: Targeting treatment to clinical phenotypes. *Curr Opin Pulm Med* 2011;17:72–78.

27. Morjaria JB, Proiti M, Polosa R. Stratified medicine in selecting biologics for the treatment of severe asthma. *Curr Opin Allergy Clin Immunol* 2011;11:58–63.

28. Ogawa Y, Calhoun WJ. The role of leukotrienes in airway inflammation. *J Allergy Clin Immunol* 2007;118:789–798.

29. Dimeloe S, Nanzer A, Ryanna K, et al. Regulatory T cells, inflammation and the allergic response: The role of glucocorticoids and Vitamin D. *J Steroid Biochem Mol Biol* 2010;120:86–95.

30. Ryanna K, Stratigou V, Safinia N, et al. Regulatory T cells in bronchial asthma. *Allergy* 2009;64:335–347.

31. Wills-Karp M, Ewart SL. Time to draw breath: Asthma susceptibility genes are identified. *Nat Rev Genet* 2004;5:376–387.

32. Scharschmidt TC, Man MQ, Hatano Y, et al. Filaggrin deficiency confers a paracellular barrier abnormality that reduces inflammatory thresholds to irritants and haptens. *J Allergy Clin Immunol* 2009;124:496–506.

33. Groschwitz KR, Hogan SP. Intestinal barrier function: Molecular regulation and disease pathogenesis. *J Allergy Clin Immunol* 2009;124:3–20.

34. Tieu DD, Peters AT, Carter RG, et al. Evidence for diminished levels of epithelial psoriasin and calprotectin in chronic rhinosinusitis. *J Allergy Clin Immunol* 2010;125:667–675.

35. Holgate ST. Epithelial dysfunction in asthma. *J Allergy Clin Immunol* 2007;120:1233–1244.

36. Grainge CL, Lau LCK, Ward JA, et al. Effect of bronchoconstriction on airway remodeling in asthma. *N Engl J Med* 2011;364:2006–2015.

37. Hilty M, Burke C, Pedro H, et al. Disordered microbial communities in asthmatic airways. *PLoS One* 2010;5:e8578.

38. Papadopoulos NG, Christodoulou I, Rohde G, et al. Viruses and bacteria in acute asthma exacerbations: A GA²LEN-DARE systematic review. *Allergy* 2011;66:458–468.

39. Jackson DJ, Gangnon RE, Evans MD, et al. Wheezing rhinovirus illnesses in early life predict asthma development in high-risk children. *Am J Respir Crit Care Med* 2008;178:667–672.

40. Holt PG, Sly PD. Interaction between adaptive and innate immune pathways in the pathogenesis of atopic asthma: Operation of a lung/bone marrow axis. *Chest* 2011;139:1165–1171.

41. Wark PA, Johnston SL, Bucchieri F, et al. Asthmatic bronchial epithelial cells have a deficient innate immune response to infection with rhinovirus. *J Exp Med* 2005;201:937–947.

42. Jartti T, Kuusipalo H, Vuorinen T, et al. Allergic sensitization is associated with rhinovirus-, but not other virus-induced wheezing in children. *Pediatr Allergy Immunol* 2010;21:1008–1014.

43. Jartti T, Korppi M. Rhinovirus-induced bronchiolitis and asthma development. *Pediatr Allergy Immunol* 2011;22:350–355.

44. Mahn K, Hirst SJ, Ying S, et al. Diminished sarco/endoplasmic reticulum Ca^{2+} ATPase (SERCA) expression contributes to airway remodeling in bronchial asthma. *Proc Natl Acad Sci USA* 2009;106:10775–10800.

45. Riccardi D, Kemp PJ. The calcium-sensing receptor beyond extracellular calcium homeostasis: Conception, development, adult physiology and disease. *Annu Rev Physiol* 2012;74:271–297.

3 Genetics and Asthma

Rebecca E. Slager, Xingnan Li, Deborah A. Meyers, and Eugene R. Bleecker

CONTENTS

CASE PRESENTATION

A 25-year-old African American patient enters her local emergency department with chest tightness, wheezing, and difficulty in breathing. As she checks in, a clinical nurse asks to speak to the patient about the Center for Personalized Medicine at the hospital. The nurse coordinator explains that the patient has the option to give consent to have her genome completely sequenced, and for her electronic medical record and any clinical samples that may be obtained during her treatment linked to this genomic information. The patient reads the material thoroughly, discusses questions with the clinical staff, and provides a detailed written consent. Blood is drawn for genome sequencing and the patient proceeds to her examination. After an initial assessment, the patient is referred to a pulmonary physician for spirometry, allergy testing, and several other biomarker measurements. The patient is diagnosed with moderately severe allergic asthma and is prescribed standard medications, including inhaled corticosteroids and an albuterol rescue inhaler. The physician also mentions that a clinical trial of a novel biologic therapy for asthma is available for enrollment. However, the physician discusses with the patient that this treatment is most effective in a group of patients with high levels of a specific serum biomarker but it can have rare adverse effects in a group of patients with a specific genetic variant. This gene variation is relatively uncommon but the patient decides to await the results of her genome sequencing to decide whether she wants to enroll in the trial. The following month, her physician receives a text message alert from the patient's medical record indicating that the patient has the most common form of the gene, so her genetic risk profile is safe. She decides to participate in the trial of the novel biologic therapy for asthma.

This personalized medicine scenario could be a reality in the near future, as many large hospitals and academic medical centers seek to link genomic information with clinical and demographic information and clinical specimens. Through an active consenting process, patients with asthma or other common diseases may soon have the majority of this information available in their electronic medical record, which can then provide immediate information to their physicians based on their genotype for specific indications (such as responsiveness to a therapy or risk of adverse effects), who can suggest safe and effective treatment choices.

INTRODUCTION

Asthma is a heterogeneous disease of related clinical phenotypes with a complex etiology based on genetic susceptibility and environmental influences. A primary aim of genetic studies in a common disease such as asthma is to identify a group of genetic variants that may interact with these environmental exposures to predict the risk for the development (susceptibility) or progression (severity) of asthma. Asthma susceptibility and severity are determined by a number of genetic variants that each contribute to the risk architecture.

Recent genome-wide association study (GWAS) approaches have identified several genes or loci that are associated with asthma susceptibility,[1–4] including the ORM1-like 3/gasdermin-like (*ORMDL3/GSDML*) region of chromosome 17q21, interleukin 33 (*IL-33*) and its receptor interleukin 1 receptor-like 1 isoform 1 (*IL-1RL1*), thymic stromal lymphopoietin (*TSLP*), the major histocompatibility (MHC) region on 6p21, and interleukin 13 (*IL-13*). Some of these genes have previously been linked to asthma or other related allergic phenotypes in earlier candidate gene or positional cloning studies, suggesting that shared inflammatory pathways may be affected. For example, the MHC region was one of the first asthma susceptibility loci identified[5] and it appears to play a major role in asthma and allergen sensitization.[3] Regulatory T cell signaling genes, such as the SMAD family member 3 (*SMAD3*), encoding a transcriptional modulator related to transforming growth factor β, may also play a critical role in the development of asthma. A number of these susceptibility genes have been replicated in some but not all populations, suggesting that there may be heterogeneity in the genetic risk in populations of different ethnic backgrounds. The results from major GWAS and meta-analyses of asthma reviewed in this chapter are summarized in Table 3.1.

Current genomic asthma research is focused on identifying the genetic factors that affect not only the disease susceptibility but also the progression and severity of asthma. Asthma severity genes may be related to specific endophenotypes, some of which are discussed in this chapter and summarized in Table 3.2: (1) genes related to pulmonary function; (2) biomarkers related to asthma progression and the risk of exacerbations; (3) pharmacogenetic interactions in which an individual may have reduced responsiveness or be resistant to a specific asthma therapy; and (4) gene–environment interactions.

GWAS OF ASTHMA SUSCEPTIBILITY

Prior to 2007, candidate genes in asthma and allergy biological pathways were tested for their association with asthma susceptibility, and family studies and positional cloning techniques identified several putative chromosomal loci related to asthma. However, many of the positive genetic associations from these earlier studies were not consistently replicated, possibly due to relatively small sample sizes, inconsistent phenotype definitions, population stratification, and lack of adequate genomic coverage. Following the transition to GWAS, the risk variants discovered in these genome-wide screens were more likely to be replicated, at least in populations of similar ethnic backgrounds. This section highlights some of the major genome-wide studies of asthma susceptibility (Table 3.1).

GWAS OF ASTHMA SUSCEPTIBILITY IN MULTIPLE ETHNIC GROUPS

Based on a doctor's diagnosis of asthma, the first asthma susceptibility GWAS was published in 2007 by the European GABRIEL consortium. This study identified variants in the *ORMDL3* gene on chromosome 17q12-21 as predictors of childhood asthma susceptibility.[1] A large follow-up study in the same cohort verified this finding[2] and many subsequent GWAS have also confirmed this result.[4] However, there is a high degree of correlation or linkage disequilibrium (LD) in this region that spans several genes and it is still not clear whether *ORMDL3* or a nearby gene is the risk gene for asthma with the causative variant(s). A splice-site mutation has been identified through sequencing, which is in strong LD with *ORMDL3* but is located on the adjacent gasdermin-like B (*GSDMB*) gene, indicating that this gene may be the actual causal risk variant for asthma.[6] This example reinforces the importance of new genetic sequencing projects and how these technologies continue to facilitate an understanding of the genetic risk for asthma.

Many of the initial asthma GWAS were carried out in non-Hispanic white discovery cohorts, although minority ethnic groups such as African Americans are more likely to experience higher asthma morbidity and mortality rates than whites.[7,8] Populations of different ancestry also have different patterns of gene variation and LD that can alter the gene-specific risk variants. Therefore, it is critical to investigate the genetic pathways that play a role in asthma in individuals of different ethnic backgrounds. Whereas the GABRIEL consortium consisted of European individuals with asthma,[1] the North American EVE meta-analysis for asthma susceptibility was established in individuals of European American, African American or Afro-Caribbean, and Latino ancestry. In EVE, five major susceptibility loci were identified in 5,416 asthma cases and replication was performed in an additional 12,649 individuals. Four of the chromosomal regions that reached genome-wide significance had been previously identified in GABRIEL or other studies: loci in the *ORMDL3* region of 17q21, the interleukin 1 receptor-like 1 isoform/interleukin 18 receptor (*IL-1RL1/IL-18R*) loci on chromosome 2q, the *TSLP* gene region on 5q22, and *IL-33* on chromosome 9p24.[4] These loci are associated with the development of asthma across ethnic groups, and a novel susceptibility locus in individuals of African descent was also identified: pyrin and HIN domain family, member 1 (*PYHIN1*) on chromosome 1q23.[4] Prior to the EVE analysis,

TABLE 3.1
Significant Asthma Susceptibility Genes from Meta-Analyses or Replicated GWAS and Primary References

Gene(s)	Chromosomal Region	Ethnic Background(s)	References
PYHIN1	1q23	African	[4]
IL-1RL1/IL-18R1	2q11	All	[2,4]
TSLP	5q22	All	[2,4,12]
IL-13	5q31	European	[2,3]
HLA-DQ/DR	6p21	All	[2,3,12,13]
IL-33	9p24	All	[2,4]
RORA	15q22	European	[2]
SMAD3	15q23	European	[2]
ORMDL3/GSDML	17q21	All	[1,2,4]

a GWAS in populations of African ancestry identified polymorphisms in the α-1B-adrenergic receptor (*ADRA1B*), the prion-related protein (PRNP), and dipeptidyl peptidase 10 (*DPP10*) as predictors of asthma risk.[9] *DPP10* had also originally been identified as an asthma gene through positional cloning in European families.[10] Ancestry association testing also recently identified a common European genetic variant on chromosome 6q14 as a risk factor for asthma in African American subjects with local European admixture (odds ratio = 2.2).[11]

Genome-wide screens for asthma risk in Asian adults and children identified genetic variants in the MHC/human leukocyte antigen (HLA) region on chromosome 6p21. In the Japanese population, 7,171 adult asthma cases and 27,912 unaffected individuals were genotyped in the discovery and replication cohorts. Five loci were associated with susceptibility to adult asthma at the genome-wide significance level, including the previously identified HLA region and the thymic stromal lymphopoietin/WD repeat domain 36 (*TSLP/WDR36*) regions, and three additional genomic regions: the ubiquitin-specific peptidase 38/GRB2-associated binding protein 1 (*USP38/GAB1*) locus on chromosome 4q31, loci on chromosome 10p14, and a region of chromosome 12q13.[12] In a separate GWAS of childhood asthma, genetic variants in the *HLA-DP* locus region on chromosome 6p21.3 were associated with the risk of pediatric asthma across Asian populations.[13] Additionally, a replication study in 710 asthma cases and 656 unaffected controls in the Chinese Han population provides further evidence that the *ORMDL3/GSDMB* locus is associated with asthma risk in multiple ethnic groups.[14]

The specific role and functional biology of novel GWAS loci such as *ORMDL3* in the pathogenesis of asthma remain unknown. However, genome-wide screens of asthma provide strong evidence of the biological importance of pathways that communicate epithelial damage to the adaptive immune system, potentially leading to airway inflammation. Moreover, epithelial cell-derived cytokines, such as *TSLP* and *IL-33*, may promote the T-helper type 2 (Th2) immune response on mast cells, Th2 cells, or regulatory T cells through *IL-1RL1* or other receptor activation.

GENETIC STUDIES OF ASTHMA SEVERITY AND RELATED PHENOTYPES

Several of the initial GWAS focused on population-based studies of childhood-onset asthma susceptibility based on somewhat limited phenotyping to accommodate large sample sizes. Therefore, whether the same genes that contribute to asthma onset also play a role in the progression and severity of the disease is not well understood. However, comprehensive studies of asthma severity require more intense, time-consuming, and costly phenotyping, often resulting in smaller cohort sizes. An analysis of asthma severity can include intermediate phenotypes, such as measures of pulmonary function, bronchial hyperresponsiveness (BHR), biomarkers, and responses to asthma therapy. Genetic studies of asthma severity also require different comparison groups

than susceptibility studies: instead of unaffected individuals, subjects with severe asthma should be compared with individuals with mild asthma, which can be an additional complexity for subject recruiting. This section will review GWAS of asthma severity and related endophenotypes, summarized in Table 3.2.

GWAS OF SEVERE, PERSISTENT ASTHMA

Bleecker and Meyers and colleagues performed a GWAS for asthma susceptibility and severity in a comprehensively phenotyped, longitudinal cohort of 473 non-Hispanic white adult asthma cases in The Epidemiology and Natural History of Asthma: Outcomes and Treatment Regimens (TENOR) study,[15] compared with publicly available controls.[3] In this analysis, several variants in the *RAD50/IL-13* region of chromosome 5q31.1 were highly associated with asthma risk, though a strong correlation between variants in this LD block makes it difficult to identify the causal variant.[3] However, this is an important example of a genome-wide study identifying a biologically relevant gene (*IL-13*), which had been

TABLE 3.2

Selected Genes Associated with Asthma Severity and Related Traits in Genome-Wide Scans

Trait	Gene(s)	References
Lung Function Measures (FEV$_1$/FVC or FEV$_1$)		
Lung function decline	TUSC3 (asthma) DLEU7 (nonasthma)	[23]
General population	HHIP, GPR126, ADAM19, AGER/PPT2, FAM13A, PTCH1, PID1, HTR4, GSTCD, TNS1, NOTCH4/AGER/PPT2, THSD4I, NTS12/GSTCD/NPNT, MFAP2, TGFB2, HDAC4, RARB, MECOM, SPATA9, ARMC2, NCR3, ZKSCAN3, CDC123, C10orf11, LRP1, CCDC38, MMP15, CFDP1, KCNE2	[18,19]
Asthma populations	HHIP, IL-6R	[20,22]
Total Serum/Plasma IgE Levels		
General population	STAT6, FCER1A, IL-13/RAD50	[24,25]
Asthma populations	HLA-DR, STAT6, FCER1A, IL-13/RAD50, C11orf30-LRRC32	[2,26]
Eosinophil Levels		
General population	IL-1RL1, IKZF2, IL-5, SH2B3	[27]
Atopic conditions	TSLP/WDR36 (eosinophilic esophagitis) WDR36, IL-33, MYB (eosinophil levels and atopic asthma)	[27,28]
Response to Asthma Therapy		
Inhaled corticosteroids	GLCCI1, T gene	[30,32]

observed in many candidate gene and animal studies of asthma and allergic inflammation.[16,17] This study also identified variants in the *HLA-DR/DQ* associated with asthma, a genomic region that has been replicated in many candidate gene studies and GWAS,[2,12,13] as discussed earlier.

LUNG FUNCTION GENES

Extensive phenotypic characterization in the National Heart, Lung, and Blood Institute (NHBLI)-sponsored Severe Asthma Research Program (SARP) cohort indicates that one of the critical determinants of asthma progression is lung function.[7,8] Therefore, identifying the genes related to pulmonary function, a statistically powerful objective measure, represents a relevant approach to defining the genes that contribute to asthma severity.

Large cross-sectional analyses for normal lung function genes were carried out in the European general population, identifying the hedgehog interacting protein (*HHIP*) gene and 11 other genomic regions associated with forced expiratory volume in 1 second (FEV_1) and/or FEV_1/forced vital capacity ratio (FEV_1/FVC) (Table 3.2).[18,19] A very large follow-up meta-analysis (approximately 90,000 European individuals in the discovery and replication cohorts) from the same consortia identified 16 additional genome-wide significant loci for normal lung function (Table 3.2), representing a number of different physiological pathways including cell growth, signaling, and migration. Because it was not clear whether these same genes or pathways were also important in lung function variation in individuals with asthma, Li and colleagues performed a meta-analysis of 14 single nucleotide polymorphisms (SNPs) in lung function candidate genes in three independent asthma cohorts.[20] This analysis identified the *HHIP/rs1512288* variant as a significant predictor of FEV_1 and FVC in asthma and an increasing number of risk variants in these lung function genes were highly associated with lower FEV_1 and increased asthma severity.[20] This approach demonstrates the close relationship between pulmonary function and asthma severity.

Another gene that could influence asthma susceptibility and severity is the interleukin 6 receptor (*IL-6R*), which was identified as a predictor of asthma risk in a GWAS of 57,800 subjects.[21] A common *IL-6R* coding variation (*Asp358Ala*) was identified as a genetic modifier of lung function in asthma, as subjects of European ancestry with asthma who inherited the *Ala358* variant had the lowest mean percent predicted FEV_1 and FEV_1/FVC, and the highest mean levels of methacholine responsiveness.[22] The functional characterization of this gene in airway cells is ongoing and there is the possibility that anti-*IL-6R* therapy could also be important in the treatment of asthma and other airway diseases.

In the first GWAS of longitudinal decline in FEV_1 or FEV_1/FVC in several European cohorts, the associated genetic variants were different between individuals with and without asthma. While none of the variants attained genome-wide significance, there was a replicated association between the height-related gene deleted in lymphocytic

leukemia 7 (*DLEU7*) and an FEV_1 decrease in individuals without asthma (discovery $P = 4.8 \times 10^{-6}$; replication $P = .03$). The most significant association for a FEV_1/FVC ratio decrease in asthma, tumor suppressor candidate 3 (*TUSC3*; $P = 5.3 \times 10^{-8}$), was not replicated and variants that were associated with pulmonary function in cross-sectional analyses were not predictive of a decline (Table 3.2).[23]

The importance of identifying gene variants that interact with lung function in asthma is that these genes appear to represent an additional risk for future lung function decline and asthma severity. It is possible that genotyping individuals with asthma earlier in the medical history of their disease could identify these patients with asthma who have an increased risk of disease progression. This genetic information could serve as a "predictive" biomarker and these at-risk asthmatics may be candidates for more aggressive therapies to prevent disease progression.

BIOMARKERS

Biomarkers such as serum immunoglobulin E (IgE) levels and blood or sputum eosinophil levels may be important in predicting the severity of asthma or the risk of exacerbations. Therefore, many asthma cohorts as well as large population-based studies have evaluated the genetic factors related to these biomarkers (Table 3.2). The GABRIEL cohort performed a GWAS for total serum IgE levels in 7087 subjects with asthma and 7667 controls, and identified one novel locus in the class II region of MHC, which was significant at the genome-wide level.[2] This study also observed several genetic variants associated with IgE levels in the *Fc* fragment of IgE, high affinity I (*FCER1A*), *IL-13*, and signal transducer and activator of transcription 6 (*STAT6*) genes. These genes were also observed in a GWAS of IgE in the general populations.[24,25] In the GABRIEL study, genes that were associated with asthma susceptibility generally did not overlap with those associated with IgE, though the authors suggest that loci strongly associated with IgE levels may contribute to the severity or progression of the disease.[2] In order to identify IgE-associated genes in asthma populations, Li and colleagues tested SNPs on chromosome 11q13.5 between the open reading frame 30 (*C11orf30*) and leucine-rich repeat containing 32 (*LRRC32*) genes, which had previously been identified in genetic analyses of related inflammatory conditions. Four SNPs in this region were significantly associated with total serum IgE levels after adjustment for multiple testing, signifying a common genetic regulation for IgE levels in atopic diseases.[26]

The asthma genes identified through GWAS have also been identified as predictors of blood eosinophil levels, an inflammatory biomarker possibly related to asthma pathogenesis and progression. For example, a large population-based GWAS of 9392 subjects in Iceland identified variants *IL-1RL1*, *WDR36*, and *IL-33* that were associated with eosinophil counts and asthma.[27] Several reports have associated the 5q22 genomic region, spanning the *TSLP* and *WDR36* genes, with asthma,[2,4] and it is also associated with an allergic disorder characterized by excess eosinophils in the esophagus.[28]

ASTHMA THERAPY AND PHARMACOGENETICS

Other genetic mechanisms that can produce more severe or difficult-to-manage asthma are the responses to asthma therapy. This section focuses on new developments in pharmacogenetics research (Table 3.2).

CORTICOSTEROID (GLUCOCORTICOID) PATHWAY

Glucocorticoid steroids are currently the most common anti-inflammatory asthma therapy. In most cases, the regular use of corticosteroids is effective and reduces mortality due to asthma. However, chronic corticosteroid use can result in side effects and there is a subset of severe asthma patients that requires high doses of inhaled and oral corticosteroids to control their symptoms and asthma exacerbations.[7,8] There is also a considerable variability in the response to inhaled corticosteroids (ICS), which is likely to have a genetic component.

The Hop protein (encoded by the stress-induced phosphoprotein 1 [*STIP1*] gene) is involved in the activation of the glucocorticoid receptor and is a novel therapeutic target in the glucocorticoid pathway. In a pharmacogenetic analysis, *STIP1* single nucleotide and haplotypic variation were related to a FEV_1 change in response to treatment with ICS. There was a heterogeneous response to corticosteroids, as approximately one-half of the *STIP1* haplotypes was associated with a reduced ICS response and the other half was associated with a greater sensitivity to ICS.[29]

A recent GWAS by Tantisira and colleagues evaluated four asthma treatment trials ($n = 935$) to identify pharmacogenetic associations related to the response to inhaled glucocorticoids. A significant, replicated association was found in two correlated SNPs in the glucocorticoid-induced transcript 1 (*GLCCI1*) gene, which confer a lung function response to inhaled glucocorticoids and reduced *GLCCI1* expression. The overall mean ($\pm$ standard error) increase in FEV_1 for ICS-treated subjects homozygous for the risk allele was significantly less than for subjects homozygous for the common allele ($3.2 \pm 1.6\%$ vs. $9.4 \pm 1.1\%$, respectively). This is an example of a replicated pharmacogenetic analysis with functional verification.[30] In addition, Tantisira et al. have also shown that a variation in the corticotrophin-releasing hormone receptor 1 gene (*CRHR1*) is associated with an improved lung function response to corticosteroids in three asthma clinical trial populations.[31] Tantisira et al. found genetic variants in the *T* gene and correlated regions associated with a FEV_1 response to ICS in an additional GWAS in the NHLBI Single-Nucleotide Polymorphism Health Association-Asthma Resource Project.[32]

BETA₂-ADRENERGIC PATHWAY

Beta-adrenergic receptor agonists or beta-agonists are commonly prescribed medications for the relief of bronchoconstriction and symptom treatment in asthma. Several pharmacogenetic studies have explored whether functional nonsynonymous *Gly16Arg* and *Gln27Glu* beta₂-adrenergic receptor (*ADRB2*) gene variants could explain the differences in bronchodilator response among asthma patients or identify a subgroup of patients with a reduced response.[33,34] However, extensive resequencing[35] of the *ADRB2* locus in African Americans and non-Hispanic whites with asthma revealed additional rare *ADRB2* polymorphisms, which may also play a role in the response to therapy. For example, African Americans with asthma and rare *ADRB2* alleles treated with a long-acting beta-agonist (LABA) demonstrated a greater percentage of sputum eosinophils when compared with those with common alleles (28% vs. 7%; $P = .02$) or those with rare alleles not treated with LABA (28% vs. 0.4%; $P = .01$).[36] Additionally, non-Hispanic whites with rare *ADRB2* alleles treated with LABA demonstrated a significantly increased number of urgent care and emergency department visits for asthma in the past year.[36] In a similar analysis among individuals with asthma treated with LABA, individuals with rare *ADRB2* variants were more likely to have asthma-related hospitalizations in the past year and to require systemic corticosteroid therapy.[37] These results suggest that rare and common gene variations modulate the responses to asthma therapy.

T-HELPER 2 PATHWAY

There are several novel asthma therapies currently under development targeting molecules in the Th2 pathway. Two clinical trials of these biologics identified specific population subgroups with improved therapeutic responses based on biomarker levels or specific genotypes. Corren and colleagues hypothesized that anti-*IL-13* therapy would benefit asthma patients with a baseline profile consistent with increased Th2 activity (based on the total IgE level and blood eosinophil counts).[38] In a clinical trial of an *IL-13* monoclonal antibody, participant subgroups were prespecified according to their Th2 status and serum periostin levels. In the overall trial, the mean increase in FEV_1 was 5.5% higher in the anti-*IL-13* group than in the placebo group ($P = .02$). However, among patients in the high periostin or the high fraction of exhaled nitric oxide (FeNO) subgroup, the increase from baseline FEV_1 was 8.2% higher in the anti-*IL-13* group than in the placebo group.[38]

Additionally, Wenzel and colleagues reported the results from a clinical trial of pitrakinra, an anti-interleukin 4 (*IL-4*) receptor antagonist. In an ICS-withdrawal, double-blind, randomized, placebo-controlled, multicenter trial, 534 participants with uncontrolled, moderate to severe asthma were randomized to 1, 3, or 10 mg of pitrakinra or a placebo twice daily for a 12-week treatment period.[39] Efficacy was not demonstrated in the overall study population; however, Slager and coworkers showed statistically significant efficacy in prespecified subpopulations including individuals with the GG genotype in IL-4 receptor (*IL-4R*) variant *rs8832*. Individuals with this genotype demonstrated the greatest relative reduction in the incidence of asthma exacerbations at the highest anti-*IL-4R* dose compared with the placebo (88%) and they also had decreased nocturnal awakenings and activities limited by asthma. There was also a significant dose-dependent reduction in exacerbations in these subjects as the frequency of exacerbations in the placebo and the 1, 3, and 10 mg treatment groups was 25%, 16%, 12%, and 3%, respectively.[40] This study represents one of the largest and most informative pharmacogenetic analysis of the Th2 pathway in patients with uncontrolled, moderate to severe asthma.

It is possible that certain biological pathways such as the Th2 immunological pathway may be more active in individuals with severe asthma. These examples are proof of the concept for personalized medicine that specific biologic therapies could be targeted at subgroups of asthma patients based on genotype or specific biomarkers, identifying an asthma subgroup with an improved response to therapy.

Issues such as statistical power, generalizability, and phenotypic characterization that are critical for all genetic studies, are especially important in pharmacogenetic studies. Identifying the appropriate replication populations also remains a challenge, due to the highly specific treatment regimens specified in clinical trials. An important step forward in this field is that GWAS are now being carried out to identify novel genetic predictors of the ICS response and other outcomes. Additionally, current pharmacogenetic analyses also represent an important step in personalized medicine, as clinical decisions for asthma patients may rely on these types of studies in the future.

GENE–ENVIRONMENT INTERACTIONS AND EPIGENETICS

Despite the importance of environmental factors in the development of asthma, very few gene–environment interactions in asthma have been consistently characterized and replicated. The challenges in genetic association studies, such as adequate statistical power, population stratification, gene coverage, and adjustment for false positives, can be compounded in gene–environment interaction studies and accurately measuring environmental factors represents additional obstacles.[41]

Traditional gene–environment studies tested a candidate gene or pathway interacting with a particular exposure for an increased risk of asthma development or severity. One of the most replicated interactions in asthma has been for the −159 promoter variant of the *CD14* gene, which encodes a subunit of the endotoxin receptor found on mononuclear cells. Many exposures have been studied for their interaction with this gene, primarily demonstrating an asthma risk for exposed subjects with the −159T allele while the −159C allele is associated with asthma in nonexposed subjects.[42]

There have also been several gene–environment studies to evaluate the interaction between genes and tobacco smoke exposure related to asthma risk, including a genetic linkage analysis in 200 Dutch families. Linkage signals for asthma and BHR were observed on chromosomes 3p and 5q, though

secondhand smoke (SHS) exposure accounted for BHR linkage to 5q.[43] Similar results were observed in U.S. families.[44] There have also been reports of a gene–environment interaction between SHS and genes in the chromosome 17q12-21 genomic region identified through GWAS.[1,2,4] Two independent, prospective cohort studies in the Netherlands assessed the interaction between *rs2305480* genotype in the *GSDML* gene and maternal smoking during pregnancy or early-life SHS exposure.[45,46] This variant was associated with wheeze and shortness of breath in children exposed to smoke during their fetal life ($P = .04$) or during their early postnatal life ($P = 5.06 \times 10^{-4}$).[46] Variants in this genomic region also interact with active smoking to modulate asthma and its related phenotypes.[47]

Perhaps even more challenging than a systematic and comprehensive evaluation of gene–environment interactions is defining how environmental exposures lead to asthma susceptibility and progression. It is likely that epigenetic mechanisms, such as methylation, regulate gene expression in response to particular exposures, ultimately affecting the disease susceptibility and severity pathways. In many cases, these mechanisms have been studied in candidate gene and genomic repeat sequence regions. For instance, Breton and colleagues investigated the methylation status of specific genomic regions in a cohort of children exposed to maternal smoking compared with those not exposed. The offspring of mothers who smoked during pregnancy had decreased methylation of the AluYb8 repeat sequence, a marker of overall DNA hypomethylation. Additionally, smoking-induced effects on the methylation of long interspersed repetitive elements-1 (LINE1) were noted in children with the glutathione-S-transferase mu 1 (*GSTM1*) null genotype only,[48] providing a putative mechanism for the interaction between epigenetic modulation and the asthma susceptibility candidate gene.

In one of the few genome-wide interaction scans for asthma and atopy, the GABRIEL study group tested genetic variants for their interaction with rural farm-related exposures in 1708 unrelated European children.[49] Overall, no significant genome-wide interactions were identified, suggesting that common genetic polymorphisms may not modulate the influence of the farming environment on childhood asthma, although rare variants could play a role.[49] This analysis also emphasizes that new statistical and measurement tools are needed to address these issues on a genome-wide scale.[41]

Despite the obvious challenges involved in gene–environment interaction studies, these analyses may account for some of the unexplained "missing heritability" observed in genome-wide scans of common diseases such as asthma. Interaction studies can also provide an insight into which environmental exposures contribute to asthma severity and the risk of exacerbations and may guide future interventions.

DISCUSSION

Since the beginning of genome-wide studies in asthma, several genes/chromosomal regions have been consistently associated with asthma susceptibility in multiple ethnic groups: *ORMDL3/GSDMB, IL-33, IL-1RL1, RAD50/IL-13, HLA-DR/DQ, TSLP,* and *SMAD3* (Table 3.1).[1,2,4] In most cases, the effect of each individual genetic variant is relatively small, suggesting that the additive effect of multiple risk variants should be evaluated. An important goal of the genetic approach in a complex disease is to identify a group of variants that will reliably predict the risk of the development (susceptibility) or progression (severity) of the disease. As the variants that contribute to susceptibility may not be the same as those that contribute to severity, it is important to characterize asthma disease heterogeneity, as different phenotypes may reflect several pathogenic pathways that have different underlying genetic architecture.[8] Improved phenotyping approaches will also improve our ability to link genotypes and phenotypes. Genes that contribute to endophenotypes such as lung function and biomarker levels provide insight into the mechanisms of asthma progression (Table 3.2).

Future genetic studies in asthma severity will also incorporate whole-genome or exome-specific sequencing to identify more common and rare genetic variants. Exome and complete genome sequencing will provide better genomic coverage than existing genotyping platforms and will discover biologically relevant causal variants. For example, resequencing the *IL-4* gene in African Americans identified an excess of private noncoding variants in asthma cases compared with unaffected individuals.[50] New genotyping technologies and comprehensive phenotyping should elucidate the genetics of asthma severity in the future. Understanding the functional biology of these novel variants that were discovered through genome-wide sequencing and how they interact with the environment will also become increasingly important. Using these variants that were identified in comprehensively phenotyped studies, we may more effectively develop a personalized therapy for all individuals with asthma.

ACKNOWLEDGMENTS

This work was funded by NHLBI grants HL69167 and HL101487. RES was supported by HL089992 and HL101487.

REFERENCES

1. Moffatt MF, Kabesch M, Liang L, et al. Genetic variants regulating ORMDL3 expression contribute to the risk of childhood asthma. *Nature* 2007;448:470–473.
2. Moffatt MF, Gut IG, Demenais F, et al. A large-scale, consortium-based genomewide association study of asthma. *N Engl J Med* 2010;363:1211–1221.
3. Li X, Howard TD, Zheng SL, et al. Genome-wide association study of asthma identifies RAD50-IL13 and HLA-DR/DQ regions. *J Allergy Clin Immunol* 2010;125:328–335.
4. Torgerson DG, Ampleford EJ, Chiu GY, et al. Meta-analysis of genome-wide association studies of asthma in ethnically diverse North American populations. *Nat Genet* 2011;43:887–892.
5. Moffatt MF, Schou C, Faux JA, et al. Association between quantitative traits underlying asthma and the HLA-DRB1 locus in a family-based population sample. *Eur J Hum Gen* 2001;9:341–346.
6. Durbin RM, Abecasis GR, Altshuler DL, et al. A map of human genome variation from population-scale sequencing. *Nature* 2010;467:1061–1073.
7. Moore WC, Bleecker ER, Curran-Everett D, et al. Characterization of the severe asthma phenotype by the National Heart, Lung, and Blood Institute's Severe Asthma Research Program. *J Allergy Clin Immunol* 2007;119:405–413.
8. Moore WC, Meyers DA, Wenzel SE, et al. Identification of asthma phenotypes using cluster analysis in the Severe Asthma Research Program. *Am J Respir Crit Care Med* 2010;181:315–323.
9. Mathias RA, Grant AV, Rafaels N, et al. A genome-wide association study on African-ancestry populations for asthma. *J Allergy Clin Immunol* 2010;125:336–346.
10. Allen M, Heinzmann A, Noguchi E, et al. Positional cloning of a novel gene influencing asthma from chromosome 2q14. *Nat Gen* 2003;35:258–263.
11. Torgerson DG, Capurso D, Ampleford EJ, et al. Genome-wide ancestry association testing identifies a common European variant on 6q14.1 as a risk factor for asthma in African American subjects. *J Allergy Clin Immunol* 2012;130:622–629.
12. Hirota T, Takahashi A, Kubo M, et al. Genome-wide association study identifies three new susceptibility loci for adult asthma in the Japanese population. *Nat Gen* 2011;43:893–896.
13. Noguchi E, Sakamoto H, Hirota T, et al. Genome-wide association study identifies HLA-DP as a susceptibility gene for pediatric asthma in Asian populations. *PLoS Genet* 2011;7:e1002170.
14. Fang Q, Zhao H, Wang A, et al. Association of genetic variants in chromosome 17q21 and adult-onset asthma in a Chinese Han population. *BMC Med Gen* 2011;12:133.
15. Haselkorn T, Fish JE, Zeiger RS, et al. Consistently very poorly controlled asthma, as defined by the impairment domain of the Expert Panel Report 3 guidelines, increases risk for future severe asthma exacerbations in The Epidemiology and Natural History of Asthma: Outcomes and Treatment Regimens (TENOR) study. *J Allergy Clin Immunol* 2009;124:895–902.
16. Howard TD, Whittaker PA, Zaiman AL, et al. Identification and association of polymorphisms in the interleukin-13 gene with asthma and atopy in a Dutch population. *Am J Respir Cell Mol Biol* 2001;25:377–384.
17. Wills-Karp M, Luyimbazi J, Xu X, et al. Interleukin-13: Central mediator of allergic asthma. *Science* 1998;282:2258–2261.
18. Hancock DB, Eijgelsheim M, Wilk JB, et al. Meta-analyses of genome-wide association studies identify multiple loci associated with pulmonary function. *Nat Gen* 2010;42:45–52.
19. Repapi E, Sayers I, Wain LV, et al. Genome-wide association study identifies five loci associated with lung function. *Nat Genet* 2010;42:36–44.
20. Li X, Howard TD, Moore WC, et al. Importance of hedgehog interacting protein and other lung function genes in asthma. *J Allergy Clin Immunol* 2011;127:1457–1465.
21. Ferreira MA, Matheson MC, Duffy DL, et al. Identification of IL6R and chromosome 11q13.5 as risk loci for asthma. *Lancet* 2011;378:1006–1014.
22. Hawkins GA, Robinson MB, Hastie AT, et al. The IL6R variation Asp(358)Ala is a potential modifier of lung function in subjects with asthma. *J Allergy Clin Immunol* 2012;130:510–515.
23. Imboden M, Bouzigon E, Curjuric I, et al. Genome-wide association study of lung function decline in adults with and without asthma. *J Allergy Clin Immunol* 2012;129:1218–1228.

24. Weidinger S, Gieger C, Rodriguez E, et al. Genome-wide scan on total serum IgE levels identifies FCER1A as novel susceptibility locus. *PLoS Genet* 2008;4:e1000166.

25. Granada M, Wilk JB, Tuzova M, et al. A genome-wide association study of plasma total IgE concentrations in the Framingham Heart Study. *J Allergy Clin Immunol* 2012;129:840–845.

26. Li X, Ampleford EJ, Howard TD, et al. The C11orf30-LRRC32 region is associated with total serum IgE levels in asthmatic patients. *J Allergy Clin Immunol* 2012;129:575–578.

27. Gudbjartsson DF, Bjornsdottir US, Halapi E, et al. Sequence variants affecting eosinophil numbers associate with asthma and myocardial infarction. *Nat Gen* 2009;41:342–347.

28. Rothenberg ME, Spergel JM, Sherrill JD, et al. Common variants at 5q22 associate with pediatric eosinophilic esophagitis. *Nat Gen* 2010;42:289–291.

29. Hawkins GA, Lazarus R, Smith RS, et al. The glucocorticoid receptor heterocomplex gene STIP1 is associated with improved lung function in asthmatic subjects treated with inhaled corticosteroids. *J Allergy Clin Immunol* 2009;123:1376–1383.

30. Tantisira KG, Lasky-Su J, Harada M, et al. Genomewide association between GLCCI1 and response to glucocorticoid therapy in asthma. *N Engl J Med* 2011;365:1173–1183.

31. Tantisira KG, Lake S, Silverman ES, et al. Corticosteroid pharmacogenetics: Association of sequence variants in CRHR1 with improved lung function in asthmatics treated with inhaled corticosteroids. *Hum Mol Genet* 2004;13:1353–1359.

32. Tantisira KG, Damask A, Szefler SJ, et al. Genome-wide association identifies the T gene as a novel asthma pharmacogenetic locus. *Am J Resp Crit Care Med* 2012;185:1286–1291.

33. Bleecker ER, Nelson HS, Kraft M, et al. Beta2-receptor polymorphisms in patients receiving salmeterol with or without fluticasone propionate. *Am J Respir Crit Care Med* 2010;181:676–687.

34. Bleecker ER, Postma DS, Lawrance RM, et al. Effect of ADRB2 polymorphisms on response to longacting beta2-agonist therapy: A pharmacogenetic analysis of two randomised studies. *Lancet* 2007;370:2118–2125.

35. Hawkins GA, Tantisira K, Meyers DA, et al. Sequence, haplotype, and association analysis of ADRbeta2 in a multiethnic asthma case-control study. *Am J Respir Crit Care Med* 2006;174:1101–1109.

36. Ortega VE, Hastie A, Sadeghnejad A, et al. Rare beta2-adrenergic receptor gene polymorphisms in asthma cases and controls from the Severe Asthma Research Program. *Am J Respir Crit Care Med* 2011;183:A1357.

37. Ortega VE, Hawkins G, Hastie AT, et al. Effects of rare β2-adrenergic receptor gene variants and long-acting beta agonists on healthcare utilization and corticosteroid use in two multi-ethnic asthma populations. *Am J Respir Crit Care Med* 2012;185:A2514.

38. Corren J, Lemanske RF, Hanania NA, et al. Lebrikizumab treatment in adults with asthma. *N Engl J Med* 2011;365:1088–1098.

39. Wenzel SE, Ind PW, Otulana BA, et al. Inhaled pitrakinra, an IL-4/IL-13 antagonist, reduced exacerbations in patients with eosinophilic asthma. *Eur Resp J* 2010;36:P3980.

40. Slager RE, Otulana BA, Hawkins GA, et al. IL-4 receptor polymorphisms predict reduction in asthma exacerbations during response to an anti-IL-4 receptor alpha antagonist. *J Allergy Clin Immunol* 2012;130:516–522.

41. Ober C, Vercelli D. Gene-environment interactions in human disease: Nuisance or opportunity? *Trends Genet* 2011;27:107–115.

42. Koppelman GH. Gene by environment interaction in asthma. *Curr Allergy Asthma Reports* 2006;6:103–111.

43. Meyers DA, Postma DS, Stine OC, et al. Genome screen for asthma and bronchial hyperresponsiveness: Interactions with passive smoke exposure. *J Allergy Clin Immunol* 2005;115:1169–1175.

44. Colilla S, Nicolae D, Pluzhnikov A, et al. Evidence for gene-environment interactions in a linkage study of asthma and smoking exposure. *J Allergy Clin Immunol* 2003;111:840–846.

45. Bouzigon E, Corda E, Aschard H, et al. Effect of 17q21 variants and smoking exposure in early-onset asthma. *N Eng J Med* 2008;359:1985–1994.

46. van der Valk RJ, Duijts L, Kerkhof M, et al. Interaction of a 17q12 variant with both fetal and infant smoke exposure in the development of childhood asthma-like symptoms. *Allergy* 2012;67:767–774.

47. Marinho S, Custovic A, Marsden P, et al. 17q12-21 Variants are associated with asthma and interact with active smoking in an adult population from the United Kingdom. *Ann Allergy Asthma Immunol* 2012;108:402–411.

48. Breton CV, Byun HM, Wenten M, et al. Prenatal tobacco smoke exposure affects global and gene-specific DNA methylation. *Am J Respir Crit Care Med* 2009;180:462–467.

49. Ege MJ, Strachan DP, Cookson WO, et al. Gene-environment interaction for childhood asthma and exposure to farming in Central Europe. *J Allergy Clin Immunol* 2011;127:138–144.

50. Haller G, Torgerson DG, Ober C, et al. Sequencing the IL4 locus in African Americans implicates rare noncoding variants in asthma susceptibility. *J Allergy Clin Immunol* 2009;124:1204–1209.

4 Endotypes and Asthma

Pranabashis Haldar and Rachid Berair

CONTENTS

CASE PRESENTATION

A 44-year-old Caucasian woman was referred to the asthma clinic with daily episodes of exertional breathlessness associated with wheeze, chest tightness, and a nonproductive cough. Two years previously, her primary care physician had diagnosed her with asthma, but her symptoms failed to respond satisfactorily to an escalating regime of asthma medication and, at the time of referral, she was prescribed a short-acting and a long-acting beta₂-adrenergic agonist,

theophylline, inhaled corticosteroids (1600 mcg beclomethasone equivalent), and maintenance oral prednisolone (10 mg). She reported no childhood or family history of asthma but had suffered previously with seasonal allergic rhinitis. She was a retired librarian and a lifelong nonsmoker. She lived alone and kept no domestic pets.

A detailed assessment at the asthma clinic identified that she was clinically obese with a body mass index (BMI) of 36 kg/m². She was a mouth breather with a respiratory *rate of 24 breaths per minute at rest. A respiratory examination demonstrated a mild expiratory wheeze with symmetrically reduced air entry. Spirometry was obstructive (forced expiratory volume in 1 second [FEV$_1$] 66% predicted, FEV$_1$/forced vital capacity [FVC] ratio of 0.6), with an 8% improvement in FEV$_1$ after 400 mcg of inhaled albuterol. She reported a high score of 28 on the Nijmegen Questionnaire, suggesting hyperventilation. Bronchial provocation testing with methacholine (PC$_{20}$) was positive at 6.4 mg/mL. Laboratory investigations, including total immunoglobulin E (IgE) and specific IgE for common allergens and molds, were unremarkable. A chest radiograph was normal. Markers of airway inflammation suggested a noneosinophilic pattern with a fractional nitric oxide concentration in exhaled breath (FeNO$_{50}$) of 8 ppb and an induced sputum quantitative cell count comprising 74% neutrophils, 24% macrophages, 2% lymphocytes, and 0% eosinophils. On this basis, her oral prednisolone dose was weaned and eventually stopped. She was referred to a dietician for weight reduction advice and was seen by a physiotherapist for breathing retraining. Serial induced sputum for quantitative cell counts remained noneosinophilic after reducing corticosteroid therapy. The patient was able to lose weight and, with time, most of her symptoms improved significantly.*

It is widely acknowledged that asthma is a heterogeneous disorder characterized by broad variability within the population for patterns of airway pathology, physiological disturbance, clinical symptoms, and response to therapy. Current asthma guidelines recommend a "one-size-fits-all" approach to management and, as this case illustrates, this is not always appropriate and can lead to poor outcomes. In this chapter, we will discuss the origins of asthma heterogeneity and the principles of classification to yield asthma phenotypes, focusing in particular on the increasing utilization of multivariate mathematical techniques for this purpose. Finally, we will review the currently accepted, important phenotypes of asthma and how they influence pathways for care.

INTRODUCTION

Surely it is hard to believe that the wheeze which comes to the young school girl for a day or two in the middle of the ragweed season is the same disease as that which develops suddenly in the tired business man or in the harassed housewife and pushes them down to the depths of depletion and despair. The problem is still wide open: the approach to it is not at all clear.

Rackemann 1948[1]

OVERVIEW OF HETEROGENEITY IN ASTHMA

Fundamentally, the absence of a disease-specific marker for asthma compromises diagnostic rigor. There are a number of accepted approaches to securing a diagnosis of asthma[2]

and the congruity between these pathways remains to be validated.

The heterogeneity in asthma is complex and multifactorial and a proposal for its basis is summarized in Figure 4.1. In broad terms, the pathogenesis of asthma includes multiple steps and its heterogeneity is recognized at each level. Its heterogeneity is further complicated by time (natural variation in disease activity) and therapy. The effect of these additional dimensions is likely underestimated in cross-sectional studies. A number of comorbidities are associated with chronic asthma. These may represent both overlapping and unrelated pathologies that coexist to either mimic or exacerbate clinical asthma symptoms. In common with other chronic diseases, the clinical expression of asthma is associated with a significant and variable psychosocial component.[3] This is frequently overlooked and may be difficult to quantify. Finally, the heterogeneity in the response to asthma pharmacotherapy is complex and multifactorial and an important component of the need for individualized therapy for patients with refractory asthma.

PROBLEMS ARISING FROM ASTHMA HETEROGENEITY

Heterogeneity is arguably the major intellectual limitation to progress in our understanding of asthma.[4] Perhaps one of the greatest barriers to the characterization of the heterogeneity of asthma has been the success of glucocorticoid therapy in the management of asthma. Glucocorticoids constitute a broad spectrum of anti-inflammatory therapies that is effective in a large proportion of patients, irrespective of the underlying pathological processes. Nevertheless, the failure of the effectiveness of conventional approaches is obvious in the subgroup of patients with difficult asthma. In this group, the heterogeneity is striking and the etiology of poor clinical control is broad and multifactorial. A systematic approach to the evaluation of these patients, together with a multidisciplinary and individualized management plan is recommended for optimizing care. More generally, there is an ambition to provide personalized therapy for all asthma sufferers.

From a scientific perspective, genetic and molecular association studies necessarily require the study of populations that are homogeneous with respect to their underlying disease pathways. The heterogeneity in such study samples increases the likelihood of type II errors. This is especially pertinent for gene-association studies where functional single nucleotide polymorphisms have a very low, independent attributable risk (less than 5%).[4] A number of novel and primarily engineered molecular therapies have been developed over the past decade, and trials with these drugs are invaluable not only for informing clinical efficacy but also for providing a novel strategy to understand elements of human asthma immunobiology *in vivo*. A meaningful interpretation of the outcomes from such studies requires a careful molecular characterization of the participating cohort.

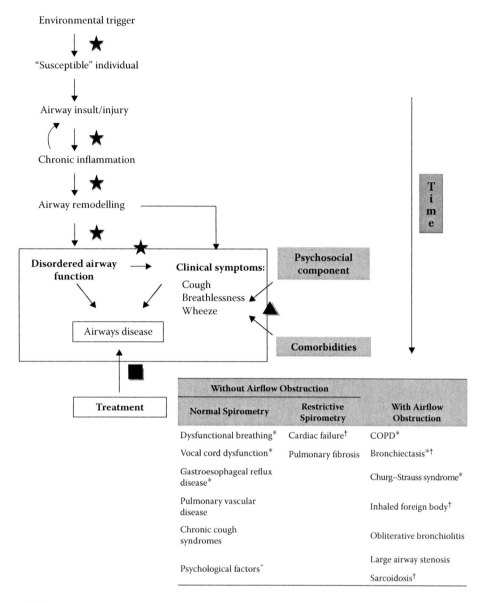

FIGURE 4.1   (See color insert) The basis of heterogeneity in asthma. Pathological heterogeneity (★) is a function of the spectrum of possible expressions at each proposed step of the disease pathogenesis. Clinical heterogeneity originates from pathological heterogeneity and is modified by a spectrum of responses to treatment (■) together with the confounding effect of comorbidities, psychosocial factors (▲), and time (long arrow). The table summarizes the commonly recognized disorders that may mimic or aggravate the clinical symptoms of asthma. *These conditions may coexist with asthma. †These conditions may be associated with normal spirometry. ^Psychological factors are also associated with behavioral traits that lead to increased disease activity in asthma. These include poor treatment adherence, failure to attend medical appointments, and smoking.

DEFINING PHENOTYPES AND ENDOTYPES

In its broadest sense, the purpose of characterizing heterogeneity in asthma is to identify and understand homogeneous subpopulations within the whole that are clinically and biologically meaningful. Increasingly, these subpopulations are described as phenotypes of asthma. In biology, a phenotype is defined as "the observable properties of an organism arising as a product of the interaction of their genotype with the environment." Endophenotypes or endotypes are more specific and refer to discrete pathogenic pathways[4] that, in theory, define a single disease process.

DISTINGUISHING PHENOTYPES AND ENDOTYPES

The difference between phenotypes and endotypes is not simply a matter of semantics. The heterogeneity in asthma has two key elements: (i) the existence of multiple pathological entities (different endotypes) and (ii) the variable influences exerted by the environment on the individual's genotype (variability within a single endotype). Fundamentally, efforts to characterize the heterogeneity of asthma need to focus on the identification of endotypes. By definition, endotypes are stable. Once these are established, the effects of the environment may be understood more clearly.

ENDOTYPES AND BIOMARKER DEVELOPMENT

A biomarker is broadly defined as any measurable characteristic that may be used as an indicator of the risk, presence, or severity of a disease state. There is considerable interest and investment in the search for novel biomarkers that may inform asthma phenotypes. In this role, biomarkers must be detectable in the presence of the disease and be independent of the disease activity and therefore the effects of therapy. However, biomarkers to date have been developed to measure disease activity. Sputum eosinophils are one example. While of clinical benefit to inform the prognosis (exacerbation risk) and the response to therapy (with corticosteroids), a clear limitation of the value of sputum eosinophilia as a phenotypic biomarker is the uncertainty arising from its variability with time and therapy.

GOALS OF CHARACTERIZING HETEROGENEITY IN ASTHMA: DIFFERENCES IN CLINICAL AND SCIENTIFIC END POINTS

The goals of asthma characterization are a product of the limitations that may be overcome by removing heterogeneity. From the discussion so far, the clinical drivers for characterizing heterogeneity differ and may even be in conflict with the scientific ideal of discovering endotypes (Table 4.1). Furthermore, discovering endotypes may require the utilization of complex, sophisticated, and expensive techniques that are far removed from the bedside tests needed for implementation in clinical practice. It is therefore likely that the evolution of the characterization of asthma will see the development of parallel models for clinical and scientific purposes that may converge as the mechanisms of the disease are better understood (Figure 4.2).

CLASSIFICATION OF ASTHMA: A HISTORICAL PERSPECTIVE

The history of asthma phenotypes provides a useful reference point for illustrating the challenges that characterizing the heterogeneity of asthma presents and the strategies that are being developed to overcome these challenges. The classification of different forms of asthma can be traced back to the seventeenth century when William Harvey suggested a distinction between asthma of bronchial and cardiac origins. Since that time, there have been several important shifts in the ideology governing the diagnosis and classification of asthma. In the nineteenth century, the recognition of "allergic excitation" together with the development of skin testing techniques encouraged a very narrow perspective of asthma as a disease that was necessarily associated with and precipitated by allergies, verifiable with skin testing. Through the diligent collection of case records, Rackemann clearly illustrated the absence of an identifiable allergic trigger in a large proportion of cases with clinical asthma.[5] He suggested a number of other associations that were significant for this group and, on this basis, he proposed a model for asthma classification. In his paper describing intrinsic asthma, Rackemann[6] summarizes this change to a broader perspective:

> In the beginning all was allergy that wheezed, and if the methods peculiar to allergy could not reveal the cause, these methods were deemed faulty. It was recognised, however, that the simple allergic process could be aggravated and continued by secondary infections. Still later, primary infections came to be regarded as the cause of asthma...

A natural consequence of a more inclusive approach to the diagnosis of asthma has been the greater heterogeneity that clinicians have sought to classify in a variety of ways (Table 4.1). The following overview illustrates a number of important points:

1. Classification was performed by clinicians with a consequent emphasis on *clinically relevant parameters.*
2. Classification was *subjective* and based on factors that the investigator deemed important.
3. Classification was usually based on a *single aspect* of the disease. A single determinant therefore defined the structure of each model and, unsurprisingly, different parameters yielded models that shared little in common.

PRINCIPLES OF CHARACTERIZING HETEROGENEITY: LESSONS FROM BIOLOGY

The reference to phenotypes of asthma is recent and significant as it acknowledges the increasing application of the taxonomic principles of biology classification. In brief, biological taxonomy is founded on the principle that the greater the number of shared characteristics between two organisms, the greater the probability that a biological relationship exists between them. A detailed physical characterization or "phenotyping" is therefore a core element of this process. Classification or taxonomy refers to the construction of models for placing phenotypes in a manner that informs their underlying relationships. Characterizing the heterogeneity is therefore a two-step process of *phenotyping* and *classification.*

Both phenotypes and classification models may change on the basis of the information gathered or available, new diagnostic techniques, and the goals that are defined. Such changes are influenced by advances in scientific understanding, and the taxonomy of any system should therefore be viewed as a dynamic process. The history of biological taxonomy illustrates this well. Although the methodological principle of grouping by observable characteristics was retained, its scope broadened over time with the development of a numerical taxonomy in the mid-twentieth century,[7] which used computer-based mathematical algorithms (cluster analysis) to measure the "evolutionary distance" between organisms on the basis of considerably larger numbers of recorded characteristics. More recently, the availability of genetic information from advances in DNA sequencing techniques has led to the replacement of a

TABLE 4.1
Historical and Modern Phenotypes of Asthma

Characteristic Measured	Author	Phenotype Description	Clinical Utility			Scientific Utility			Stable with Time and Therapy
			Informs Therapy	Informs Risk/ Prognosis	Informs Management	Informs Pathobiology	Yields Biomarkers	Associated Genetic Polymorphisms	
Classical Phenotypes									
Trigger based	Rackemann (1928)	Extrinsic/intrinsic asthma	++	+	+	+	+	Unknown	+
	Burge (1992)	Occupational asthma[a]	±	+	++	+	–	Unknown	–
Variable airflow obstruction (peak flow)	Samter (1968)	Aspirin sensitive	+	+	+	+	–	Unknown	+
	Ayres (1998)	Types I and II brittle asthma	+	+	+	Unknown	+	Unknown	–
	Turner–Warwick (1977)	Brittle/morning dipper/ irreversible/drifter	+	+	–	Unknown	+	Unknown	–
Treatment requirement	GINA (1995), ATS (2000)	Refractory (severe asthma/difficult asthma)	NA	++	+	Unknown	–	Unknown	±
Asthma outcome	Boulet (1995)	Fixed airflow obstruction	–	+	–	Unknown	–	+	+
Modern Phenotypes									
Inflammatory	Pavord (1999)	Eosinophilic/ noneosinophilic	++	+	+	+	+	Unknown	–
Early-onset atopic	Multiple authors	Synonymous with extrinsic asthma	++	+	+	+	+	Unknown	+
Late-onset eosinophilic	Wenzel (2006)	Aspirin sensitive/ inflammation predominant	++	+	+	+	+	Unknown	±
Obesity-related asthma	Haldar (2008)	Late onset, female predominant, and noneosinophilic	+	+	+	Unknown	+	Unknown	Unknown

Note: GINA, Global Initiative for Asthma; ATS, American Thoracic Society.

[a] Occupational asthma is a stable phenotype in that a defined trigger predictably causes and aggravates asthma in a susceptible individual; however, early avoidance of the occupational agent may prevent chronic asthma from developing at all.

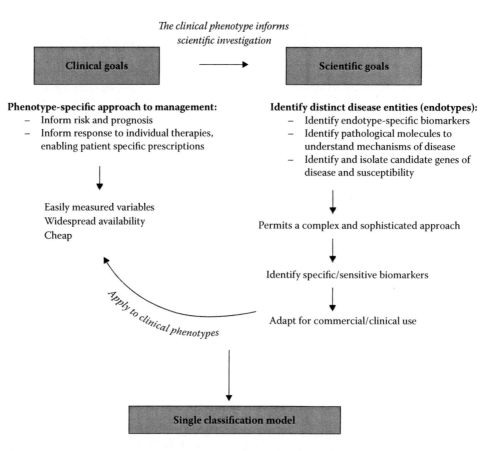

FIGURE 4.2 The dynamics of asthma classification. The schema illustrates the differences in the focus for the development of classification models of clinical and scientific interest. Such models may develop in parallel to inform each other and may converge with time.

phenotype-based numerical taxonomy with phylogenetics to compare genetic data from organisms past and present, using predictive mathematical models to construct evolutionary trees. Thus, the "evolution" of taxonomy is dependent on developments in many fields, and the terms *systems biology* and *systems medicine* have been coined to underline the need for a coordinated and multidisciplinary approach to the ongoing refinement of the taxonomy of different biological systems.

MULTIVARIATE MATHEMATICAL TECHNIQUES

The development of technologies enabling the high throughput and high efficiency output of molecular and genetic data is yielding large and complex data sets for analysis. Methodologically, classical analysis techniques alone are insufficient and not well suited to address the scientific questions posed by such data. In particular, such techniques are not designed to explore the underlying pattern structure, and between-group comparisons are undermined by the uncertainty of how to define statistical significances after multiple comparisons.[8]

MULTIVARIATE TECHNIQUES APPLIED TO ASTHMA

Characterizing heterogeneity on the basis of multiple aspects of a disease is biologically appealing. First, it incorporates a broader spectrum of observable characteristics, increasing

the likelihood of identifying meaningful (biological) relationships. Secondly, it defines each phenotype on the basis of the relationship expressed between different domains of the disease rather than the absolute expression of a single aspect of the disease. In biological terms, examining relationships between domains is likely to better delineate the underlying processes and pathways. Additionally, this will be associated with greater phenotypic stability. As an example, "noneosinophilic asthma" (discussed further later) may indicate either a distinct phenotype or eosinophilic asthma with good inflammatory control. The two are indistinguishable on the basis of inflammatory characteristics alone. The inclusion of clinical symptom expression as a characteristic may distinguish these groups by revealing concordance of expression (few symptoms) with well-controlled eosinophilic asthma, and discordance with the true noneosinophilic phenotype. Furthermore, such a system would correctly classify poorly controlled eosinophilic asthma (high levels of eosinophilic inflammation + high symptoms) together with well-controlled eosinophilic asthma (noneosinophilic + few symptoms) as the same phenotype across a spectrum of severity.

MULTIVARIATE TECHNIQUES USED IN ASTHMA: CLUSTER ANALYSIS AND FACTOR ANALYSIS

The past decade has witnessed an increasing use of factor analysis and cluster analysis as multivariate techniques for characterizing asthma heterogeneity. Although conceptually similar, the two groups of techniques differ in the algorithms that they employ, with implications for their respective suitability to different classification tasks. Both seek to identify patterns within data and these patterns inform the likely underlying structure of the data that forms the basis of their classification. Each group of techniques comprises a number of algorithms that differ in the mathematical rules governing pattern recognition and classification processes. This can lead to considerable variability in the interpretation of the data structure. An understanding of the underlying principles of these techniques is therefore a necessary prerequisite for their appropriate use in research practice.

FACTOR ANALYSIS

Overview

Factor analysis includes a group of algorithms that are primarily used to identify patterns of variability and the correlation between variables within a data set. In brief, variables that group together are represented by a factor, which is mathematically the vectorial sum of the contributions from each component variable. The factor, therefore, represents a weighted sum of data from all the grouping variables, and may be used in place of the individual variables in a further analysis without a significant loss of information (Figure 4.3).

Methodology

Factor analysis techniques use a two-step algorithm to classify patterns of expression (Figure 4.3). The first step is primarily a data reduction step. In this step, a factor "axis" is constructed that maximizes the representation of the common variability within the data (in effect, linear regression). A second factor is then constructed to specifically account for the variability that is *not* included in the first step. This factor is, therefore, mathematically independent of the first and will be represented geometrically by an axis that is perpendicular to the first factor axis. Iterations continue until all of the variability within the data set is accounted for by independent factors. The second step of the algorithm is an optimization step. The factor axes are rotated to maximize their representation of the variability for groups of variables rather than the whole data set. With rotation, the relationships between each factor axis and the individual variables will change; however, the proportion of variance of the data set accounted for by the factor remains constant. Rotation is important for changing the emphasis of the factors from a data reduction model that is representative of the whole data set to a structural model in which individual factors define the clustering variables. The rotated factor solution is believed to yield "invariant factors," that is, the factor model is less sensitive to the removal or the addition of one or a few data set items.

Uses

The main uses of factor analysis are data reduction and the identification of groups of variables sharing related patterns of expression. Data reduction is invaluable to help overcome the problems associated with the application of classical statistical tests to complex data sets. This is achieved using either the factor score for each factor (weighted sum of the contribution of all variables to the factor) or a single representative variable (with a high loading coefficient to the factor, implying a majority contribution to the factor score) for further analysis. As a technique that identifies relationships between groups of variables, factor analysis makes statistical inferences that can contribute to identifying and understanding underlying mechanisms and processes. However, the relationships defined by factor analysis are mathematical and not biological. The identified patterns are *hypothesis generating* and can help direct further study; factor analysis should not be used in isolation to draw biological conclusions.

Application in Asthma

The properties of factor analysis make it a powerful tool for characterizing heterogeneity. A large number of measurable characteristics are routinely recorded as part of a clinical assessment of asthma. Yet, little is known about the relationship and redundancy that exist between these variables and whether the information that is gathered may be organized in a structured manner. Factor analysis lends itself to tackling these questions. Rosi and colleagues[9] performed a factor analysis of eight measured characteristics recorded in 99 consecutive patients with asthma. The authors identified three factors associated with the eight measurements and, based on the loading patterns, these factors could be identified as being representative of lung function (FEV_1, FVC, inspiratory vital capacity [IVC]); airway dysfunction (bronchodilator reversibility, airway hyperresponsiveness); and eosinophilic airway inflammation (sputum eosinophils, eosinophil cationic protein [ECP]), respectively. Conceptually, the factor model presents a view of the independent components or domains that make up the clinical phenotype of asthma.

CLUSTER ANALYSIS

Overview

Cluster analysis is a generic term for a broad range of numerical methods that is designed primarily to identify groups or clusters of homogeneous observations within heterogeneous multivariate data sets.[10] In mathematical terms, a cluster refers to a collection of items that exhibits "internal cohesion" (within-group homogeneity) and "external isolation" (between-group separation). Cluster analysis algorithms are designed to fulfill both conditions. Whereas factor analysis classifies the patterns of expression of *variables*, cluster analysis is more appropriately utilized to perform the classification of the *population* based on patterns of expression for specified variables.

Methodology

Cluster analysis techniques are broadly of two types: (i) hierarchical and (ii) nonhierarchical or optimization clustering techniques. Broadly speaking, clustering techniques follow a two-step algorithm. The first step involves quantifying

	Factor Analysis	**Cluster Analysis**
Plotting data for reduction	The population sum for each variable is calculated and plotted as a vector in space	The geometrical position of each data point is computed from the vectorial sum of the clustering variables
Measuring similarity	Angular relationship between constructed vectors	Geometrical distance in space between plotted data point(s)
Grouping	Defined according to the angular relationship between vectors and constructed factor axes	*Hierarchical methods:* Either group together or divide preformed groups according to threshold distances between pairs of data point(s)
		Nonhierarchical methods: Construct a prespecified number of cluster centers. Clusters are defined according to the geometrical distance between data point(s) and cluster centers
Outcome	Useful for characterising relationships between variables within a data set	Useful for grouping cases within a data set on the basis of shared similarity for chosen variables

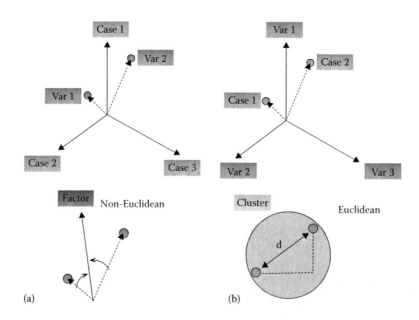

FIGURE 4.3 **(See color insert)** An overview and a comparison of (a) factor analysis and (b) cluster analysis.

the similarity between cases. This is a geometrical distance in space. The second step involves placing cases into groups on the basis of their measured similarity. Group allocation is an iterative process (Figure 4.3). Similarity may be defined on the basis of one (monothetic) or several (polythetic) variables and is generally measured as the geometric distance between two cases plotted in space. Several geometric measures of distance are available with differing influences on the outcome. For polythetic clustering, the number of variables used determines the dimensionality of the distance calculation; this calculation assumes that all dimensions are statistically independent. An increasing dimensionality requires larger sample sizes to identify the cluster structure, and Formann[11] suggests a minimum sample size of 2^k, where k is the number of variables used for clustering. Within the

families of hierarchical and nonhierarchical cluster analysis, various algorithms exist that differ according to the mathematical functions that are used for measuring similarity and grouping cases into clusters. For a given data set, these differences can lead to considerable variability in the cluster structure.

Uses

As previously discussed, cluster analysis is used to inform the taxonomic structure. In psychiatry, cluster analysis has played a useful role in both informing and validating aspects of the disease nomenclature.[12] The technique has also been applied to risk stratify subgroups within a heterogeneous population of attempted suicide cases.[13] Conceptually, the identification of risk *groups* rather than risk *factors* in this way may be a better approach for studying complex and multifactorial outcomes.

LIMITATIONS OF MULTIVARIATE METHODS

Multivariate techniques have a growing application in the applied sciences. However, the idea that these numerical approaches yield results that are objective and free of a priori bias should not be considered dogma. Applying multivariate techniques to biological disciplines relies appropriately on subject-specific expertise for deciding the factors for inclusion in an analysis and the interpretation of the results obtained. Both of these aspects have a significant subjective weighting. In an exploratory context, multivariate techniques are, perhaps, better considered as quantitative approaches to a qualitative solution. From a methodological perspective, there is no accepted standardized approach, and far from being "black-box" techniques, analyses can be customized in accordance with the study and the subject-specific aims. Until a validated and standardized methodology is available, conclusions derived from the outcomes of such studies require cautious interpretation. Variability is also compounded by differences in the composition of the populations sampled. The results obtained in a single population would require replication at other centers for validation.

CONCLUSIONS

Despite the limitations, factor and cluster analyses offer a novel approach for tackling the complexity of asthma heterogeneity. The two groups of methods provide complementary information and may be used in tandem: factor analysis can be used to define the distinct domains or dimensions that make up the asthma phenotype and cluster analysis may be used to study distinct patterns of domain coexpression in the asthma population (Figure 4.3).

CLASSIFICATION OF ASTHMA AND RECOGNIZED PHENOTYPES

OVERVIEW

Studies suggest that asthma phenotypes may differ between adults and children. Many phenotypes of childhood wheeze do not progress to asthma and are not considered further here. True endotypes of asthma are yet to be characterized. The most likely candidates are phenotypes described on the basis of defined triggers. For these, one may hypothesize a clear genetic susceptibility to the trigger that is associated with the clinical manifestation of the disease and this relationship is invariant of time and therapy. Although they are not endotypes of the disease, molecular associations with the response to specific therapies have been identified. Targeted gene studies have identified polymorphisms of the $beta_2$-adrenoceptor as being associated with the heterogeneity in the response to short-acting beta-agonists but not long-acting beta-agonists,[14] and polymorphisms of the 5-lipoxygenase

biosynthetic and receptor pathway are associated with a differential response to montelukast.[15]

There is some debate about whether severe asthma constitutes a phenotype of asthma. In some ways, this is analogous to the argument of whether old age is a phenotype of man. Like age, severity is a descriptive term applied to qualify phenotypic expression, with no independent significance for examining phylogenetic relationships. However, old age has prognostic importance and may help inform the factors associated with the mechanisms of aging. Similarly, severe asthma is prognostically significant and further, it is proposed that specific genetic factors associated with "severity" may only be identified by characterizing severe asthma as a phenotype.[4]

Phenotyping on the basis of asthma outcomes is also an approach that has been used. From a methodological viewpoint, outcomes should be a product of, and be predicted by the phenotype. It remains a matter of debate whether working backward in this way is correct. Nevertheless, outcomes have an accepted objective definition that provides a suitable reference for classification and are clinically relevant to construct models that inform risk associations.

The current literature identifies a number of phenotypes of adult asthma, which were characterized using both single- and multidimensional approaches. Here, we discuss the most influential phenotypes in current practice that have been recognized and validated by studies in a number of different populations using different approaches. The relationship between different phenotypes is complex (Figure 4.4). Although multidimensional phenotypes frequently identify more homogeneous subgroups of larger unidimensional phenotypes, independent phenotypes may be recognized in this way.

UNIDIMENSIONAL CLASSIFICATION: INFLAMMATORY PHENOTYPES OF ASTHMA

Eosinophilic Asthma

Eosinophilic airway inflammation was one of the earliest recognized pathological characteristics of asthma. Although previously considered the primary pathological disturbance in all cases of asthma, noneosinophilic variants of asthma are now widely recognized (discussed later). Consequently, eosinophilic asthma is more appropriately considered an important disease phenotype with distinct clinical properties.

Definition of Phenotype

Eosinophilic asthma is defined by the demonstration of greater than normal eosinophil numbers in the lower airways. This is quantified in population-based studies using the noninvasive technique of sputum induction as >2% of the viable sputum cell count.[16] Eosinophilic inflammation is effectively ameliorated with glucocorticoid therapy (see later). The phenotype may therefore be undetermined without serial testing in patients receiving regular inhaled corticosteroids.

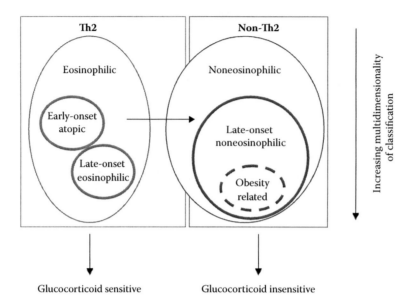

FIGURE 4.4 The probable relationship between currently characterized phenotypes of asthma. The specificity of the phenotypes increases with greater dimensionality, improving the scope for identifying endotypes. With available biomarkers, the phenotypes characterized are not stable and will be affected by numerous factors. In broad terms, the eosinophilic or Th2 phenotype is significantly more likely to be responsive to glucocorticoids.

Pathology: Eosinophilic Asthma and the "T-Helper Type 2 (Th2) Phenotype"?

Eosinophilic inflammation represents one terminal pathway of a broader network of cellular activity that occurs as part of the Th2 immune response. In this context, it may itself be viewed as a biomarker of a broader phenotype of "Th2-driven" asthma. At a molecular level, IL-5-driven eosinophilic inflammation is accompanied by the upregulation of other Th2 cytokines, classically IL-4 (B-cell isotype switching to IgE) and IL-13 (airway hyperresponsiveness and mucus cell hypersecretion). Indeed, the expression of three genes inducible with IL-13 (*POSTN, CLCA1,* and *SERPINB2*) has been utilized to provide molecular validation of the Th2 phenotype.[17] However, the significant heterogeneity in the coexpression of Th2 cytokines is increasingly recognized, suggesting that eosinophilic asthma itself is not an endotype. This is supported by the differences in clinical expression: eosinophilic bronchitis, a disease characterized by eosinophilic airway inflammation without airway hyperresponsiveness typically expresses IL-5 but not IL-13[18]; among patients with airway hyperresponsiveness, subgroups with high and low IgE titers are well recognized, contributing to the characterization of other important asthma phenotypes described here.

Important Clinical Characteristics

Eosinophilic Inflammation and Response to Glucocorticoid Therapy A number of studies have reported the presence of underlying eosinophilic airway inflammation to be a critical determinant of the clinical responsiveness to glucocorticoid therapy.[19] Moreover, this pattern of responsiveness has been reported in chronic obstructive pulmonary disease (COPD)[20] and also in subjects without a specific respiratory diagnosis, presenting with new symptoms of airways disease.[21] In this context, eosinophilic inflammation may be viewed as a phenotypic determinant for airways disease more generally.

Eosinophilic Airway Inflammation and Severe Exacerbations A consistent and compelling body of evidence supports an association between the extent of eosinophilic airway inflammation, quantified with sputum induction and the pathogenesis of severe exacerbations. There are two aspects to this:

1. Uncontrolled eosinophilic inflammation predates severe exacerbation events and may be used as a biomarker of risk to guide therapy. Studies using a glucocorticoid withdrawal protocol to induce exacerbations in previously well-controlled participants have shown an association between the risk of exacerbation and both the eosinophil counts and the products of eosinophil degranulation in sputum that are either high at baseline or rise significantly with time and treatment withdrawal.[22] Conversely, serial sputum inductions for patients treated with oral prednisolone during asthma exacerbations demonstrated a significant inverse correlation

between the change (fall) in the sputum eosinophil count and the lung function with therapy.[23] As a corollary to these observations, three randomized studies have demonstrated benefits with a strategy of glucocorticoid therapy delivered to ameliorate eosinophilic airway inflammation in sputum, for lowering the frequency of severe exacerbations, compared with the usual clinical practice in adult patients with asthma.[24–26]

2. Eosinophils have an effector role in the pathogenesis of severe exacerbations. Targeted, specific anti-eosinophil therapies may be effective for preventing severe exacerbations in patients with severe eosinophilic asthma. Two recently conducted studies reported a significant (~50%) reduction in exacerbation frequency following treatment with the anti-IL-5 monoclonal antibody, mepolizumab, a specific anti-eosinophil therapy, in patients with severe asthma of an eosinophilic phenotype.[27,28] Importantly, early studies with mepolizumab that were not confined to eosinophilic asthma failed to identify a similar clinical benefit,[29] underlining the importance of phenotype-driven patient selection for drug trials of specific molecular therapies.

Biomarkers of the Phenotype

Two biomarkers of eosinophilic asthma have been widely utilized in both research and clinical settings: (i) the sputum eosinophil count, obtained with sputum induction; and (ii) the fractional exhaled nitric oxide (FeNO). Of these, the sputum eosinophil count is widely accepted as the gold standard with the strongest evidence base. FeNO is used as a surrogate for sputum eosinophils but it may be raised in several conditions that are not necessarily associated with eosinophilic airway inflammation.[30] Although a less specific biomarker of the eosinophilic phenotype, FeNO has comparable utility as a marker of the clinical response to glucocorticoid therapy,[31,32] with effectiveness in longitudinal studies of asthma management for guiding the titration of corticosteroid doses.[33] In contrast, only sputum eosinophil counts have been reliably shown to guide corticosteroid therapy for reducing the frequency of severe asthma exacerbations.[34] These findings may be in keeping with the view that eosinophils have a more direct effector role in the pathogenesis of exacerbations while glucocorticoid responsiveness is more closely associated with Th2 activity per se that is reliably informed by FeNO. Recent data suggest that the blood eosinophil count may be a reliable biomarker for predicting the response to mepolizumab and could be used to identify the phenotype in this context.[35]

Noneosinophilic Asthma

Definition

The accepted criteria for diagnosing noneosinophilic asthma include: (i) the presence of typical symptoms; (ii) the objective evidence of significant variable airflow obstruction or airway hyperresponsiveness; (iii) the consistent absence of sputum eosinophilia; and (iv) the exclusion of an alternative

diagnosis.[36] The phenotype of noneosinophilic asthma is confounded significantly by anti-inflammatory asthma therapy. Cross-sectional population studies using sputum induction have reported normal sputum eosinophil counts (cutoff <1.9%) in up to 25% of patients with *untreated* symptomatic asthma[37] and in over 50% of patients (cutoff <2.5%) treated with high doses of inhaled corticosteroids.[38] In a survey of several asthma studies reporting inflammatory cell counts using either induced sputum or bronchoscopic methods, 49% of the participants with asthma had a noneosinophilic (<2% eosinophils) phenotype.[39]

A significant limitation of the point prevalence figures for noneosinophilic asthma based on cross-sectional studies is the absence of information on the longitudinal stability of the phenotype. However, studies have identified the noneosinophilic phenotype in subjects with symptomatic asthma not receiving glucocorticoid therapy[40] and it has also been a stable finding during the serial evaluation of subjects followed longitudinally, both during scheduled visits[41] and at the time of exacerbation.[42]

Pathology

Noneosinophilic asthma defines a heterogeneous phenotype of cellular profiles in sputum that are broadly categorized[43] as: (i) neutrophilic (sputum neutrophil count >61%) and (ii) paucigranulocytic (no dominant cell type). It has been suggested that the different inflammatory profiles are due to the different patterns of antigen exposure in the airways.[44] Neutrophil-predominant inflammation is thought to be driven primarily by innate and cell-mediated immune responses. Numerous etiological factors are believed to evoke responses along these immune pathways, particularly through the direct activation of macrophages.[45] Important examples include endotoxins, viral and bacterial infections, the constituents of cigarette smoke, and many occupational agents. While useful, this model is likely to be an oversimplification. There is an increasing recognition of considerable cross talk between the Th1 and Th2 pathways, with cytokines such as tumor necrosis factor alpha (TNFα) playing an important role in the augmentation of both types of immunity. Thus, although a viral etiology is identified most often during asthma exacerbations,[46] the pattern of airway inflammation (either eosinophilic or noneosinophilic) is far more heterogeneous, but it is reported to exhibit within-subject consistency at successive exacerbation episodes.[42] It is therefore likely that eosinophilic and noneosinophilic phenotypes differ not only in their pattern of exposure and their susceptibility to specific antigens but also in the type of responses they evoke to a given antigen. It is also worth remembering that the noneosinophilic phenotype does not necessarily imply a non-Th2 process. A phenotype of symptom-predominant asthma reported by Haldar et al. was characterized by early-onset atopic disease (high IgE titers) without sputum eosinophilia.[47] Moreover, the prevalence of a noneosinophilic phenotype of Th2 asthma is likely to increase as the exogenous blockade of IL-5 activity with specific anti-eosinophil therapies becomes available.

40 Clinical Asthma: Theory and Practice

Important Clinical Characteristics

Impaired Response to Glucocorticoid Therapy As a corollary to the observations in eosinophilic asthma, noneosinophilic asthma is associated with an impaired clinical response to glucocorticoid therapy[48] and such treatment does not modify the exacerbation risk. Much of the morbidity associated with refractory asthma is attributable to the side effects of high-dose glucocorticoid therapy and a clear implication of these observations is that identifying the noneosinophilic phenotype can help to identify a group in which glucocorticoids may be safely titrated down. This view is supported by the findings of a *post hoc* analysis by Haldar et al., which demonstrated that a strategy of glucocorticoid therapy titrated to the sputum eosinophil count achieved a significant reduction in the daily dose of regular glucocorticoid therapy (mean reduction 1829 mcg beclometasone dipropionate [BDP] equivalent) for patients with uncontrolled noneosinophilic asthma, without adversely affecting asthma control, compared with a traditional symptom-driven algorithm of care.[45]

Macrolide Therapy for Neutrophilic Asthma The neutrophilic subtype of noneosinophilic asthma shares immunopathological characteristics with other forms of airways disease, including bronchiectasis and COPD. Macrolides have been identified as modulators of innate immunity and have been shown to lower the burden of neutrophilic inflammation.[49] In practice, this may improve the clinical outcomes as pilot studies suggest benefits in patients with bronchiectasis.[50]

Biomarkers of the Phenotype

There are no specific biomarkers to identify noneosinophilic asthma. In contrast with its uncertain positive predictive value, a low FeNO level is a useful biomarker in clinical practice for identifying patients that are unlikely to benefit from glucocorticoid treatment.[21]

MULTIDIMENSIONAL PHENOTYPES OF ASTHMA

Overview

In addition to the pattern of airway inflammation, aspects of the disease that appear to contribute significantly to the clinical phenotypes of asthma include: (i) age of disease onset, (ii) variability of airflow obstruction, (iii) gender, and (iv) BMI. All or some of these phenotypic domains in different combinations have been included in different asthma populations using multivariate techniques to define phenotypes. Some studies have also included postbronchodilator FEV_1 in their analyses to identify the phenotypes associated with fixed airflow obstruction as a specific end point.[51] Although strongly associated with the recognized phenotypes of asthma, the atopic status was not a significant independent determinant of phenotypic structure in either mild to moderate or more severe asthma.[47,51] It is likely that the atopic status correlates with the age of onset, with the latter having a more dominant effect.

Early-Onset Atopic Asthma

Features

This phenotype is characterized by onset in childhood (usually <12 years) and has a strong association with allergen sensitization and related atopic diseases, typically allergic rhinitis and eczema. This is the classical asthma phenotype and is synonymous with the phenotype of "extrinsic asthma" characterized by Rackemann.[5] This is the most prevalent phenotype of asthma, particularly in groups with mild to moderate disease. Indeed, the identification of this acknowledged phenotype using unsupervised multivariate mathematical techniques has been argued to validate their role in this field.[47]

Pathology

The association of this phenotype with atopy is supported by the finding of high IgE titers and eosinophilic airway inflammation, implying a pathology driven by Th2 immune pathways.

Clinical Characteristics

In a cross-sectional analysis, it has been suggested that significant concordance exists between the level of underlying eosinophilic airway inflammation and the clinical symptoms for this group. Thus, a traditional symptom-led approach to asthma pharmacotherapy is likely to be effective in this group and is probably the reason for the persistence with and the success of such algorithms in clinical practice.

Allergen exposure is thought to play an important role in driving the disease pathology. Although allergen avoidance studies have shown a variable effect on asthma control, it remains uncertain how effective strategies to exclude ubiquitous allergens from daily life can be best achieved and sustained. Importantly, omalizumab, a monoclonal antibody against IgE, currently remains the only specific molecular therapy that is approved for use in asthma. The treatment eligibility for this drug requires that specific criteria be met, which generally place candidates within this asthma phenotype.

Late-Onset Eosinophilic Asthma

Features

This phenotype is characterized by onset in adulthood. Patients have eosinophilic airway inflammation without evidence of atopic associations, and serum IgE titers are often normal or low. Severe asthma of this phenotype has been associated with nasal polyps and recurrent sinopulmonary infections.[52] This form occurs more frequently in females and overlaps with the historical phenotype of Samter's triad (nasal polyps, severe asthma, and aspirin sensitivity), or aspirin exacerbated respiratory disease (AERD). A male "inflammation-predominant" form of late eosinophilic asthma has also been described and is characterized by a relative paucity of symptoms in the presence of severe eosinophilic airway inflammation.[44]

Pathology

In contrast with the early-onset phenotype, late-onset eosinophilic asthma forms a heterogeneous group. A low IgE titer and the absence of an association with allergic triggers suggest that differences with the early-onset phenotype are likely in patterns of Th2 cytokine expression. Interestingly, the inflammation-predominant form described in males shares the demographic characteristics of idiopathic hypereosinophilic syndrome (HES). Whether some cases of inflammation-predominant asthma overlap with a mild form of single-organ HES is not known, but it provides a mechanism for the discordant expression of Th2 cytokines.

Clinical Characteristics

Severe forms of late-onset eosinophilic asthma can exhibit considerable resistance to treatment, requiring high doses of maintenance oral glucocorticoids to retain control. The avoidance of aspirin and other nonsteroidal anti-inflammatory drugs should be advised, particularly if nasal polyposis is identified or there is a history of chronic sinusitis. As mentioned earlier, there may be significant discordance between the symptoms and the level of eosinophilic inflammation. Poor perception of bronchoconstriction and an abnormal chemoreceptor response to hypoxia[53] are factors that are associated with severe eosinophilic airway inflammation and may be relevant in this group. Symptom-guided therapy may underestimate the disease activity, with the consequent risk of severe or life-threatening exacerbations and an inflammation-guided approach, as described earlier, has been shown to significantly lower the frequency of severe exacerbation events.[47]

Obesity-Related Asthma

Features

Although a relationship between obesity and asthma has been proposed, the application of multivariate techniques has enabled the formal recognition of this phenotype in multiple cohorts. The phenotype is characterized by late-onset (adult) asthma in predominantly female patients with a high BMI (usually >35 kg/m²). This phenotype is distinct from early-onset asthma progressing to adulthood in patients with a high BMI. The former is usually noneosinophilic and is associated with a high burden of symptoms but only modest airway inflammation and preserved lung function.

Pathology

The mechanism of obesity-related asthma is unclear. The mechanical effects of a high BMI are likely to contribute to the expression of symptoms. A relationship between BMI and airway hyperresponsiveness has been reported.[54] The specific association of this phenotype with the female gender suggests that hormonal factors may play a role. Obesity is recognized to be a proinflammatory state; however, studies examining the relationship between airway inflammation and BMI have failed to identify a significant association.[55]

Clinical Characteristics

In the absence of significant eosinophilic airway inflammation, escalating doses of glucocorticoids to treat the symptoms of this phenotype should be avoided because they are likely to be ineffective (noneosinophilic phenotype) and may promote further weight gain. Studies report an improvement in asthma-related symptoms that correlates with the magnitude of the weight loss that is achieved. This is likely to reflect an improvement in respiratory mechanics as well as better fitness levels. Interestingly, weight loss has been shown to promote Th2 immune pathways[56] and this may be associated with greater responsiveness to conventional glucocorticoid pharmacotherapy.

CONCLUSIONS

The systematic characterization of asthma heterogeneity is critical for furthering our understanding of the important pathological determinants that may eventually inform the development and delivery of personalized asthma treatment plans for all. In this chapter, we have explored and discussed the multidimensional complexity of asthma heterogeneity and the rationale of the strategies that are being developed to address this heterogeneity. More generally, promoting a multidisciplinary "systems approach" that brings together diverse expertise with a common objective is likely to be effective.

REFERENCES

1. Rackemann F. A working classification of asthma. *Am J Med* 1947;3(5):601–606.
2. British Thoracic Society Scottish Intercollegiate Guidelines Network. British Guideline on the Management of Asthma. *Thorax* 2008;63(Suppl 4):iv1–iv121.
3. Harrison BD. Psychosocial aspects of asthma in adults. *Thorax* 1998;53(6):519–525.
4. Anderson GP. Endotyping asthma: New insights into key pathogenic mechanisms in a complex, heterogeneous disease. *Lancet* 2008;372(9643):1107–1119.
5. Rackemann FM. Studies in asthma: A clinical survey of 1074 patients with asthma followed for 2 years. *J Lab Clin Med* 1927;12:1185–1197.
6. Rackemann FM. Intrinsic asthma. *Postgrad Med* 1950;8(2):134–140.
7. Sneath PH, Sokal RR. Numerical taxonomy. *Nature* 1962;193:855–860.
8. Chen JJ, Roberson PK, Schell MJ. The false discovery rate: A key concept in large-scale genetic studies. *Cancer Control* 2010;17(1):58–62.
9. Rosi E, Ronchi MC, Grazzini M, et al. Sputum analysis, bronchial hyperresponsiveness, and airway function in asthma: Results of a factor analysis. *J Allergy Clin Immunol* 1999;103(2 Pt 1):232–237.
10. Everitt BS, Landau S, Leese M. *Cluster Analysis*, 4th edn. London: Arnold, 2001.
11. Formann AK, Kohlmann T. Latent class analysis in medical research. *Stat Methods Med Res* 1996;5(2):179–211.
12. Paykel ES. Classification of depressed patients: A cluster analysis derived grouping. *Brit J Psychiat* 1971;118(544):275–288.

13. Kurz A, Moller HJ, Baindl G, et al. Classification of para-suicide by cluster analysis. Types of suicidal behaviour, therapeutic and prognostic implications. *Brit J Psychiat* 1987;150:520–525.

14. Hawkins GA, Weiss ST, Bleecker ER. Clinical consequences of ADRbeta2 polymorphisms. *Pharmacogenomics* 2008;9(3):349–358.

15. Klotsman M, York TP, Pillai SG, et al. Pharmacogenetics of the 5-lipoxygenase biosynthetic pathway and variable clinical response to montelukast. *Pharmacogenet Genom* 2007;17(3):189–196.

16. Spanevello A, Confalonieri M, Sulotto F, et al. Induced sputum cellularity. Reference values and distribution in normal volunteers. *Am J Respir Crit Care Med* 2000;162(3 Pt 1):1172–1174.

17. Woodruff PG, Boushey HA, Dolganov GM, et al. Genome-wide profiling identifies epithelial cell genes associated with asthma and with treatment response to corticosteroids. *Proc Natl Acad Sci USA* 2007;104(40):15858–15863.

18. Park SW, Jangm HK, An MH, et al. Interleukin-13 and interleukin-5 in induced sputum of eosinophilic bronchitis: Comparison with asthma. *Chest* 2005;128(4):1921–1927.

19. Szefler SJ, Martin RJ, King TS, et al. Significant variability in response to inhaled corticosteroids for persistent asthma. *J Allergy Clin Immunol* 2002;109(3):410–418.

20. Brightling CE, McKenna S, Hargadon B, et al. Sputum eosinophilia and the short term response to inhaled mometasone in chronic obstructive pulmonary disease. *Thorax* 2005;60(3):193–198.

21. Smith AD, Cowan JO, Brassett KP, et al. Exhaled nitric oxide: A predictor of steroid response. *Am J Respir Crit Care Med* 2005;172(4):453–459.

22. Deykin A, Lazarus SC, Fahy JV, et al. Sputum eosinophil counts predict asthma control after discontinuation of inhaled corticosteroids. *J Allergy Clin Immunol* 2005;115(4):720–727.

23. Pizzichini MM, Pizzichini E, Clelland L, et al. Sputum in severe exacerbations of asthma: Kinetics of inflammatory indices after prednisone treatment. *Am J Respir Crit Care Med* 1997;155(5):1501–1508.

24. Green RH, Brightling CE, McKenna S, et al. Asthma exacerbations and sputum eosinophil counts: A randomised controlled trial. *Lancet* 2002;360(9347):1715–1721.

25. Chlumsky J, Striz I, Terl M, et al. Strategy aimed at reduction of sputum eosinophils decreases exacerbation rate in patients with asthma. *J Int Med Res* 2006;34(2):129–139.

26. Jayaram L, Pizzichini MM, Cook RJ, et al. Determining asthma treatment by monitoring sputum cell counts: Effect on exacerbations. *Eur Respir J* 2006;27(3):483–494.

27. Haldar P, Brightling CE, Hargadon B, et al. Mepolizumab and exacerbations of refractory eosinophilic asthma. *N Engl J Med* 2009;360(10):973–984.

28. Nair P, Pizzichini MM, Kjarsgaard M, et al. Mepolizumab for prednisone-dependent asthma with sputum eosinophilia. *N Engl J Med* 2009;360(10):985–993.

29. Leckie MJ, ten Brinke A, Khan J, et al. Effects of an interleukin-5 blocking monoclonal antibody on eosinophils, airway hyper-responsiveness, and the late asthmatic response. *Lancet* 2000;356(9248):2144–2148.

30. Abba AA. Exhaled nitric oxide in diagnosis and management of respiratory diseases. *Ann Thorac Med* 2009;4(4):173–181.

31. Smith AD, Cowan JO, Brassett KP, et al. Exhaled nitric oxide: A predictor of steroid response. *Am J Respir Crit Care Med* 2005;172(4):453–459.

32. Pérez-de-Llano LA, Carballada F, Castro Añón O, et al. Exhaled nitric oxide predicts control in patients with difficult-to-treat asthma. *Eur Respir J* 2010;35(6):1221–1227.

33. Smith AD, Cowan JO, Brassett KP, et al. Use of exhaled nitric oxide measurements to guide treatment in chronic asthma. *N Engl J Med* 2005;352(21):2163–2173.

34. Petsky HL, Cates CJ, Lasserson TJ, et al. A systematic review and meta-analysis: Tailoring asthma treatment on eosinophilic markers (exhaled nitric oxide or sputum eosinophils). *Thorax* 2012;67:199–208.

35. Pavord ID, Korn S, Howarth P, et al. Mepolizumab for severe eosinophilic asthma (DREAM): A multicentre, double-blind, placebo-controlled trial. *Lancet* 2012;380(9842):651–659.

36. Haldar P, Pavord ID. Noneosinophilic asthma: A distinct clinical and pathologic phenotype. *J Allergy Clin Immunol* 2007;119(5):1043–1052.

37. Green RH, Brightling CE, Woltmann G, et al. Analysis of induced sputum in adults with asthma: Identification of subgroup with isolated sputum neutrophilia and poor response to inhaled corticosteroids. *Thorax* 2002;57(10):875–879.

38. Gibson PG, Simpson JL, Saltos N. Heterogeneity of airway inflammation in persistent asthma: Evidence of neutrophilic inflammation and increased sputum interleukin-8. *Chest* 2001;119(5):1329–1336.

39. Douwes J, Gibson P, Pekkanen J, et al. Non-eosinophilic asthma: Importance and possible mechanisms. *Thorax* 2002;57(7):643–648.

40. Berry M, Morgan A, Shaw DE, et al. Pathological features and inhaled corticosteroid response of eosinophilic and non-eosinophilic asthma. *Thorax* 2007;62(12):1043–1049.

41. Simpson JL, Scott R, Boyle MJ, et al. Inflammatory subtypes in asthma: Assessment and identification using induced sputum. *Respirology* 2006;11(1):54–61.

42. D'silva L, Cook RJ, Allen CJ, et al. Changing pattern of sputum cell counts during successive exacerbations of airway disease. *Respir Med* 2007;101(10):2217–2220.

43. Gibson PG. Inflammatory phenotypes in adult asthma: Clinical applications. *Clin Respir J* 2009;3(4):198–206.

44. Wardlaw AJ, Brightling CE, Green R, et al. New insights into the relationship between airway inflammation and asthma. *Clin Sci* 2002;103(2):201–211.

45. Medzhitov R, Janeway Jr. C. Innate immunity. *N Engl J Med* 2000;343(5):338–344.

46. Johnston SL, Pattemore PK, Sanderson G, et al. Community study of role of viral infections in exacerbations of asthma in 9–11 year old children. *BMJ* 1995;310(6989):1225–1229.

47. Haldar P, Pavord ID, Shaw DE, et al. Cluster analysis and clinical asthma phenotypes. *Am J Respir Crit Care Med* 2008;178(3):218–224.

48. Pavord ID, Brightling CE, Woltmann G, et al. Non-eosinophilic corticosteroid unresponsive asthma. *Lancet* 1999;353(9171):2213–2214.

49. Simpson JL, Powell H, Boyle MJ, et al. Clarithromycin targets neutrophilic airway inflammation in refractory asthma. *Am J Respir Crit Care Med* 2008;177(2):148–155.

50. Cymbala AA, Edmonds LC, Bauer MA, et al. The disease-modifying effects of twice-weekly oral azithromycin in patients with bronchiectasis. *Treat Respir Med* 2005;4(2):117–122.

51. Moore WC, Meyers DA, Wenzel SE, et al. Identification of asthma phenotypes using cluster analysis in the Severe Asthma Research Program. *Am J Respir Crit Care Med* 2010;181(4):315–323.

52. Miranda C, Busacker A, Balzar S, et al. Distinguishing severe asthma phenotypes: Role of age at onset and eosinophilic inflammation. *J Allergy Clin Immunol* 2004;113(1):101–108.

53. Kikuchi Y, Okabe S, Tamura G, et al. Chemosensitivity and perception of dyspnea in patients with a history of near-fatal asthma. *N Engl J Med* 1994;330(19):1329–1334.

54. Rasmussen F, Hancox RJ, Nair P, et al. Associations between airway hyperresponsiveness, obesity, and lipoproteins in a longitudinal cohort. *Clin Respir J* 2012;7(3):268–275.

55. Sideleva O, Suratt BT, Black KE, et al. Obesity and asthma: An inflammatory disease of adipose tissue not the airway. *Am J Respir Crit Care Med* 2012;186(7):598–605.

56. Dixon AE, Pratley RE, Forgione PM, et al. Effects of obesity and bariatric surgery on airway hyperresponsiveness, asthma control, and inflammation. *J Allergy Clin Immunol* 2011;128(3):508–515.

Section II

Diagnosis of Asthma

5 Guidelines in Asthma

Louis-Philippe Boulet

CONTENTS

INTRODUCTION

Since the early 1980s, national and international asthma guidelines have been published to address deficiencies in asthma care and provide guidance on how to deliver the best care. These guides are generally considered useful to synthesize current knowledge and propose to the clinician what is considered to be the optimal management of asthma based on the available evidence. Their production process has been improved in the last decade, and new methods have been developed to ensure high-quality, evidence-based reports proposing unbiased recommendations. However, the implementation of these guidelines is still suboptimal and barriers and facilitators to their application in care have been identified. The "implementability" of the guidelines should be improved, and clinicians should be offered tools and strategies to help translate their key recommendations into current care, in specific environments, and with different types of resources available. This chapter provides a succinct overview of the production of asthma guidelines over the last decades, their main recommendations, and how they can help practitioners to improve care delivery, in addition to providing suggestions on how to facilitate their implementation.

EXAMPLE OF INTEGRATION OF GUIDELINES RECOMMENDATIONS INTO CARE

A 35-year-old man with a previous diagnosis of asthma consults for persistent respiratory symptoms despite the use of an inhaled corticosteroid (ICS) and "on-demand" inhaled salbutamol. Using a summary of the most recent asthma guideline as a reminder, the physician notes that the patient never had objective proof of the asthma diagnosis. He notes the various ways to confirm such a diagnosis and requests spirometry before and after bronchodilators. This test comes back normal so a methacholine challenge is obtained, which shows a moderate degree of airway hyperresponsiveness, consistent with the diagnosis of asthma. According to the guideline's asthma control criteria, the patient's asthma is uncontrolled and after looking at the list of items to determine the possible cause of such a lack of control (environmental, inhaler technique, adherence, etc.), the physician notes that the guideline recommendations on treatment are not commensurate with the objective findings. After an adjustment of therapy to a combination of ICS and long-acting beta$_2$-adrenergic agonists (LABA), which was determined to be the minimal treatment required to achieve good asthma control, he consults the guideline to produce an action plan for the management of asthma exacerbations in addition to scheduling regular follow-up visits to assess ongoing asthma control and adherence to the recommendations.

EXAMPLE OF GUIDELINES IMPLEMENTATION INITIATIVES: CASE PRESENTATION

In order to improve adherence to the Canadian emergency department (ED) asthma management guidelines and improve patient outcomes, a standardized ED asthma care pathway (ACP) was developed for adults.[1] Ten Ontario hospital EDs (five interventions, five controls) took part in a 5-month pre-post intervention study. At the intervention sites, the ACP was used in 26.4% of 383 visits (ranging from 6% to 60% among the sites). When compared with the control sites, the use of metered-dose inhalers (MDIs), ICSs, referrals, oxygen, and documentation of teaching and patient recollection of teaching were significantly improved (all end points $P \leq .001$). An increase in the peak expiratory flow (PEF) documentation and systemic corticosteroid use in the ED and on discharge was only found in patients who were on the ACP at the intervention sites. Admissions to the intervention sites increased from 3.9% to 9.4% in contrast to the control sites, where they remained fairly stable ($P = .016$), but did not differ with ACP use. There were no statistically significant differences in repeat ED visits. This example shows how small changes in care delivery could result in a significant improvement in care delivery and it also illustrates the difficulties in changing practice behaviors and integrating tools to help implement guidelines and standardize care. As with many initiatives, however, the net result on patient morbidity and health-care use should be assessed, as an analysis of the results of these interventions could help to improve asthma management to make it more effective, particularly in looking at barriers to their implementation and to the effect of their specific components.

Another similar initiative was aimed at introducing the Pediatric Acute Asthma Management Guideline (PAMG) to the ED of a pediatric tertiary care hospital. The medical charts of 278 retrospective ED visits and 154 prospective visits were reviewed.[2] During the implementation of the PAMG, patients who visited the ED were more likely to receive oral corticosteroids ($P < .0001$) and oxygen saturation reassessment before ED discharge ($P < .0001$). Improvements in asthma education and discharge planning were noted, but the changes were not statistically significant. After the implementation of an evidence-based guideline reminder card, medication treatment for acute asthma in the ED was significantly improved. However, asthma education and discharge planning remained unchanged; therefore, efforts to promote guideline-based practice in the ED should emphasize these components.

HISTORICAL BACKGROUND

Clinical practice guidelines have been developed over the last few decades in many fields of medicine to optimize health care according to current evidence and then, hopefully, decrease the morbidity and mortality associated with various conditions. In regard to asthma, the development of these documents was further promoted following an increase in asthma-related mortality and morbidity associated with industrialized countries during the 1970s. The first initiatives came from Australia, New Zealand, Canada, the United Kingdom, and the United States.[3-6] These were followed by the development of the international report, Global Initiative for Asthma (GINA), inaugurated in 1993, which aimed at developing a program to reduce asthma prevalence, morbidity, and mortality worldwide.[7] Since then, the GINA reports have been revised regularly (www.ginasthma.com). Updates of national guidelines are also regularly produced.

PRODUCTION OF GUIDELINES AND GRADING THE EVIDENCE

Over the last two decades, the methods for producing guidelines have been improved, and quality standards have been developed. For example, the AGREE tool, originally developed in 2001[8] and since revised, offers a standard tool for guideline development, reporting, and evaluation.[9] It includes 23 items grouped in 6 domains: scope and purpose, stakeholder involvement, rigor of development, clarity of presentation, applicability, and editorial independence. Furthermore, grading the evidence has evolved and tools such as the Grades of Recommendation, Assessment, Development, and Evaluation[10] system are now widely used.[11] As reported by Guyatt,[12] this tool has been developed by a widely representative group of international guideline developers, establishing a clear separation between the quality of the evidence and the strength of the recommendations, and providing an explicit evaluation of the importance of the outcomes of alternative management strategies. Furthermore, it provides explicit, comprehensive criteria for downgrading and upgrading the quality of the evidence ratings, a transparent process of moving from evidence to recommendation, an explicit acknowledgment of values and preferences, and a clear, pragmatic interpretation of strong versus weak recommendations for clinicians, patients, and policy makers (Figure 5.1). This tool can be useful for systematic reviews and health technology assessments, as well as guidelines.

ARE GUIDELINES USEFUL?

Following a review of 59 evaluations that met rigorous scientific criteria, Grimshaw and Russell concluded that almost all of the guidelines on various conditions including asthma were associated with an improvement in medical practice, while the size of the improvements in performance varied from one intervention to another.[13]

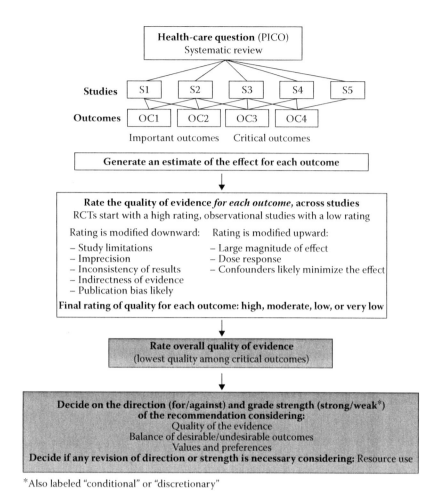

FIGURE 5.1   Schematic view of the GRADE process for developing recommendations. Abbreviation: RCT, randomized controlled trials. (Reproduced from Guyatt, G.H., Oxman, A.D., Schünemann, H.J., Tugwell, P., and Knottnerus, A., *J. Clin. Epidemiol.*, 64, 383–394, 2011. With permission.)

Nonetheless, there is evidence that guidelines and the initiatives developed to implement their recommendations have significantly reduced the severity and mortality of asthma in countries and regions where management plans have been implemented.[14–18] Otherwise, improved prescription practices have been reported, such as a reduction in rescue medications and increased prescriptions for ICS.[19] However, the impact of therapeutic guidelines on the clinical outcome of asthma requires better documentation, particularly following different implementation strategies, in different settings and addressing specific asthma management care gaps (Table 5.1).

DO PHYSICIANS KNOW AND COMPLY WITH GUIDELINES?

Wide variations have been observed in the translation of current guidelines into care, particularly primary care, and various care gaps persist.[20,21] Although an improvement in guideline implementation has been noted in the last decade, some recommendations remain problematic. We previously reported significant discrepancies between the Canadian asthma guidelines and the practice of physician, for example, in regard to the use of short-acting beta₂-adrenergic agonists,

the provision of asthma action plans, or the referral for asthma education.[22] Discrepancies were also found between prescriptions for asthma medications in children and the published asthma consensus guidelines, particularly with regard to anti-inflammatory therapy.[23]

A previous study on the Third Brazilian Consensus on Asthma Management showed that there was poor implementation of these guidelines in the public health-care system.[24] Most asthma patients did not receive treatment consistent with the consensus guidelines, particularly with regard to the underuse of ICS, possibly due to the lack of access to and inappropriate use of medications, the low adherence to treatment, the lack of patient knowledge regarding the disease/ principles of treatment/procedures for using inhaled medications, and the lack of education being mentioned as possible causes.

More recently, we looked at the recommendations of the main Canadian asthma and chronic obstructive pulmonary disease (COPD) guidelines for primary care physicians using a standardized questionnaire, the Physician Practice Assessment Questionnaire (PPAQ).[25] The most poorly implemented recommendations (in less than 50% of the physicians' patients) were, for both asthma and COPD, referral for

TABLE 5.1
Common Asthma Management Care Gaps

Management Care Gap	Barriers to Reducing the Gap (Example)	Possible Implementation Strategy	Process and Outcome Measures
Overdiagnosis/underdiagnosis/lack of early recognition of asthma	Unavailability of pulmonary function tests	Identification of nearby PFT facilities	Percentage of patients for whom PFTs are done
Not considering asthma when symptoms present	Insufficient awareness of asthma	Increase awareness	Prevalence of new asthma diagnoses
Physician's nonadherence to guidelines	Insufficient knowledge/motivation to implement guideline	Improved dissemination/interactive workshops	Assessment of recommendations and implementation into care
Patient–doctor communication	Insufficient time/communication skills	System changes—asthma educator referral	Degree of patient satisfaction with communication
Inadequate assessment of asthma control	Lack of knowledge of criteria	Education/CME	Survey of criteria use
Insufficient environmental/preventative measures	Lack of time to explain	Increase access to educator. Involve patients as educators	Survey implementation of intervention
Lack of individualized pharmacotherapy	Insufficient knowledge of guideline	Education/CME	Assessment of treatment (e.g., audit)
Lack of education and guided self-management	Unavailability of educators	Increase access to educator. Involve patients as educators in the process	Percentage of patients offered education
Absence or nonuse of an action plan for the management of exacerbations	Not enough time to produce and explain	Increase access to educator. Provide simple printed formats for clinicians	Number of patients receiving a written action plan
No assessment of techniques (inhalers, peak flow measurement)	Lack of time or knowledge	Systematic assessment at visits	Percentage of patients for whom this is checked
No assessment of adherence to therapy	Not integrated into practice	Reminders	Percentage of patients for whom this is checked
No regular follow-up—discontinuity of care	Lack of follow-up arrangements	Improved management	Survey on regular follow-up
Inadequate management of acute asthma	Lack of knowledge and resources	Adherence to guidelines. Improve ED staff training/asthma management	Regular survey of hospital admissions and deaths
Variable/insufficient access to care—nonavailability of asthma controllers	Insufficient resources	Increase resources—revise process	Assess continuity of care
Poor communication between various groups of health-care personnel	Lack of willingness to change	Organize joint sessions on asthma care	Focus group assessing this aspect of care

Source: Adapted from Boulet, L.P., FitzGerald, J.M., Levy, M.L., Cruz, A.A., Pedersen, S., Haahtela, T., and Bateman, E.D., *Eur. Respir. J.*, 39, 1220–1229, 2012. With permission.

Note: For some of these care gaps, more evidence on the effectiveness of the implementation strategies is required. However, the recommendations provided are based on current recommendations. CME = continuing medical education; PFT = pulmonary function testing.

patient education, provision of a written asthma action plan, and regular assessment of inhaler technique. In addition, for asthma, referral to a specialist for difficult-to-control asthma or uncertain diagnosis was poorly implemented.

A recent Italian study looked at the implementation of GINA recommendations among Italian pulmonary specialists (PSs) using a detailed questionnaire that was sent to 296 respiratory units (RUs) in Italy; 25% of the questionnaires were returned and analyzed.[26] Spirometry was available in more than 90% of RUs, but was performed in no more than 50% of patients in most units. Asthma treatment concurred with GINA recommendations in most RUs. Only a few RUs offered individual educational sessions or "asthma school."[26]

WHY ARE GUIDELINES NOT ALWAYS IMPLEMENTED?

Specialists are usually well aware of the current guidelines but primary care physicians less so. This may be due to the number and format of the guidelines (too lengthy or complex), in addition to socioeconomic and organizational factors.[27,28] The translation of recommendations into care by practitioners is influenced by their level of knowledge and their attitudes, skills, beliefs, and values. Guidelines recommendations should be adapted according to the cultural and socioeconomic contexts in which they are applied. Clinicians may consider that the recommendations cannot be applied in their practice due to the lack of time or resources or the type of patient that they treat. They may consider that the potential benefit expected does not justify a change in their practice.

The implementation of recommendations also depends on the patient's acceptance of the suggestions, and there is a need for adequate communication between the patient and the caregiver. In this regard, a "shared decision-making" process may help improve patient adherence to recommendations.[29]

Despite suboptimal implementation, practitioners usually recognize that guidelines help to standardize medical practice and benefit the patient. However, they need guidance on how to implement guidelines and they must have sufficient time and access to sufficient resources (e.g., medication and educators).

HOW TO IMPROVE GUIDELINES IMPLEMENTATION

The dissemination of guidelines through medical/scientific publications, mailings, continuing professional development (CPD), workshops, and symposia is generally considered insufficient to change medical practice.[30] Many publications have addressed the question of how to improve the implementation of guidelines; interactive strategies, practice aids, reminders, algorithms, and summaries, particularly using new electronic tools, should help facilitate the translation of guideline recommendations into day-to-day care.[20,31,32] A multidisciplinary approach is required to achieve this goal, which involves all health-care providers, with articulated interventions and a common message to the patient. The implementation of guidelines should be tailored to the environment and the resources available[33] (Table 5.2). Knowledge translation models, such as the Knowledge-to-Action framework, can be useful to structure the interventions[34] (Figure 5.2). Furthermore, tools such as the Guideline Implementability Appraisal (GLIA) can help assess the implementability of guidelines [www.openclinical.org/applInstrument_glia.html]. In a recent publication, we summarized how to implement guidelines such as the GINA strategy and this can be applied to any guidelines.[35]

CONTENT OF CURRENT ASTHMA GUIDELINES

An exhaustive discussion of the guidelines-based management of asthma is beyond the scope of this chapter and other sections of this book will discuss those various components. Although the reader should consult the respective guidelines, herein we will stress some general principles and commonalities of the current guidelines.[36-39]

Definition of Asthma and Diagnosis

The definition of asthma provided by the current guidelines has not changed significantly in the last two decades and indicates that it is a chronic inflammatory disorder of the airways characterized by variable airway obstruction and airway hyperresponsiveness, which manifest in the form of various respiratory symptoms—dyspnea, wheezing, cough,

TABLE 5.2

A Plan for a Guideline Implementation Program

1. Identify stakeholders and form a working group
2. Select the guideline to be implemented and determine if it needs adaptation
3. Perform a needs assessment and review the current status of care and the main care gaps
4. Select the main care gaps to be addressed and the key messages to be conveyed
5. Develop and prioritize implementation strategies
6. Develop and agree on specific indicators of change and targets for each outcomes in the initiative
7. Ensure that the resources needed are available
8. Produce a step-by-step implementation plan
9. Plan initial interventions and evaluate their effects
10. Review the project in light of pilot projects and other information gathered
11. Determine how the current interventions could be improved/evaluate the feasibility of implementing the project
12. Plan continuation/expansion of the initiative and its long-term evaluation: ensure long-term planning

Source: Reproduced from Boulet, L.P., FitzGerald, J.M., Levy, M.L., Cruz, A.A., Pedersen, S., Haahtela, T., and Bateman, E.D., *Eur. Respir. J.*, 39, 1220–1229, 2012. With permission.

chest tightness, and phlegm production. Specific criteria have been reported to establish what constitutes significant variability/reversibility of airway obstruction and what is considered significantly increased airway responsiveness.[36-39] An assessment of the diagnosis in young children is considered more complex as respiratory symptoms are frequent in nonasthmatic children and pulmonary function tests are not usually reliable before 6 years of age. Therefore, a diagnosis of asthma in a child is mostly based on a history of recurrent asthmalike symptoms, a family history of asthma or atopy, maternal smoking, and other risk factors for asthma; specific criteria are currently suggested by asthma guidelines.[36,40]

Goal of Therapy: A Shift from Severity to Control of Asthma

As there is no cure for asthma, we should try to reduce the consequences of asthma as much as possible. Furthermore, as stressed by Cockcroft, asthma control should be differentiated from its severity, where "control" reflects the degree to which asthma manifestations are kept to a minimum with treatment, while severity mostly refers to the intrinsic mechanisms of the disease, evidenced by the level of treatment required to achieve control.[41] The former is also more closely associated with the risk of asthma events.[42] So, as Canadian asthma guidelines have suggested since the 1990s, in the last decade, most guidelines have adopted a "control-driven" approach for the management of asthma, and recommend that management should be based on achieving and maintaining complete asthma control[37-40] (Table 5.3). Furthermore, the

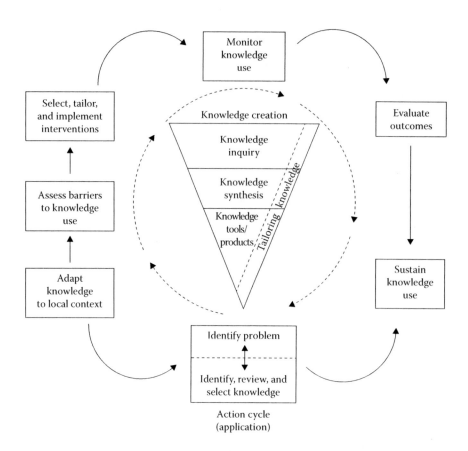

FIGURE 5.2 Knowledge-to-Action Model. (From Graham, I.D., Logan, J., Harrison, M.B., Straus, S.E., Tetroe, J., Caswell, W., et al., *J. Contin. Educ. Health. Prof.*, 26, 13–24, 2006. With permission.)

TABLE 5.3
Definition of Asthma Control

Guideline	GINA 2012[a]	Canadian 2012	BTS 2012
Daytime symptoms	None (twice or less/week)	<4 times/week	The last version of the BTS/SIGN
Nocturnal symptoms/awakening	None	<Once/week	guideline suggests assessing control by
Emergency visits	—[b]	None	using one of the available composite
Beta$_2$-agonist need	None (twice or less/week)	<4 times/week[e]	measurement tools[d]
Activities (including exercise)	No limitation	Normal physical activities[e]	
Exacerbations	—[b]	Mild, infrequent	
Expiratory flows (FEV$_1$, PEF)	Normal	≥90% best	
PEF variability (diurnal variation)	—	<10%–15%	

Note: FEV$_1$, forced expiratory volume in 1 second; PEF, peak expiratory flow.

[a] All of the following.

[b] Global control includes an assessment of the future risk of exacerbations, instability, rapid decline in lung function and side effects, as reflected by poor clinical control, frequent exacerbations in the past year, ever admission to critical care for asthma, low FEV$_1$, exposure to cigarette smoke, and high-dose medications.

[c] No absenteeism from work or school.

[d] http://www.brit-thoracic.org.uk/Portals/0/Guidelines/AsthmaGuidelines/sign101%20Jan%202012.pdf.

[e] Including doses taken before exercise.

risk of acute/severe events should be differentiated from current control.[42]

Guideline-defined asthma control criteria can be achieved in most patients through patient education, environmental control, and individualized pharmacotherapy (Table 5.3).

Patient Education

All consensus reports stress the importance of educating asthmatic patients and their families about the disease and its management, and ensure that they have adequate self-management skills. There is now ample evidence that adequate asthma education is pivotal in achieving and maintaining asthma control.[43] It should include notions about asthma and its management, drug utilization and their mode of action, triggers, and proper inhaler use while addressing key elements such as adherence to therapy, how to assess asthma control, and a discussion of an asthma action plan for the management of exacerbations. The treatment of comorbidities and monitoring control (including, for some, occasional PEF measures) should also be addressed with an emphasis on regular outpatient follow-up.

Environmental Control and Lifestyle

Guidelines suggest avoiding contact with triggering factors whenever possible (except exercise, which is to be promoted). The identification of sensitizers that should be avoided at home, at school, and in the workplace should be performed. Respiratory "irritants" (e.g., indoor or outdoor pollutants), aspirin and other anti-inflammatory agents for asthmatic individuals intolerant to those drugs, should also be avoided. Many guidelines suggest measures to reduce the effects of environmental triggers, although the level of evidence to establish their beneficial effects on asthma is often low or uncertain.

Specific asthma phenotypes have been reported in smoking and in obese asthmatic patients, and these last two groups seem to be more resistant to therapy.[44,45] Smoking cessation is a key measure in asthmatic subjects who smoke and weight loss should be part of the recommendations for obese persons.

Pharmacological Treatment

Treatment "steps" are often recommended, although some guidelines, including the Canadian guidelines, consider treatment as a continuum.[36–39,41] A reduction of airway inflammation and an improvement in symptom control with added bronchodilators when ICS are insufficient are the basis of asthma therapy. Medications categorized as *relievers* (or *rescue/quick-relief medications*) include short-acting bronchodilators, long-acting bronchodilators with a rapid onset of action such as formoterol, and rarely, in patients intolerant to beta$_2$-agonists, ipratropium bromide. Otherwise, *preventers* (*controllers* or *long-term preventative medications*) include ICS and oral corticosteroids, LABA, leukotriene-receptors antagonists (LTRAs), and more rarely, mainly in some severe asthmatic patients, sustained-release theophylline and anti-cholinergics, and in severe allergic asthma, monoclonal antibodies such as omalizumab.

Rapid-acting beta$_2$-agonists are considered the drugs of choice in children and adults for the relief of acute symptoms. Long-acting inhaled beta$_2$-agonists, including formoterol and salmeterol, should not be used as monotherapy in asthma as these medications do not appear to influence airway inflammation in asthma. Occasionally, rapid-acting beta$_2$-agonists can also be used to prevent exercise-induced asthma although their need for this purpose should be minimal if the asthma is sufficiently controlled. They should be kept to a minimum frequency, usually less than three to four times per week according to the different guidelines, as the need for a bronchodilator is considered to reflect the degree of asthma control.

ICS are considered the mainstay of anti-inflammatory medication for asthma. They generally improve lung function and airway responsiveness, reduce and prevent asthma symptoms, and prevent exacerbations.[46]

LABAs are generally considered as add-on therapy when ICS are insufficient to control asthma, and are a preferred alternative to doubling the dose of ICS in adults.[47] These agents do not significantly reduce airway inflammation and should *always* be used with an anti-inflammatory medication such as ICS.[48]

LTRAs are considered as a second choice for initial anti-inflammatory therapy of asthma, and as a second-choice add-on therapy to ICS.[36–41,49] Sustained-relief theophylline is considered as a third-line add-on controller medication.

Monitoring of Asthma

Often, asthma control is poorly assessed, which can lead to undertreatment and an increased risk of severe events. This is often due to the poor use of control criteria and objective measures that assess airflow obstruction.[50] Spirometry should be regularly measured, ideally at each visit and at least once a year. If spirometry is not available, PEF measurements with devices such as the Mini-Wright peak flow meter should be utilized. Measures of airway inflammation (i.e., induced sputum and exhaled nitric oxide) have been proposed, particularly for moderate to severe asthma, to titrate the treatment, and these measures have resulted in the reduction of exacerbations.

Management of Exacerbations: The Asthma Action Plan

Since the late 1980s, consensus reports recognize that asthma is a chronic disease whose seriousness can fluctuate on a daily basis and that asthmatics should know how to modify their treatment accordingly. Written action plans are recommended for all asthmatic patients, indicating when and how to intensify their anti-inflammatory therapy according to asthma control criteria, when to introduce oral corticosteroids, and when to seek medical advice. Action plans based on symptoms are as effective as those that are based on PEF monitoring.[51] Although much remains to be evaluated in regard to the optimal action plan, the most important strategies to include in action plans have recently been formally evaluated.[36]

Treatment of Associated Conditions

Rhinosinusitis, obesity, gastroesophageal reflux, or other associated respiratory conditions such as smoking-induced COPD should be identified and the required treatment measures addressed.[52]

UPDATING CURRENT GUIDELINES

Most national and international guidelines are regularly updated, although the process usually takes from a few months up to 1 or 2 years. Sometimes, the whole document is revised with regard to potential new topics or the need to update recommendations according to the reviewers of the current evidence. As an example, in the most recent Canadian guidelines, four clinical questions were identified (PICO questions) as a focus to update the guidelines, including (1) the role of noninvasive measurements of airway inflammation, such as induced-sputum analysis, for the adjustment of therapy; (2) how to initiate add-on therapy to ICS for uncontrolled asthma; (3) the role of a combination ICS and a LABA combination as a reliever and as a reliever and a controller; and, finally, (4) how to increase controller medication when asthma control is acutely lost as part of a self-management action plan for exacerbations. The strength of the recommendations is based on the GRADE tool.

With respect to the GINA strategy, this guideline is reviewed every 6–12 months and changes are highlighted in its introduction. Recent grading has been performed according to the GRADE tool. The British Thoracic Society's (BTS) asthma guidelines have been revised almost every year over the last 5 years, in collaboration with the Scottish Intercollegiate Guidelines Network (SIGN). It uses a grading system from 1+ to 4+ based on the level of evidence and from A to D based on the grades of recommendation.

SUMMARIES OF GUIDELINES

For Health-Care Professionals

Guidelines developers have now produced summaries of their guidelines and of key recommendations (e.g., "Slim Jims" of Canadian Guidelines, GINA's "Pocket Guide for Asthma Management and Prevention," and others). These documents can help find the main features of a guideline while referencing the core document if needed (www.respiratoryguidelines.ca).

For Patients

Patients' guideline summaries are becoming increasingly available as offered by the recent BTS-SIGN guideline.[53,54]

FUTURE OF ASTHMA GUIDELINES

Further research is still required to optimize the implementation of guidelines, but more resources should be made available to accomplish this task, as they are currently mainly allocated to their production and dissemination. Interventions to help translate guidelines into care should be offered and improved. New communications tools such as intelligent telephones, handheld computers, and user-friendly websites offer innovative ways of communicating guideline recommendations.[20] Web-based social networks, communities of practice, and other means of interacting are increasingly available. Electronic health records can also possibly help improve access to recommendations at the site of care.[55] Forums such as the Guidelines International Network (G-I-N)[56] can help exchange ideas on the best methods to effectively translate guidelines.

CONCLUSIONS

Evidence-based guidelines can help optimize medical practice, but more effort should be made to better implement them. Methods to produce, assess, and translate guidelines more effectively have been developed. Asthma guidelines have been among the first guidelines produced and current recommendations have become more consistent from one guideline to another. Asthma management now universally resides on confirming the diagnosis by objective means, achieving and maintaining asthma control according to a set of criteria, and using nonpharmacological and pharmacological interventions to achieve this goal. Particular attention should be given to persistent care gaps, such as asthma education, inhaler technique demonstration, and the provision/use of asthma action plans for the management of exacerbations.

REFERENCES

1. Lougheed MD, Olajos-Clow J, Szpiro K, Moyse P, Julien B, Wang M, Day AG; Ontario Respiratory Outcomes Research Network. Multicentre evaluation of an emergency department asthma care pathway for adults. *CJEM* 2009;11:215–229.
2. To T, Wang C, Dell SD, Fleming-Carroll B, Parkin P, Scolnik D, Ungar WJ; PAMG Team. Can an evidence-based guideline reminder card improve asthma management in the emergency department? *Respir Med* 2010;104:1263–1270.
3. Boulet LP. Asthma guidelines and outcomes. Chapter 70. In: Adkinson NF Jr, Yunginger JW, Busse WW, Bochner BS, Holgate ST, Simons FER (eds). *Middleton's Allergy: Principles and Practice*, 6th edn, Vol. 2. Philadelphia: Mosby, pp. 1283–1301, 2003.
4. Hargreave FE, Dolovich J, Newhouse JT. The assessment and treatment of asthma conference report. *J Allergy Clin Immunol* 1990;85:1089–1090.
5. National Asthma Education and Prevention Program. Expert Panel Report: Guidelines for the diagnosis and management of asthma. Bethesda, MD: National Institutes of Health, 1991, NIH Publication no.91-3642.
6. Guidelines for management of asthma in adults: I—Chronic persistent asthma. Statement by the British Thoracic Society, Research Unit of the Royal College of Physicians of London, King's Fund Centre, National Asthma Campaign. *BMJ* 1990;301:651–653.
7. National Heart, Lung and Blood Institute and World Health Organization. Global initiative for Asthma. Bethesda, MD: National Institutes of Health, 1995, NIH Publication no.95-3659.
8. AGREE. Advancing the science of practice guidelines. Enterprise website 2010-2013. http://www.agreetrust.org/.
9. Brouwers MC, Kho ME, Browman GP, Burgers JS, Cluzeau F, Feder G, et al. Development of the AGREEII, Part 1: Performance, usefulness and areas for improvement. *CMAJ* 2010;182:1045–1052.
10. The GRADE working group 2005-2013. http://www.gradeworkinggroup.org/.
11. Guyatt GH, Oxman AD, Vist GE, Kunz R, Falck-Ytter Y, Alonso-Coello P, Schünemann HJ. GRADE: An emerging consensus on rating quality of evidence and strength of recommendations. *BMJ* 2008;336:924–926.
12. Guyatt GH, Oxman AD, Schünemann HJ, Tugwell P, Knottnerus A. GRADE guidelines: A new series of articles in the Journal of Clinical Epidemiology. *J Clin Epidemiol* 2011;64:380–382.

13. Grimshaw JM, Russell IT. Effect of clinical guidelines on medical practice: A systematic review of rigorous evaluations. *Lancet* 1993;342:1317–1322.

14. Woolf SH, Grol R, Hutchinson A, Eccles M, Grimshaw J. Clinical guidelines: Potential benefits, limitations, and harms of clinical guidelines. *BMJ* 1999;318:527–530.

15. FitzGerald JM, Quon B. The impact of asthma guidelines. *Lancet* 2010;376:751–753.

16. Bousquet J, Clark TJ, Hurd S, Khaltaev N, Lenfant C, O'Byrne P, Sheffer A. GINA guidelines on asthma and beyond. *Allergy* 2007;62:102–112.

17. Haahtela T, Tuomisto LE, Pietinalho A, Klaukka T, Erhola M, Kaila M, et al. A 10 year asthma programme in Finland: Major change for the better. *Thorax* 2006;61:663–670.

18. Souza-Machado C, Souza-Machado A, Franco R, Ponte EV, Barreto ML, Rodrigues LC, et al. Rapid reduction in hospitalizations after an intervention to manage severe asthma. *Eur Respir J* 2010;35:515–521.

19. Grol R, Grimshaw J. From best evidence to best practice: Effective implementation of change in patients' care. *Lancet* 2003;362:1225–1230.

20. Boulet LP, Becker A, Bowie D, Hernandez P, McIvor A, Rouleau M, et al. Implementing practice guidelines: A workshop on guidelines dissemination and implementation with a focus on asthma and COPD. *Can Respir J* 2006;13(Suppl A):5–47.

21. Partridge MR. Translating research into practice: How are guidelines implemented? *Eur Respir J* 2003;39(Suppl):23s–29s.

22. Jin R, Choi BC, Chan BT, McRae L, Li F, Cicutto L, et al. Physician asthma management practices in Canada. *Can Resp J* 2000;7:456–465.

23. Thompson R, Dixon F, Watt J, Crane J, Beasley R, Burgess C, et al. Prescribing for childhood asthma in the Wellington area comparison with international guidelines. *NZ Med J* 1993;106:81–83.

24. Mattos W, Grohs LB, Roque F, Ferreira M, Mânica G, Soares E. Asthma management in a public referral center in Porto Alegre in comparison with the guidelines established in the III Brazilian Consensus on Asthma Management. *J Bras Pneumol* 2006;32:385–390.

25. Boulet LP, Devlin H, O'Donnell DE. The Physicians' Practice Assessment Questionnaire on asthma and COPD. *Respir Med* 2011;105:8–14.

26. Bacci E, Melosini L, Novelli F, Marinaro S, Pala AP, Angino A, Dente FL, Paggiaro P. Are Italian pulmonologists aware of the guidelines for asthma management and do they know how to apply them? *Monaldi Arch Chest Dis* 2011;75:120–125.

27. Baiardini I, Braido F, Bonini M, Compalati E, Canonica GW. Why do doctors and patients not follow guidelines? *Curr Opin Allergy Clin Immunol* 2009;9:228–233.

28. Kitson AL, Strauss S. Identifying the knowledge-to-action gaps. In: Straus S, Tetroe J, Graham I. (eds.), *Knowledge Translation in Health Care: Moving from Evidence to Practice*. Oxford: Wiley-Blackwell Publishing, 2009.

29. Légaré F, Ratté S, Stacey D, Kryworuchko J, Gravel K, Graham ID, Turcotte S. Interventions for improving the adoption of shared decision making by health care professionals. *Cochrane Db Syst Rev* 2010;(5):CD006732.

31. Burgers J, Grol R, Eccles M. Clinical guidelines as a tool for implementing change in patient care. In: Grol R, Wensing M, Eccles M. (eds.), *Improving Patient Care. The Implementation of Change in Clinical Practice*, pp. 71–92. Oxford: Butterworth-Heinemann, 2005.

32. Tomaszewski W. Computer-based medical decision support system based on guidelines, clinical pathways and decision nodes. *Acta Bioeng Biomech* 2012;14:107–116.

33. Harrison MB, Légaré F, Graham ID, Fervers B. Adapting clinical practice guideline stolocal context and assessing barriers to their use. *CMAJ* 2010;182:E78–E84.

34. Graham ID, Logan J, Harrison MB, Straus SE, Tetroe J, Caswell W, et al. Lost in knowledge translation: Time for a map? *J Contin Educ Health Prof* 2006;26:13–24.

35. Boulet LP, FitzGerald JM, Levy ML, Cruz AA, Pedersen S, Haahtela T, Bateman ED. A guide to the translation of the Global Initiative for Asthma (GINA) strategy into improved care. *Eur Respir J* 2012;39:1220–1229.

36. Lougheed MD, Lemiere C, Ducharme FM, Licskai C, Dell SD, Rowe BH, Fitzgerald M, Leigh R, Watson W, Boulet LP; Canadian Thoracic Society Asthma Clinical Assembly. Canadian Thoracic Society 2012 guideline update: Diagnosis and management of asthma in preschoolers, children and adults. *Can Respir J* 2012;19:127–164.

37. Bateman ED, Hurd SS, Barnes PJ, Bousquet J, Drazen JM, FitzGerald M, et al. Global strategy for asthma management and prevention: GINA executive summary. *Eur Respir J* 2008;31:143–178. (updates of GINA can be found at www.ginasthma.com).

38. The British Thoracic Society Scottish Intercollegiate Guidelines Network. Guideline on the Management of Asthma. Quick Reference Guide, May 2008, revised May 2011; http://www.sign.ac.uk/pdf/qrg101.pdf.

39. National Heart, Lung, and Blood Institute. National Asthma Education and Prevention Program. Expert Panel Report 3: Guidelines for the Diagnosis and Management of Asthma. Full Report. 2007. http://www.nhlbi.nih.gov/guidelines/asthma/asthgdln.pdf.

40. The Global Initiative for Asthma (GINA). www.ginasthma.org/guidelines-global-strategy-for-the-diagnosis.html.

41. Cockcroft DW, Swystun VA. Asthma control versus asthma severity. *J Allergy Clin Immunol* 1996;98:1016–1018.

42. Bateman ED, Harrison TW, Quirce S, Reddel HK, Buhl R, Humbert M, et al. Overall asthma control achieved with budesonide/formoterol maintenance and reliever therapy for patients on different treatment steps. *Respir Res* 2011;12:38.

43. McDonald VM, Gibson PG. Asthma self-management education. *Chron Respir Dis* 2006;3:29–37.

44. Fitch KD, Sue-Chu M, Anderson SD, Boulet LP, Hancox RJ, McKenzie DC, et al. Asthma and the elite athlete: Summary of the International Olympic Committee's consensus conference, Lausanne, Switzerland, January 22–24, 2008. *J Allergy Clin Immunol* 2008;122:254–260.

45. Boulet LP. Asthma and obesity. *Clin Exp Allergy* 2013;43:8–21.

46. Barnes PJ. Efficacy of inhaled corticosteroids in asthma. *J Allergy Clin Immunol* 1998;102:531–538.

47. O'Byrne PM, Gauvreau GM, Murphy DM. Efficacy of leukotriene receptor agonists and synthesis inhibitors in asthma. *J Allergy Clin Immunol* 2009;124:397–403.

48. Sears MR. Safe use of long-acting β-agonists: What have we learnt? *Expert Opin Drug Saf* 2011;10:767–778.

49. Montuschi P, Peters-Golden ML. Leukotriene modifiers for asthma treatment. *Clin Exp Allergy* 2010;40:1732–1741.

50. Schatz M. Predictors of asthma control: What can we modify? *Curr Opin Allergy Clin Immunol* 2012;12:263–268.

51. Gibson PG, Wlodarczyk J, Hensley MH, Murree-Allen K, Olson LG, Saltos N. Using quality-control analysis of peak expiratory flow recordings to guide therapy for asthma. *Ann Intern Med* 1995;123:488–492.

52. Boulet LP, Boulay ME. Asthma-related comorbidities. *Expert Rev Respir Med* 2011;5:377–393.

53. SIGN 1993-2013: Scottish Intercollegiate Guidelines Network, Healthcare Improvement Scotland, www.sign.ac.uk.

54. The Global Initiative for Asthma (GINA). www.ginasthma.org/patient-guide.html.

55. Lougheed MD, Minard J, Dworkin S, Juurlink MA, Temple WJ, To T, Koehn M, Van Dam A, Boulet LP. Pan-Canadian REspiratory STandards Initiative for Electronic Health Records (PRESTINE): 2011 national forum proceedings. *Can Respir J* 2012;19:117–126.

56. Guidelines International Network (G-I-N). http://www.g-i-n.net/.

6 Diagnosis of Asthma in Preschool-Age Children

Chris Cleveland, Lora Stewart, Bradley Chipps, and Joseph D. Spahn

CONTENTS

CASE PRESENTATION

AW is an 18-month-old female who comes to see you for an evaluation of her food allergies and eczema. She was breast-fed until 8 months when a soy-based formula was introduced. At 1 year, and after cow's milk was introduced, AW broke out in hives and vomited immediately after ingesting milk. AW was diagnosed with eczema shortly after birth. It was initially confined to her face but it has progressively spread to include her entire body. She has never had a wheezing illness, but her father has asthma. You perform percutaneous skin testing for the foods that account for the majority of food allergies in early childhood. AW has positive skin tests to peanut, soy, milk, and egg. She is placed on an elemental formula.

AW returns to your clinic 6 months later. She has done well on an elemental diet and her eczema is well controlled. AW is here today because she has had several episodes of cough and wheeze over the past 3 months, with the most recent episode requiring an emergency room visit and a course of oral steroids. Currently, she is being treated with nebulized albuterol, which she requires up to several times a day to treat episodes of cough and wheeze. There is no environmental tobacco smoke exposure and no pets in her home, although she is exposed to a dog three times a week while being cared for at her grandparents' home. You perform

percutaneous skin testing for a limited panel of aeroallergens and find that she is sensitized to dog dander.

The parents have several questions regarding their daughter's respiratory symptoms:

   1. Does AW have asthma?
   2. If so, will she outgrow it?
   3. Does AW need to be on a daily medication to treat her symptoms?
   4. If so, what are the choices? And are they safe when given long term?

INTRODUCTION

Although great strides have been made in our understanding of the mechanisms and management of asthma over the past couple decades, a great deal needs to be learned regarding the origin and treatment of early-onset asthma. This is of major importance as the burden of asthma is greatest in preschool-age children. The rates of emergency department visits and hospitalizations for children under the age of 4 years are much greater than those for other age groups.[1] In addition, the cumulative prevalence of asthma is as high as 22% by the age of 4 years.[2,3] Lastly, many issues are unique to this age group, such as the difficulty in diagnosing asthma and assessing its severity and control;

the presence of confounding factors and disease masqueraders, which require treatment with daily controller medications; and deciding when therapy should be instituted, what medications to use, and how best to deliver these medications. This chapter will focus on how to diagnose asthma in this challenging group of children with recurrent cough and wheeze.

Diagnosing asthma in a preschool-age child can be a challenging endeavor. First and foremost, many preschool-age children with recurrent episodes of wheezing will "outgrow" their asthma. Large birth cohorts have shown that approximately 50% of preschool-age children with recurrent wheezing have a transient condition that resolves by grade school (6 years of age).[4] In addition, the difficulties inherent in diagnosing asthma in older children and adults are magnified in the preschool-age child. Diagnostic studies such as spirometry, bronchial challenge testing, and exhaled nitric oxide (FeNO) that are used to support the diagnosis of asthma are often not feasible in the preschool-age child. Thus, when considering an asthma diagnosis in younger children, one must rely on many aspects of their current and past medical history, their family and environmental history, and the findings of physical examinations.

IMPORTANT ASPECTS OF THE HISTORY OF PRESENT ILLNESS

Recurrent or persistent respiratory symptoms often prompt consideration of a diagnosis of asthma. The most frequent presenting symptom is recurrent wheeze.[4] Because many parents confuse wheeze with upper airway congestion or noise, previous physician-documented wheezing is helpful in confirming the presence of true wheeze. Often, wheezing has only been associated with previous viral respiratory tract infections, but it is important to clarify if any wheezing has been appreciated independent of obvious respiratory infections. Additional triggers of wheeze and other respiratory symptoms such as cough and shortness of breath include exercise or activity, exposure to furred or feathered animals, and environmental tobacco smoke.

Cough is another important symptom that is often reported by caregivers, and persistent cough can be a sign of an active disease. Unfortunately, cough is a nonspecific symptom, as most children cough during childhood, especially those with viral respiratory tract illnesses. The characteristic asthma cough is described as dry and it will often respond to bronchodilator therapy. Additionally, persistent cough apart from a viral illness, especially nocturnal cough, is consistent with a diagnosis of asthma and a frequent nocturnal cough may be associated with a more severe disease.[5] Finally, cough associated with physical activity such as exercise, laughing, or tickling is often related to asthma.[6] Furthermore, a history of tachypnea, respiratory distress, or hypoxia is very helpful in assessing the severity of an episode and may help to distinguish a simple upper respiratory infection (URI) from an episode of bronchospasm associated with asthma.

IMPORTANT ASPECTS OF PAST MEDICAL HISTORY

It is important to clarify birth history, specifically prematurity and a history of oxygen requirement and/or mechanical ventilation, in patients undergoing an evaluation for recurrent respiratory symptoms. Patients born prematurely often develop chronic lung disease or bronchopulmonary dysplasia (BPD) and many also have airway hyperresponsiveness, a characteristic feature of asthma.[7] Some studies have shown a lack of persistent inflammation in former premature infants with current asthma, and the condition may be different in this population compared with former term infants with current asthma.[8] That being said, former premature infant status is associated with an increased risk of asthma, especially when presented with additional risk factors such as a very low birth weight, prolonged mechanical ventilation, and prolonged oxygen requirement.[9] Premature status does not appear to be associated with an increased risk of allergies, and there is some controversy as to whether late prematurity (34–36 weeks estimated gestational age) is associated with asthma in later years.[10–12]

It is important to clarify the details regarding the child's respiratory status during viral URIs and when the child is well. Children who have a history of cough or wheeze between episodes of URIs are more likely to have persistent wheezing in the future compared with children with symptoms associated only with viral URIs. Additionally, children with frequent episodes of recurrent wheeze or cough (more than three per year) are more likely to have persistent disease.[4]

The number of unscheduled visits to the primary physician, emergency or urgent care center visits, and hospitalizations secondary to wheezing episodes can help determine the severity of the symptoms. Finally, a good response to previous therapies, including bronchodilators and inhaled and systemic corticosteroids, is helpful in assessing the etiology of respiratory symptoms because simple URIs without associated bronchospasm will not be improved with the use of bronchodilator therapy or systemic corticosteroids.

PRESENCE OF ATOPIC DERMATITIS

Infants and young children who have both atopic dermatitis (AD) and a recurrent respiratory wheeze are at an increased risk for developing asthma. In the Tucson birth cohort, the presence of eczema was found to be a major risk factor in predicting the likelihood of persistent disease.[13] Based on this cohort, the Asthma Predictive Index (API) was developed as listed in Table 6.1. This tool uses a combination of clinical and easily available laboratory data to help identify preschool-age children at risk for developing persistent asthma. The index requires recurrent wheezing in the first 3 years, plus one major (parental history of asthma or physician-diagnosed AD) or two of three minor (eosinophilia [≥4%], wheezing unrelated to a viral URI, and/or allergic rhinitis) risk factors. Children with a positive API were up to

TABLE 6.1
API versus the Modified API

Asthma Predictive Index[13]	Modified Asthma Predictive Index[14]
Major Criteria	
• Parental history of asthma	• Parental history of asthma
• Physician-diagnosed atopic dermatitis	• Physician-diagnosed atopic dermatitis
	• Allergic sensitization to ≥1 aeroallergen
Minor Criteria	
• Physician-diagnosed allergic rhinitis	• Allergic sensitization to egg, milk, or peanut
• Wheezing apart from colds	• Wheezing apart from colds
• Blood eosinophilia (>4%)	• Blood eosinophilia (>4%)

10 times more likely to have active asthma at some time during grade school compared with those with a negative API. In addition, both the negative predictive value and the specificity for the API were greater than 80%, indicating that the vast majority of preschool-age children with recurrent wheeze and a negative API will not have asthma at school age.[13]

The API has recently been modified based on a large early intervention study called Prevention of Early Asthma in Kids (PEAK).[14] In this study, 2- to 3-year-old children with recurrent wheeze who were also at risk of developing persistent asthma were enrolled to receive 2 years of an inhaled glucocorticoid or a matching placebo. The entry criteria included the presence of one of three major criteria (parental history of asthma, physician-diagnosed AD, or allergic sensitization to ≥1 aeroallergen) or two minor criteria (allergic sensitization to milk, egg, or peanut; wheezing unrelated to URIs; or blood eosinophils ≥4%). As both AD and asthma are often manifestations of atopy, many children initially present with eczema with or without food allergies, then develop asthma, and finally allergic rhinitis. This sequence of developing one atopic condition after another has been called the "atopic march."[15]

EARLY SENSITIZATION TO AEROALLERGENS

An important publication by the German Multicentre Allergy Study (MAS) provides further insight into the pivotal role of atopy in the development of persistent asthma.[16] In this large birth cohort study of over 1300 children, the authors sought to determine the onset of allergen sensitization, and the role that allergen exposure plays in the development of asthma in childhood. To accomplish this, sensitization to food and aeroallergens was measured serially from 1 to 10 years, while exposure to dust mites and cat allergens was serially measured from 6 months to 5 years. Spirometry was also measured at 7, 10, and 13 years, while bronchial hyperresponsiveness to histamine was determined at 7 years.

Wheezing children who had developed allergic sensitization by 3 years were defined as having an "atopic wheeze," while those who did not develop allergic sensitization were

considered to have a "nonatopic wheeze." There was no difference in either the frequency or the severity of the wheeze episodes between those with an atopic wheeze compared with those with a nonatopic wheeze during the first 5 years of life. However, from 6 to 13 years, the percentage of children with persistent wheeze progressively declined in those with nonatopic wheeze, so that by 13 years of age, 90% had no evidence of active asthma and their lung function was normal. In contrast, 44% of the children with atopic wheeze had active asthma at age 13 and they developed impaired lung function. The children with asthma who were at greatest risk of lung function impairment were both sensitized and exposed to high concentrations of indoor aeroallergens.[16]

RESPIRATORY VIRAL INFECTIONS EARLY IN LIFE

Studies have shown that severe bronchiolitis early in life necessitating hospitalization and/or oxygen requirement is an independent risk factor for the development of asthma.[17,18] The most commonly recovered organisms from these severe infections are respiratory syncytial virus (RSV) and rhinovirus (RV). It remains to be determined whether the infection itself results in the development of asthma, or whether the infection is the inciting event in children destined to have asthma. Historically, RSV infection has held a strong association with predicting future asthma; however, more recent studies have emphasized the role of RV infection in predicting future asthma, and in some some studies, it has actually held a stronger association with the presence of persistent asthma than RSV.[19,20] This highlights the need for continued vigilant monitoring of children with severe disease even when they are RSV-negative.

IMPORTANT ASPECTS OF FAMILY HISTORY

The evaluation of children with recurrent respiratory symptoms should include thorough reviews of their family medical history. As discussed earlier, physician-diagnosed parental asthma is one of the two major risk factors in the API for persistent wheezing in a preschool-age child.[13,14] Reviewing the family history for the presence of other atopic diseases, such as allergic rhinitis, food allergy, and eczema, will help establish a potential atopic genetic background for the patient.

IMPORTANT ASPECTS OF ENVIRONMENTAL HISTORY

An environmental history should be obtained in order to determine the presence of potential perennial allergens in the home such as dust mites and pets.[21] As noted earlier, the MAS study identified early sensitization and exposure to an indoor aeroallergen such as dog or cat dander, dust mites, mold, or cockroach allergens as among the strongest predictors of subsequent persistent asthma in preschool-age children with recurrent wheeze.[16] Thus, information such as the types of family pets, both furred and feathered, whether the pets are indoor or outdoor, and if they sleep in the child's bedroom should be ascertained. In dust mite-endemic regions, the use of mattress and pillow covers, the frequency and manner of cleaning bedding, and the presence of carpeting, curtains, upholstered furniture, and stuffed animals should be included in an environmental history.[22] Additional questions should address the age of the home and dampness, relating to the presence of mold. Sensitization to mold species such as *Aspergillus* and *Penicillium* has been shown to be associated with an asthma diagnosis.[23] Dampness in general unrelated to mold sensitization has been found to be associated with increased upper and lower respiratory symptoms in children. A recent meta-analysis assessing the health effects of indoor dampness or mold exposure in 31,742 children from 8 ongoing European birth cohorts revealed that a home environment with mold in early life is associated with an increased risk of asthma in young children and allergic rhinitis symptoms in school-age children.[24]

Previous studies have shown that children who are sensitized to house-dust mite allergens and to the mold *Alternaria* are more likely to have asthma as documented by bronchial hyperresponsiveness.[25] Details on the presence of other potential irritants such as tobacco smoke, fireplaces, or wood-burning stoves; on the type of heating and air-cooling systems; and on the proximity to road traffic should be noted as studies have related the exposure to traffic-related air pollution and biomass smoke with persistent asthma.[26,27]

IMPORTANT ASPECTS OF PHYSICAL EXAMINATION

There are several portions of the physical examination that may support atopic disease in young children with recurrent wheeze. An examination of the nose will often reveal edema and rhinorrhea, but unfortunately, it is nearly impossible to differentiate allergic rhinitis from viral upper respiratory illnesses. When performing a lung examination on a child who appears well, the examination, including the respiratory rate, inspiratory to expiratory phase ratio, oxygen saturation, and auscultation, will likely be normal. As such, a normal lung examination during a time when a child is well does not rule in or rule out the diagnosis of asthma. During an acute episode, a lung examination will be most helpful. The documentation of wheezing, tachypnea, retractions, and/or hypoxia is important in characterizing the symptoms and the severity of an episode. A skin examination is important in determining whether the child has any concomitant AD, specifically looking for erythema, excoriations, thickening, or lichenification. In the preschool age group, the distribution of eczema may include the face and the extensor regions as seen in infancy or it may be transitioning to the flexor regions as seen in the older age groups.

TESTING OPTIONS IN YOUNGER CHILDREN

LUNG FUNCTION TESTING

In older children, lung function tests such as spirometry and lung volume measurements (body plethysmography) are often helpful in confirming or excluding a diagnosis of asthma. An improvement in airflow limitation by $\geq 12\%$ following albuterol inhalation in a patient with respiratory symptoms is strongly suggestive of asthma.[28] Unfortunately, these tests require both cooperation and coordination to complete. In preschool-age children, lung function testing is possible, but its regular application is limited by the requirement for sedation, costly equipment, and specialized personnel.

In younger children, several techniques are available to quantitate the lower airway function. Currently, most of the techniques are used in research settings and normative values are available in the American Thoracic Society/ European Respiratory Society (ATS/ERS) guidelines; however, the standardization of the techniques is lacking and the results may be difficult to interpret.[29] The available techniques include standard spirometry, maximal flow referenced to functional residual capacity, impulse oscillometry (IOS), interrupter resistance (Rint), plethysmography, gas dilution techniques, and gas mixing indices.[29] These tests may be used in clinical situations such as: (1) unexplained tachypnea, cough, hypoxemia, or respiratory distress where a definitive diagnosis is not clear; (2) children with lower airway symptoms who are not responding to standard therapy; (3) determining the severity of lower airway obstruction and providing a basis for follow-up after intervention; and (4) better defining the course of diseases and the response to therapy in research studies. It is hoped that further advances will allow for a wider application of this technology as the equipment becomes more affordable and easier to use, and better normative standards become available.

IMPULSE OSCILLOMETRY

IOS is a technology that utilizes small-amplitude pressure oscillations to determine the resistance of the airway. It is largely effort independent and does not require coordination, but it does require the cooperation of the child, which is a limiting factor for routine use.[30] To perform IOS, the child holds a mouthpiece in place over a 30 second period of time while breathing normally (tidal breathing). Sound impulses of various frequencies from 5 to 35 Hz are applied to the airway through the mouthpiece with the total respiratory system resistance (Rrs) and reactance (Xrs) determined at the various frequencies. IOS has been studied in young children with suspected asthma and conflicting results have been obtained. Some investigators have not found IOS to be useful in differentiating recurrent wheezers from healthy preschool-age children, while others have found significant differences in both the baseline Rrs and the change in Rrs following the inhalation of a beta-agonist in asthmatic compared with nonasthmatic children.[31,32] Lastly, young children at risk for asthma have been shown to display a significant change in Rrs following bronchodilator therapy compared with age-matched control children.[33,34] Thus, IOS has the potential to be a useful lung function measure in young children with suspected asthma, but currently it remains largely a research tool.

In older children and adults who are able to complete spirometry, a bronchial challenge (methacholine, histamine, or exercise) demonstrating airway hyperresponsiveness is strongly supportive of a diagnosis of asthma.[35] Because younger children are unable to perform spirometry, bronchial challenge testing has been modified by incorporating auscultation and pulse oximetry monitoring. Currently, the presence of wheeze, significant tachypnea, and/or a 5% or more decrease in oxygen saturation from baseline constitutes a positive challenge.[36] Unfortunately, the test is not standardized and there has been dispute as to what is the best parameter to confirm positivity. These issues aside, there is evidence that more severe degrees of airway hyperresponsiveness are correlated with an increased likelihood of disease development and persistence.[37]

OTHER TESTS

Radiographic studies such as chest x-rays and chest computed tomography (CT) scans of young children with a history of recurrent wheezing or cough are not routinely obtained during periods when the child is well. The usefulness of radiographic studies during acute wheezing episodes has been debated and are usually reserved for patients with significant tachypnea, localized findings on auscultation, associated fever, or significant hypoxemia.[38] Additionally, chest radiographs can be useful when concern exists about a foreign body (FB) or the presence of an anatomical abnormality.

The demonstration of specific immunoglobulin E (IgE) either by percutaneous skin prick testing or by a serum-specific IgE measurement can confirm atopy in a child. Because it often takes several seasons to develop sensitization to seasonal aeroallergens such as trees, grass, or weed pollen, skin testing in the preschool-age child is often limited to perennial allergens (dust mite and cockroach allergens, mold, and pet dander) or food allergens if this is a concern for an individual patient. Documented early sensitization to an allergen(s) is a risk factor for persistent disease with over 60% of 2- to 3-year-old children with recurrent wheezing having a positive modified API with sensitization to either food or aeroallergens.[14] Unfortunately, negative testing in a young child does not rule out atopy. It merely confirms that there is currently no sensitization to the allergens tested. In fact, a negative test at a young age does not predict whether or not the child might develop allergic sensitization in the future.[39,40]

Additional laboratory results such as an elevated circulating eosinophil count or an elevated serum IgE level may suggest atopy, but are much less specific. With that said, an elevated eosinophil count is considered a minor criterion for predicting the persistence of wheeze as defined by the API and the modified API.[13,14]

In patients in whom there is concern for recurrent infection as the etiology of recurrent wheeze or cough, a screening immune system evaluation may be warranted, including quantitative immunoglobulin levels (IgG, IgM, and IgA) and assays for functional antibodies. Typically, patients with an underlying immunodeficiency have additional signs and

symptoms apart from recurrent wheeze or cough, such as a recurrent fever, failure to thrive, and documented bacterial infections.[41]

Cystic fibrosis (CF) must also be considered in any young child presenting with a history of recurrent or persistent respiratory symptoms. Classically, CF presents with additional symptoms of failure to thrive or evidence of pancreatic insufficiency, but milder variants of CF exist and these can be ruled out by a normal sweat test or by the demonstration of the absence of a CF DNA mutation. The presence of bilateral nasal polyps is highly suspicious for CF. The reference ranges for infants under 6 months of age are: ≤29 mmol/L, CF unlikely; 30–59 mmol/L, intermediate; and ≥60 mmol/L, indicative of CF. The recommended reference values for a change in sweat chloride after 6 months of age are: ≤39 mmol/L, CF unlikely; 40–59 mmol/L, intermediate; and ≥60 mmol/L, indicative of CF.[42]

Some patients present with recurrent episodes of choking or aspiration or a history of gastroesophageal reflux symptoms in addition to recurrent wheeze or cough. These patients warrant an evaluation for a swallowing dysfunction, and aspiration or gastroesophageal reflux disease (GERD) by barium swallow and/or a pH probe study. These problems are not infrequently found in combination with underlying bronchial hyperresponsiveness and the treatment of GERD, often resulting in an improvement of both problems.[43]

Finally, in patients with a history of inspiratory stridor or wheeze, or in patients who have failed to respond to bronchodilator therapy or a short course of systemic steroids, tracheomalacia must be considered. Although a diagnosis can often be made clinically, the diagnosis and severity assessment are best made by bronchoscopy.[44]

DIFFERENTIAL DIAGNOSIS OF RECURRENT WHEEZE IN PRESCHOOL-AGE CHILDREN

When evaluating a preschool-age child with suspected asthma, one must rule out other respiratory diseases that present with cough and wheeze. The differential diagnosis of recurrent cough and wheeze is quite extensive, but it can be narrowed down based on a thorough history and physical examination (Table 6.2). Additionally, one should focus first on common conditions such as GERD, and upper airway diseases such as rhinitis and sinusitis, unless the evaluation supports pursuing rare etiologies.

GERD is commonly diagnosed in young children. Often, this age group does not complain of the classic symptoms of heartburn or abdominal pain, but rather presents with excess burping or emesis, coughing after meals, or nocturnal cough or wheeze.[45] A diagnosis can be clinically suspected and confirmed with a positive response to an empiric therapy with an acid suppression regimen. Alternatively, a pH/impedance probe to document increased or prolonged events of acid and nonacid stomach contents in the esophagus, or radiographic studies such as a tailored barium swallow/upper gastrointestinal (GI) series may be utilized before treatment is started. Because GERD and asthma symptoms may coexist,

TABLE 6.2
Differential Diagnosis of Recurrent Wheezing

Upper Airway Conditions
1. Allergic rhinitis
2. Sinusitis
3. Adenoidal hypertrophy

Large Airway Conditions
1. Laryngotracheomalacia
2. Foreign body aspiration
3. Vascular rings, laryngeal webs
4. Tracheoesophageal fistula
5. Vocal cord paresis/paralysis
6. External mass compressing airway (e.g., tumor, enlarged lymph nodes, or congenital heart disease)
7. Vocal cord dysfunction (rare in young children)

Small Airway Conditions
1. Viral bronchiolitis (e.g., RSV and RV)
2. Gastroesophageal reflux
3. Bronchopulmonary dysplasia
4. Bronchiolitis obliterans
5. Diseases associated with bronchiectasis
   a. Cystic fibrosis
   b. B-cell immune deficiency
   c. Alpha-1-antitrypsin deficiency
   d. Primary ciliary dyskinesia

a diagnosis of one or the other is not mutually exclusive. There are conflicting studies regarding whether the treatment of GERD results in improved asthma symptoms and a decreased need for asthma medication.[46–47]

Chronic sinusitis or rhinitis with associated postnasal drip may contribute to persistent cough in the preschool-age patient. Typically, patients have evidence of persistent nasal congestion or drainage in association with the cough. The cough is more likely to be wet and/or productive and is worse at night or early morning. This type of cough will not improve with bronchodilator or inhaled corticosteroid therapy, but often improves with the treatment of the underlying condition. The treatment can be started empirically, but a sinus CT may also be useful if considering a prolonged antibiotic course.[48]

Tracheomalacia is a common anatomical defect seen in young children. Patients with tracheomalacia often present with recurrent episodes of stridor, wheeze, or barky cough, which are worsened by crying, and a concurrent respiratory infection.[49,50] The respiratory symptoms often subside while sleeping, in contrast to asthma symptoms that often worsen at night. In many patients, the symptoms are present between episodes of infection, but mild cases may only be symptomatic with infection or vigorous crying. Additionally, treatment with a bronchodilator results in no change or even worsens the symptoms because it results in diminished airway tone in the presence of malacia. Glucocorticoids, both systemic and inhaled, are also ineffective. For the majority of patients, the symptoms associated with tracheomalacia

resolve by age 2, but more persistent disease can occur. An evaluation for less common etiologies, including a tracheo-esophageal fistula (TEF), a vascular ring, or an underlying connective tissue disorder, should be pursued for severe or persistent presentations. A bronchoscopy is the examination of choice in the diagnosis and assessment of tracheomalacia.

Mechanical airway compression due to congenital cardiac anomalies should be considered in a patient with recurrent respiratory symptoms that have failed to improve with bronchodilator or corticosteroid therapy. Anatomic compression is obviously a less common etiology for recurrent wheeze compared with asthma, but it is often unrecognized in this age group. Compression can occur due to vascular rings or slings (right-sided or double aortic arch, anomalous innominate artery, or pulmonary artery sling) or due to an enlargement of the cardiac and/or pulmonary vasculature (dilated pulmonary arteries, left atrial enlargement, or massive cardiomegaly). A classic presentation includes recurrent respiratory difficulties with wheezing and stridor. Many patients have associated dysphagia or apnea. The symptoms are usually aggravated by crying and concurrent respiratory viral infections. The severity of the symptoms is dependent on the location and the degree of the anomaly. When this diagnosis is suspected, a chest x-ray should be obtained with close attention to the side of the aortic arch, the size and shape of the cardiac silhouette, and for the presence of tracheal deviation or constriction. Esophagrams are often used to evaluate for vascular rings and slings, but are nonspecific and may be normal despite the presence of an anomaly if that anomaly does not compress the esophagus. Of note, bronchoscopy is not diagnostic; rather magnetic resonance imaging (MRI) of the chest or multidetector CT (MDCT) is employed to confirm the diagnosis.[51] Finally, congestive heart failure in young children rarely presents with wheezing, but it may present with a history of increased work of breathing.

The rare H-type TEF may need to be considered in a patient with recurrent respiratory symptoms, especially recurrent pneumonia or persistent infiltrates on a chest radiograph. These patients will not respond to conventional therapies, including bronchodilators and corticosteroids. The vast majority of patients with TEF have additional birth anomalies. This type of TEF may be difficult to demonstrate by conventional radiographic studies, but a high-resolution CT is often used for the diagnosis. Bronchoscopy may also be useful.[52]

In a preschool-age patient with an acute onset of wheeze, cough, or both, FB aspiration must be considered. On physical examination, the wheezing will often be unilateral or localized. A forced expiratory chest radiograph may demonstrate air trapping behind the FB. The diagnosis is confirmed by bronchoscopy and removal of the FB. Typically, patients present with acute respiratory symptoms, but chronic symptoms or a history of infiltrate or pneumonia that fails to clear can also occur.[53]

Patients with CF classically present with a history of recurrent respiratory symptoms in association with systemic symptoms of failure to thrive, diarrhea, and recurrent sinus and ear infections. Additionally, there are many more mild variants of classic CF that may not have associated systemic symptoms. Therefore, in patients with recurrent pneumonia or those that have failed to respond to conventional therapies, one should consider CF in the differential diagnosis.[54]

Immunodeficiency presenting with recurrent wheeze, cough, or both without superimposed infections, diarrhea, rash, or failure to thrive is quite rare. Immunodeficiency should not be considered in the initial differential diagnosis of a young child with only recurrent wheeze, cough, or both.

SUMMARY

The diagnosis of asthma in childhood is primarily based on the frequency, quality, variability, and severity of the symptoms in addition to a family history and other allergic comorbidities (Table 6.1). Although predicting the likelihood of persistent asthma in a preschool-age child with recurrent or persistent respiratory symptoms is difficult, the presence of several risk factors including a personal history of eczema or allergic rhinitis, a parental history of asthma, positive allergy skin tests, and the persistence of symptoms without viral illnesses will aid in the diagnosis. The response to therapy can be especially helpful in younger children where pulmonary function testing may not be feasible. The differential diagnosis of recurrent wheezing is large especially in younger children and testing to rule out other conditions should be performed in a thoughtful manner (Table 6.2). Alternative diagnoses or comorbid conditions such as GERD, tracheomalacia, or CF must be appropriately evaluated and treated. Finally, a number of tests are available to support a diagnosis of asthma and the risk of future asthma, such as skin prick testing, blood work documenting atopy (eosinophilia or elevated IgE levels), or even documentation of bronchial hyperresponsiveness.

The keys to the diagnosis of asthma in children include a high index of suspicion as 80% of asthma starts before the age of 5 years.[55] The clinical course will reflect the variability of childhood asthma with some patients having long periods of quiescent symptoms. This should not prevent appropriate diagnoses and treatment when supported by the appropriate clinical presentation.

REFERENCES

1. Akinbami LJ, Moorman JE, Garbe PL, et al. Status of childhood asthma in the United States, 1980–2007. *Pediatrics* 2009;123:S131–S145.
2. Croner S, Kjellman N-I. Natural history of bronchial asthma in childhood. *Allergy* 1992;47:150–157.
3. Tariq SM, Matthews SM, Hakim EA, et al. The prevalence of and risk factors for atopy in early childhood: A whole population birth cohort study. *J Allergy Clin Immunol* 1998;101:587–593.
4. Martinez FD, Wright AL, Taussig LM, et al. Asthma and wheezing in the first six years of life. *N Engl J Med* 1995;332:133–138.
5. Meijer GG, Postma DS, Wempe JB, et al. Frequency of nocturnal symptoms in asthmatic children attending a hospital out-patient clinic. *Eur Respir J* 1995;8(12):2076–2080.
6. Liangas G, Morton JR, Henry RL. Mirth-triggered asthma: Is laughter really the best medicine? *Pediatr Pulmonol* 2003;36(2):107–112.
7. Lum S, Kirkby J, Welsh L, et al. Nature and Severity of lung function abnormalities in extremely pre-term children at 11 years of age. *Eur Respir J* 2011;37:1199–1207.
8. Kim do K, Choi SH, Yu J, et al. Bronchial responsiveness to methacholine and adenosine 5-monophosphate in preschool children with bronchopulmonary dysplasia. *Pediatr Pulmonol* 2006;41(6):538–543.
9. Jaakkola J, Ahmed P, Ieromnimon A, et al. Preterm delivery and asthma: A systematic review and meta-analysis. *J Allergy Clin Immunol* 2006;118:823–830.
10. Siltanen M, Wehkalampi K, Hovi P, et al. Preterm birth reduces the incidence of atopy in adulthood. *J Allergy Clin Immunol* 2011;127(4):935–942.
11. Goyal NK, Fiks AG, Lorch SA. Association of late-preterm birth with asthma in young children: Practice-based study. *Pediatrics* 2011;128(4):e830–e838.
12. Abe K, Shapiro-Mendoza CK, Hall LR, et al. Late preterm birth and risk of developing asthma. *J Pediatr* 2010;157(1):74–78.
13. Castro-Rodriguez JA, Holberg CJ, Wright AL, et al. A clinical index to define risk of asthma in young children with recurrent wheezing. *Am J Respir Crit Care Med* 2000;162:1403–1406.
14. Guilbert TW, Morgan WJ, Zeiger RS, et al. Atopic characteristics of children with recurrent wheezing at high risk for the development of childhood asthma. *J Clin Immunol* 2004;114:1282–1287.
15. Wahn, U. What drives the allergic march? *Allergy* 2000;55:591–599.
16. Illi S, Von Mutius E, Niggemann B, et al. Perennial allergen sensitization early in life and chronic asthma in children: A birth cohort study. *Lancet* 2006;368:763–770.
17. Sigurs N, Bjarnason R, Sigurbergsson F, et al. Respiratory syncytial virus bronchiolitis in infancy is an important risk factor for asthma and allergy at age 7. *Am J Respir Crit Care Med* 2000;161:1501–1507.
18. Henderson J, Hilliard TN, Sherriff A, et al. Hospitalization for RSV bronchiolitis before 12 months of age and subsequent asthma, atopy and wheeze: A longitudinal birth cohort study. *Pediatr Allergy Immunol* 2005;16:386–392.
19. Lemanske RF, Jackson DJ, Gangnon RE, et al. Rhinovirus illnesses during infancy predict subsequent childhood wheezing. *J Allergy Clin Immunol* 2005;116:571–577.
20. Midulla F, Pierangeli A, Cangiano G, et al. Rhinovirus bronchiolitis and recurrent wheezing: 1-year follow-up. *Eur Respir J* 2012;39:396–402.
21. McHugh B, MacGinnitie AJ. Indoor allergen sensitization and the risk of asthma and eczema in children in Pittsburgh. *Allergy Asthma Proc* 2011;32:372–376.
22. Platts-Mills TA, Vervloet D, Thomas WR, et al. Indoor allergens and asthma: Report of the Third International Workshop. *J Allergy Clin Immunol* 1997;100:S2–S24.
23. Reponen T, Lockey J, Bernstein DI, et al. Infant origins of childhood asthma associated with specific molds. *J Allergy Clin Immunol* 2012;130(3):639–644.
24. Tischer CG, Hohmann C, Thiering E, et al. Meta-analysis of mould and dampness exposure on asthma and allergy in eight European birth cohorts: An ENRIECO initiative. *Allergy* 2011;66(12):1570–1579.

25. Halonen M, Stern DA, Wright AL, et al. Alternaria as a major allergen for asthma in children raised in a desert environment. *Am J Respir Crit Care Med* 1997;155:1356–1361.

26. Herr M, Just J, Nikasinovic L, et al. Risk factors and characteristics of respiratory and allergic phenotypes in early childhood. *J Allergy Clin Immunol* 2012;130:389–396.

27. Lambauch RJ, Kipen HM. Respiratory health effects of air pollution: Update on biomass smoke and traffic pollution. *J Allergy Clin Immunol* 2012;129:3–11.

28. Pellegrino R, Viegi G, Brusasco V, et al. Interpretative strategies for lung function tests. *Eur Respir J* 2005;26(5):948–968.

29. Beydon N, Davis SD, Lombardi E, et al. An official American Thoracic Society/European Respiratory Society statement: Pulmonary function testing in preschool children. *Am J Respir Crit Care Med* 2007;175:1304–1345.

30. Komarow HD, Skinner J, Young M, et al. A study of the use of impulse oscillometry in the evaluation of children with asthma: Analysis of lung parameters, order effect, and utility compared with spirometry. *Pediatr Pulmonol* 2012;47:18–26.

31. Bailly C, Crenesse D, Albertini M. Evaluation of impulse oscillometry during bronchial challenge testing in children. *Pediatr Pulmonol* 2011;46:1209–1214.

32. Wilson NM, Bridge P, Phagoo SB, et al. The measurement of methacholine responsiveness in 5-year old children: Three methods compared. *Eur Respir J* 1995;8:364–370.

33. Marotta A, Klinnert MD, Price MR, et al. Impulse oscillometry provides an effective measure of lung dysfunction in 4-year-old children at risk for persistent asthma. *J Allergy Clin Immunol* 2003;112:317–322.

34. Schulze J, Smith HJ, Fuchs J, et al. Methacholine challenge in young children as evaluated by spirometry and impulse oscillometry. *Respir Med* 2012;106:627–634.

35. National Heart, Lung, and Blood Institute. Expert Panel Report 3: Guidelines for the Diagnosis and Management of Asthma. NIH Publication 07-4051. Bethesda, MD: National Institutes of Health; August 2007.

36. Springer C, Godfrey S, Picard E, et al. Efficacy and safety of methacholine bronchial challenge performed by auscultation in young asthmatic children. *Am J Respir Crit Care Med* 2000;162:857–860.

37. Cohen S, Avital A, Hevroni A, et al. Predictive value of Adenosine 5'-monophosphate challenge in preschool children for the diagnosis of asthma 5 years later. *J Pediatr* 2012;161(1):156–159.

38. Gershel JC, Goldman HS, Stein RE, et al. The usefulness of chest radiographs in first asthma attacks. *N Engl J Med* 1983;309:336–339.

39. Kjaer HF, Eller E, Andersen KE, et al. The association between early sensitization patterns and subsequent allergic disease. The DARC birth cohort study. *Pediatr Allergy Immunol* 2009;20:726–734.

40. Silvestri M, Rossi GA, Cozzani S, et al. Age-dependent tendency to become sensitized to other classes of aeroallergens in atopic asthmatic children. *Ann Allergy Asthma Immunol* 1999;83:335–340.

41. Bonilla FA, Bernstein IL, Khan DA, et al. Practice parameter for the diagnosis and management of primary immunodeficiency. *Ann Allergy Asthma Immunol* 2005;94:S1–S63.

42. Farrell PM, Rosenstein BJ, White TB, et al. Cystic Fibrosis Foundation. Guidelines for diagnosis of cystic fibrosis in newborns through older adults: Cystic Fibrosis Foundation consensus report. *J Pediatr* 2008;153:S4–S14.

43. Ghezzi M, Silvestri M, Guida E, et al. Acid and weakly acid gastroesophageal refluxes and type of respiratory symptoms in children. *Respir Med* 2011;105:972–978.

44. Saglani S, Nicholson AG, Scallon M, et al. Investigation of young children with severe recurrent wheeze: Any clinical benefit? *Eur Respir J* 2006;27:29–35.

45. Borrelli O, Marabotto C, Mancini V, et al. Role of gastroesophageal reflux in children with unexplained chronic cough. *J Pediatr Gastroenterol Nutr* 2011;53:287–292.

46. Kiljander TO, Junghard O, Beckman O, et al. Effect of esomeprazole 40 mg once or twice daily on asthma: A randomized, placebo-controlled study. *Am J Respir Crit Care Med* 2010;181:1042–1048.

47. Writing Committee for the American Lung Association Asthma Clinical Research Centers. Lansoprazole for children with poorly controlled asthma: A randomized controlled trial. *JAMA* 2012;307:373–381.

48. Wald ER. Beginning antibiotics for acute rhinosinusitis and choosing the right treatment. *Clin Rev Allergy Immunol* 2006;30:143–152.

49. Doshi J, Krawiec M. Clinical manifestations of airway malacia in young infants. *J Allergy Clin Immunol* 2007;120:1276–1278.

50. Boogaard R, Huijsmans S, Pijnenberg M, et al. Tracheomalacia and bronchomalacia in children: Incidence and patient characteristics. *Chest* 2005;128:3391–3397.

51. McLaren CA, Elliot MJ, Roebuck DJ. Vascular compression of the airway in children. *Paediatr Resp Rev* 2008;9:85–94.

52. Hajjar WM, Iftikhar A, Al Nassar SA, et al. Congenital tracheoesophageal fistula: A rare and late presentation in adult patient. *Ann Thorac Med* 2012;7:48–50.

53. Saliba J, Mijovic T, Daniel S, et al. Asthma: The great imitator in foreign body aspiration? *J Otolaryngol Head Neck Surg* 2012;41:200–206.

54. Hamosh A, Corey M. Correlation between genotype and phenotype in patients with cystic fibrosis. The Cystic Fibrosis Genotype-Phenotype Consortium. *N Engl J Med* 1993;329:1308–1313.

55. Ydunginger JW, Reed CE, O'Connell EJ, et al. A community based study of the epidemiology of asthma. *Am Rev Respir Dis* 1992;146:888–894.

7 Diagnosis of Asthma in Older Children and Adults

Paul M. O'Byrne

CONTENTS

CASE PRESENTATION

A 52-year-old man presented with a 1-year history of shortness of breath on exertion, being limited to less than two flights of stairs, a chronic cough that was generally nonproductive and was most troublesome at night, and intermittent chest tightness. He denied any wheezing or chest pain. His symptoms were worsened when exposed to extremes of temperature. He was previously a smoker, having smoked 25 pack-years, but had stopped smoking 4 years before, at which time he had presented to the emergency department with an acute myocardial infarction, which was managed with coronary angioplasty. His current medications were a beta-blocker, a statin, and daily low-dose aspirin. He had no history of atopic disease, nor any relevant family history. He had been told that he had episodes of "bronchitis" as a young child, but he remembers very little detail about these episodes.

Initial investigations included a chest x-ray (CXR), which was normal, and spirometry, which showed a forced expiratory volume in 1 second (FEV_1) and a forced vital capacity (FVC) of 1.9 and 4.4 L, respectively (ratio 43%) with normal values of 3.9/4.7 L. After inhaled beta$_2$-agonist treatment, the values were 2.0/4.5 L, showing no acute reversibility in airflow obstruction. Skin prick testing to common environmental allergens showed a positive response to house-dust mites and grass pollen. Blood tests included a complete blood count and electrolytes, which were normal (no increase in blood eosinophils) and his total immunoglobulin E (IgE) was slightly elevated at 230. Thus, the patient presented with severe airflow obstruction and a long previous smoking history, atopy, and a history in childhood consistent with mild asthma.

A decision was made to begin treatment with a course of oral corticosteroids (prednisolone 50 mg/day) for 3 weeks and a combination inhaler containing an inhaled corticosteroid (ICS) and a long-acting inhaled beta$_2$-agonist (LABA) administered twice daily. At his return clinic visit, his symptoms had markedly improved; his cough was no longer troublesome at night and his spirometry demonstrated values of 3.0/4.6 L (a 58% improvement in FEV_1). The diagnosis was established as asthma, but with residual airflow obstruction, possibly related to his history of cigarette smoking. The prednisolone was discontinued, he was switched from a beta-blocker to an angiotensin receptor antagonist, and the combination inhaler was continued. He was left on low-dose aspirin, as he had no history of worsening symptoms while taking this medication. At the next follow-up visit, 3 months later, he remained largely symptom free and his spirometry values were 2.9/4.4 L.

COMMENT

This case demonstrates a patient who was suspected of having chronic obstructive pulmonary disease (COPD) because of his long smoking history, and who had no acute reversibility after inhaled beta$_2$-agonists, but who demonstrated largely reversible airflow obstruction after treatment with corticosteroids, confirming a diagnosis of asthma.

INTRODUCTION

Asthma is a chronic inflammatory disease of the airways that is characterized by recurrent respiratory symptoms of dyspnea, wheezing, chest tightness, and/or cough, and is associated with variable airflow obstruction.[1] Another clinical characteristic of asthma is airway hyperresponsiveness, which is identified by an exaggerated response of the airways to a variety of stimuli.[2] Asthma usually begins in childhood, although sometimes the initial symptoms begin much later in life. Establishing the diagnosis can often be straightforward, particularly in older children, but it can be troublesome in preschool children and older adults because of the difficulty in obtaining objective evidence of variable airflow obstruction in younger children, and because of the possible presence of other diseases, which can present with symptoms similar to asthma, in older adults.

ROLE OF MEDICAL HISTORY IN ESTABLISHING A DIAGNOSIS

Patients with asthma seek medical attention because of respiratory symptoms. A typical feature of asthma symptoms is their variability. These symptoms are wheezing, chest tightness, episodic shortness of breath, and/or cough.[1] Importantly, however, none of these symptoms are diagnostic of asthma, because similar symptoms can be present with other respiratory or even cardiac diseases (Table 7.1). It is important to elicit whether the symptoms are triggered or worsened by factors such as exercise, exposure to allergens, viral infections, and emotions, which would suggest a diagnosis of asthma. In some asthmatics (particularly children), wheezing and chest tightness are absent, and the only symptom that the patient complains of is chronic cough. This has been labeled *cough-variant asthma*[3]; however, this terminology is not often used now because, with a careful history, other symptoms consistent with asthma are often elicited. Since the symptoms of asthma are nonspecific, the differential diagnosis is quite extensive, and the main goal for the physician is to consider and exclude other possible diagnoses (Table 7.1). The lack of specificity of the symptoms of asthma also makes it essential that the diagnosis is made using objective measures of airflow obstruction. This is even more important if the response to a trial of therapy has been negative.

Asthma clusters in families and its genetic determinants appear to be linked to those of other allergic IgE-mediated diseases.[4] Thus, a personal or a family history of asthma and/or allergic rhinitis, atopic dermatitis, or eczema increases the likelihood of a diagnosis of asthma.

Physical activity is an important cause of symptoms for most asthma patients, particularly children, and for some it is the only cause. Exercise-induced bronchoconstriction does not usually develop during exercise, but 5–10 minutes afterward, and it resolves spontaneously within 30–45 minutes.[5] The prompt relief of symptoms after the use of an inhaled beta$_2$-agonist, or their prevention by pretreatment with an inhaled beta$_2$-agonist before exercise, supports a diagnosis of asthma.

The important aspects of a personal history are exposure to agents that are known to worsen asthma in the home, such as dusty environments, forced air heating systems, or exposure to allergens (e.g., pets, house-dust mites, and cockroaches) to which the patient is sensitized; workplace conditions, environmental tobacco smoke, or even the general environment (e.g., fumes from traffic). In adult patients, a careful occupation history is essential to decide whether there is a possible occupational sensitizer that is responsible for the onset of asthma. Several hundred different agents have been recognized to cause occupational asthma[6], only some of which are classical allergens, causing asthma through IgE-dependent mechanisms.

PHYSICAL EXAMINATION

In mild asthma, a physical examination is usually not helpful, as it is normal under stable conditions, but becomes characteristically abnormal during asthma exacerbations. Typical physical signs during an asthma exacerbation are wheezing on auscultation, cough, and signs of acute hyperinflation (e.g., poor diaphragmatic excursion at percussion and use of the accessory muscles of respiration). In some asthmatics, wheezing may only be detectable on forced expiration, or it may even be absent in the presence of very severe airflow obstruction. In these patients, however, the severity of their asthma is mostly indicated by other signs, such as cyanosis, drowsiness, difficulty in speaking, tachycardia, a hyperinflated chest, use of the accessory muscles, and intercostal recession.

TABLE 7.1
Differential Diagnosis of Asthma

Pulmonary	COPD
	Sarcoidosis
	Eosinophilic bronchitis
	Pulmonary eosinophilia
	Cystic fibrosis
	Bronchiectasis
Neoplastic	Lung cancer
	Endobronchial tumors
	Lymphoma with hilar adenopathy
Cardiovascular	Left ventricular failure
	Pulmonary embolism
Other pathologies	Gastroesophageal reflux/aspiration
	Inhaled foreign body
	Vocal cord dysfunction
	Medication (e.g., angiotensin-converting enzyme [ACE] inhibitors)

LUNG FUNCTION TESTS

While respiratory symptoms suggest asthma, the sine qua non for the diagnosis of asthma is the presence of reversible airflow obstruction and/or airway hyperresponsiveness or increased peak expiratory flow (PEF) variability in subjects without airways obstruction.[1]

Spirometry

Lung function tests play a critical role in both the diagnosis and follow-up of patients with asthma. Spirometric measurements, FEV_1 and slow vital capacity (VC) or FVC, are the standard means for assessing airflow limitation (Figure 7.1). FEV_1, FVC, and the ratio of these two numbers are the measurements most widely used to document airflow obstruction. This is because they are the most reliable (reproducible and responsive) of all the measurements of lung function. The American Thoracic Society and the European Respiratory Society have published guidelines on the standardization of the measurement of spirometry and its interpretation.[7] The measurements, however, are mainly a reflection of larger airways obstruction. Other measurements that can be obtained from a spirogram include flows at lower lung volumes, such as the forced expiratory flow 25%–75% (FEF_{25-75}), which may better reflect smaller airways obstruction; however, these measurements are much less reliable than FEV_1, and are not often used clinically for this reason. In addition, almost all of the studies that have related lung function measurements to other clinical outcomes, morbidity, quality of life, or even mortality in patients with airflow obstruction have used FEV_1 as the reference measurement. Spirometry is recommended at the time of initial diagnosis and for the assessment of the severity of asthma.[1] It should be repeated to monitor the

disease and when there is a need for a reassessment, such as during exacerbations. Spirometry can usually be reliably performed in children as young as 7 years, and sometimes even younger than that age.[8]

The airflow limitation is usually defined by the absolute reduction of a postbronchodilator FEV_1/FVC ratio of <0.7. However, because this parameter decreases with aging, it should be confirmed by postbronchodilator FEV_1/VC values below the lower limit of age-corrected normal values. Other pulmonary function measurements, such as the measurement of lung volumes and the gas transfer capacity, may be useful in determining the degree of hyperinflation and/or enlargement of the airspaces, and these may help in the differential diagnosis with COPD, but are not necessary for the diagnosis or the assessment of the severity of asthma.

Peak Expiratory Flow

If spirometry does not reveal airflow limitation at the time of the initial assessment of the patient, then home monitoring of PEF for 2 weeks may help to detect an increased variability of the airway caliber, and assist in making the diagnosis of asthma.[9] Daily monitoring of PEF (at least in the morning on awakening and in the evening hours, preferably both before and after bronchodilator inhalation) is also useful to assess the severity of asthma and its response to treatment, and it can help patients to detect early signs of asthma deterioration. Diurnal variability is calculated as follows:

$$\frac{PEF_{max} - PEF_{min} \times 100}{PEF_{max} + PEF_{min} / 2}$$

A diurnal variability of PEF of more than 20% is diagnostic of asthma, and the magnitude of the variability is broadly proportional to the disease severity.[10] PEF monitoring may be of use not only in establishing a diagnosis of asthma and assessing its severity but also in uncovering an occupational cause for asthma.[11] When used in this way, PEF should be measured more frequently than twice daily and special attention should be paid to changes occurring in and outside the workplace.

REVERSIBILITY TO BRONCHODILATORS

As already discussed, the demonstration of reversible airflow obstruction is required for a diagnosis of asthma and a single demonstration of reversibility, defined as >12% reversibility and >200 mL in FEV_1 after bronchodilator inhalation, can establish the diagnosis[1,12] (Figure 7.1). However, reversibility is often not present, particularly in patients on treatment, and thus the absence of reversibility does not exclude the diagnosis. Repeated testing of the reversibility of both clinical features and functional abnormalities may be useful in obtaining the best level of asthma control achievable and/or the best lung function for individual patients. Achieving and maintaining lung function at the best possible level is one of the objectives of asthma management.[1,12]

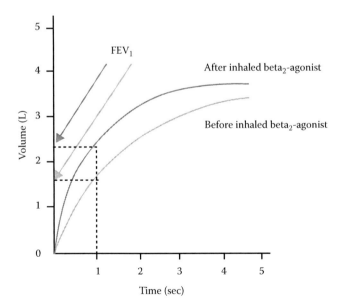

FIGURE 7.1 (See color insert) Measurements of FEV_1 before and 10 minutes after an inhaled beta$_2$-agonist in an asthmatic patient. The FEV_1 value was 1.7 L before and 2.3 L after the inhaled beta$_2$-agonist. This reversibility is consistent with a diagnosis of asthma.

Airway Hyperresponsiveness

Airway hyperresponsiveness is an increased sensitivity of the airways to constrictor agonists, as indicated by the smaller concentration of a constrictor agonist needed to initiate the bronchoconstrictor response, a steeper slope of the dose–response curve, and a greater maximal response to the agonist[2] (Figure 7.2). In asthmatic subjects, airway hyperresponsiveness is present to many chemical or physical stimuli, such as inhaled histamine,[13] or the inhaled cholinergic agonist methacholine,[14] as well as physical stimuli such as exercise,[15] hyperventilation of cold dry air,[16] and both hypotonic and hypertonic solutions, such as mannitol.[17] The methacholine inhalation challenge is the most widely used test to document airway hyperresponsiveness, and an abnormal methacholine challenge test can be demonstrated in almost all patients with current symptomatic asthma.[2] However, defining an exact level of airway responsiveness, which would distinguish asthmatic subjects from nonasthmatic subjects, is not possible because of a continuous distribution of airway responsiveness in the general population, with asthmatic subjects in one tail of this distribution. In addition, even subjects with a normal methacholine airway responsiveness can develop symptomatic asthma if they are exposed to a specific stimuli to which they are sensitized, such as an inhaled allergen.[18] The severity of airway hyperresponsiveness correlates with the severity of asthma, as determined by the amount of treatment needed to control asthma,[14] with a variability in PEF,[19] and an improvement in FEV_1 after an inhaled bronchodilator.[19]

Other challenge tests that are used to clinically document airway hyperresponsiveness include inhaled mannitol,[20] exercise,[5] and eucapnic voluntary hyperpnea,[5] which are considered "indirect" challenge procedures, causing

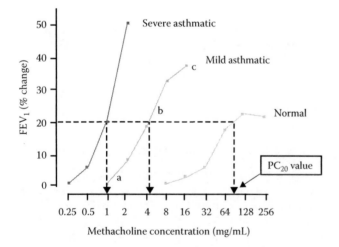

FIGURE 7.2 **(See color insert)** Dose–response curves obtained during inhalation challenges with methacholine in a severe asthmatic, a mild asthmatic, and a normal subject. The response to increasing inhaled doses of methacholine is measured by a change in FEV_1 from baseline. Asthmatics have (a) a lower threshold, (b) a steeper slope of the dose–response curve, and (c) a greater maximal response to inhaled methacholine. The response is expressed as the provocative concentration of methacholine causing a 20% fall in FEV_1 (PC_{20}).

bronchoconstriction by releasing bronchoconstrictor mediators from inflammatory cells in the airways.

The measurements of airway hyperresponsiveness are particularly useful in patients with a normal airway caliber in whom a diagnosis of asthma is being considered; however, they are not useful in the presence of an irreversible airflow limitation, thereby aiding in the differential diagnosis between asthma and COPD. Another important application of measuring airway responsiveness is the diagnosis of occupational asthma.[21] Lastly, the measurement of airway responsiveness may be useful in determining the optimal treatment requirements in asthma.[22]

Allergy Tests

The presence of allergic disorders in a patient's family history should be investigated in all patients with symptoms of asthma. Such a history provides important information about the patient's lifestyle and occupation, both of which influence the patient's exposure to allergens and the time and factors possibly involved in the onset and exacerbations of asthma.[4] Skin tests with all relevant allergens present in the geographic area in which the patient lives are the primary diagnostic tool in determining the allergic status of the patient. The main limitation of the methods to assess the patient's allergic status is that a positive test does not necessarily mean that asthma is allergic in nature or that it is causing asthma, as some individuals have specific IgE antibodies without any symptoms and allergy may not be causally involved. The relevant exposure and its relation to the symptoms must be confirmed by patient history.

ADDITIONAL TESTS

While the diagnosis and assessment of the severity of asthma can be fully established on the basis of a clinical history and lung function tests, additional tests are sometimes helpful to better characterize individual patients.

Imaging

While chest radiography may be useful to exclude diseases that may mimic asthma (Table 7.1), it is not required in the confirmation of the diagnosis of asthma. The utility of chest radiography is to exclude other conditions that may imitate or complicate asthma. Examples include pneumonia, cardiogenic pulmonary edema, pulmonary thromboembolism, tumors (especially those that result in airway obstruction with resulting peripheral atelectasis), and pneumothorax.

Assessment of Airway Inflammation

While airway biopsies and bronchoalveolar lavage may provide useful information in research protocols, they are considered too invasive for the diagnosis or staging of asthma. In contrast, noninvasive markers of airway inflammation have been increasingly used, particularly to differentiate asthma from COPD, and to measure the response to treatment. These noninvasive measurements include induced sputum and exhaled nitric oxide (FeNO). Induced sputum is not helpful in the diagnosis of asthma, but it can be very useful in the management of severe asthma.[23] In particular, induced sputum helps to identify the persistence of airway eosinophilia or airway neutrophilia in patients with difficult-to-treat asthma, which can be useful in deciding the appropriate doses of ICSs and in reducing the risks of severe asthma exacerbations.[24] FeNO is increased in atopic asthma,[25] but less so in nonatopic asthma. A normal level of FeNO in a patient not using an ICS may be helpful in excluding an asthma diagnosis.[25] FeNO measurements can also be helpful in monitoring adherence to ICSs,[26] as it is effectively reduced by ICSs, but not by bronchodilators.

DIFFERENTIATING BETWEEN ASTHMA AND COPD

In adult patients, the most difficult diagnostic issue in patients with airflow obstruction, in past or current smokers, is differentiating between asthma and COPD. In most patients, their clinical presentation and history provide the strongest diagnostic criteria to distinguish these conditions (Table 7.2). The results of pulmonary function tests, particularly spirometric measurements that show a nearly complete reversibility of airflow limitation, will confirm a diagnosis of asthma, and measurements that show poorly reversible airflow limitation may help to confirm the diagnosis of COPD (Table 7.2). The differential diagnosis between asthma and COPD becomes more difficult in elderly patients, in whom some features may overlap, such as smoking and atopy, and when the patient has airflow limitation that is poorly reversible after treatment. In these cases, symptoms, lung function, airway responsiveness, imaging, and even pathological findings may overlap and thus may not provide solid information to establish the diagnosis. Because an accurate diagnosis is needed to provide better treatment, it is important in these cases to undertake an individual approach and to perform additional tests. Reversibility

to corticosteroids alone or in combination with long-acting bronchodilators, measurements of lung volumes and diffusion capacity, an analysis of sputum and FeNO, and imaging of the chest may demonstrate whether asthma or COPD is the predominant cause of airflow limitation (Table 7.3).

CONCLUSIONS

The diagnosis of asthma in older children and adults is made by the presence of symptoms consistent with asthma and the demonstration of variable airflow obstruction. The presence of the characteristic symptoms alone is not sufficient for an accurate diagnosis, as these are not specific for asthma. Variable airflow obstruction is usually documented by demonstrating changes in spirometry, particularly FEV_1 and VC, and the ratio of these numbers. The currently accepted definition of an improvement in FEV_1 that is consistent with asthma is >12% and >200 mL. This is often demonstrated within 10–30 minutes after the inhalation of a beta$_2$-agonist, such as salbutamol. In some instances, however, an improvement in FEV_1 is only demonstrated after a more prolonged period of treatment with inhaled or oral corticosteroids (as in the case presentation). In patients with mild asthma, or those on an effective treatment, spirometry can be normal. In these situations, measurements of PEF over several weeks, or the documentation of airway hyperresponsiveness to inhaled chemical mediators, such as methacholine, or bronchoconstriction after exercise or inhaled mannitol, can establish the diagnosis.

Making the diagnosis of asthma can be challenging in patients (particularly younger children) who cannot reproducibly perform spirometry, and in adults with a smoking history and in whom there is fixed airflow obstruction (not reversible even after optimal treatment has been administered for a period of time). The presence of fixed airflow obstruction suggests a diagnosis of COPD, but this should be confirmed with ancillary testing, which may include

TABLE 7.2

History, Symptoms, and Results of Pulmonary Function Tests in the Differential Diagnosis between Asthma and COPD

	Asthma	COPD
Onset	Often in childhood	Mid- to late-adult life
Smoking	Often nonsmokers	Usually smokers
Daily cough and sputum	Often absent	Frequent (chronic bronchitis)
Dyspnea on effort	Variable and reversible with treatment	Constant, poorly reversible, and progressive
Nocturnal symptoms	Relatively common	Relatively uncommon
Airflow limitation	Increased diurnal variability	Normal diurnal variability
Response to bronchodilator	Good	Poor
Airway hyperresponsiveness	In most patients, with or without airflow limitation	In most patients with airflow limitation

TABLE 7.3

Ancillary Tests in the Differential Diagnosis between Stable Asthma and COPD

Ancillary Test	Asthma	COPD
Reversibility to bronchodilator and/or glucocorticosteroids	Usually present	Usually absent
Lung volumes, residual volume, total lung capacity	Usually normal or, if increased, reversible	Usually irreversibly increased
Diffusion capacity	Normal	Decreased
Airway hyperresponsiveness	Increased	Usually not measurable due to airflow limitation
Allergy tests	Often positive	Often negative
Imaging of the chest	Usually normal	Usually abnormal
Sputum	Eosinophilia	Neutrophilia
Exhaled NO	Increased	Usually normal

measurements of lung volumes, diffusing capacity, and chest imaging. Measurements of inflammatory cells in the blood or sputum or of FeNO are often not helpful in differentiating between asthma and COPD.

Making a correct diagnosis of asthma is an essential step prior to the development of an asthma management plan. Unfortunately, this step is sometimes not completed, either because the managing health-care professional is convinced by the patient history or because the ability to document variable airflow obstruction is not readily available. This lack of precision in making the diagnosis is a reasonably common cause of patients being referred for specialist assessment, because the asthma treatment recommended is ineffective.

REFERENCES

1. Bateman ED, Hurd SS, Barnes PJ, Bousquet J, Drazen JM, Fitzgerald M, et al. Global strategy for asthma management and prevention: GINA executive summary. *Eur Respir J* 2008;31(1):143–178.
2. O'Byrne PM, Inman MD. Airway hyperresponsiveness. *Chest* 2003;123(3 Suppl):411S–416S.
3. Irwin RS, Baumann MH, Bolser DC, Boulet LP, Braman SS, Brightling CE, et al. Diagnosis and management of cough executive summary: ACCP evidence-based clinical practice guidelines. *Chest* 2006;129(1 Suppl):1S–23S.
4. Bousquet J, Khaltaev N, Cruz AA, Denburg J, Fokkens WJ, Togias A, et al. Allergic Rhinitis and its Impact on Asthma (ARIA) 2008 update (in collaboration with the World Health Organization, GA(2)LEN and AllerGen). *Allergy* 2008;63(86 Suppl):8–160.
5. Anderson SD. Provocative challenges to help diagnose and monitor asthma: Exercise, methacholine, adenosine, and mannitol. *Curr Opin Pulm Med* 2008;14(1):39–45.
6. Malo JL, Chan-Yeung M. Agents causing occupational asthma. *J Allergy Clin Immunol* 2009;123(3):545–550.
7. Miller MR, Hankinson J, Brusasco V, Burgos F, Casaburi R, Coates A, et al. Standardisation of spirometry. *Eur Respir J* 2005;26(2):319–338.
8. Beydon N, Davis SD, Lombardi E, Allen JL, Arets HG, Aurora P, et al. An official American Thoracic Society/ European Respiratory Society statement: Pulmonary function testing in preschool children. *Am J Respir Crit Care Med* 2007;175(12):1304–1345.
9. Reddel HK, Marks GB, Jenkins CR. When can personal best peak flow be determined for asthma action plans? *Thorax* 2004;59(11):922–924.
10. Reddel HK. Peak flow monitoring in clinical practice and clinical asthma trials. *Curr Opin Pulm Med* 2006;12(1):75–81.
11. Huggins V, Anees W, Pantin C, Burge S. Improving the quality of peak flow measurements for the diagnosis of occupational asthma. *Occup Med* 2005;55(5):385–388.
12. British Thoracic Society and Scottish Intercollegiate Guidelines Network. British Guideline on the Management of Asthma: A National Clinical Guideline. *BMJ* 2009;63(Suppl. 4):1–121.
13. Cockcroft DW, Killian DN, Mellon JJ, Hargreave FE. Bronchial reactivity to inhaled histamine: A method and clinical survey. *Clin Allergy* 1977;7(3):235–243.
14. Juniper EF, Frith PA, Hargreave FE. Airway responsiveness to histamine and methacholine: Relationship to minimum treatment to control symptoms of asthma. *Thorax* 1981;36(8):575–579.
15. Anderson SD, Daviskas E. The mechanism of exercise-induced asthma is … *J Allergy Clin Immunol* 2000;106(3):453–459.
16. O'Byrne PM, Ryan G, Morris M, McCormack D, Jones NL, Morse JL, et al. Asthma induced by cold air and its relation to nonspecific bronchial responsiveness to methacholine. *Am Rev Respir Dis* 1982;125(3):281–285.
17. Anderson SD, Charlton B, Weiler JM, Nichols S, Spector SL, Pearlman DS. Comparison of mannitol and methacholine to predict exercise-induced bronchoconstriction and a clinical diagnosis of asthma. *Respir Res* 2009;10:4.
18. Boulet LP, Cartier A, Thomson NC, Roberts RS, Dolovich J, Hargreave FE. Asthma and increases in nonallergic bronchial responsiveness from seasonal pollen exposure. *J Allergy Clin Immunol* 1983;71(4):399–406.
19. Ryan G, Latimer KM, Dolovich J, Hargreave FE. Bronchial responsiveness to histamine: Relationship to diurnal variation of peak flow rate, improvement after bronchodilator, and airway calibre. *Thorax* 1982;37(6):423–429.
20. Brannan JD, Anderson SD, Perry CP, Freed-Martens R, Lassig AR, Charlton B. The safety and efficacy of inhaled dry powder mannitol as a bronchial provocation test for airway hyperresponsiveness: A phase 3 comparison study with hypertonic (4.5%) saline. *Respir Res* 2005;6:144.
21. Cartier A, Bernstein IL, Burge PS, Cohn JR, Fabbri LM, Hargreave FE, et al. Guidelines for bronchoprovocation on the investigation of occupational asthma. Report of the subcommittee on bronchoprovocation for occupational asthma. *J Allergy Clin Immunol* 1989;84(5 Pt 2):823–829.
22. Sont JK, Willems LN, Bel EH, van Krieken JH, Vandenbroucke JP, Sterk PJ. Clinical control and histopathologic outcome of asthma when using airway hyperresponsiveness as an additional guide to long-term treatment. The AMPUL Study Group. *Am J Respir Crit Care Med* 1999;159(4 Pt 1):1043–1051.
23. Hargreave FE. Quantitative sputum cell counts as a marker of airway inflammation in clinical practice. *Curr Opin Allergy Clin Immunol* 2007;7(1):102–106.
24. Wardlaw AJ, Brightling CE, Green R, Woltmann G, Bradding P, Pavord ID. New insights into the relationship between airway inflammation and asthma. *Clin Sci* 2002;103(2):201–211.
25. Pedrosa M, Cancelliere N, Barranco P, Lopez-Carrasco V, Quirce S. Usefulness of exhaled nitric oxide for diagnosing asthma. *J Asthma* 2010;47(7):817–821.
26. Lim KG, Mottram C. The use of fraction of exhaled nitric oxide in pulmonary practice. *Chest* 2008;133(5):1232–1242.

8 United Airways
Managing Patients with Allergic Rhinitis and Asthma

Glenis K. Scadding and Guy Scadding

CONTENTS

CASE PRESENTATION

Stephen is 10 years old. He loves to play football. He suffers from hay fever in the summer, for which he takes an occasional antihistamine, but he still has an itchy, runny nose that blocks up, and red, sore eyes. He always wheezes on running and is supposed to use salbutamol for this, but he usually forgets to take it. His legs become red and itchy when he walks through long grass.

One summer evening, Stephen is playing football in the park despite having a slight cold. He becomes wheezy, but he has no salbutamol, so he tries to play on. His asthma becomes much worse and he collapses, almost unable to breathe. Fortunately, his friend gives him his own salbutamol and calls for an emergency ambulance on his cell phone, and Stephen is saved after rapid transfer to a nearby hospital.

WHY DID STEPHEN HAVE SUCH A BAD ASTHMA ATTACK? IS THIS UNUSUAL?

There are multiple potential causative factors:

1. *Rhinitis that is uncontrolled.*
2. *Exposure to a high allergen load ...*
3. *... at multiple sites—nose, eyes, chest, and skin.*
4. *Undertreated asthma.*
5. *Exercise.*
6. *Intercurrent viral infection.*
7. *Food-related, exercise-induced anaphylaxis. This was discounted in Stephen's case as he had not eaten for several hours prior to the attack.*

Seasonal asthma exacerbations, which can be severe, are not uncommon. Unfortunately, asthma deaths include a

TABLE 8.1

Evidence for a Link between Rhinitis and Asthma and Postulated Mechanisms of Their Interaction

Evidence	References
Epidemiological	
Approximately 20%–60% of patients with allergic rhinitis have clinical asthma, whereas >80% of patients with allergic asthma have concomitant rhinitis symptoms.	8,14–16
The presence of rhinitis predicts the onset of asthma.	15
Worsening rhinitis negatively affects the course of asthma.	8,11–13,31
Treating rhinitis reduces the incidence of asthma exacerbations.	33–35
Pathological	
Allergic rhinitis patients have evidence of subclinical airways obstruction and inflammation even in the absence of overt asthma.	19,20
Asthmatic patients have evidence of upper airway inflammation even in the absence of overt rhinitis.	22
Allergen challenge specifically in the nasal or bronchial airways leads to marked inflammatory responses in the upper and lower airways, respectively.	6,23–25
Allergens and aspirin can trigger exacerbations of both asthma and rhinitis and lead to inflammatory responses, involving increased expression of Th2 cytokines.	5,7,26
Nasal allergen challenge leads to the production of circulating Th2 effector cells responsible for promoting lower airways inflammation in mice.	7
Treating the upper airway with intranasal steroids reduces bronchial hyperresponsiveness.	9,10

Possible Mechanisms of Upper and Lower Airway Interaction

Absence of nasal functions—filtering, warming, and humidifying inspired air—allows direct contact of cold, polluted air with the lower airway epithelium.

Spread of inflammation from one site to another via airways or systemically.

Reflex activation of nerves by inflammation.

Alteration of nitric oxide levels in nose may affect the larynx and bronchi.

Postnasal dripping of infected material, cytokines, and mediators passes to the stomach so they are unlikely to affect the lungs.

Source: Adapted from Scadding, G., Walker, S., *Prim. Care Respir. J.*, 21, 222, 2012.[63]

---

proportion of people like Stephen whose asthma has previously been mild and largely ignored.[1] This chapter explores the links between rhinitis and asthma.

Table 8.1 shows evidence for an association between rhinitis and asthma and the postulated mechanisms of their interaction.

As the majority of the literature related to rhinitis and asthma focuses on the allergic phenotype, the term rhinitis used in this chapter is referring to "allergic rhinitis" unless stated otherwise.

ALLERGIC RHINITIS

Hay fever (seasonal allergic rhinitis [SAR]) is a form of rhinitis that is frequently undiagnosed and undertreated.[2,3] Seasonal allergen triggers vary geographically around the world, with grass pollen being the most common trigger in the United Kingdom. For example, the highest grass pollen levels in the United Kingdom are at the end of June (early summer). As the air cools in the evening, pollen descends and the levels inspired can be very high, particularly when exercising. Rhinitis is defined by the presence of two or more of the following nasal symptoms: rhinorrhea, congestion, itching, and sneezing. It can be allergic, nonallergic, infective, or a combination of these.[4] In children, allergy accounts for the majority of rhinitis cases; while in adults, allergy

causes approximately one-third of cases. It is estimated that 25% of young people in the United Kingdom have rhinitis, which is similar to the prevalence of allergic rhinitis in other westernized countries.

Allergic rhinitis is associated with a biphasic immunologic response to an allergen, similar to that seen in allergic asthma. An early-phase reaction occurs almost immediately after an allergen exposure due to immunoglobulin E (IgE)-mediated mast cell degranulation and the release of chemical mediators such as histamine, leukotrienes, and prostaglandins. The late-phase reaction occurs several hours later, lasting for 12–24 hours, and is associated with the activation of T cells and the recruitment, activation, and prolonged survival of eosinophils in the nasal mucosa.[5] The resulting immediate symptoms in the nose are itching, sneezing, and rhinorrhea. The late phase gives rise to nasal obstruction, a reduced sense of smell, and general hyperreactivity, which can extend throughout the respiratory tract.[6,7]

Asthma tends to be more severe in patients with perennial allergic rhinitis.[8] Allergic rhinitis induced bronchial hyperreactivity can be reduced by the use of nasal corticosteroids.[9,10] Concurrent rhinitis in asthma patients is associated with more asthma-related primary care visits and hospital referrals, and higher costs.[11–13]

Epidemiological and pathophysiological studies show that rhinitis and asthma frequently coexist with over 80% of asthma patients having a coexisting upper airways disease.[14,15] Rhinitis, allergic or nonallergic, often precedes the development of asthma and is one of the strongest independent risk factors for asthma.[14–17] This can be seen most clearly in the context of occupational asthma where the greatest risk for developing asthma is in the year after the onset of rhinitis.[18] Many rhinitis patients without an overt diagnosis of asthma demonstrate subclinical changes such as inflammation in the lower airways and impaired lung function.[19,20] Equally, asthmatics may have upper airway inflammation, even in the absence of symptoms.[21] There is proportionality between the extent of eosinophilia at both sites,[22] probably explained by the fact that an allergen challenge at either site causes inflammation in both the upper and the lower airways.[23–25] Rhinitis and asthma are thus considered by many as manifestations of the same "united" airway disease, interlinked by a common mucosa and nerve supply via the systemic circulation.[26,27]

Most asthma exacerbations begin in the upper airway. Rhinovirus upper respiratory tract infections are the major precipitating factor for asthma exacerbations in both children and adults.[28] Moreover, viral colds are more frequent and last longer in children and adults with allergic rhinitis.[29,30] As there is synergy between virus-induced and allergy-induced inflammations, not only is rhinovirus infection strongly associated with current wheezing, but also the greatest risk is seen in children who also have high levels of IgE antibodies to dust mites.[31] In particular, asthmatic children who are sensitized to an allergen, and then subsequently suffer combined exposure to that allergen and a naturally acquired viral upper respiratory tract infection, are nearly 20 times more likely to be hospitalized for asthma.[32]

Retrospective studies show that patients with asthma whose rhinitis is treated have fewer emergency visits and hospital admissions than those with untreated rhinitis, independent of asthma treatment.[33–35] The WHO Allergic Rhinitis and Its Impact on Asthma (ARIA) guidelines can be helpful in diagnosing and treating rhinitis.[36] These guidelines recommend that people with asthma are assessed for rhinitis and vice versa so that they can be optimally managed. Useful diagnostic questionnaires are available at www.whiar.org.

DIAGNOSIS OF RHINITIS

TAKING A SPECIFIC HISTORY

Rhinitis can be broadly divided into three categories: allergic, infective, and nonallergic. Sneezing, an itchy nose and palate, and eye involvement suggest allergic rhinitis, although symptoms alone cannot differentiate between allergic and nonallergic subtypes. The personal and family history of any allergic disease makes a diagnosis of allergic rhinitis more likely. The symptoms on exposure to relevant triggers such as pets, mold, and seasonal or occupational allergens may give a further indication of the probable causes.[4] To guide subsequent treatment, it is important to ask if the symptoms are intermittent or persistent, and mild or moderate to severe[36] (Figure 8.1). A previous study demonstrated that patients with

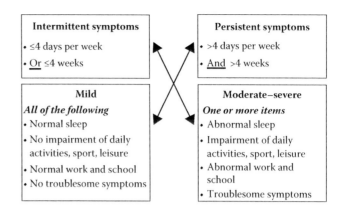

FIGURE 8.1 ARIA classification of allergic rhinitis. (Adapted from Bousquet, J., Khaltaev, N., Cruz, A., et al., *Allergy*, 63, 8–160, 2008. With permission.)

rhinitis symptoms beginning later in life (age >35), no family history of allergies, no seasonality, and no symptoms around furry pets or odorants such as fragrances and perfumes had a greater than 98% likelihood of having nonallergic rhinitis before allergy skin and/or serology-specific IgE testing.[37]

PHYSICAL EXAMINATION

Observation of the patient for signs of sniffing, nose rubbing, reduced nasal airflow, mouth breathing, and a transverse skin crease across the dorsum of the nose is helpful in determining the presence of rhinitis. Patients with rhinitis may have erythematous eyes and "allergic shiners," which are a manifestation of chronic venous congestion. It is important to examine the nasal mucosa using a speculum and a head-mounted lamp, an endoscope if available, or simply use an otoscope with the largest earpiece. The nasal mucosa in allergic rhinitis is typically watery, swollen, and a slightly blue-gray shade of red. Additional features suggesting alternative diagnoses include the presence of nasal polyps (pale, shiny, white-gray, grapelike structures, often originating close to the middle turbinate), crusting, bleeding, septal perforation, mucopurulent discharge, and, from external observation, the presence of nasal bridge collapse or lupus pernio. The latter findings may warrant further assessment to rule out conditions such as Wegener's granulomatosis or relapsing polychrondritis among other structural problems.

ALLERGEN IDENTIFICATION: SKIN PRICK TESTS/SERUM IgE

A good medical history should include a thorough environmental history of the home and workplace to identify likely allergens and other nonallergic triggers that could be causing or aggravating the patient's symptoms. To assess the patient's atopic status, skin prick testing or serum-specific IgE testing to seasonal and perennial allergens should be performed. Patients with classical hay fever, with typical symptoms and seasonal timing, can often be diagnosed by their medical history alone. The British Society of Allergy and Clinical Immunology (BSACI) guidelines[4] recommend that skin prick tests are routinely used in secondary care in order to confirm or exclude underlying IgE sensitivity to common aeroallergens (atopy) and to provide objective information to support the clinical history concerning an underlying allergic basis. In primary care, if skin prick tests are not available, serum-specific IgE tests may be requested. It should be kept in mind that both skin and serum tests alone identify allergic "sensitization"; however, a diagnosis of allergy requires positive tests to correlate with the patient's clinical history. Therefore, performing numerous screening tests in the absence of a compatible history is not recommended. Recently, a large, cross-sectional study used an irritant index questionnaire to reclassify patients with a physician diagnosis of allergic, nonallergic, or mixed rhinitis. The study found that both allergic and nonallergic rhinitis patients with a high-irritant burden had a significantly greater likelihood of having a diagnosis of asthma compared with allergic and nonallergic rhinitis patients with a low-irritant burden. This study indicates that quantifying the irritant burden in rhinitis patients results in distinct, "more severe" rhinitis phenotypes that may represent the "difficult-to-treat" rhinitis patient.[38]

Additional investigations that may aid in the diagnosis and identification of the cause of rhinitis refractory to conventional treatment include:

- Complete blood count, erythrocyte sedimentation rate (ESR), and differential white cell count
- C-reactive protein, if chronic infection is suspected
- Thyroid function tests
- Urine toxicology—if cocaine abuse is suspected

Peak expiratory flow measurements and spirometry should be considered for all patients with anything more than mild, intermittent rhinitis to screen for an airway obstruction since allergic rhinitis is a risk factor for asthma. A diagnosis of asthma is more complicated and may be confused by symptoms of cough caused by rhinitis and postnasal drip, leading to either an inaccurate diagnosis or overtreatment of asthma. Few self-administered questionnaires are currently available for the assessment of both disorders.[39] RHINASTHMA is a 30-item questionnaire, which differentiates between patients with rhinitis and patients with comorbid rhinitis and asthma, as well as controlled and uncontrolled asthma in asthmatic patients with symptomatic or nonsymptomatic rhinitis.[40]

MANAGEMENT OF PATIENTS WITH COMORBID RHINITIS AND ASTHMA

Increasing evidence suggests that the better management of rhinitis may result in decreased asthma comorbidity and an improved quality of life.[33–35,41] This includes:

- Allergen and irritant identification and avoidance
- Pharmacological treatment
- Immunotherapy
- Patient education

ALLERGEN AVOIDANCE

To date, the results of meta-analyses of allergen avoidance studies, particularly for house-dust mites, have been disappointing.[42] However, this may, in part, be due to methodological problems related to many of the published studies. If sufficient avoidance can be achieved, for example by relocating patients to a high altitude,[43] improvements in symptoms, lung function, and allergen-induced bronchial hyperreactivity can be demonstrated. In real-life settings, allergen avoidance can be effective: one inner-city study of children with asthma, involving multiple intervention measures, proved effective,[44] whereas another study utilizing a single intervention measure with allergen-impregnable bedcovers proved ineffective.[45] There is evidence for a reduction of nose and eye symptoms by: nasal air filters compared with placebo filters in a pollen season study[46]; another placebo-controlled study demonstrated a reduction of both asthma and rhinitis symptoms using a nocturnal laminar airflow device, which removes particulate matter, including allergens, from the patients' breathing space[47]; and saline nasal douching, which reduces symptoms and inflammatory mediators simply by washing allergens out of the nose.[48,49]

PHARMACOTHERAPY

Intranasal Corticosteroids

The current guidelines recommend the treatment of rhinitis according to an algorithm based on symptom frequency and severity (Figures 8.2 and 8.3). For any form of allergic rhinitis that is more than mild and intermittent, topical intranasal corticosteroids (INCS) are the first-line medication of choice. Meta-analyses have demonstrated these drugs to be more effective than antihistamines (oral or topical), antileukotrienes, and the combination of antihistamine plus antileukotriene.[50–53] Topical corticosteroids reduce all nasal symptoms, including nasal obstruction, and they have also been shown to be beneficial for associated eye symptoms.[54]

Systemic absorption is very low with nasal mometasone and fluticasone, with good long-term safety data in children and adults, but it is high for nasally administered betamethasone and dexamethasone.[55] Although INCS may have a fast onset of action (within 6–8 hours), the maximal improvement in symptoms may not occur for at least 2 weeks. Minor nose bleeding may occur in 5%–8% of patients and result in the need for discontinuation. This adverse effect can be reduced by judicious use of the spray, aiming the nozzle placed just inside the nose toward the lateral wall of the nasal cavity and spraying in two different directions; upward and backward. Sniffing should be avoided as this pulls the spray straight back to the posterior pharynx and triggers swallowing. Very rarely, hypothalamic–pituitary axis suppression may occur with long-term use and guidelines advise monitoring growth in children.

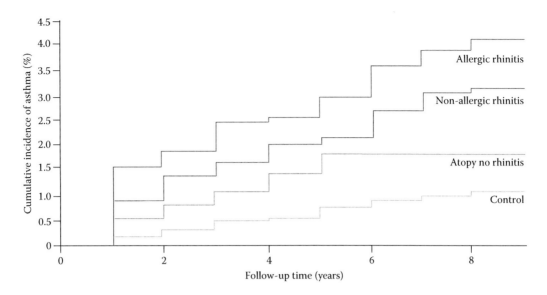

FIGURE 8.2 **(See color insert)** Association of rhinitis with the onset and incidence of asthma. (From Shaaban, R., Zureik, M., Soussan, D., et al., *Am. J. Respir. Crit. Care Med.*, 176, 659–666, 2007. With permission.)

Antihistamines

Antihistamines are useful for mild symptoms, either intermittent or persistent. In the latter case, regular daily use is advisable because when they are withdrawn the histamine receptor becomes more active and the symptoms can increase. Antihistamines are active against sneezing, rhinorrhea, and nasal itch, but are inferior to nasal corticosteroids in reducing nasal congestion. Most second-generation oral antihistamines (loratidine, cetirizine, fexofenadine, desloratidine, levocetirizine, misolastine, rupatadine) reduce symptoms within 1 hour and are used once daily. Acrivastine is an exception to this rule; it has a rapid onset of action, but lasts only 8 hours. Topical nasal antihistamines are available as azelastine and olopatadine, which have a 15-minute onset of action.

First-generation antihistamines, such as chlorphenamine, may cause sedation with a resultant reduction in work and school performance; therefore, these should be avoided.[56] Second-generation antihistamines, especially fexofenadine, have a very low potential for sedation. All have few major drug interactions. Grapefruit impairs fexofenadine absorption and therefore should be avoided. The adverse effects of azelastine include local irritation and taste disturbance.

Combination Therapy

If the symptoms of rhinitis persist despite the use of antihistamines or topical INCS alone, it is important to review the diagnosis, check concordance with the treatment, and check the nasal spray technique. If the response remains poor, then most practitioners would recommend combined treatment with both a topical nasal corticosteroid and a nonsedating antihistamine, either oral or topical.[4] A spray containing both fluticasone propionate and azelastine is superior to either alone and is now available in the United States and the United Kingdom.

OTHER TREATMENT OPTIONS (FIGURE 8.4)

- In cases of nasal blockage, the short-term use (i.e., <10 days) of an intranasal decongestant (e.g., ephedrine, xylometazoline, or oxymetazoline) may be beneficial. Regular prolonged use of topical decongestants leads to chronic nasal obstruction through tachyphylaxis and should therefore be avoided. However, recent studies have demonstrated that topical decongestants are well tolerated and do not cause rhinitis medicamentosa (nasal congestion rebound) when used in conjunction with an INCS. Oral decongestants, such as phenylephrine, show poor efficacy and cause adverse effects, and therefore are not recommended for long-term use.[57,58]
- Oral leukotriene receptor antagonists (LTRAs) may be beneficial in patients with mild rhinitis, particularly in patients with comorbid asthma.
- Topical anticholinergic preparations such as ipratropium bromide may be beneficial in reducing rhinorrhea, particularly in the treatment of nonallergic (vasomotor) or allergic rhinitis.
- Topical sodium cromoglicate is modestly effective but it needs to be used three to four times a day. It is used by clinicians in the treatment of small children.
- Cromone and antihistamine-containing eye drops can be used alone or in combination with oral/topical nonsedating antihistamines and INCS for ocular symptoms if required.
- Systemic corticosteroids should rarely be used, but they have a role in severe nasal obstruction as a short-term rescue medication, particularly for important life events. The BSACI guideline recommends 0.5 mg/kg orally for 5–10 days in combination with a topical nasal corticosteroid, taken in the morning with food.[4]

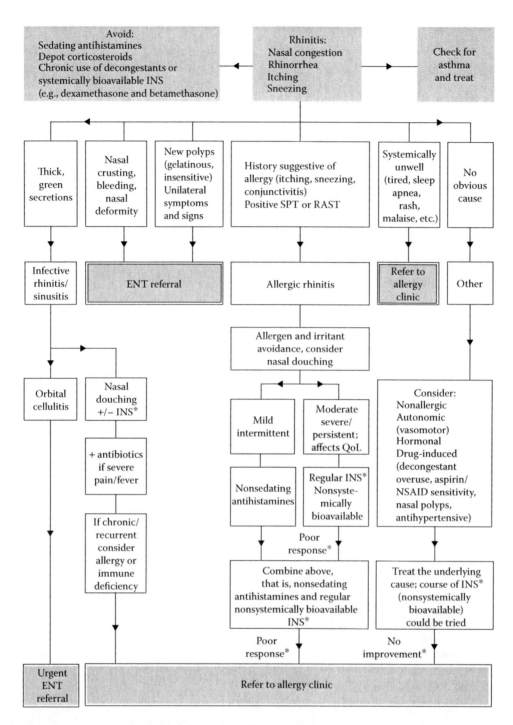

FIGURE 8.3 Management of rhinitis. (From e-guidelines. http://www.eguidelines.co.uk/eguidelinesmain/guidelines/summaries/eye_ear_nose_throat/bsaci_rhinitis.php. With permission.) *Notes:* NS, intranasal corticosteroids; SPT, skin prick test; RAST, radioallergosorbent test; QoL, quality of life; NSAID, nonsteroidal antiinflammatory drugs.

Concordance with all treatments should be monitored regularly until patients reach a level of optimal symptom control.

Allergen Immunotherapy

Allergen immunotherapy is the only treatment that is able to alter the course of a disease and it probably prevents progression from rhinitis to asthma.[59] Previously only performed by subcutaneous injection, the recent

confirmation of the efficacy and safety of sublingual immunotherapy (SLIT) for SAR in Europe has opened this avenue of therapy to a wider group of patients.[60] Schedules for both approaches typically involve a 3-year treatment program and, depending on the allergen and formulation, use either weekly upwardly titrated dosing schedules followed by maintenance injections every 4–6 weeks; 4–9 preseasonal injections; or a daily sublingual tablet. Chronic,

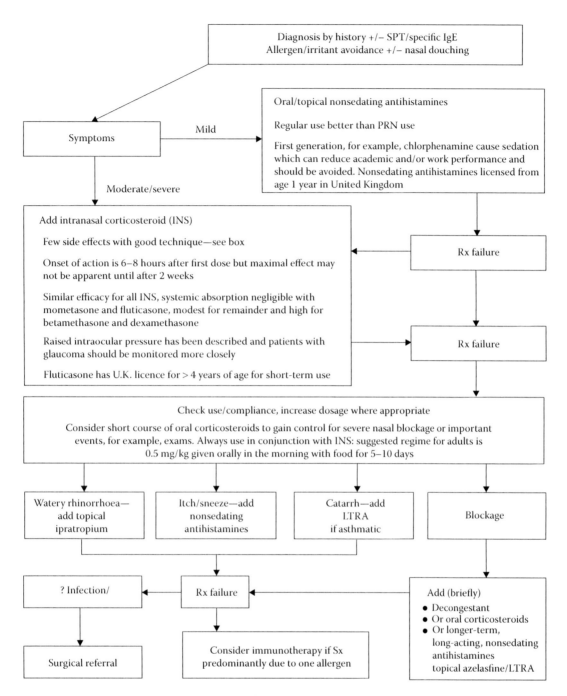

FIGURE 8.4 Treatment of allergic rhinitis. (Adapted from Scadding, G.K., Durham, S., Mirakian, R., et al., *Clin. Exp. Allergy*, 38, 19–42, 2008.)

perennial asthma is a contraindication and systemic reactions (particularly in patients with asthma) including urticaria, angioedema, bronchospasm, and anaphylaxis can occur. For these reasons and also to ensure the appropriate targeting of the treatment to those patients most likely to benefit, immunotherapy is restricted to specialist allergy clinics. SLIT has the advantage of self-administration by the patient at home, following supervision of the first dose in the clinic. This route is currently underused in the United Kingdom; however, in the future, it should reduce overall treatment costs by reducing the need for the repeat

clinic visits that are required for injection immunotherapy. Whether the therapeutic responses with SLIT will be as robust as subcutaneous immunotherapy (SCIT) remains to be determined.

Education and Prevention

The BSACI guideline[4] emphasizes the importance of education, particularly with regard to the negative effect that rhinitis may have on quality of life. Relevant allergen avoidance should be discussed. The patient should be provided with information about the potential complications of rhinitis, such as asthma, sinusitis, and eustachian tube dysfunction. Information about therapy should be given, including a demonstration of the nasal spray technique where prescribed. Occupational rhinitis is considered a risk factor for occupational asthma and usually predates the onset of asthma. Of particular relevance to the workplace is primary prevention, particularly through the use of non-powdered or nonlatex gloves, and the avoidance of other occupational allergens known to cause sensitization (see Chapter 24). The superior efficacy and safety of the new-generation topical corticosteroids should be highlighted for those patients who are reluctant to use these drugs. Patients may be reluctant to use corticosteroids at more than one site, the nose as well as the lungs, but the contribution to the total corticosteroid load from INCS is minute compared with that from bronchial inhalers. Conversely, the contribution from untreated rhinitis to the overall disease burden can be considerable. In some asthmatic patients, the addition of nasal therapy allows a reduction in the inhaled dose.

SPECIAL CONSIDERATIONS

TREATMENT IN PREGNANCY

Pregnancy-associated rhinitis is self-limiting and treatment should only be initiated if the benefit of the treatment outweighs the risk to the fetus.[61] Saline nasal douching is safe and may help. For allergic rhinitis, the INCS budesonide is pregnancy category B, but other INCS, such as beclometasone and fluticasone, have been widely used by pregnant women and are therefore considered safe. The second-generation antihistamines, cetirizine, loratidine, and levocetirizine, are pregnancy category B, but other agents including fexofenadine, desloratidine, and the first-generation antihistamines chlorphenamine and diphenhydramine have been used in pregnancy without reported adverse effects. Montelukast and zafirlukast are both pregnancy category B and are therefore considered safe to take during pregnancy. Conversely, decongestants have been associated with teratogenic effects and should be avoided. Immunotherapy should not be initiated, but it can be continued during pregnancy (see Chapter 27).

TREATMENT IN CHILDREN

The therapy for children includes antihistamines and nasal corticosteroids. Those with the lowest systemic bioavailability (budesonide, fluticasone, and mometasone) at the lowest dose for effective symptom control should be used, with monitoring of growth if the treatment is given long term.

REFERRAL

Treatment failure, which occurs in some 20% of rhinitis patients,[62] should prompt a referral to either an allergist to assess whether the patient has allergic, nonallergic, or mixed rhinitis, and/or to an otolaryngologist to rule out structural abnormalities. The circumstances prompting referral to an allergist include:

- Inadequate control of symptoms
- Recurrent nasal polyps
- Patient systemically unwell as a result of rhinitis
- Need for allergen or trigger identification or diagnosis
- Consideration of immunotherapy
- Presence of a multisystem allergy (e.g., rhinitis with asthma, eczema, or food allergy)
- Occupational rhinitis

Referral to an ear, nose, and throat (ENT) clinic should be made if there is/are:

- Unilateral symptoms and signs, such as nasal obstruction (which may be due to a nasal tumor), nasal perforation, or ulceration
- Thick, green nasal secretions, suggesting an acute or recurrent infective rhinosinusitis
- Periorbital cellulitis (an emergency warranting an urgent ENT referral)
- New-onset nasal polyps
- Significant nasal septal deviation or very enlarged turbinates in someone who is unresponsive to treatment; surgical management may be required to improve the nasal airway for access of topical medications
- Evidence of persistent nasal crusting, nasal collapse, or bleeding from the nostrils, which may be signs of systemic disorders such as sarcoidosis or Wegener's granulomatosis

CONCLUSIONS

Rhinitis and asthma frequently occur as comorbid conditions in adults and children as manifestations of the same inflammatory disease continuum. Rhinitis is a predictor of future asthma. It impacts negatively on asthma, leading to more severe disease, worse asthma control, and impaired quality of life, despite adherence to asthma treatment. Good treatment of rhinitis is likely to improve asthma control and outcomes. The WHO-ARIA recommendation is that patients with asthma and rhinitis should be treated for both conditions. Relevant allergens and triggers should be sought and excluded. The combination of intranasal and inhaled corticosteroids for persistent rhinitis and asthma should be considered, with the addition of other drugs including antihistamines, cromones, and LTRAs as appropriate. The overall corticosteroid load should be reviewed on a regular basis to prevent unwanted side effects. Allergen-specific immunotherapy for allergic rhinitis has the potential to prevent the development of asthma.

REFERENCES

1. Anagnostou K, Harrison B, Iles R, et al. Risk factors for childhood asthma deaths from the UK Eastern Region Confidential Enquiry 2001–2006. *Prim Care Respir J* 2012;21(1):71–77.
2. Ryan D, Grant-Casey J, Scadding G, et al. Management of allergic rhinitis in UK primary care: Baseline audit. *Prim Care Respir J* 2005;14(4):204–209.
3. Maurer M, Zuberbier T. Under-treatment of rhinitis symptoms in Europe: Findings from a cross-sectional questionnaire survey. *Allergy* 2007;62(9):1057–1063.
4. Scadding GK, Durham S, Mirakian R, et al. BSACI guidelines for the management of allergic and non-allergic rhinitis. *Clin Exp Allergy* 2008;38(1):19–42.
5. Durham SR. Mechanisms of mucosal inflammation in the nose and lungs. *Clin Exp Allergy* 1998;28(Suppl 2):11–16.
6. Corren J, Adinoff AD, Irvin CG. Changes in bronchial responsiveness following nasal provocation with allergen. *J Allergy Clin Immunol* 1992;89:611–618.
7. KleinJan A, Willart M, van Nimwegen M, et al. United airways: Circulating Th2 effector cells in an AR model are responsible for promoting lower airways inflammation. *Clin Exp Allergy* 2010;40:494–504.
8. Magnan A, Meunier JP, Saugnac C, et al. Frequency and impact of AR in asthma patients in everyday general medical practice: A French observational cross-sectional study. *Allergy* 2008;63:292–298.
9. Agondi RC, Machado ML, Kalil J, et al. Intranasal corticosteroid administration reduces nonspecific bronchial hyperresponsiveness and improves asthma symptoms. *J Asthma* 2008;45(9):754–757.
10. Foresi A, Pelucchi A, Gherson G, et al. Once daily intranasal fluticasone propionate (200 micrograms) reduces nasal symptoms and inflammation but also attenuates the increase in bronchial responsiveness during the pollen season in allergic rhinitis. *J Allergy Clin Immunol* 1996;98(2):274–282.
11. Clatworthy J, Price D, Ryan D, et al. The value of self-report assessment of adherence, rhinitis and smoking in relation to asthma control. *Prim Care Respir J* 2009;18:300–305.
12. Brandão HV, Cruz CS, Pinheiro MC, et al. Risk factors for ER visits due to asthma exacerbations in patients enrolled in a program for the control of asthma and allergic rhinitis in Feira de Santana, Brazil. *J Bras Pneumol* 2009;35:1168–1173.
13. Price D, Zhang Q, Kocevar VS, et al. Effect of a concomitant diagnosis of AR on asthma-related health care use by adults. *Clin Exp Allergy* 2005;35:282–287.
14. Linneberg A, Henrik Nielsen N, Frolund L, et al. The link between AR and allergic asthma: A prospective population-based study. The Copenhagen Allergy Study. *Allergy* 2002;57:1048–1052.
15. Leynaert B, Neukirch F, Demoly P, et al. Epidemiologic evidence for asthma and rhinitis comorbidity. *J Allergy Clin Immunol* 2000;106(Suppl 5):S201–S205.
16. Shaaban R, Zureik M, Soussan D, et al. Allergic rhinitis and onset of bronchial hyperresponsiveness: A population-based study. *Am J Respir Crit Care Med* 2007;176(7):659–666.
17. Shaaban R, Zureik M, Soussan D, et al. Rhinitis and onset of asthma: A longitudinal population-based study. *Lancet* 2008;372:1049–1057.
18. Fishwick D, Barber CM, Bradshaw LM, et al. Standards of care for occupational asthma: An update. *Thorax* 2012;67(3):278–280.
19. Ciprandi G, Capasso M. Association of childhood perennial allergic rhinitis with subclinical airflow limitation. *Clin Exp Allergy* 2010;40(3):398–402.
20. Brown JL, Behndig AF, Sekerel BE, et al. Lower airways inflammation in allergic rhinitics: A comparison with asthmatics and normal controls. *Clin Exp Allergy* 2007;37(5):688–695.
21. Braunstahl G-J, Fokkens W. Nasal involvement in allergic asthma. *Allergy* 2003;58:1235–1243.
22. Gaga M, Lambrou P, Papageorgiou N, et al. Eosinophils are a feature of upper and lower airway pathology in non-atopic asthma, irrespective of the presence of rhinitis. *Clin Exp Allergy* 2000;30(5):663–669.
23. Inal A, Kendirli SG, Yilmaz M, et al. Indices of lower airway inflammation in children monosensitized to house dust mite after nasal allergen challenge. *Allergy* 2008;63(10):1345–1351.
24. Bonay M, Neukirch C, Grandsaigne M, et al. Changes in airway inflammation following nasal allergic challenge in patients with seasonal rhinitis. *Allergy* 2006;61:111–118.
25. Braunstahl GJ, Kleinjan A, Overbeek SE, et al. Segmental bronchial provocation induces nasal inflammation in AR patients. *Am J Respir Crit Care Med* 2000;161:2051–2057.
26. Simons FER. Allergic rhinobronchitis: The asthma-AR link. *J Allergy Clin Immunol* 1999;104:534–540.
27. Togias A. Mechanisms of nose-lung interaction. *Allergy* 1999;54(Suppl 57):94–105.
28. Busse WW, Lemanske RF Jr, Gern JE. Role of viral respiratory infections in asthma and asthma exacerbations. *Lancet.* 2010;376(9743):826–834.
29. Ciprandi G, Tosca MA, Fasce L. Allergic children have more numerous and severe respiratory infections than non-allergic children. *Pediatr Allergy Immunol* 2006;17(5):389–391.
30. Cirillo I, Marseglia G, Klersy C, et al. Allergic patients have more numerous and prolonged respiratory infections than non allergic subjects. *Allergy* 2007;62(9):1087–1090.
31. Soto-Quiros M, Avila L, Platts-Mills TA, et al. High titres of IgE antibodies to dust mite allergen and risk for wheezing among asthmatic children infected with rhinovirus. *J Allergy Clin Immunol* 2012;129:1499–1505.
32. Murray CS, Poletti G, Kebadze T, et al. Study of modifiable risk factors for asthma exacerbations: Virus infection and allergen exposure increase the risk of asthma hospital admissions in children. *Thorax* 2006;61(5):376–382.
33. Crystal-Peters J, Neslusan C, Crown WH, et al. Treating allergic rhinitis in patients with comorbid asthma: The risk of asthma-related hospitalizations and emergency department visits. *J Allergy Clin Immunol* 2002;109(1):57–62.
34. Adams RJ, Fuhlbrigge AL, Finkelstein JA, et al. Intranasal steroids and the risk of emergency department visits for asthma. *J Allergy Clin Immunol* 2002;109(4):636–642.
35. Corren J, Manning B, Thompson S, et al. Rhinitis therapy and the prevention of hospital care for asthma: A case-control study. *J Allergy Clin Immunol* 2004;113(3):415–419.
36. Bousquet J, Khaltaev N, Cruz A, et al; World Health Organization; GA2(2) LEN; AllerGen. Allergic Rhinitis and its Impact on Asthma (ARIA) 2008 update (in collaboration with the World Health Organization, GA(2)LEN and AllerGen). *Allergy* 2008;63(Suppl 86):8–160.
37. Brandt D, Bernstein JA. Questionnaire evaluation and risk factor identification for nonallergic vasomotor rhinitis. *Ann Allergy Asthma Immunol* 2006;96(4):526–532.
38. Bernstein JA, Levin LS, Al-Shuik E, Martin VT. Clinical characteristics of chronic rhinitis patients with high vs low irritant trigger burdens. *Ann Allergy Asthma Immunol* 2012;109(3):173–178.

39. Demoly P, Bozonnat MC, Dacosta P, et al. The diagnosis of asthma using a self-questionnaire in those suffering from AR: A pharmaco-epidemiological survey in everyday practice in France. *Allergy* 2006;61:699–704.

40. Baiardini I, Pasquali M, Giardini A, et al. Rhinasthma: A new specific QoL questionnaire for patients with rhinitis and asthma. *Allergy* 2003;58(4):289–294.

41. Braido F, Baiardini I, Balestracci S, et al. Does asthma control correlate with quality of life related to upper and lower airways? A real life study. *Allergy* 2009;64:937–943.

42. Sheikh A, Hurwitz B, Nurmatov U, et al. House dust mite avoidance measures for perennial allergic rhinitis. *Cochrane Db Syst Rev* 2010;(7):CD001563.

43. Peroni DG, Boner AL, Vallone G, et al. Effective allergen avoidance at high altitude reduces allergen-induced bronchial hyperresponsiveness. *Am J Respir Crit Care Med* 1994;149(6):1442–1446.

44. Morgan WJ, Crain EF, Gruchalla RS, et al. Results of a home-based environmental intervention among urban children with asthma. *N Engl J Med* 2004;351(11):1068–1080.

45. Woodcock A, Forster L, Matthews E, et al. Control of exposure to mite allergen and allergen-impermeable bed covers for adults with asthma. *N Engl J Med* 2003;349(3):225–236.

46. O'Meara TJ, Sercombe JK, Morgan G, et al. The reduction of rhinitis symptoms by nasal filters during natural exposure to ragweed and grass pollen. *Allergy* 2005;60(4):529–532.

47. Boyle RJ, Pedroletti C, Wickman M, et al. Nocturnal temperature controlled laminar airflow for treating atopic asthma: A randomised controlled trial. *Thorax* 2012;67(3):215–221.

48. Garavello W, Romagnoli M, Sordo L, et al. Hypersaline nasal irrigation in children with symptomatic seasonal allergic rhinitis: A randomized study. *Pediatr Allergy Immunol* 2003;14(2):140–143.

49. Georgitis JW. Nasal hyperthermia and simple irrigation for perennial rhinitis. Changes in inflammatory mediators. *Chest* 1994;106(5):1487–1492.

50. Weiner JM, Abramson MJ, Puy RM. Intranasal corticosteroids versus oral H1 receptor antagonists in allergic rhinitis: Systematic review of randomised controlled trials. *BMJ* 1998;317(7173):1624–1629.

51. Yáñez A, Rodrigo GJ. Intranasal corticosteroids versus topical H1 receptor antagonists for the treatment of allergic rhinitis: A systematic review with meta-analysis. *Ann Allergy Asthma Immunol* 2002;89(5):479–484.

52. Di Lorenzo G, Pacor ML, Pellitteri ME, et al. Randomized placebo-controlled trial comparing fluticasone aqueous nasal spray in mono-therapy, fluticasone plus cetirizine, fluticasone plus montelukast and cetirizine plus montelukast for seasonal allergic rhinitis. *Clin Exp Allergy* 2004;34(2):259–267.

53. Wilson AM, O'Byrne PM, Parameswaran K. Leukotriene receptor antagonists for allergic rhinitis: A systematic review and meta-analysis. *Am J Med* 2004;116(5):338–344.

54. Bernstein DI, Levy AL, Hampel FC, et al. Treatment with intranasal fluticasone propionate significantly improves ocular symptoms in patients with seasonal allergic rhinitis. *Clin Exp Allergy* 2004;34(6):952–957.

55. Demoly P. Safety of intranasal corticosteroids in acute rhinosinusitis. *Am J Otolaryngol* 2008;29(6):403–413.

56. Walker S, Khan-Wasti S, Fletcher M, et al. Seasonal allergic rhinitis is associated with a detrimental effect on examination performance in United Kingdom teenagers: Case-control study. *J Allergy Clin Immunol* 2007;120(2):381–387.

57. Vaidyanathan S, Williamson P, Clearie K, Khan F, Lipworth B. Fluticasone reverses oxymetazoline-induced tachyphylaxis of response and rebound congestion. *Am J Respir Crit Care Med* 2010;182(1):19–24.

58. Baroody FM, Brown D, Gavanescu L, DeTineo M, Naclerio RM. Oxymetazoline adds to the effectiveness of fluticasone furoate in the treatment of perennial allergic rhinitis. *J Allergy Clin Immunol* 2011;127(4):927–934.

59. Jacobsen L, Niggemann B, Dreborg S, et al. Specific immunotherapy has long-term preventive effect of seasonal and perennial asthma: 10-year follow-up on the PAT study. *Allergy* 2007;62(8):943–948.

60. Radulovic S, Wilson D, Calderon M, et al. Systematic reviews of sublingual immunotherapy (SLIT). *Allergy* 2011;66(6):740–752.

61. Demoly P, Piette V, Daures J-P. Treatment of allergic rhinitis during pregnancy. *Drugs* 2003;63(17):1813–1820.

62. Bousquet J, Bachert C, Canonica GW, et al. Unmet needs in severe chronic upper airway disease (SCUAD). *J Allergy Clin Immunol* 2009;124(3):428–433.

63. Scadding G, Walker S. Poor asthma control? – then look up the nose. The importance of co-morbid rhinitis in patients with asthma. *Prim Care Respir J* 2012;21(2):222–228.

Section III

Asthma Triggers

9 Viral Infections in Asthma

Joy Hsu and Pedro C. Avila

CONTENTS

CASE PRESENTATION

A 2-year-old boy is referred to the clinic for three episodes of wheezing since he was 18 months old. His wheezing episodes began in the fall and seem to be triggered by a respiratory viral illness. He does not wheeze in between respiratory viral illnesses. The patient has not required oral corticosteroids, emergency department evaluation, or hospitalization to treat his wheezing. During his most recent wheezing episode 2 months earlier, his pediatrician prescribed him daily inhaled corticosteroid (ICS) therapy. His past medical history is notable for the absence of atopic dermatitis and allergic rhinitis. His family history is notable for a paternal history of physician-diagnosed asthma. Since starting ICS therapy 2 months ago, the patient has not had a respiratory viral illness or another wheezing episode. His parents ask the following questions:

- *What is this patient's risk of developing asthma?*
- *Will ICS therapy reduce his risk of developing asthma?*
- *Why do other children in his day-care center not wheeze with the same respiratory illness?*

INTRODUCTION

Respiratory virus infections are the most common infections among infants, children, and adults, and these play an important role in the development and onset of asthma.[1–4] Knowledge in these areas is rapidly growing due to the recent advances in virus detection methods, the discovery of new viruses, and birth cohort studies.[1,2] This chapter will focus on our current understanding of how respiratory viruses may contribute to asthma inception and asthma exacerbations, as well as identify areas in need of further study.

ADVANCES IN THE DETECTION OF RESPIRATORY VIRUSES

Advances in detecting respiratory viruses have provided important insights into the relationship between viruses and asthma. Conventional methods, including viral culture, antigen detection using labeled antibodies, and serological conversion, are insensitive for identifying viruses, yielding detection rates of 30%–50%.[2] The advent of molecular detection techniques, including polymerase chain reaction (PCR), reverse-transcriptase PCR, gene sequencing, and microarrays, has yielded far superior viral detection rates (as high as 90% of acute respiratory infections [ARI]).[2,5] This advancement has resulted in the identification of viruses as the main etiology of infant wheezing and asthma exacerbations;[2,3] the discovery of new classes of viruses, including human metapneumoviruses (hMPVs), bocaviruses (hBoVs), and polyomaviruses (PyVs); the discovery of new species of viruses such as human rhinovirus (HRV) C; and the discovery of new strains of viruses such as the severe acute respiratory syndrome (SARS) coronavirus.[1–3] Many of these recently identified viruses are difficult or impossible to grow in the available tissue culture systems, which explains why they have only been identified using molecular diagnostics.[2] These newly discovered viruses have also been linked to wheezing illnesses and asthma exacerbations (see Table 9.1).[1,3,6] In summary, the molecular methods for virus detection have greatly advanced our knowledge of respiratory viruses, and research employing these techniques in asthma patients and birth cohorts has provided new insights in our understanding of asthma etiopathogenesis.

TABLE 9.1

Families of Respiratory Viruses Linked to Asthma Inception or Exacerbation

Family

Picornaviridae
Human rhinoviruses (HRVs)
Enteroviruses
Orthomyxoviridae
Influenza viruses (IFVs)
Paramyxoviridae
Respiratory syncytial virus (RSV)
Parainfluenza viruses (PIV)
Human metapneumovirus (hMPV)
Coronaviridae
Human coronaviruses (HCoVs)
Adenoviridae
Adenoviruses (AdVs)
Parvoviridae
Human bocaviruses (HBoVs)
Polyomaviridae
Polyomaviruses (PyVs)

VIRUSES AND ASTHMA INCEPTION

VIRUS-INDUCED WHEEZING AND SUBSEQUENT ASTHMA

Respiratory virus infections are universal in early childhood.[6] Up to one-half of children wheeze with a lower respiratory tract illness (LRTI) at least once before school age,[6] and respiratory viruses are the most frequent pathogens associated with these wheezing illnesses.[7] Based on data from the Tucson Children's Respiratory Study (TCRS), a U.S. prospective birth cohort of over 1000 children, the timing and the persistence of wheezing LRTIs in early life appear predictive of a subsequent asthma risk.[6,8,9] Over 60% of this cohort were "transient wheezers," who began wheezing before 3 years of age, but ceased to have wheezing exacerbations by age 6, and they were no more likely to wheeze at age 11 than those who never wheezed before age 3.[6] In contrast, "persistent wheezers" began wheezing before 3 years of age and continued to wheeze at school age. These children had reduced lung function at 6 years of age that persisted at least through their teenage years.[6,10] A German birth cohort of 1314 children found similar results.[5]

Based on the TCRS data, study investigators have developed an index to predict the risk of developing asthma in children who have recurrent wheezing ($\geq$3 episodes of wheezing in 1 year by age 3).[8,9] The Asthma Predictive Index (API) uses several criteria to predict the risk of asthma (see Table 9.2).[8,9] A child is given a positive API score if he or she has recurrent wheezing and at least one major criterion or at least two minor criteria of the API. In the TCRS, a positive API score by age 3 was associated with a 77% chance of active asthma from ages 6 to 13, while children with a negative API score at age 3 had less than a 3% chance of active asthma during school age.[9] Since the development of the API,

TABLE 9.2
Asthma Predictive Index (API) from Tucson Children's Respiratory Study

Major Criteria

1. Parental history of physician-diagnosed asthma
2. Physician diagnosis of atopic dermatitis (in age 2 or 3 years)

Minor Criteria

1. Physician diagnosis of allergic rhinitis (in age 2 or 3 years)
2. Wheezing apart from colds
3. Eosinophilia ≥4%

Source: Castro-Rodriguez, J.A., *The Journal of Allergy and Clinical Immunology*, 126, 212–216, 2010; Castro-Rodriguez, J.A., Holberg, C.J., Wright, A.L., and Martinez, F.D., *American Journal of Respiratory and Critical Care Medicine*, 162, 1403–1406, 2000.

Note: Positive API = early recurrent wheezer (≥3 episodes of wheezing by age 3 years) and ≥1 major criterion or ≥2 minor criteria.

other asthma indices using birth cohorts from other nations have been developed.[8]

DAY CARE AND VIRUS-INDUCED WHEEZING

The Childhood Origins of Asthma (COAST) study, a U.S. prospective birth cohort of 285 children, found an association between day-care attendance and an increased risk of ARI due to HRV and respiratory syncytial virus (RSV), as well as an increased risk of HRV-induced wheezing in infants.[11] TCRS investigators also reported an association between day care and wheezing,[12] but other studies have either found no such association[13] or they have found an inverse association.[14]

Host differences may explain some of these discrepant findings. For example, genetic variants in the genes *TLR2*, *FCER1B*, and interleukin (*IL*)-*4RA* may modulate the risk of atopy and of wheezing associated with day care.[15,16]

RSV AND ASTHMA INCEPTION

RSV, of the family Paramyxoviridae, is a common cause of bronchiolitis and the leading cause of hospitalization for children younger than 1 year old.[2,3,5] A RSV infection is seasonal, peaking during the winter months in the United States.[2] Most children are infected with RSV by 2 years of age,[17] but fewer than one-half of children develop clinically recognized bronchiolitis, and only a small fraction develop bronchiolitis severe enough to require hospitalization.[17]

RSV bronchiolitis in early life, especially the form of the illness that is severe enough to require emergency department care or hospitalization, has been identified as a risk factor for asthma in multiple studies.[5,17,18] A retrospective study of over 95,000 infants enrolled in the Tennessee Medicaid program found that children born 120 days before the peak of the RSV season had the highest risk of hospitalization for LRTI, as well as the highest risk of asthma between 4 and 5.5 years of age. In the COAST study, the development of RSV bronchiolitis between birth and age 3 was associated with an odds ratio (OR) of 2.6 for asthma at age 6.[19] This association between RSV bronchiolitis and subsequent asthma has been replicated in multiple prospective cohorts.[5,17,19,20] However, the results from other studies argue against an association[2,5] or indicate that RSV-associated asthma may subside by 13 years of age.[21] Taken together, the relationship between RSV and asthma inception remains controversial[2,5] because severe RSV bronchiolitis may reflect a host phenotype that is already predisposed to future asthma, rather than a causal relationship between RSV and asthma. Indeed, an inherited susceptibility to bacterial and viral infections throughout an individual's lifetime may be a hallmark of asthma, as has been extensively reviewed recently.[22]

HRVs AND ASTHMA INCEPTION

HRVs, in the genus *Enterovirus* of the Picornaviridae family, are the predominant cause of the common cold in both children and adults.[3–5] Unlike RSVs, HRV infections may occur throughout the year, and are the leading cause of bronchiolitis outside of the winter RSV season.[5] HRVs are also more frequently associated with wheezing than are RSVs, even in infants.[3] Based on virus genome sequences, HRVs were initially divided into two groups (A and B), but a novel species of HRV, called HRV group C (HRV-C),[1,2] has been identified by molecular techniques and linked to wheezing illnesses.[1–3]

Studies have linked HRV-associated wheezing illnesses in infancy to the development of asthma,[3,5,19] and they have also shown that HRV-associated wheezing is a stronger predictor of asthma inception than RSV-associated wheezing.[3,5,19] For example, the COAST study[17] found that HRV-associated wheezing during the first year of life was the most significant predictor of wheezing at age 3 (OR = 10) and asthma at age 6 (OR = 9.8);[19,23] these children also had impaired lung function at both time points.[24] In the COAST study, the relationship between the risk of asthma and HRV-associated wheezing in early life appeared to increase with each year of age, such that subjects who had developed HRV-associated wheezing by age 3 had an OR of 25.6 for developing asthma by age 6.[19] In contrast, an RSV-associated wheezing illness by age 3 in the COAST study had an OR of 2.6 for developing asthma by age 6.[19] Similarly, a Tennessee study indicated that bronchiolitis during the HRV-predominant months was associated with a 25% increased risk for childhood asthma over bronchiolitis during the RSV-predominant months.[25]

Some evidence suggests that the risk of asthma following HRV-associated wheezing may be influenced by the patient's atopic status. In an Australian birth cohort of 263 children, Kusel et al.[26] found that a relationship between HRV-associated wheezing in early life and the risk of asthma at age 5 was only significant in subjects who had demonstrable atopy (by skin prick test) by age 2 (OR = 3.2), and not in subjects who developed atopy after 2 years of age or who did not develop atopy during their 5-year study period. Thus, host factors such as atopy may modulate the risk of asthma following HRV-associated wheezing episodes in early life.

INFLUENZA VIRUSES AND ASTHMA INCEPTION

Influenza viruses (IFVs) from the Orthomyxoviridae family are well known for their associated annual epidemics and the risk of pandemics.[1,3] IFVs are associated with wheezing in children and adults,[1,3] but hospitalizations for IFV-associated wheezing in children are relatively rare compared with RSV- and HRV-associated wheezing.[7] All three types of IFVs (i.e., IFV-A, IFV-B, and IFV-C) can cause ARIs in humans, but IFV-A and IFV-B are the most prominent in the annual "flu season," which occurs during the winter months.[1]

Experimental evidence suggests that IFV-A may predispose individuals to atopy and asthma.[18,27] Al-Garawi et al.[27] infected neonatal mice with IFV-A and exposed them to the house-dust mite (HDM). The neonatal mice exhibited a slight immune response to HDM in the absence of IFV-A infection, but when HDM allergen exposure occurred concurrently with IFV-A infection, these mice displayed robust allergen-specific immunity, allergic inflammation, lung remodeling, and impaired lung function.[18,27] Lung remodeling persisted into early adulthood for these mice, long after the HDM allergen exposure had ceased.[27] These data suggest a relationship between IFV and asthma in a mouse model, but whether this relationship exists in humans remains unknown.

OTHER RESPIRATORY VIRUSES AND ASTHMA INCEPTION

Less is known regarding the role of other respiratory viruses and the risk of developing asthma.[1,7] Parainfluenza viruses (PIVs), of the same Paramyxoviridae family as RSV, have been associated with approximately 10% of wheezing illnesses in children, and a possible association between PIV infection and asthma was reported in a Canadian birth cohort study.[28] Other studies have found adenoviruses (AdVs), human bocaviruses (HBoVs), hMPVs, human coronaviruses (HCoVs), and PyVs to be associated with childhood wheezing and bronchiolitis, but their role in the pathogenesis of asthma is not yet known. The potential roles of HBoVs and PyVs in the risk of asthma remain especially unclear, since these viruses are frequently codetected with other viruses such as rhinoviruses and influenza.[1,3,7]

MECHANISMS BY WHICH VIRUSES MAY CAUSE ASTHMA

DIMINISHED T-HELPER TYPE 1 (TH1) HOST IMMUNE RESPONSE

Evidence suggests that a diminished antiviral immune response may predispose individuals to asthma after a respiratory virus infection.[5] Interferons (IFNs) are important in the human Th1 immune response to a virus infection, and respiratory viruses are known to upregulate IFN-responsive genes during an infection.[29] Studies have shown that a diminished host production of IFN (IFN-α, IFN-β, IFN-γ, and IFN-λ) correlated with wheezing and asthma following a viral infection.[5,30–32] For example, the differences at birth in the peripheral blood mononuclear cell (PBMC) production of IFN-γ in response to HRV and RSV have been shown to correlate with wheezing in infancy, preschool age, and school age.[30,31] Recent data have linked deficient IL-15 production, a cytokine that helps connect innate immunity to adaptive immunity during a viral infection, to the deficient IFN response associated with asthma (Table 9.3).[33]

BIASED T-HELPER TYPE 2 (TH2) HOST IMMUNE RESPONSE

Th2 ("allergic") inflammation is often associated with asthma, and studies suggest that a host predisposition toward an allergic Th2 immune response may also contribute to the development of asthma after a respiratory virus infection.[5] For instance, the COAST study found a stable production of IL-13 (a key Th2 cytokine) by PBMC stimulated with phytohemagglutinin over the first year of life in children who wheezed with virus infections compared with those who did not wheeze with colds.[30] More recently, another U.S. prospective cohort study found that the strongest determinant of asthma following RSV bronchiolitis was an elevated level of nasal epithelial chemokine (C-C motif) ligand 5 (CCL5) (also known as regulated upon activation, normal T-cell expressed and secreted chemokine [RANTES]), a Th2 chemokine.[20]

OTHER HOST FACTORS THAT MAY PREDISPOSE TO ASTHMA

Other components of the host immune system may contribute to the risk of asthma following a respiratory virus infection. At 1 year of age, fewer host regulatory T cells ("Tregs"), which suppress Th1 and Th2 inflammation, have been linked to the risk of allergic sensitization at 1 and 2 years of age and may also mediate the risk of asthma.[34] An impaired epithelial barrier (e.g., due to a diminished expression of the barrier protein filaggrin) is associated with atopic dermatitis, but it may also increase the risk of asthma in certain individuals,[5] although filaggrin is not expressed in the airways. Aside from the epithelial barrier, other aspects of innate immunity, such as Toll-like receptors (TLRs), may also play a role.[15]

TABLE 9.3
Mechanisms by Which Viruses May Cause Asthma

Host Factors

Diminished Th1 immune response
Biased Th2 immune response
Fewer T regulatory cells
Altered innate immunity (including epithelial barrier)
Differences in airway repair and remodeling

Virus Factors

Affect airway repair and remodeling
Drive Th2 immune response

Finally, host differences in airway repair and remodeling may also influence the risk of asthma following respiratory virus infections.[35]

VIRUS FACTORS THAT MAY PREDISPOSE TO ASTHMA

Respiratory viruses may increase the risk of asthma through several pathways. *In vitro* experiments using human airway epithelial cells have shown that a HRV infection increased the production of factors involved in airway remodeling, including amphiregulin, activin A, and vascular endothelial growth factor (VEGF).[5] *In vivo*, VEGF increases in the nasal lavage fluid during a natural human HRV infection.[36] These effects may ultimately lead to changes in the airway smooth muscle, which are characteristic of asthma. Studies of humans and mice also suggest that paramyxoviruses (such as RSV) may drive a Th2 immune response via the increased production of IL-4.[37,38]

"TWO-HIT" HYPOTHESIS

As described previously, both host factors and virus factors may contribute to asthma inception after a respiratory virus infection. Hence, a "two-hit" hypothesis has been proposed, in which children with immune dysregulation (e.g., a diminished Th1 response, a biased Th2 response, altered innate immunity, and/or aberrant airway remodeling) who acquire a viral LRTI during a critical time in their life will develop airway inflammation, damage, and remodeling that, together with allergic sensitization, will subsequently lead to the development of asthma.[5,17] However, this hypothesis needs confirmation and elucidation of the detailed mechanism of the interaction between virus infections and allergic sensitization.

THERAPIES THAT MAY DECREASE RISK OF ASTHMA INCEPTION AFTER INFECTION WITH RSV OR HRV

THERAPIES THAT MAY DECREASE RISK OF ASTHMA INCEPTION AFTER RSV INFECTION

To modify the risk of asthma after RSV infection, several therapies have been investigated (Table 9.4). A small Finnish retrospective study that involved children hospitalized for RSV-induced wheezing found that oral prednisolone only decreased the risk of subsequent recurrent wheezing in subjects with atopic dermatitis.[39] A U.S. retrospective study of children with a physician's diagnosis of chronic lung disease or bronchopulmonary dysplasia found that subjects who had received a monthly prophylaxis with RSV immune globulin in infancy had better spirometry values and fewer asthma attacks during school age compared with subjects who had not received RSV immune globulin.[18] While the rates of bronchial hyperreactivity, asthma diagnosis, and asthma medication use did not differ significantly between the two groups, a trend toward benefit was seen in the group treated

TABLE 9.4

Interventions That May Decrease Risk of Asthma after Respiratory Virus Infection

Intervention	Significant Effect Found?
RSV	
Oral prednisolone after RSV infection	No
RSV immune globulin	Yes
Anti-RSV monoclonal antibody	Yes
Rhinovirus	
Oral prednisolone	Yes
Nonvirus specific	
Inhaled fluticasone (PEAK study) [41]	No

with RSV immune globulin.[18] Prospective studies are needed to further evaluate the role of systemic corticosteroids and RSV immune globulin in reducing the risk of asthma in such patients.

One European prospective controlled study has examined the effect of the anti-RSV monoclonal antibody (mAb) palivizumab on the risk of asthma in premature infants (<36 weeks gestational age) who had received palivizumab as routine care for prematurity.[40] The rates of RSV infection in the palivizumab group were not tracked, although documented RSV infection was accounted for in selecting the control subjects.[40] Palivizumab decreased the risk of recurrent wheezing in nonatopic children by 80%, but showed no benefit for children with a personal or a family history of atopy.[40] These investigators concluded that palivizumab was effective in reducing the risk of recurrent wheezing in nonatopic children, and suggested that RSV may predispose individuals to asthma through an atopy-independent pathway.[40]

THERAPIES THAT MAY DECREASE RISK OF ASTHMA INCEPTION AFTER HRV INFECTION

Currently, there is no strategy available for the successful prevention of ARI caused by HRV.[2] Finnish investigators evaluated prednisolone therapy in 40 children (mean age 1.38 years) hospitalized for their first or second episode of HRV-associated wheezing, and found that oral prednisolone decreased the risk of recurrent wheezing in the following year compared with a placebo (OR 0.19; 95% confidence interval [CI] 0.05–0.71; see also Table 9.4).[39] Larger studies are needed to confirm this benefit. The efficacy of ICS in decreasing the risk of asthma was explored in the Preventing Early Asthma in Kids (PEAK) study.[41] In the PEAK study, preschool children at high risk of asthma (i.e., with a positive API score) were randomized to 2 years of a placebo or inhaled fluticasone propionate, which were continued throughout any wheezing illnesses that the subjects experienced during the 2 years of intervention. There was no change in the rate of the development of asthma symptoms or in lung function values between the placebo and the ICS groups after these interventions were discontinued during the third treatment-free year.[41] HRV was not studied specifically in the PEAK study, but it is well known that HRV is the most frequently isolated respiratory virus in preschool-age children.[3] These data suggest that ICS therapy during HRV infections in preschoolers does not appear to decrease the risk of asthma development.

ANTENATAL VIRUSES AND ASTHMA INCEPTION

While most research into the relationship between viruses and the development of asthma has focused on viral infections in early childhood, a few studies have investigated whether antenatal viruses (i.e., respiratory viruses that infect a mother while a child is in utero) predispose these children to developing wheezing or asthma.[42,43] In a questionnaire-based cohort study of 8088 Finnish children conducted by Xu et al.,[43] self-reported maternal febrile illness during pregnancy (especially in the first and second trimesters) correlated with offspring asthma (by parent report) (adjusted OR for any maternal febrile illness during pregnancy 1.65; 95% CI 1.25–2.18). Unfortunately, the authors did not describe the causes of the maternal febrile illnesses (e.g., whether they were respiratory illnesses). A British study conducted by Hughes et al.[42] did examine maternal respiratory illnesses in a case-control study of 200 asthmatic children (ages 5–16) and 200 age-matched controls: ARIs during pregnancy (derived from primary care records) were significantly associated with asthma in the offspring (OR 1.69; 95% CI 1.05–2.77), even after adjustment for multiple variables.[42] The lack of virological data is a limitation of this study, and the mechanism underlying this possible relationship remains unclear. Several studies have suggested that the neonatal immune system is affected by antenatal exposures,[44–46] including vaccination with IFV,[47] but a direct link between maternal respiratory virus illnesses and the development of postnatal asthma has yet to be established. With the advent of molecular methods for viral detection since the publication of the aforementioned studies, further research should utilize these new methods to determine the relationship between antenatal respiratory viral infections and the risk for subsequent asthma.

VIRUSES AND ASTHMA EXACERBATIONS

VIRUSES ASSOCIATED WITH ASTHMA EXACERBATIONS

For over 40 years, respiratory viruses have been associated with asthma exacerbations.[1,3,4] With the advent of molecular techniques to identify viruses, viruses have been detected in approximately 80%–85% of wheezing episodes in school-age children, and in approximately 50%–75% of acute wheezing episodes in adults. HRV is the most frequent virus isolated in acute exacerbations of asthma, but IFV and RSV are also important pathogens. HRV infections can occur year-round but are most common in the spring and fall, whereas RSV, IFV, and hMPV are typically limited to the winter and early spring months. RSV-associated wheezing is especially important in infants hospitalized with bronchiolitis, as well as in adults over age 65. RSV may account for up to 7% of hospitalizations for asthma in adults over age 65.[48] hMPV has been associated with wheezing in young children, although its role in asthma exacerbations in older patients remains unclear. AdVs seem to play a minor role in asthma exacerbations overall, but they can be associated with near-fatal asthma. HCoVs appear to have a minor, if any, contribution to asthma exacerbations. The role of HBoVs, PyVs, and enteroviruses (other than HRV) remains unclear.[1,3,4]

MECHANISMS BY WHICH VIRUSES MAY EXACERBATE ASTHMA

Patients with asthma are not at greater risk of ARIs, having the same frequency of illnesses as people without asthma. However, when asthmatic individuals get colds, they experience more severe and prolonged lower respiratory tract symptoms and greater reductions in lung function compared with nonasthmatics.[4,49] The mechanisms underlying this discrepancy remain poorly understood, but ex vivo experiments suggest that HRV replicates more efficiently in asthmatic bronchial epithelial cells (BECs) than in BECs from controls,[50] although this is not a consistent finding.[35,51] As previously mentioned, asthmatic individuals may be deficient in their IFN responses (IFN-α, IFN-β, IFN-λ, and IFN-γ) upon viral infection.[4,32,50]

VIRUS–ATOPY AND VIRUS–BACTERIA INTERACTIONS

A growing body of evidence suggests that respiratory viruses interact with atopic responses in asthma exacerbations. Sensitization and exposure to high levels of the relevant allergen increase the risk of exacerbations when atopic asthmatics develop rhinovirus infections.[52–54] Attempts to simulate this interaction by challenging asthmatic individuals with allergens before rhinovirus inoculation have failed to support this epidemiological observation,[55,56] indicating that virus–allergen interactions are complex.

In contrast to virus–atopy interactions, the observation that respiratory tract viral infections often precede bacterial infections is well described. Recent evidence is now starting to delineate the mechanisms that may underlie this relationship. Oliver et al.[57] found that viruses impaired human alveolar macrophage secretion of IL-8 and tumor necrosis factor (TNF) after stimulation with lipopolysaccharide and lipoteichoic acid, two common components of bacteria. IL-8 is key to neutrophil chemotaxis and activation in the setting of an infection, and TNF has many proinflammatory effects that upregulate the host immune response.[58,59] In these experiments, a decreased secretion of IL-8 and TNF was independent of IL-10, prostaglandin E2, and TLR2,[57] but the exact mechanism remains unclear. This virus-induced impairment in the antibacterial host defense may facilitate bacterial superinfection during a viral respiratory illness. Because of the increased risk for invasive pneumococcal disease in asthmatic patients, the CDC Advisory Committee on Immunization Practices (ACIP) has advised pneumococcal vaccination for all asthmatic patients aged 19 years and older.[60]

THERAPIES THAT MAY DECREASE RISK OF ASTHMA EXACERBATION DUE TO RESPIRATORY VIRUSES

VACCINATION

IFV vaccination (including vaccination against pandemic H1N1 IFV) for asthma patients is strongly recommended, and several studies (though not all) suggest that IFV vaccination reduces asthma exacerbations.[61] Currently, no effective vaccine exists for HRV infection, the most common cause of asthma exacerbations, due to the antigenic diversity of approximately 200 rhinovirus strains.

ANTIVIRAL AGENTS

Antiviral agents such as oseltamivir can reduce asthma exacerbations precipitated by IFV.[62] New antiviral agents for rhinovirus infections are being developed and tested for their ability to reduce the risk for rhinovirus-induced asthma exacerbations (see later).

CURRENTLY AVAILABLE ASTHMA CONTROLLER THERAPIES

ICS has been shown to decrease virus-induced asthma exacerbations in children, and in adults with intermittent or persistent asthma. Studies of both children and adults also suggest that a combination of ICS and long-acting beta-agonist (LABA) is more effective in reducing asthma exacerbations compared with ICS alone.[63] Mechanistic experiments have demonstrated that ICS (budesonide) suppressed HRV-induced BEC expression of proinflammatory cytokines (IL-6) and chemokines (CCL5, CXCL8, and CXCL10) as well as remodeling-associated mediators (VEGF and fibroblast growth factor). Other data suggest that the combination of ICS with LABA synergistically suppresses BEC secretion of rhinovirus-induced chemokines. Leukotriene receptor antagonists such as montelukast may also reduce asthma exacerbations in patients with mild asthma.[4]

mABS

Several mAbs have been studied in asthma, but specific information about respiratory viruses is largely unavailable in these studies. Omalizumab (mAb against immunoglobulin E [IgE], the key immunoglobulin involved in atopic and Th2 immune responses) decreases the rate of asthma exacerbations in adults and children compared with ICS alone. In addition to mAb anti-IgE, mAbs targeting other molecules in the Th2 inflammatory pathway have been investigated in clinical trials of asthmatic individuals, including mAbs anti-cytokines IL-4, IL-5, and IL-13; soluble receptor blockers for IL-4 showed potential to decrease asthma exacerbations, but larger studies did not confirm the initial results. Mepolizumab (mAb against IL-5) decreased asthma exacerbations in a study involving severe steroid-refractory asthmatics with sputum eosinophilia. Studies are ongoing to confirm its effectiveness

in severe asthmatics with sputum eosinophilia. Similarly, lebrikizumab (mAb against IL-13) reduced asthma exacerbations in a "Th2-high" subgroup, characterized by elevated levels of periostin (an IL-13-induced protein). In contrast, golimumab (mAb against the proinflammatory cytokine TNF) showed no benefit in asthma exacerbations, and the study was stopped early due to adverse side effects, including concerns for an increased occurrence of malignancies. While little information is available regarding the identification of respiratory viruses in these studies, the efficacy of these mAbs in preventing virus-induced asthma exacerbations can be inferred from previous observations that the majority of asthma exacerbations appear to be associated with viruses.[4]

MACROLIDES

Macrolides are known to have immunomodulatory effects in addition to antimicrobial properties. Mechanistic studies using airway epithelial cell cultures have shown that macrolides attenuate rhinovirus-induced epithelial inflammatory responses. Clinical trials suggest that macrolides may be beneficial in controlling asthma and reducing asthma exacerbations, but the current evidence is not strong enough to recommend macrolides for this use.[64]

POTENTIAL FUTURE THERAPIES

Given the aforementioned experimental evidence implicating IFN-β deficiency in asthmatic susceptibility to HRV infection,[50] clinical studies are under way to test whether inhaled IFN-β (SNG001, Synairgen Research Ltd.) may attenuate virus-induced asthma exacerbations. mAbs against the pro-Th2 cytokines IL-25 and IL-33 are being tested in animal models and a mAb against thymic stromal lymphopoeitin (another potent Th2-skewing cytokine) is currently in development (AMG157). Inhibitors of kinases and phosphodiesterases are also under investigation to prevent asthma exacerbations.

FUTURE DIRECTIONS: MICROBIOME AND ASTHMA

Microorganisms are known to live inside and on the skin of humans (microbiota), and the collective genomes of these microbiota (microbiome) and the emerging evidence suggest that the composition of individual microbiomes may mediate the risk of diseases including asthma[2] (see also Chapter 27). A study by Bisgaard et al. suggests that early colonization (at age 1 month) with *Streptococcus pneumoniae*, *Haemophilus influenzae*, and *Moraxella catarrhalis* was associated with an increased risk of asthma at age 5.[65] Similar studies in older children and adults have shown that *Haemophilus* spp. and other microorganisms (including members of the Comamonadaceae, Sphingomonadaceae, and Oxalobacteraceae families) correlate with asthma, lung function, and airway hyperresponsiveness. Albeit distant from the bronchial tree, gut microbiota may also direct a Th2 immune response leading to allergy and asthma.[2]

The role of respiratory viruses in the microbiome and asthma is relatively understudied compared with bacteria. PyVs are known to establish latency in humans, but as previously mentioned, their contribution to asthma pathogenesis and exacerbations remains unclear. HBoVs have been detected in asymptomatic humans, but their relevance in asthma is also not well understood. Although chronic infection with HRV only occurs with immunosuppression, HRV has also been identified in asymptomatic asthma subjects. However, HRV RNA may be detected several weeks following an ARI, so further study is needed to determine if the detection of HRV (and other common respiratory viruses) in asymptomatic asthmatics reflects resolving the infection versus an altered microbiome in asthma.[1-3]

CONCLUSION

Respiratory viruses cause asthma exacerbations and are associated with an increased risk of developing asthma. Common respiratory viruses such as HRV and RSV are most frequently implicated, but many additional respiratory viruses have recently been identified using newer molecular virus detection methods. Additional research is needed to further elucidate the relationship between respiratory viruses and asthma inception, to characterize the clinical significance of recently identified respiratory viruses in asthma, and to evaluate interventions that may decrease asthma prevalence, morbidity, and mortality associated with respiratory virus infections.

CONCLUSION TO CASE PRESENTATION

This patient has had recurrent wheezing (defined as more than three episodes of wheezing in 1 year). The factors that determine virus-induced wheezing and asthma inception after a respiratory virus infection remain under active investigation, but research suggests that individual differences in innate immunity, antiviral IFN response, the degree of Th2 ("allergic") inflammation, allergen exposure, and airway remodeling and repair are all factors that contribute to the development of virus-induced wheezing and asthma in this patient and not other children.

This child's risk of developing asthma can be predicted using the API (see Table 9.2). The patient's parental history of physician-diagnosed asthma is one of the major criteria of the API. Because this patient had recurrent wheezing and he meets a major criterion of the API, he has a positive API score. A positive API score by age 3 is associated with a 77% chance of active asthma from ages 6 to 13, according to the TCRS birth cohort.

ICS therapy reduces respiratory symptoms but does not appear to reduce the risk of developing asthma after virus-induced wheezing, according to the PEAK study. In the PEAK study, preschool children with a positive API score were randomized to 2 years of a placebo or ICS (fluticasone propionate), but inhaled fluticasone did not prevent the development of asthma nor did it improve lung function after 2 years of therapy and during a third, treatment-free year.[41]

LIST OF ABBREVIATIONS

Abbreviation	Significance
AdV	Adenovirus
API	Asthma predictive index
ARI	Acute respiratory infection
BEC	Bronchial epithelial cell
CI	Confidence interval
COAST	Childhood origins of asthma
HBoV	Human bocavirus
HCoV	Human coronavirus
HDM	House dust mite
HRV	Human rhinovirus
hMPV	Human metapneumovirus
ICS	Inhaled corticosteroid
IFN	Interferon
IFV	Influenza virus
IL	Interleukin
LABA	Long-acting beta-agonist
LTRI	Lower respiratory tract illness
mAb	Monoclonal antibody
OR	Odds ratio
PBMC	Peripheral blood mononuclear cell
PCR	Polymerase chain reaction
PEAK	Preventing early asthma in kids
PIV	Parainfluenza virus
PyV	Polyomavirus
RSV	Respiratory syncytial virus
SARS	Severe acute respiratory syndrome
TCRS	Tucson children's respiratory study
TLR	Toll-like receptor
TNF	Tumor necrosis factor
VEGF	Vascular endothelial growth factor

REFERENCES

1. McErlean P, Greiman A, Favoreto Jr, S, Avila PC. Viral diversity in asthma. *Immunology and Allergy Clinics of North America.* 2010;30(4):481–495.
2. Rosenthal LA, Avila PC, Heymann PW, Martin RJ, Miller EK, Papadopoulos NG, et al. Viral respiratory tract infections and asthma: The course ahead. *The Journal of Allergy and Clinical Immunology.* 2010;125(6):1212–1217.
3. Papadopoulos NG, Christodoulou I, Rohde G, Agache I, Almqvist C, Bruno A, et al. Viruses and bacteria in acute asthma exacerbations: A GA(2) LEN-DARE systematic review. *Allergy.* 2011;66(4):458–468.
4. Jackson DJ, Sykes A, Mallia P, Johnston SL. Asthma exacerbations: Origin, effect, and prevention. *The Journal of Allergy and Clinical Immunology.* 2011;128(6):1165–1174.
5. Jackson DJ, Lemanske Jr RF. The role of respiratory virus infections in childhood asthma inception. *Immunology and Allergy Clinics of North America.* 2010;30(4):513–522.
6. Martinez FD, Wright AL, Taussig LM, Holberg CJ, Halonen M, Morgan WJ. Asthma and wheezing in the first six years of life. The Group Health Medical Associates. *The New England Journal of Medicine.* 199519;332(3):133–138.

7. Jartti T, Lehtinen P, Vuorinen T, Osterback R, van den Hoogen B, Osterhaus AD, et al. Respiratory picornaviruses and respiratory syncytial virus as causative agents of acute expiratory wheezing in children. *Emerging Infectious Diseases.* 2004;10(6):1095–1101.

8. Castro-Rodriguez JA. The Asthma Predictive Index: A very useful tool for predicting asthma in young children. *The Journal of Allergy and Clinical Immunology.* 2010;126(2):212–216.

9. Castro-Rodriguez JA, Holberg CJ, Wright AL, Martinez FD. A clinical index to define risk of asthma in young children with recurrent wheezing. *American Journal of Respiratory and Critical Care Medicine.* 2000;162(4 Pt 1):1403–1406.

10. Morgan WJ, Stern DA, Sherrill DL, Guerra S, Holberg CJ, Guilbert TW, et al. Outcome of asthma and wheezing in the first 6 years of life: Follow-up through adolescence. *American Journal of Respiratory and Critical Care Medicine.* 2005;172(10):1253–1258.

11. Copenhaver CC, Gern JE, Li Z, Shult PA, Rosenthal LA, Mikus LD, et al. Cytokine response patterns, exposure to viruses, and respiratory infections in the first year of life. *American Journal of Respiratory and Critical Care Medicine.* 2004;170(2):175–180.

12. Taussig LM, Wright AL, Holberg CJ, Halonen M, Morgan WJ, Martinez FD. Tucson Children's Respiratory Study: 1980 to present. *The Journal of Allergy and Clinical Immunology.* 2003;111(4):661–675.

13. Caudri D, Wijga A, Scholtens S, Kerkhof M, Gerritsen J, Ruskamp JM, et al. Early daycare is associated with an increase in airway symptoms in early childhood but is no protection against asthma or atopy at 8 years. *American Journal of Respiratory and Critical Care Medicine.* 2009;180(6):491–498.

14. Ball TM, Castro-Rodriguez JA, Griffith KA, Holberg CJ, Martinez FD, Wright AL. Siblings, day-care attendance, and the risk of asthma and wheezing during childhood. *The New England Journal of Medicine.* 2000;343(8):538–543.

15. Custovic A, Nicolaou N. Peanut allergy: Overestimated in epidemiology or underdiagnosed in primary care? *The Journal of Allergy and Clinical Immunology.* 2011;127(3):631–632.

16. Hoffjan S, Nicolae D, Ostrovnaya I, Roberg K, Evans M, Mirel DB, et al. Gene–environment interaction effects on the development of immune responses in the 1st year of life. *American Journal of Human Genetics.* 2005;76(4):696–704.

17. Lemanske Jr RF. The childhood origins of asthma (COAST) study. *Pediatric Allergy and Immunology.* 2002;13(Suppl 15):38–43.

18. Martinez FD. New insights into the natural history of asthma: Primary prevention on the horizon. *The Journal of Allergy and Clinical Immunology.* 2011;128(5):939–945.

19. Jackson DJ, Gangnon RE, Evans MD, Roberg KA, Anderson EL, Pappas TE, et al. Wheezing rhinovirus illnesses in early life predict asthma development in high-risk children. *American Journal of Respiratory and Critical Care Medicine.* 2008;178(7):667–672.

20. Bacharier LB, Cohen R, Schweiger T, Yin-Declue H, Christie C, Zheng J, et al. Determinants of asthma after severe respiratory syncytial virus bronchiolitis. *The Journal of Allergy and Clinical Immunology.* 2012;130(1):91–100.

21. Stein RT, Sherrill D, Morgan WJ, Holberg CJ, Halonen M, Taussig LM, et al. Respiratory syncytial virus in early life and risk of wheeze and allergy by age 13 years. *Lancet.* 1999;354(9178):541–545.

22. James KM, Peebles Jr RS, Hartert TV. Response to infections in patients with asthma and atopic disease: An epiphenomenon or reflection of host susceptibility? *The Journal of Allergy and Clinical Immunology.* 2012;130(2):343–351.

23. Lemanske Jr RF, Jackson DJ, Gangnon RE, Evans MD, Li Z, Shult PA, et al. Rhinovirus illnesses during infancy predict subsequent childhood wheezing. *The Journal of Allergy and Clinical Immunology.* 2005;116(3):571–577.

24. Guilbert TW, Singh AM, Danov Z, Evans MD, Jackson DJ, Burton R, et al. Decreased lung function after preschool wheezing rhinovirus illnesses in children at risk to develop asthma. *The Journal of Allergy and Clinical Immunology.* 2011;128(3):532–538.

25. Carroll KN, Wu P, Gebretsadik T, Griffin MR, Dupont WD, Mitchel EF, et al. Season of infant bronchiolitis and estimates of subsequent risk and burden of early childhood asthma. *The Journal of Allergy and Clinical Immunology.* 2009;123(4):964–966.

26. Kusel MM, de Klerk NH, Kebadze T, Vohma V, Holt PG, Johnston SL, et al. Early-life respiratory viral infections, atopic sensitization, and risk of subsequent development of persistent asthma. *The Journal of Allergy and Clinical Immunology.* 2007;119(5):1105–1110.

27. Al-Garawi A, Fattouh R, Botelho F, Walker TD, Goncharova S, Moore CL, et al. Influenza A facilitates sensitization to house dust mite in infant mice leading to an asthma phenotype in adulthood. *Mucosal Immunology.* 2011;4(6):682–694.

28. Lee KK, Hegele RG, Manfreda J, Wooldrage K, Becker AB, Ferguson AC, et al. Relationship of early childhood viral exposures to respiratory symptoms, onset of possible asthma and atopy in high risk children: The Canadian Asthma Primary Prevention Study. *Pediatric Pulmonology.* 2007;42(3):290–297.

29. Proud D, Turner RB, Winther B, Wiehler S, Tiesman JP, Reichling TD, et al. Gene expression profiles during in vivo human rhinovirus infection: insights into the host response. *American Journal of Respiratory and Critical Care Medicine.* 2008;178(9):962–968.

30. Gern JE, Brooks GD, Meyer P, Chang A, Shen K, Evans MD, et al. Bidirectional interactions between viral respiratory illnesses and cytokine responses in the first year of life. *The Journal of Allergy and Clinical Immunology.* 2006;117(1):72–78.

31. Stern DA, Guerra S, Halonen M, Wright AL, Martinez FD. Low IFN-gamma production in the first year of life as a predictor of wheeze during childhood. *The Journal of Allergy and Clinical Immunology.* 2007;120(4):835–841.

32. Gill MA. The role of dendritic cells in asthma. *The Journal of Allergy and Clinical Immunology.* 2012;129(4):889–901.

33. Holt PG, Strickland DH, Sly PD. Virus infection and allergy in the development of asthma: What is the connection? *Current Opinion in Allergy and Clinical Immunology.* 2012;12(2):151–157.

34. McLoughlin RM, Calatroni A, Visness CM, Wallace PK, Cruikshank WW, Tuzova M, et al. Longitudinal relationship of early life immunomodulatory T cell phenotype and function to development of allergic sensitization in an urban cohort. *Clinical and Experimental Allergy.* 2012;42(3):392–404.

35. Bochkov YA, Hanson KM, Keles S, Brockman-Schneider RA, Jarjour NN, Gern JE. Rhinovirus-induced modulation of gene expression in bronchial epithelial cells from subjects with asthma. *Mucosal Immunology.* 2010;3(1):69–80.

36. Leigh R, Oyelusi W, Wiehler S, Koetzler R, Zaheer RS, Newton R, et al. Human rhinovirus infection enhances airway epithelial cell production of growth factors involved in airway remodeling. *The Journal of Allergy and Clinical Immunology.* 2008;121(5):1238–1245.

37. Pala P, Bjarnason R, Sigurbergsson F, Metcalfe C, Sigurs N, Openshaw PJ. Enhanced IL-4 responses in children with a history of respiratory syncytial virus bronchiolitis in infancy. *European Respiratory Journal.* 2002;20(2):376–382.

38. Siegle JS, Hansbro N, Herbert C, Rosenberg HF, Domachowske JB, Asquith KL, et al. Early-life viral infection and allergen exposure interact to induce an asthmatic phenotype in mice. *Respiratory Research.* 2010;11:14.

39. Lehtinen P, Ruohola A, Vanto T, Vuorinen T, Ruuskanen O, Jartti T. Prednisolone reduces recurrent wheezing after a first wheezing episode associated with rhinovirus infection or eczema. *The Journal of Allergy and Clinical Immunology.* 2007;119(3):570–575.

40. Simoes EA, Carbonell-Estrany X, Rieger CH, Mitchell I, Fredrick L, Groothuis JR. The effect of respiratory syncytial virus on subsequent recurrent wheezing in atopic and nonatopic children. *The Journal of Allergy and Clinical Immunology.* 2010;126(2):256–262.

41. Guilbert TW, Morgan WJ, Zeiger RS, Mauger DT, Boehmer SJ, Szefler SJ, et al. Long-term inhaled corticosteroids in preschool children at high risk for asthma. *The New England Journal of Medicine.* 2006;354(19):1985–1997.

42. Hughes CH, Jones RC, Wright DE, Dobbs FF. A retrospective study of the relationship between childhood asthma and respiratory infection during gestation. *Clinical and Experimental Allergy.* 1999;29(10):1378–1381.

43. Xu B, Pekkanen J, Jarvelin MR, Olsen P, Hartikainen AL. Maternal infections in pregnancy and the development of asthma among offspring. *International Journal of Epidemiology.* 1999;28(4):723–727.

44. Devereux G, Barker RN, Seaton A. Antenatal determinants of neonatal immune responses to allergens. *Clinical and Experimental Allergy.* 2002;32(1):43–50.

45. Vanderbeeken Y, Sarfati M, Bose R, Delespesse G. In utero immunization of the fetus to tetanus by maternal vaccination during pregnancy. *American Journal of Reproductive Immunology Microbiology.* 1985;8(2):39–42.

46. Babik JM, Cohan D, Monto A, Hartigan-O'Connor DJ, McCune JM. The human fetal immune response to hepatitis C virus exposure in utero. *Journal of Infectious Diseases.* 2011;203(2):196–206.

47. Rastogi D, Wang C, Mao X, Lendor C, Rothman PB, Miller RL. Antigen-specific immune responses to influenza vaccine in utero. *Journal of Clinical Investigation.* 2007;117(6):1637–1646.

48. Falsey AR. Respiratory syncytial virus infection in elderly and high-risk adults. *Experimental Lung Research.* 2005;31(Suppl. 1):77.

49. Corne JM, Marshall C, Smith S, Schreiber J, Sanderson G, Holgate ST, et al. Frequency, severity, and duration of rhinovirus infections in asthmatic and non-asthmatic individuals: A longitudinal cohort study. *Lancet.* 2002;359(9309):831–834.

50. Wark PA, Johnston SL, Bucchieri F, Powell R, Puddicombe S, Laza-Stanca V, et al. Asthmatic bronchial epithelial cells have a deficient innate immune response to infection with rhinovirus. *Journal of Experimental Medicine.* 2005;201(6):937–947.

51. Lopez-Souza N, Favoreto S, Wong H, Ward T, Yagi S, Schnurr D, et al. In vitro susceptibility to rhinovirus infection is greater for bronchial than for nasal airway epithelial cells in human subjects. *The Journal of Allergy and Clinical Immunology.* 2009;123(6):1384–1390.

52. Rakes GP, Arruda E, Ingram JM, Hoover GE, Zambrano JC, Hayden FG, et al. Rhinovirus and respiratory syncytial virus in wheezing children requiring emergency care. IgE and eosinophil analyses. *American Journal of Respiratory and Critical Care Medicine.* 1999;159(3):785–790.

53. Green RM, Custovic A, Sanderson G, Hunter J, Johnston SL, Woodcock A. Synergism between allergens and viruses and risk of hospital admission with asthma: Case–control study. *British Medical Journal.* 2002;324(7340):763.

54. Murray CS, Poletti G, Kebadze T, Morris J, Woodcock A, Johnston SL, et al. Study of modifiable risk factors for asthma exacerbations: Virus infection and allergen exposure increase the risk of asthma hospital admissions in children. *Thorax.* 2006;61(5):376–382.

55. Avila PC, Abisheganaden JA, Wong H, Liu J, Yagi S, Schnurr D, et al. Effects of allergic inflammation of the nasal mucosa on the severity of rhinovirus 16 cold. *The Journal of Allergy and Clinical Immunology.* 2000;105(5):923–932.

56. de Kluijver J, Evertse CE, Sont JK, Schrumpf JA, van Zeijl-van der Ham CJ, Dick CR, et al. Are rhinovirus-induced airway responses in asthma aggravated by chronic allergen exposure? *American Journal of Respiratory and Critical Care Medicine.* 2003;168(10):1174–1180.

57. Oliver BG, Lim S, Wark P, Laza-Stanca V, King N, Black JL, et al. Rhinovirus exposure impairs immune responses to bacterial products in human alveolar macrophages. *Thorax.* 2008;63(6):519–525.

58. Commins SP, Borish L, Steinke JW. Immunologic messenger molecules: Cytokines, interferons, and chemokines. *The Journal of Allergy and Clinical Immunology.* 2010;125(2 Suppl. 2):S53–S72.

59. Mukaida N. Interleukin-8: An expanding universe beyond neutrophil chemotaxis and activation. *International Journal of Hematology.* 2000;72(4):391–398.

60. Centers for Disease C, Prevention, Advisory Committee on Immunization P. Updated recommendations for prevention of invasive pneumococcal disease among adults using the 23-valent pneumococcal polysaccharide vaccine (PPSV23). *Morbidity and Mortality Weekly Report.* 2010;59(34):1102–1106.

61. Cates CJ, Jefferson TO, Rowe BH. Vaccines for preventing influenza in people with asthma. *Cochrane Database of Systematic Reviews.* 2008;(2):CD000364.

62. Johnston SL, Ferrero F, Garcia ML, Dutkowski R. Oral oseltamivir improves pulmonary function and reduces exacerbation frequency for influenza-infected children with asthma. *The Pediatric Infectious Disease Journal.* 2005;24(3):225–232.

63. Ducharme FM, Ni Chroinin M, Greenstone I, Lasserson TJ. Addition of long-acting beta2-agonists to inhaled corticosteroids versus same dose inhaled corticosteroids for chronic asthma in adults and children. *Cochrane Database of Systematic Reviews.* 2010;(5):CD005535.

64. Johnston SL, Blasi F, Black PN, Martin RJ, Farrell DJ, Nieman RB, et al. The effect of telithromycin in acute exacerbations of asthma. *The New England Journal of Medicine.* 2006;354(15):1589–1600.

65. Bisgaard H, Hermansen MN, Buchvald F, Loland L, Halkjaer LB, Bonnelykke K, et al. Childhood asthma after bacterial colonization of the airway in neonates. *The New England Journal of Medicine.* 2007;357(15):1487–1495.

10 Asthma and Allergens

James L. Friedlander, Sachin Baxi, and Wanda Phipatanakul

CONTENTS

CASE PRESENTATION

Kiara is a 10-year-girl who was diagnosed with asthma at the age of 3. She initially presented with multiple episodes of wheezing associated with viral upper respiratory infections in infancy. Around school age, she began to have more persistent symptoms of wheezing, which necessitated frequent albuterol use, and she was placed on a daily maintenance treatment with inhaled corticosteroid treatments. Despite the addition of a controller medication, she continued to have difficulty with asthma exacerbations, especially during the winter and spring months. She was referred to an allergist for further evaluation. A further history was elicited, which included a clear nasal discharge present on most days and the development of itchy red eyes and frequent sneezing while at her grandmother's home, which has two cats. She had tried over-the-counter antihistamine therapy for these symptoms with limited results. There was no history of food allergies, but she did have eczema as an infant. An environmental history revealed the presence of mice and cockroaches in the home.

A physical examination showed injected conjunctivae and the presence of Denny's lines. The nasal turbinates were edematous, pale, and boggy with clear rhinorrhea. There was a "cobblestone" appearance of her posterior pharynx. Her lungs were clear bilaterally with good aeration. A cardiac and abdominal examination was unremarkable. Her skin was significant for scattered eczematous patches along the flexural areas of her upper and lower extremities.

Kiara underwent skin prick testing to an inhalant environmental allergen panel including common indoor and outdoor allergens with positive histamine and negative saline controls. The testing revealed sensitization to dust mites, cats, mice, and cockroaches, along with multiple tree and grass pollens. The testing was negative to dogs, weeds, and molds.

Appropriate allergen avoidance and integrative pest management (IPM) strategies were discussed with Kiara's family. She was started on a leukotriene antagonist, a long-acting daily antihistamine, and a steroid nasal spray. The possibility of allergen immunotherapy was also discussed with her family.

INTRODUCTION

Asthma is a heterogeneous disease that is influenced by multiple factors including the environment, genetics, pollution, infection, and diet. Atopy, defined as a predisposition to developing allergic sensitization, is a strong predisposing factor for the development of asthma, and for over two decades, there has been increasing evidence that specific allergens can have a causative role in the development of asthma.[1,2] Environmental allergen sensitivity can also play an important role in the severity and treatment of asthma. The percentage of patients with asthma sensitized to ≥1 environmental allergen approaches 80%, and atopy may be the causative factor in over 50% of asthma cases.[3] An increased exposure to allergens in sensitized individuals can lead to more asthma morbidity and increased health-care utilization.[4–6] While many allergens are found indoors, the primary aeroallergens to which asthmatics are sensitized include house-dust mites, cats, dogs, mice, cockroaches, and mold (Table 10.1). This chapter will describe specific indoor allergens, highlighting their roles in asthma, and discuss strategies for their avoidance and environmental remediation.

BRIEF IMMUNOLOGICAL PRINCIPLES

In allergic asthma, individuals are sensitized to a variety of allergens. On reexposure to an offending inhaled allergen,

TABLE 10.1
Indoor Allergen Classification

Common Name	Taxonomic Name	Major Allergen(s)	Molecular Weight (kD)
House-dust mite	*Dermatophagoides pteronyssinus* and *D. farina*	Der p 1, Der f 1	24, 27
Cat	*Felis domesticus*	Fel d 1	17
Dog	*Canis familiaris*	Can f 1, 2	23, 19
Cockroach	*Blatella germanica* and *Periplaneta americana*	Bla g 1, Bla g 2, Per a 1	46, 36, 45
Mouse	*Mus musculus*	Mus m 1, 2	19,16

cross-linking of a specific immunoglobulin E (IgE) occurs on the surfaces of mast cells and triggers a rapid release of inflammatory mediators from the mast cells, including histamine, tryptase, and chymase. Within several hours, a late-phase reaction occurs, which is characterized by the release of leukotrienes, prostaglandins, and cluster of differentiation 4 (CD4+) type 2 helper T cell cytokines, such as interleukin (IL)-3, IL-4, IL-5, and IL-13. IL-4 is the major stimulus for IgE production, whereas IL-5 promotes the recruitment of eosinophils. An inflammatory mediator release causes increased vascular permeability, bronchial smooth muscle contraction, mucous secretion, and connective tissue matrix remodeling. The end result is chronic inflammation of the airways.

HOUSE-DUST MITE

House-dust mites are microscopic arachnids that thrive in the indoor environment and are prevalent in warm, humid home environments. They are commonly found in bedding (mattresses and pillows) and other products with woven or stuffed material, including stuffed animals. The most common species are *Dermatophagoides pteronyssinus* and *D. farinae*. Of the six major groups of dust mite allergens, the primary allergens are Der p 1 and Der f 1. Proteases found in the dust mite's gut and fecal particles are potent inducers of allergic disease.

The association between house-dust mite allergy and asthma has been well characterized.[1,6] In 1921, Kern first reported positive skin testing to house-dust mites in asthmatics using dust from patients' homes.[7] House-dust mite sensitization is present in over 50% of asthmatics and is a known risk factor for the development of childhood asthma.[8] A study by Sporik et al. showed that the relative risk of developing asthma was approximately five times greater in subjects with high levels of dust mite allergen exposure (>10 μg/g).[2] A more recent study by Celedon et al. demonstrated that early exposure to house-dust mites was associated with an increased risk of asthma and late-onset wheezing.[9]

There are several approaches to house-dust mite remediation (Table 10.2), and experts agree that a comprehensive strategy is best. This would include the use of dust mite encasings for mattresses and pillows,[10] washing linens weekly in hot water greater than 130°F, the removal of carpeting especially

TABLE 10.2
Dust Mite Allergen Avoidance and Patient Education

Basic Education Principles
- Assess home environment.
- Provide a general description of mites (including sources of food; human skin scales).
- Avoid conditions for optimal dust mite growth (keep humidity <50%).
- Identify local areas of dust mite growth (pillows, mattresses, box springs, carpet, upholstered furniture, draperies, stuffed animals).

Priorities for Mite/Allergen Avoidance
Bedroom
- Encase pillows (<10 μm pore fine-woven or vapor-permeable cover).
- Encase mattress in vapor-permeable or plastic cover.
- Encase box spring in vinyl or plastic.
- Wash bedding weekly in hot water (>130°F).

Floor
- Vacuum weekly (wear mask; leave room for 20 min after cleaning).
- Ensure vacuum cleaner has good-quality bags (double thickness) and/or high efficiency particulate air (HEPA) filter on air outlet.
- Clean smooth floors by vacuuming plus damp mopping.
- Loose rugs may be washed intermittently to remove allergens.

Furnishings
- If possible, replace with cleanable items that do not retain dust.
- Possible compromise may be regularly washing loose covers of tight-weave cloth.

Long-Term Changes
- Reduce indoor relative humidity (air conditioning [A/C], dehumidifier, open windows).
- Replace carpets with polished flooring (wood, vinyl, tile) if possible.
- Replace upholstered furniture with leather, vinyl, or wood.
- Replace draperies with shades or blinds that can be wiped down.
- Avoid living in basements.

in the bedroom, keeping humidity levels in the home to less than 50%, and using a high-efficiency particulate air (HEPA) filter vacuum on a weekly basis. Platts-Mills et al. looked at the long-term effects of avoiding house-dust mite allergens in nine asthmatics.[11] Clinical symptoms and morning peak flow measurements improved in all subjects, and five subjects tolerated significant increases in the concentration of histamine necessary to provoke a 30% fall in forced expiratory volume in 1 s (FEV_1).

CAT AND DOG

Domestic animal allergies are common in people with asthma. The primary cat allergen is Fel d 1, which is found in saliva, dander, and hair, and is produced in the sebaceous, salivary, and anal glands. The cat allergen can take several months to degrade once the primary source is removed from an indoor environment, and this allergen has been found in dust samples taken from environments without cat exposure, including schools and day cares.[12,13] The major dog allergen is Can f 1, which is also found in hair, saliva, and dander. Both cat and dog allergens consist of small particles that are capable of rapid dispersal in the air.

The role of pet allergen exposure and sensitization is unclear, as there is controversy over whether early, frequent exposure to pets will lead to sensitization or induce tolerance. Several recent studies suggest protective effects in reducing allergic sensitization in infants exposed to pet allergens.[14–16] Ingram et al., however, reported a strong correlation between asthma and children sensitized and exposed to increased levels of cat and dog allergens.[17] Overall, there is a general agreement that cat and dog allergens in sensitized asthmatic individuals can be problematic. Cat allergen exposure in sensitized individuals is also associated with decreased lung function in young children.[18]

The avoidance measures for pet allergens are summarized in Table 10.3. While the best way to eliminate a pet allergen is to remove the pet from the home, this is often difficult for families. If the pet remains, it is generally recommended to remove the pet from the bedroom and confine it to one area of the home as much as possible. Other effective strategies include the removal of all carpeting, the use of allergen-proof encasings for mattresses and pillows, and the use of HEPA filters and HEPA filter vacuums.

COCKROACH

The primary indoor species of cockroach are *Blattella germanica* (German cockroach) and *Periplaneta americana* (American cockroach). The major allergens are Bla g 1, Bla g 2, and Per a 1, which are found in fecal material, saliva, secretions, and debris. A cockroach infestation is associated with an urban, inner-city environment, a high population density, and a low socioeconomic status.

TABLE 10.3
Avoidance Measures for Pet Allergens

Basic Principles
- Emphasis is on control using allergy-proof encasings, furnishings (cleanable), carpets (removal/cleanable surfaces), and clothing (change if contaminated, wash regularly).
- Low confidence on methods that rely on chemicals.
- Focus on air filtration as a pet allergen is airborne for prolonged periods of time.

Control of Source
- Encourage the eviction of the animal, particularly where clinical effects are obvious and sensitization is present.
- If not possible, families can limit the animal's territory to indoor cleanable areas (kitchen) and confine it to the outdoors at other times.
- Note that an allergen is very persistent and can last many months, and its control may require aggressive cleaning and the removal of heavily contaminated items.

Additional Comments
- Measures may be required to prevent the significant transport of an allergen to houses without pets from houses with furred pets and from public buildings.
- Production varies widely between animals and over time, it is not well understood, and it is unlikely that truly allergen-free breeds of cats or dogs exist.

Rosenstreich et al. investigated home cockroach allergen exposure and asthma morbidity in urban home environments in inner-city children.[19] This study utilized the National Cooperative Inner-City Asthma Study (NCICAS), a cohort of 1528 children with asthma from 8 major inner-city areas in the United States. It was demonstrated that children who were sensitized to cockroaches and had evidence of elevated cockroach antigen levels in their homes had increased asthma morbidity. Specifically, children with asthma who were sensitized to cockroaches and had high cockroach allergen exposure levels in their homes had significantly higher rates of asthma-related hospitalization, more unscheduled medical visits per year, more days of wheezing, more school absences, more nights with lost sleep, and more disruption of their caregiver's plans. Rosenstreich's study highlighted the importance of the cockroach allergen as a unique and modifiable inner-city exposure, and led to further research focusing on cockroaches and other urban allergen exposures and their effects on asthma.[20,21] Exposure to the cockroach allergen in the home has also been associated with incident doctor-diagnosed asthma and recurrent wheezing.[22]

The cockroach allergen is also prevalent in schools. Over 66% of collected dust samples from urban Baltimore elementary schools had detectable levels of the cockroach allergen.[13] A similar study found detectable levels in 77% of 11 urban high schools in the northeastern United States.[23] Research is ongoing regarding the association of the cockroach allergen and asthma morbidity in the school setting.

Controlling a cockroach infestation is best accomplished with a comprehensive approach. This would include the use of insecticides, pesticides, and bait traps, along with sealing holes and cracks in the home. Eggleston et al. demonstrated a 51% reduction in the cockroach allergen by using education, extermination, HEPA filters, and bed encasings.[24] Cockroach management and control strategies are summarized in Table 10.4.

TABLE 10.4
Cockroach Management and Control Procedures

- Perform a careful inspection to detect insect hiding places and travel routes, and to identify food sources (grease, cooking debris).
- Remove sources of food and household food wastes (do not keep garbage cans inside, avoid exposed pet food and snack food containers).
- Remove or repair leaking faucets or condensation on pipes.
- Before applying an insecticide, perform a good general cleaning so that the insects are more likely to eat the gels or baits.
- Apply insecticides using gels or baits, in selected areas. In the kitchen, apply gel spots to cracks, crevices, the junctures of cupboards or walls with floors, and counters. Bait traps are just as effective as gel baits if they are used properly.
- Perform a section treatment after 1 or 2 weeks.
- After 1 week following the application of an insecticide, perform a thorough house cleaning, removing grease and other food debris.
- Wash bedding, curtains, and clothing.
- Consider the same principles for rodent or other pest management.

MOUSE

The major mouse allergens include mus m 1 and mus m 2, which are found in mouse urine, dander, and hair follicles. Similar to cockroaches, mouse infestations are more prevalent in urban, high population density environments, as well as high-rise apartments and homes with physical damage.

Studies by Phipatanakul and Matsui have highlighted the relationship between the mouse allergen and asthma.[25–28] Phipatanakul demonstrated detectable mouse allergen levels in 95% of homes in 499 subjects from the NCICAS, and also demonstrated that high mouse allergen levels can lead to sensitization. Homes with higher mouse allergen levels in this study had significantly higher rates of mouse sensitization.[28] In the Boston Home Allergens and Asthma Study, which included 500 infants of atopic parents, a significant association was seen between current mouse exposure and current wheeze through age 7. Early mouse exposure in infancy was predictive of atopy, but did not predict the presence of asthma or wheeze at age 7.[26] Matsui found that in mouse-sensitized, inner-city children, exposure to the mouse allergen may be an important cause of asthma morbidity.[27]

POLLEN AND MOLD

Detailed descriptions of the complexities involved in pollen and mold species are beyond the scope of this chapter. However, pollen and mold spore exposures can trigger asthma exacerbations or worsen the symptoms in sensitized individuals. Pollen's role in nature is to transport the male gamete (i.e., DNA) to the female part of a flower through wind or insect dispersal. In most parts of the United States, trees pollinate in the spring, grass pollinates from late spring to early summer, and weeds pollinate in late summer through fall. In tropical climates, these seasons can be longer.

Trees are either seed bearing (gymnosperms) or flowering (angiosperms), and most allergenic trees are in the flowering group.[29] Birch, oak, elm, and maple trees are common in the northeast and less prevalent in the southwest.[30] A single birch tree flower cluster can produce 6 million pollen grains. Tree pollens range in size from 20 to 50 μm.

Ragweed pollen is released in the morning and peaks by noon.[31] A single ragweed plant can expel a million pollen grains in a day. Species such as ragweed, lamb's quarter, and plantain are found throughout the United States. Weed pollens range in size from 10 to 20 μm.

Grass pollen is a common cause of springtime allergies. It is a larger pollen around 50 μm in size. Northern grasses in the United States include timothy, orchard, meadow, rye, Kentucky, redtop, and vernal, while southern grasses include Bermuda, Bahia, and Johnson.

Fungal spores are responsible for both seasonal and perennial allergy symptoms. Outdoor spores peak in mid-summer and diminish with the first hard frost in regions that experience cold winter seasons. Dry-air spores, including *Alternaria*, *Cladosporium*, and *Epicoccum*, peak in the afternoon hours under low humidity. Wet-air spores peak during the predawn hours with high humidity and include ascospores and basidiospores (mushrooms, puffballs). *Alternaria* is the most prevalent mold in dry, warm climates. It is commonly found in soil, seeds, and plants. Several studies have shown associations between *Alternaria* and severe asthma.[32–35] *Cladosporium* is the most prevalent spore in temperate regions and is the most commonly identified outdoor fungus. It is found on dead plants or vegetable matter. *Aspergillus* is often isolated from house dust. It is also found in compost heaps and dead vegetation. *Penicillium* is found in soil, food and grains, and house dust. It grows in water-damaged buildings, wallpaper, and decaying fabrics, giving a green "mildew" color. All of these molds induce allergic rhinitis, asthma, and hypersensitivity pneumonitis.

Pollen and fungal spore counts are collected the previous day and then counted; therefore, the reports that we see on television or on websites are a day late. The National Allergy Bureau (NAB) is part of the American Academy of Allergy, Asthma, and Immunology and it supplies the public with estimates of pollen and spore counts (www.aaaai.org/nab). The most common type of sampling devices is volumetric samplers that draw pollens and mold spores from the air. Studies have shown that there is a variation in pollen counts even between locations in the same city.[36,37] Therefore, one pollen count may not represent the entire city, but the information does inform people when their pollen season begins and pollen counts roughly correlate with the severity of symptoms.

Intact pollens range from 10 to 100 μm, though most have diameters between 20 and 35 μm, while fungal spores range from 2 to 50 μm.[38] These large particles are removed by the nasal mucosa and upper tracheobroncial passages. However, particles <5 μm generally reach the alveoli of the lungs.[39] An intact pollen is too large to reach the alveoli, but studies have shown that submicronic pollen-derived bioaerosols can reach the alveoli. For example, ryegrass pollen ruptures on contact with water and releases microscopic starch particles (0.5–2.5 μm) containing a major grass allergen. Such bioaerosols have been shown to be expulsed from pollens and mold spores.[40–43] While rain can wash pollen grains or spores from the air, the expulsed bioaerosols can trigger asthma exacerbations. Bioaerosols are thought to be associated with thunderstorm asthma epidemics.[39,40–43] In Melbourne, in 1987, there was a fivefold increase in asthma emergency department (ED) visits in a 24-h period after a thunderstorm. In 1989, there was a tenfold increase with 277 ED visits.[39,44] In 1994, in London, 40 patients presented with asthma flares within 24 h of a storm.[45,46]

A number of studies describe morbidity secondary to fungal exposure. *Alternaria* sensitivity has been found to be a risk factor for severe asthma attacks and epidemic asthma.[32,33] Targonski et al. demonstrated that Chicago asthma deaths were more than two times higher on days when there were 1000 spores per cubic meter.[34] Dales et al. studied the association between daily ED visits for asthma to a children's hospital and concentrations of pollen grains and fungal spores during a 5-year period.[47] The authors found that the concentration of fungal spores and not grass pollen significantly correlated

TABLE 10.5

Mold Management and Control Measures

Locate mold-contaminated items and remove them.

Clean moist areas as these are prone to mold growth.

Repair leaks.

Reduce humidity to <50%.

Consider the same principles in pollen avoidance for outdoor mold.

with ED visits. Sears et al. reported similar findings in a group of New Zealand children followed from birth to 13 years of age. The most common allergen sensitization was grass; however, a relative risk analysis demonstrated that sensitivity to house-dust mites, cats, dogs, and indoor mold was a highly significant risk factor associated with current asthma whereas sensitivity to grass was not a significant risk factor.[35]

Strategies for mold management are listed in Table 10.5 and include reducing humidity levels to less than 50% and promptly repairing leaks. It is not possible to control the pollen or mold spore level outside the home, but one can control the amount of allergen that gets inside the house. Two major components of control are keeping windows and doors closed during high counts and bathing to remove allergens in the hair and on the body (Table 10.4). HEPA filters can reduce pollen in the home.[48] Sensitized individuals with allergen-induced asthma can benefit from immunotherapy. A number of trials have shown that immunotherapy is beneficial in treating allergen-induced asthma.[49–54] Abramson et al. conducted a meta-analysis for the Cochrane Database of 20 published prospective, randomized, placebo-controlled trials of immunotherapy for asthma between 1960 and 1990, and concluded that immunotherapy reduces asthma symptoms and the use of asthma medications, and improves bronchial hyperreactivity.[50]

CURRENT AND FUTURE RESEARCH

While continuing to examine the role of indoor allergens in the home environment, research has recently been expanded to examine the role of indoor allergen exposure in other commonly encountered childhood environments such as schools and day-care centers.[55] Sheehan et al. found detectable levels of the mouse allergen in 89% of dust samples obtained from inner-city schools.[56] Permaul et al. recently investigated allergens in inner-city schools.[57] Over 400 airborne and settled dust samples from 12 inner-city schools were compared with 118 samples from the homes of asthmatic children attending these schools. The results showed substantial mouse allergen levels as well as increased levels of dog and cat allergens in the schools compared with the homes. The study concluded that mouse allergens in inner-city school classrooms may be a significant source of exposure for students.

The identification of urban allergen exposures such as cockroaches and mice, and their associations with allergen sensitization and asthma morbidity led to intervention strategies termed *integrative pest management*. This comprehensive approach involves education, extermination,

maintaining proper food storage, use of air filters, and sealing of holes and cracks in the home. IPM has been shown to significantly reduce mouse allergen levels in the homes of asthmatic children with mouse sensitization.[58] Ongoing studies are attempting to understand the role of interventions to reduce urban allergen exposures in homes and asthma morbidity. Furthermore, an understanding of allergen exposures, including mice[59–61] and mold,[62] in urban environments outside of the home, such as schools, is ongoing, and may prove to be important targets for effective and efficient intervention strategies to reduce allergenic triggers.

CONCLUSION

In atopic individuals, environmental allergens can play a significant role in asthma development and asthma morbidity. Patients with asthma, as in our patient case, can benefit from skin testing to identify common environmental inhalant allergens. Once the culprit allergens are identified in susceptible patients, the focus should shift to appropriate environmental remediation strategies, including education, avoidance, carpet removal, allergy-proof encasings, air filtration, HEPA filter vacuums, and IPM. The ongoing primary prevention trials are needed to determine whether the early reduction of indoor allergen exposures will decrease the risk of asthma development.

REFERENCES

1. Sears MR, Herbison GP, Holdaway MD, Hewitt CJ, Flannery EM, Silva PA. The relative risks of sensitivity to grass pollen, house dust mite and cat dander in the development of childhood asthma. *Clinical and Experimental Allergy.* 1989;19(4):419–424.
2. Sporik R, Holgate ST, Platts-Mills TA, Cogswell JJ. Exposure to house-dust mite allergen (Der p I) and the development of asthma in childhood. A prospective study. *The New England Journal of Medicine.* 1990;323(8):502–507.
3. Arbes Jr. SJ, Gergen PJ, Vaughn B, Zeldin DC. Asthma cases attributable to atopy: Results from the Third National Health and Nutrition Examination Survey. *Journal of Allergy and Clinical Immunology.* 2007;120(5):1139–1145.
4. Platts-Mills T, Leung DY, Schatz M. The role of allergens in asthma. *American Family Physician.* 2007;76(5):675–680.
5. Platts-Mills TA, Vervloet D, Thomas WR, Aalberse RC, Chapman MD. Indoor allergens and asthma: Report of the Third International Workshop. *Journal of Allergy and Clinical Immunology.* 1997;100(6 Pt 1):S2–S24.
6. Squillace SP, Sporik RB, Rakes G, Couture N, Lawrence A, Merriam S, Zhang J, Platts-Mills AE. Sensitization to dust mites as a dominant risk factor for asthma among adolescents living in central Virginia. Multiple regression analysis of a population-based study. *American Journal of Respiratory and Critical Care Medicine.* 1997;156(6):1760–1764.
7. Kern RA. Dust sensitization in bronchial asthma. *Journal of Immunology.* 1921;10:465.
8. Peat JK, Tovey E, Toelle BG, Haby MM, Gray EJ, Mahmic A, Woolcock AJ. House dust mite allergens. A major risk factor for childhood asthma in Australia. *American Journal of Respiratory and Critical Care Medicine.* 1996;153(1):141–146.

9. Celedon JC, Milton DK, Ramsey CD, Litonjua AA, Ryan L, Platts-Mills TA, Gold DR. Exposure to dust mite allergen and endotoxin in early life and asthma and atopy in childhood. *Journal of Allergy and Clinical Immunology.* 2007;120(1):144–149.

10. Halken S, Host A, Niklassen U, Hansen LG, Nielsen F, Pedersen S, Osterballe O, Veggerby C, Poulsen LK. Effect of mattress and pillow encasings on children with asthma and house dust mite allergy [Comment]. *Journal of Allergy and Clinical Immunology.* 2003;111(1):169–176.

11. Platts-Mills TA, Tovey ER, Mitchell EB, Moszoro H, Nock P, Wilkins SR. Reduction of bronchial hyperreactivity during prolonged allergen avoidance. *Lancet.* 1982;2(8300):675–678.

12. Instanes C, Hetland G, Berntsen S, Lovik M, Nafstad P. Allergens and endotoxin in settled dust from day-care centers and schools in Oslo, Norway. *Indoor Air.* 2005;15(5):356–362.

13. Amr S, Bollinger ME, Myers M, Hamilton RG, Weiss SR, Rossman M, Osborne L, et al. Environmental allergens and asthma in urban elementary schools. *Annals of Allergy, Asthma and Immunology.* 2003;90(1):34–40.

14. Perzanowski MS, Chew GL, Divjan A, Johnson A, Goldstein IF, Garfinkel RS, Hoepner LA, Platts-Mills TA, Perera FP, Miller RL. Cat ownership is a risk factor for the development of anti-cat IgE but not current wheeze at age 5 years in an inner-city cohort. *Journal of Allergy and Clinical Immunology.* 2008;121(4):1047–1052.

15. Ownby DR, Johnson CC. Does exposure to dogs and cats in the first year of life influence the development of allergic sensitization? *Current Opinion in Allergy and Clinical Immunology.* 2003;3(6):517–522.

16. Ownby DR, Johnson CC, Peterson EL. Exposure to dogs and cats in the first year of life and risk of allergic sensitization at 6 to 7 years of age. *JAMA.* 2002;288(8):963–972.

17. Ingram JM, Sporik R, Rose G, Honsinger R, Chapman MD, Platts-Mills TA. Quantitative assessment of exposure to dog (Can f 1) and cat (Fel d 1) allergens: relation to sensitization and asthma among children living in Los Alamos, New Mexico. *Journal of Allergy and Clinical Immunology.* 1995;96(4):449–456.

18. Lowe LA, Woodcock A, Murray CS, Morris J, Simpson A, Custovic A. Lung function at age 3 years: Effect of pet ownership and exposure to indoor allergens. *Archives of Pediatrics and Adolescent Medicine.* 2004;158(10):996–1001.

19. Rosenstreich DL, Eggleston P, Kattan M, Baker D, Slavin RG, Gergen P, Mitchell H, et al. The role of cockroach allergy and exposure to cockroach allergen in causing morbidity among inner-city children with asthma. *New England Journal of Medicine.* 1997;336(19):1356–1363.

20. Gruchalla RS, Pongracic J, Plaut M, Evans III R, Visness CM, Walter M, Crain EF, et al. Inner City Asthma Study: Relationships among sensitivity, allergen exposure, and asthma morbidity. *Journal of Allergy and Clinical Immunology.* 2005;115(3):478–485.

21. Chew GL, Perzanowski MS, Canfield SM, Goldstein IF, Mellins RB, Hoepner LA, Ashby-Thompson M, Jacobson JS. Cockroach allergen levels and associations with cockroach-specific IgE. *Journal of Allergy and Clinical Immunology.* 2008;121(1):240–245.

22. Litonjua AA, Carey VJ, Burge HA, Weiss ST, Gold DR. Exposure to cockroach allergen in the home is associated with incident doctor-diagnosed asthma and recurrent wheezing. *Journal of Allergy and Clinical Immunology.* 2001;107(1):41–47.

23. Chew GL, Correa JC, Perzanowski MS. Mouse and cockroach allergens in the dust and air in northeastern United States inner-city public high schools. *Indoor Air.* 2005;15(4):228–234.

24. Eggleston PA, Butz A, Rand C, Curtin-Brosnan J, Kanchanaraksa S, Swartz L, Breysse P, et al. Home environmental intervention in inner-city asthma: A randomized controlled clinical trial. *Annals of Allergy, Asthma and Immunology.* 2005;95(6):518–524.

25. Phipatanakul W. Rodent allergens. *Current Allergy and Asthma Reports.* 2002;2(5):412–416.

26. Phipatanakul W, Celedon JC, Sredl DL, Weiss ST, Gold DR. Mouse exposure and wheeze in the first year of life. *Annals of Allergy, Asthma and Immunology.* 2005;94(5):593–599.

27. Matsui EC, Eggleston PA, Buckley TJ, Krishnan JA, Breysse PN, Rand CS, Diette GB. Household mouse allergen exposure and asthma morbidity in inner-city preschool children. *Annals of Allergy, Asthma and Immunology.* 2006;97(4):514–520.

28. Phipatanakul W, Eggleston PA, Wright EC, Wood RA. Mouse allergen. II. The relationship of mouse allergen exposure to mouse sensitization and asthma morbidity in inner-city children with asthma. *Journal of Allergy and Clinical Immunology.* 2000;106(6):1075–1080.

29. Esch R, Bush, RK. Aerobiology of outdoor allergens. In: Adkinson NF, Yunginger, JW, Busse WW, eds. *Middleton's Allergy Princliples & Practice.* Philadelphia, PA: Mosby, 2003.

30. Kagen S, Lewis W, Levetin E. *Aeroallergen PhotoLibrary of North America,* Ark Studies, Appleton, WI, 2004.

31. Barnes C, Pacheco F, Landuyt J, Hu F, Portnoy J. Hourly variation of airborne ragweed pollen in Kansas City. *Annals of Allergy, Asthma and Immunology.* 2001;86(2):166–171.

32. Pulimood TB, Corden JM, Bryden C, Sharples L, Nasser SM. Epidemic asthma and the role of the fungal mold Alternaria alternata. *Journal of Allergy and Clinical Immunology.* 2007;120(3):610–617.

33. O'Hollaren MT, Yunginger JW, Offord KP, Somers MJ, O'Connell EJ, Ballard DJ, Sachs MI. Exposure to an aeroallergen as a possible precipitating factor in respiratory arrest in young patients with asthma. *New England Journal of Medicine.* 1991;324(6):359–363.

34. Targonski PV, Persky VW, Ramekrishnan V. Effect of environmental molds on risk of death from asthma during the pollen season. *Journal of Allergy and Clinical Immunology.* 1995;95(5 Pt 1):955–961.

35. Sears MR, Herbison GP, Holdaway MD, Hewitt CJ, Flannery EM, Silva PA. The relative risks of sensitivity to grass pollen, house dust mite and cat dander in the development of childhood asthma. *Clinical and Experimental Allergy.* 1989;19(4):419–424.

36. Katelaris CH, Burke TV, Byth K. Spatial variability in the pollen count in Sydney, Australia: can one sampling site accurately reflect the pollen count for a region? *Annals of Allergy, Asthma and Immunology.* 2004;93(2):131–136.

37. Frenz DA. Interpreting atmospheric pollen counts for use in clinical allergy: Spatial variability. *Annals of Allergy, Asthma and Immunology.* 2000;84(5):481–489.

38. Portnoy J, Barnes C. Clinical relevance of spore and pollen counts. *Immunology and Allergy Clinics of North America.* 2003;23(3):389–410.

39. Suphioglu C. Thunderstorm asthma due to grass pollen. *International Archives of Allergy and Immunology.* 1998;116(4):253–260.

40. Taylor PE, Flagan RC, Miguel AG, Valenta R, Glovsky MM. Birch pollen rupture and the release of aerosols of respirable allergens. *Clinical and Experimental Allergy.* 2004;34(10):1591–1596.

41. Taylor PE, Flagan RC, Valenta R, Glovsky MM. Release of allergens as respirable aerosols: A link between grass pollen and asthma. *Journal of Allergy and Clinical Immunology.* 2002;109(1):51–56.

42. Taylor PE, Jonsson H. Thunderstorm asthma. *Current Allergy and Asthma Reports.* 2004;4(5):409–413.

43. Grote M, Vrtala S, Niederberger V, Valenta R, Reichelt R. Expulsion of allergen-containing materials from hydrated rye grass (*Lolium perenne*) pollen revealed by using immunogold field emission scanning and transmission electron microscopy. *Journal of Allergy and Clinical Immunology.* 2000;105(6 Pt 1):1140–1145.

44. Bellomo R, Gigliotti P, Treloar A, Holmes P, Suphioglu C, Singh MB, Knox B. Two consecutive thunderstorm associated epidemics of asthma in the city of Melbourne. The possible role of rye grass pollen. *Medical Journal of Australia.* 1992;156(12):834–837.

45. Davidson AC, Emberlin J, Cook AD, Venables KM. A major outbreak of asthma associated with a thunderstorm: Experience of accident and emergency departments and patients' characteristics. Thames Regions Accident and Emergency Trainees Association. *British Medical Journal.* 1996;312(7031):601–604.

46. Celenza A, Fothergill J, Kupek E, Shaw RJ. Thunderstorm associated asthma: A detailed analysis of environmental factors. *British Medical Journal.* 1996;312(7031):604–607.

47. Dales RE, Cakmak S, Burnett RT, Judek S, Coates F, Brook JR. Influence of ambient fungal spores on emergency visits for asthma to a regional children's hospital. *American Journal of Respiratory and Critical Care Medicine.* 2000;162(6):2087–2090.

48. Sublett JL, Seltzer J, Burkhead R, Williams PB, Wedner HJ, Phipatanakul W. Air filters and air cleaners: Rostrum by the American Academy of Allergy, Asthma & Immunology Indoor Allergen Committee. *Journal of Allergy and Clinical Immunology.* 2009.

49. Cox L, Li JT, Nelson H, Lockey R. Allergen immunotherapy: A practice parameter second update. *Journal of Allergy and Clinical Immunology.* 2007;120(3 Suppl):S25–S85.

50. Abramson MJ, Puy RM, Weiner JM. Allergen immunotherapy for asthma. *Cochrane Database Systematic Review.* 2003(4):CD001186.

51. Durham SR, Walker SM, Varga EM, Jacobson MR, O'Brien F, Noble W, Till SJ, Hamid QA, Nouri-Aria KT. Long-term clinical efficacy of grass-pollen immunotherapy. *New England Journal of Medicine.* 1999;341(7):468–475.

52. Moller C, Dreborg S, Ferdousi HA, Halken S, Host A, Jacobsen L, Koivikko A, et al. Pollen immunotherapy reduces the development of asthma in children with seasonal rhinoconjunctivitis (the PAT-study). *Journal of Allergy and Clinical Immunology.* 2002;109(2):251–256.

53. Walker SM, Varney VA, Gaga M, Jacobson MR, Durham SR. Grass pollen immunotherapy: Efficacy and safety during a 4-year follow-up study. *Allergy.* 1995;50(5):405–413.

54. Walker SM, Pajno GB, Lima MT, Wilson DR, Durham SR. Grass pollen immunotherapy for seasonal rhinitis and asthma: A randomized, controlled trial. *Journal of Allergy and Clinical Immunology.* 2001;107(1):87–93.

55. Salo PM, Sever ML, Zeldin DC. Indoor allergens in school and day care environments. *Journal of Allergy and Clinical Immunology.* 2009;124(2):185–192.

56. Sheehan WJ, Rangsithienchai PA, Muilenberg ML, Rogers CA, Lane JP, Ghaemghami J, Rivard DV, et al. Mouse allergens in urban elementary schools and homes of children with asthma. *Annals of Allergy, Asthma and Immunology.* 2009;102(2):125–130.

57. Permaul P, Hoffman E, Fu C, Sheehan W, Baxi S, Gaffin J, Lane J, et al. Allergens in urban schools and homes of children with asthma. *Pediatrics Allergy and Immunology.* 2012;23(6):543–549.

58. Phipatanakul W, Cronin B, Wood RA, Eggleston PA, Shih MC, Song L, Tachdjian R, Oettgen HC. Effect of environmental intervention on mouse allergen levels in homes of inner-city Boston children with asthma. *Annals of Allergy, Asthma and Immunology.* 2004;92(4):420–425.

59. Permaul P, Hoffman E, Fu C, Sheehan W, Baxi S, Gaffin J, Lane J, et al. Allergens in urban schools and homes of children with asthma. *Pediatrics Allergy and Immunology.* 2012;23(6):543–549.

60. Permaul P, Petty C, Sheehan W, Baxi S, Gaffin J, Kopel L, Kanchongkittiphan W, et al. Mouse allergen exposure in urban schools and its effect on childhood asthma morbidity. *Journal of Allergy and Clinical Immunology.* 2013;131(2):AB503.

61. Sheehan WJ, Rangsithienchai PA, Muilenberg ML, Rogers CA, Lane JP, Ghaemghami J, Rivard DV, et al. Mouse allergens in urban elementary schools and homes of children with asthma. *Annals of Allergy, Asthma and Immunology.* 2009;102(2):125–130.

62. Baxi S, Petty C, Fu C, Sheehan W, Permaul P, Rogers C, Muilenberg M, DR Gold, Phipatanakul W. Classroom fungal spore exposure and asthma morbidity in inner-city school children. *Journal of Allergy and Clinical Immunology.* 2013;131:AB54 (*in press*).

11 Air Pollutants

Neil E. Alexis and Chris Carlsten

CONTENTS

CASE PRESENTATION

A 38-year-old professor moved from a rural community to a dense urban environment. She had long enjoyed bicycle commuting to work, and recalled the calming effect of her rides along a flat and quiet bike path to the small college campus of her former employment. Her new bicycle route to work would logically take her through streets with the most prominent vehicular traffic, in order to pursue the most direct path to her office. Within weeks of settling into her new environment, she noted wheezing toward the end of her 30-min ride to the university. She had asthma as a child but had been asymptomatic since her teenage years. Her new physician recommended that she obtain peak flow readings throughout both her commuting workdays and weekend days (during which she did not exercise). She recorded such readings four times daily for 4 weeks during April and demonstrated that peak flows were generally above 500 L/sec throughout the weekend days and in the mornings of workdays, but they dropped intermittently below 400 L/sec at the midmorning and early afternoon weekday readings. The midmorning reading was performed shortly after her arrival at work, at the end of her bicycle commute but before she entered her office. The lowest readings were associated with wheezing but were unassociated with the daily temperature or humidity. However, the overall pattern (lower average readings on workdays with her bike commute than on weekends when she generally stayed at home) became more obvious and severe toward the end of the month of data gathering.

With this information, her physician suspected that traffic-related air pollution was exacerbating her asthma, previously quiescent during her recent decades in a small, rural academic community. He further suspected that she had an allergy to trees that had not been prominent in her last community and that these tree allergens were interacting with the traffic-related particulate matter (PM) to augment the adverse effect on her asthma.

A referral to an allergist who tested her to aeroallergens revealed that she was sensitized to birch pollen by skin prick testing. The professor's bicycling route was analyzed in terms of the proportion of time that she spent on or within 300 m of major roadways (with four lines of traffic) and it was noted that 70% of her commute was in such proximity to high-traffic byways.

On advice from her physician, the professor was able to map out an alternate route by which only 15% of her time was within 300 m of a major roadway, and after a trial she noted that the duration of her commute increased by only 4 min in each direction. Following this new route over the next month, the frequency of her wheezing and peak flow readings below 400 L/min decreased dramatically.

INTRODUCTION

Asthma is a disease characterized by intermittent broncho-constriction due to increased airway responsiveness to both allergic and nonallergic stimuli. Airways inflammation is a key underlying feature of this disease. Epidemiological evidence from the last two decades has shown that environmental pollutants such as ozone, PM, diesel exhaust (DE), and biological/microbial agents contribute significantly to the morbidity associated with asthma, including increasing exacerbation frequency.[1–4] More recently, some pollutants, such as ozone, are now being implicated as causal agents in the development of new-onset asthma. Of note, the association between asthma exacerbation and air pollution has been reported at pollutant levels below the current ambient air quality standard. Moreover, studies have now focused on certain exposure locations, such as living near busy roadways or high traffic areas, as places of particularly high risk to suffer the deleterious effects of air pollution.[5] As noted in the preceding case study, daily (Monday to Friday) exercise (bicycling) exposure near a busy urban roadway in combination with exposure to high levels of a specific allergen (birch pollen), was the likely cause of enhanced asthma exacerbations in a patient who, prior to this routine exposure, was symptomatically quiescent. Furthermore, in the absence of this exposure routine on weekends, her frequency of symptoms was significantly reduced. This case study draws our attention to the fact that air pollution may be affecting the airway's host defense capability to allergens or equally feasible, and according to recent evidence,[6] it may even augment exposure to airborne allergens.

The public health concern regarding the effect of air pollution on asthma is valid. It is estimated that over 120 million people in the United States live in areas that are not in compliance with current air pollutant standards. Therefore, poor air quality in many places remains a significant problem for patients with asthma. This chapter will review our current understanding of asthma and air pollution by examining recent findings in the context of association-based evidence provided by epidemiological and cohort studies, as well as effects-based evidence generated from controlled chamber studies.

MODIFYING FACTORS

At the outset, it is prudent to recognize that a myriad of factors must be considered when discussing the impact of air pollution on asthma. These factors can all contribute to the heterogeneity in the results often observed when examining this complex area. These factors are typically related to: (a) subject phenotype such as age (childhood vs. adult asthma), race, gender, body mass index (BMI), and asthma inflammatory phenotype and genotype; (b) differences in study design and analysis techniques, that is, the proximity to exposure versus the estimation of exposure by using land-use regression modeling; (c) implementation of different exposure matrices; and (d) use of a range of methods to measure clinical and biological outcomes. For example, studying asthma exacerbation in existing asthmatics is quite different from assessing whether a pollutant is causing new-onset asthma. Likewise, the measurement and sampling techniques for inflammatory biomarkers in patients are not necessarily interchangeable or comparable; for example, the use of induced sputum examines cellular and biochemical markers of inflammation on the surfaces of the central airways[7] compared with bronchoalveolar lavage, which reflects events in the more distal airways. Therefore, caution must be used when making direct study comparisons or including studies in meta-analyses where different measurement and analysis methodologies have been used.

AIR POLLUTION AND ASTHMA EXACERBATION

It is widely accepted that air pollution can exacerbate asthma in those individuals who already have the condition. Many studies from the past several years have reported significant associations between exposure to air pollution (ozone, PM, diesel exhaust particles [DEPs], mold/fungal spores) and asthma exacerbations, and in the case of certain pollutants such as ozone, a lag time of 1–2 days following exposure is correlated with increased admissions to emergency departments (ED) for respiratory complaints.[8–13] Recent studies continue to support the association between air pollution and asthma. For example, Glad et al.[14] examined ED visits for asthma (a specific metric for asthma exacerbation) over a period of 3 years (2003–2005) in 6979 individuals. They reported a 2.5% increase in asthma ED visits for each 10 ppb increase in the 1 h maximum ozone level on day 2 after exposure, which was associated with a significant odds ratio (OR = 1.025, $P < .05$). PM2.5 (coarse size PM) also had a significant effect (OR = 1.036, $P < .05$) on ED visits on day 1 after exposure in the total population examined and on days 1, 2, and 3 in the African American population but not the Caucasian population. These more current epidemiological data continue to support the long-held view that there is a clear association between air pollution and asthma exacerbation. Several meta-analyses have been conducted on cohort studies that examined specific communities living in close proximity to traffic-related pollutants in order to define their specific impact on asthma morbidity. These studies generally agree that an association exists between asthma prevalence (the number of existing cases of asthma) and exposure to traffic, particularly in children.[15,16] A recent meta-analysis of 19 studies conducted by Gasana and colleagues[16] concluded that exposure to the traffic-related pollutants nitrogen dioxide ([NO$_2$] meta-OR: 1.05; 95% confidence interval [CI]: 1.0–1.1), nitrous oxide (meta-OR: 1.02; 95% CI: 1.0–1.04), and carbon monoxide (meta-OR: 1.06; 95% CI: 1.0–1.02) was positively associated with a higher prevalence of childhood asthma. Indeed, even more specific components of the traffic exposure matrix have begun to emerge as important. For example, Eckel and colleagues[17] recently reported that the length of a roadway was the only significant indicator of residential traffic-related pollution exposure associated with airway inflammation in children with asthma. The relationship between asthma and air pollution, however, has been more difficult to establish when analyzing beyond individual communities. In other words, the relationship does not appear to hold when the analysis is expanded to the community level. For example, Anderson and colleagues,[18] using satellite-based estimates of ambient air pollution and global variations in childhood asthma prevalence, reported no evidence of a positive association between air pollution levels and childhood asthma prevalence.

AIR POLLUTION AND NEW-ONSET ASTHMA

Evidence has been emerging over the last 3–4 years that air pollution, specifically traffic-related air pollutants, may be contributing to new-onset asthma. One of the early reports from Islam and colleagues[19] from Southern California showed that functional polymorphisms in the genes regulating antioxidant defense capability were related to asthma onset in children, and this effect was dependent on living in a high-ozone or a low-ozone environment. A year later, Jarrett et al.[20] reported on a prospective cohort study in children using personal exposure measurements (Southern California Children's Health Study). In models controlling for confounders, "incident" (new-onset) asthma was positively associated with traffic pollution, with a hazard ratio (HR) of 1.29 (95% CI, 1.07–1.56) across the average within-community interquartile range of 6.2 ppb in annual residential NO_2. McConnell[21] also reported that modeled exposure to nonfreeway traffic-related pollutants both at home and in school increased the risk of children developing new-onset asthma. There is quite a lot of evidence (some of it methodologically stronger than others) that there is a weak association, particularly with exposure to traffic within cities. In contrast, when traffic within whole cities is compared, there is generally no (ecological) association with asthma prevalence.[22,23] Two recent reviews of meta-analyses examining the association between asthma incidence and air pollution were conducted by Gasana[16] in South Florida and Gowers[15] in the United Kingdom. Both analyses concluded that there is a positive association between the prevalence of asthma symptoms and possible asthma incidence and traffic-related pollutants. Specifically, the U.S. study identified the exposure to NO_2 as having a positive association with childhood asthma incidence (meta-OR: 1.14; 95% CI: 1.06–1.24). The influence of traffic-related pollutants (DEPs) on very early-age groups was assessed in the Cincinnati Childhood Allergy and Air Pollution Study (CCAAPS) birth cohort. That study concluded that the proximity to stop-and-go traffic with high bus and truck concentrations predicted persistent wheeze during infancy and DEP exposure was significantly associated with wheeze at age 1 and persistent wheeze at age 3.[24] An additional longitudinal follow-up of this population is necessary to confirm whether persistent wheezing in this population represents the development of asthma. The evidence suggests that in addition to air pollution acting as an exacerbating agent, air pollutants, particularly traffic-related ones, may be contributing to the development of new-onset asthma.

Epidemiological studies and cohort studies can highlight the association between disease and exposure, but they cannot assess how individual pollutants affect the biology and physiology of asthma. To address these questions, chamber exposure studies are used in which individuals (asthmatic and nonasthmatics) are exposed to selected pollutants under carefully controlled conditions, such as exposure duration, pollutant concentration, and ventilation or breathing rate. Clinical and biological outcome measures are obtained both before and after exposure. Much evidence has been acquired from these types of controlled exposure studies to further our understanding of how pollutants are exerting their effects on the biology and physiology of asthma.

EFFECT OF AIR POLLUTANTS ON ASTHMA BIOLOGY

To understand how oxidant pollutants such as ozone, or biological/bacterial-based pollutants such as endotoxin affect the biology of asthma, it is important to appreciate the constitutive state of the asthmatic airway prior to exposure in terms of inflammation, immunology, and physiology. This will allow a better appreciation of how the asthmatic airway is predisposed to respond to a particular air pollutant, especially since pollutants differ in their mechanisms of action. For example, pollutants such as ozone or PM[25,26] will induce oxidative stress responses, whereas pollutants with biological components adhered to their surface, such as bacterial endotoxin on coarse size PM (PM2.5–10) or peptidoglycan/gram-positive bacteria on swine dust,[27] may exert their effects primarily or initially through innate immune mechanisms. In terms of airways inflammation, there are different asthma phenotypes to be recognized (eosinophilic, neutrophilic, paucigranulocytic) and these differ according to the stability of the disease (stable vs. acute) and whether it is present in children or adults. For acute asthma, the eosinophilic phenotype predominates in children (50%), while in adults, the neutrophilic phenotype predominates (82%) and is negatively correlated with lung function and airflow obstruction.[28,29] For stable asthma, the paucigranulocytic phenotype appears to be the most common in both children and adults. In terms of microbial presence, it has now become clear that more severe asthmatics have increased microbial colonization of the airways[30,31] and, in fact, they have an increased risk of invasive pneumococcal disease.[32,33] A recent study conducted in Sao Paulo, Brazil, reported that indoor levels of NO_2 and personal exposure to ozone were significantly associated with the prevalence of pneumonia ($P = .02$) in asthmatic children.[34] In general, asthmatic patients have increased lower respiratory tract symptoms, greater impairment of their lung function, and increased bronchial hyperresponsiveness. However, pertinent to how they may respond to inhaled pollutants, asthmatics have a diminished innate immune response capability and depleted levels of antioxidants.[35,36] Several years ago, Alexis showed that sputum macrophages from eosinophilic asthmatics had decreased expression of the innate immune cell-surface marker cluster of differentiation 64 (CD64) and decreased phagocytic capacity (Figure 11.1a), where the latter effect was positively correlated with markers of asthma severity (PC_{20,FEV_1}; forced expiratory volume in 1 s [FEV_1] percentage; eosinophils percentage) (Figure 11.1b).[35]

More recently, Newcomb and Peebles[37] showed that asthmatics have muted interferon gamma (IFNγ) and interleukin (IL)-10 responses following a challenge with an experimental rhinovirus infection, while Brickey[38] recently reported that asthmatics have decreased inflammasome gene expression, arguably making them more susceptible to the deleterious effects of inhaled pollutants. Kongerud et al.[36] also showed that asthma patients have deficient levels of the potent antioxidant ascorbic acid in their airways, thus making them more susceptible to inhaled environmental oxidants such as ozone,

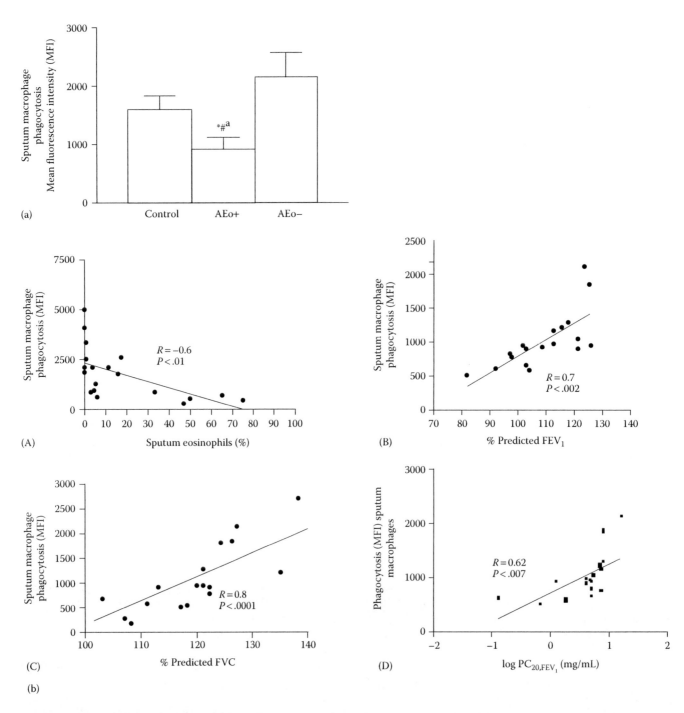

FIGURE 11.1 (a) Sputum macrophage phagocytosis of IgG-opsonized yeast (in the presence of human serum) expressed as the mean fluorescence intensity (MFI) in healthy controls, eosinophilic asthmatics (AEo+), and noneosinophilic asthmatics (AEo−). Compared with healthy controls and AEo− subjects, AEo+ subjects demonstrated decreased phagocytosis. *Significantly different from AEo− subjects; #significantly different from control; [a]$P < .01$. (b) Linear regression analysis of sputum macrophage phagocytosis (expressed as mean fluorescence intensity) and sputum eosinophils (%) in all asthmatics. (A) A significant ($P = .01$) negative correlation ($R = −0.6$) was observed between phagocytosis and the percentage of sputum eosinophils. (B) and (C) Linear regression analyses of sputum macrophage phagocytosis (MFI) and the percentage of predicted forced expiratory volume in 1 s (FEV$_1$; B) and forced vital capacity (FVC; C) in all asthmatics. Significant positive linear correlations were observed between sputum macrophage phagocytosis and the percentage of predicted FEV$_1$ ($R = 0.7$, $P < .002$) and FVC ($R = 0.8$, $P < .0001$). (D) Linear regression analysis of sputum macrophage phagocytosis (MFI) and nonspecific airway responsiveness (provocative concentration that produces a 20% fall in FEV$_1$ [PC$_{20,\text{FEV}_1}$]) in all asthmatics. A significant ($P < .007$) positive correlation ($R = 0.6$) was observed between sputum macrophage phagocytosis and PC$_{20,\text{FEV}_1}$. (From Alexis, N.E., Soukup, J., Nierkens, and S., Becker, S., *Am. J. Physiol. Lung Cell Mol. Physiol.*, 280, L369–L375, 2001. With permission.)

and less able to neutralize endogenously derived free radicals produced from activated inflammatory cells.

OZONE

Asthmatics have been studied for several years following controlled inhalation challenges with pollutants such as ozone, endotoxin, PM, and DEPs. Among these pollutants, ozone has been the most extensively examined. Following a controlled exposure to ozone, the most noted and consistent effects observed in both asthmatics and nonasthmatics are symptoms such as pain on deep inspiration, decrements in lung function (FEV_1), increased neutrophil levels, and elevated proinflammatory cytokines (IL-8, IL-6) in the airways. Other less consistent effects that have been reported include increased airway reactivity and increased airway eosinophil levels in atopic individuals. In terms of ozone-induced changes in their lung function and airways inflammation, it

is, in fact, debatable whether asthmatics have an enhanced response compared with nonasthmatics. Hernandez et al.[39] examined spirometric and inflammatory responses to 2 h 0.4 ppm ozone exposure in both allergic asthmatics and healthy volunteers. They reported equivalent nociceptive decreases in lung function and neutrophil influx to the airways, but did observe that asthmatics had significantly increased expression of CD23, FcεRI, and TLR4 on sputum macrophages (Figure 11.2), increased levels of proinflammatory cytokines IL-6, IL-8, and IL-1b, and decreased levels of IL-10 before and after ozone exposure.

Furthermore, Hernandez reported that the gene expression profiles of the airway cells from asthmatics had increased immune signaling and upregulated expression of the human epidermal growth factor receptor 2 (HER-2) gene network compared with nonasthmatics, suggesting in the case of HER-2, an inability to limit epithelial cell proliferative responses following ozone-induced oxidative stress.[40] Together, these

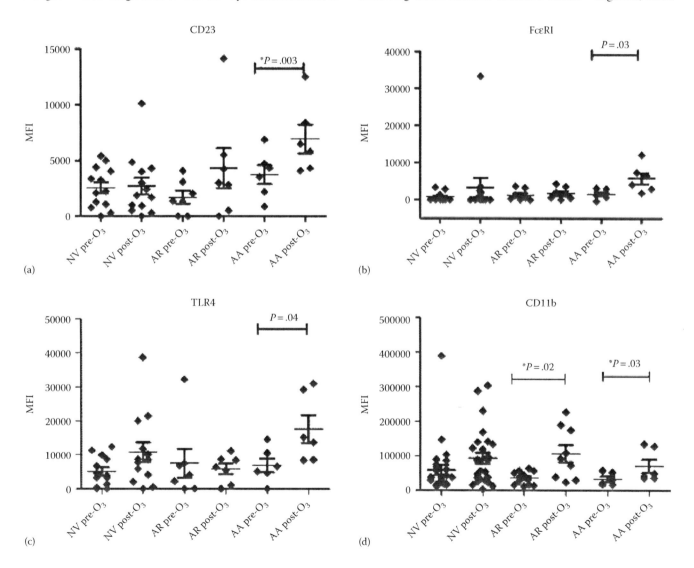

FIGURE 11.2 (a–d) Changes in cell-surface marker expression (mean fluorescent intensity [MFI]) on induced sputum macrophages: $n = 13$ healthy volunteers (NV), 7 atopic subjects (AR), and 6 atopic asthmatic subjects (AA). Lines depict means and SEMs. (From Hernandez, M.L., Lay, J.C., Harris, B., Esther Jr, C.R., Brickey, W.J., Bromberg, P.A., Diaz-Sanchez, D., et al., *J. Allergy Clin. Immunol.*, 126, 537–544, 2010. With permission.)

data suggest that, following acute ozone exposure, asthmatics may be primed for enhanced innate and acquired (immunoglobulin E [IgE]-mediated) immune responses to subsequently inhaled pollutants. Potentially, biomarkers may be useful in predicting which individual asthmatics may have an exaggerated inflammatory response to ozone, thereby making them more susceptible to subsequently inhaled allergenic stimuli. Indeed, Alexis et al.[41] showed that CD11b expression on circulating monocytes may be a useful biomarker, as it was found to be positively associated with the magnitude of the neutrophil response following inhaled ozone exposure in asthmatics. To this end, Svendsen et al.[42] also reported that asthmatic children without a measurable CD14 expression on circulating neutrophils had significant decrements in their lung function not observed in children with CD14 expression, which were associated with exposure to ambient PM2.5 and PM2.5–10.

ENDOTOXIN

Although perhaps not generally considered an air pollutant by classic definition, endotoxin or lipopolysaccharide (LPS) is ubiquitous in nature, an active component of PM-induced airway cell toxicity,[43] and an active component of both house dust and occupational dust.[44–46] Endotoxin is a known enhancing factor for asthma severity[47] and can act as an adjuvant for the subsequent response to inhaled allergens in the nasal[48] and lower airways.[49] These data suggest that atopy plays an important role in how endotoxin exerts its effect in asthma. Indeed, significant associations have been reported between the magnitude of the LPS-induced polymorphonuclear neutrophil (PMN) response (PMN per milligram) and constitutive levels of the LPS receptor (CD14), in both its soluble form (sCD14) and its membrane-bound form (mCD14).[50] Alexis showed that baseline levels of airway eosinophils were positively correlated with sCD14 and the magnitude of the PMN response to LPS, suggesting that atopy plays an important role in the sensitivity of asthmatics to LPS.[50] Moreover, Alexis[51] further showed that blunting eosinophil levels in asthmatics with a corticosteroid (fluticosone proprionate [FP]) pretreatment decreased monocytic cell mCD14 expression before and after LPS inhalation, and it decreased the magnitude of the PMN response to inhaled LPS (Figure 11.3a and 11.3b).

Although not the case for ozone, LPS appears to induce opposite responses in asthmatics depending on whether the dose is relatively high (>30,000 EU) or quite low (10,000 EU). At high doses (>30,000 EU), endotoxin will induce lung function decline, symptoms such as malaise, fever, chills, and neutrophil influx to the airways, as measured by an increase in the percentage of neutrophils in the sputum.[52–55] But, in general, LPS appears to cause an overall reduction in immunoinflammatory activity both locally in the airway and systemically. Hernandez[40] recently reported a reduction in the total number of inflammatory cells recruited to the airways, as well as a muted expression of CD11b, while others have reported a blunted phagocytic ability on the sputum

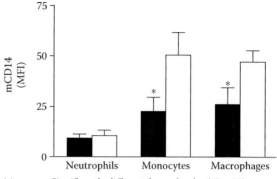

(a)   Significantly different from placebo (*P = .03)

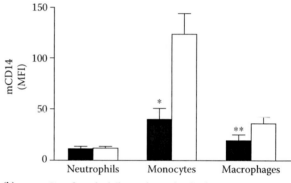

(b)   Significantly different from placebo (*P = .001; **P = .04)

FIGURE 11.3 (a) Effect of FP (*solid bar*) and placebo (*open bar*) on mCD14 expression on sputum neutrophils, monocytes, and macrophages 48 h before LPS (5 μg) inhalation challenge in 12 subjects with atopic asthma. (b) Effect of FP (*solid bar*) and placebo (*open bar*) on mCD14 expression on sputum neutrophils, monocytes, and macrophages 6 h after LPS (5 μg) inhalation challenge in 12 subjects with atopic asthma. (From Alexis, N.E. and Peden, D.B., *J. Allergy Clin. Immunol.*, 108, 577–580, 2001. With permission.)

and circulating phagocytes.[41] Compared with nonasthmatics, the levels of IL-1b and IL-18 and the expression of TLR2 and TLR4 remained stable after LPS (30,000 EU) inhalation, but were elevated in nonasthmatics.[40] In contrast, at low LPS levels (10,000 EU), asthmatics demonstrated significant upregulation of the cell-surface markers associated with innate immunity and antigen presentation (CD14, CD11b, CD16, HLA-DR, CD86, FceR1), and an increased expression of the genes that modulate antigen presentation (HLA-DR, MCP1), immune activation (CD14, IL-1β), and inflammation (ICAM1, iκBα).[56] *In vitro* evidence also shows that small concentrations of endotoxin (<1 ng/mL) activate alveolar macrophages causing the release of several proinflammatory mediators,[57] again suggesting that low-dose endotoxin is an innate immune stimulant or primer. Although the dose–response effect of endotoxin is also present in nonasthmatics, it may be more significant in susceptible populations such as asthmatics. For example, it has been established that asthmatics require a lower dose of LPS to elicit bronchoconstriction and inflammation than that required by nonasthmatics.[56,58] Overall, the evidence suggests that the effect of dose is clearly important when describing the toxic effects of endotoxin on asthma. Other pollutants such as PM have additional factors to consider when analyzing their relative toxicity and asthma. Particle size and origin are two important modifying factors for PM when it comes to contributing to asthma morbidity. Wagner[59] recently showed in an allergic asthma rat model that despite inhalation exposure to the same mass concentration (yet different chemical composition and size distribution) of urban PM2.5, disparate health effects could be induced in the airways of sensitized rats, suggesting that chemical components and PM size are important factors associated with PM toxicity.[59] Others have also demonstrated similar associations in children, where fine-sized and coarse-sized PM have significant associations with asthma morbidity.[60]

DIESEL EXHAUST AND DIESEL EXHAUST PARTICLES

The epidemiology surrounding the effects of DE or DEP on asthma has been discussed earlier in the chapter in terms of traffic-related pollutants, with a number of studies documenting a worsening of asthma following exposure to DEP. A number of years ago, a handful of nasal exposure studies with DEP were conducted by Diaz-Sanchez et al.[61–63] They showed that DEP had adjuvant properties that promoted IgE-mediated sensitization, induced the production of T-helper cell type 2 (Th2) cytokines and IgE following a nasal allergen challenge, and increased histamine levels in nasal lavage fluid following a mite challenge.[61–63] More recently, a small number of controlled chamber exposure studies to DE and DEP in asthmatics have been conducted. While one study reported increased airway responsiveness and airway resistance, as well as elevated levels of sputum IL-6,[64] all three studies failed to show DE- or DEP-induced (300 $\mu g/m^3$, 1 h; 108 $\mu g/m^3$, 2 h; 100 $\mu g/m^3$, 2 h) increases in markers of allergic (eosinophilic, myeloperoxidase [MPO]) or nonallergic (neutrophilic, IL-6) inflammation that were greater in asthmatics compared with healthy nonasthmatics.[64–66] In general, these exposure studies have shown a lack of inflammatory response to DE or DEP in the lower airways of asthmatics.

BIOMASS FUELS

About 2.4 billion persons live in households in which biomass fuels (BMFs) are the primary fuel for cooking, heating, or both,[67,68] with more than 90% of subjects in rural areas in less-developed countries (LDCs) using BMFs. BMFs for indoor cooking stoves include wood, charcoal, dung, and crop residues. Biomass emissions, however, can also technically include cigarette smoke. All of these are important sources of indoor air pollution, particularly in developing countries and LDCs. Unlike the positive association with BMF and respiratory infection in children[69] and chronic obstructive pulmonary disease (COPD) in women,[70] the association between the exposure to BMF and asthma is not clear or definitive. The results are mixed, with some studies showing an association between asthma prevalence and BMF,[71] while others, including a recent meta-analysis, concluding that there is no overall increased risk of asthma in women and children exposed to BMF.[70,72] The success of the measures to reduce exposure to

BMF has begun to be assessed for their effect on respiratory health outcomes. Again, the data appear to generate mixed results. One study reported an improvement in respiratory symptoms and lung function in households supplied with a cleaner stove,[73] while another study found only an improvement in the diagnosis of severe pneumonia.[74]

SUMMARY AND FUTURE DIRECTION

Evidence from epidemiology and cohort-based studies establishes a clear link between exposure to air pollution and asthma exacerbation, and supports a growing trend that traffic-related air pollutants can act as causal agents in the development of new-onset asthma. Controlled exposure studies have provided evidence that pollutants such as ozone or PM affect the biology of asthma by increasing inflammation in the airways and modifying the innate immune capability of the airways. The constitutive state of the asthmatic airway in terms of inflammation, innate immune responsiveness, and antioxidant defense capability are all important factors to consider when analyzing how a particular pollutant may be exerting its effect on the biology of asthma. Additional modifying factors, not discussed in this chapter, require careful attention as to their role in the effect of air pollution on asthma. They include a genetic predisposition (polymorphisms of the glutathione S-transferase [GST] and tumor necrosis factor alpha [TNFα] genes), obesity, gender, and age. Future studies will have to include these factors into an already complex equation as we move forward with emerging evidence.

REFERENCES

1. Peden DB. Air pollution in asthma: Effect of pollutants on airway inflammation. *Ann Allergy Asthma Immunol.* 2001;87(6 Suppl. 3):12–17.
2. McDonnell WF, Abbey DE, Nishino N, Lebowitz MD. Long-term ambient ozone concentration and the incidence of asthma in nonsmoking adults: The AHSMOG Study. *Environ Res.* 1999;80(2 Pt 1):110–121.
3. Bates DV. Observations on asthma. *Environ Health Perspect.* 1995;103(Suppl. 6):243–247.
4. Thurston GD, Ito K, Hayes CG, Bates DV, Lippmann M. Respiratory hospital admissions and summer time haze air pollution in Toronto, Ontario: Consideration of the role of acid aerosols. *Environ Res.* 1994;65(2):271–290.
5. Peden DB. The epidemiology and genetics of asthma risk associated with air pollution. *J Allergy Clin Immunol.* 2005;115(2):213–219.
6. Eckl-Dorna J, Klein B, Reichenauer TG, Niederberger V, Valenta R. Exposure of rye (Secale cereale) cultivars to elevated ozone levels increases the allergen content in pollen. *J Allergy Clin Immunol.* 2010;126:1315–1317.
7. Alexis NE, Hu SC, Zeman K, Alter T, Bennett WD. Induced sputum derives from the central airways: Confirmation using a radio labeled aerosol bolus delivery technique. *Am J Respir Crit Care Med.* 2001;164(10 Pt 1):1964–1970.
8. Delfino RJ, Coate BD, Zeiger RS, Seltzer JM, Street DH, Koutrakis P. Daily asthma severity in relation to personal ozone exposure and outdoor fungal spores. *Am J Respir Crit Care Med.* 1996;154:633–641.

9. Delfino RJ. Epidemiologic evidence for asthma and exposure to air toxics: Linkages between occupational, indoor, and community air pollution research. *Environ Health Perspect.* 2002;110(Suppl. 4):573–589.

10. Pope III CA. Respiratory hospital admissions associated with PM10 pollution in Utah, Salt Lake, and Cache Valleys. *Arch Environ Health.* 1991;46:90–97.

11. Schwartz J, Slater D, Larson TV, Pierson WE, Koenig JQ. Particulate air pollution and hospital emergency room visits for asthma in Seattle. *Am Rev Respir Dis.* 1993;147:826–831.

12. Peters A, Dockery DW, Heinrich J, Wichmann HE. Short-term effects of particulate air pollution on respiratory morbidity in asthmatic children. *Eur Respir J.* 1997;10:872–879.

13. Mortimer KM, Neas LM, Dockery DW, Redline S, Tager IB. The effect of air pollution on inner-city children with asthma. *Eur Respir J.* 2002;19(4):699–705.

14. Glad JA, Brink LL, Talbott EO, Lee PC, Xu X, Saul M, Rager J. The relationship of ambient ozone and PM(2.5) levels and asthma emergency department visits: Possible influence of gender and ethnicity. *Arch Environ Occup Health.* 2012;67(2):103–108.

15. Gowers AM, Cullinan P, Ayres JG, Anderson HR, Strachan DP, Holgate ST, Mills IC, Maynard RL. Does outdoor air pollution induce new cases of asthma? Biological plausibility and evidence; a review. *Respirology.* 2012;17(6):887–898.

16. Gasana J, Dillikar D, Mendy A, Forno E, Ramos Vieira E. Motor vehicle air pollution and asthma in children: A meta-analysis. *Environ Res.* 2012;117:36–45.

17. Eckel SP, Berhane K, Salam MT, Rappaport EB, Linn WS, Bastain TM, Zhang Y, Lurmann F, Avol EL, Gilliland FD. Residential traffic-related pollution exposures and exhaled nitric oxide in the children's health study. *Environ Health Perspect.* 2011;119(10):1472–1477.

18. Anderson HR, Butland BK, van Donkelaar A, Brauer M, Strachan DP, Clayton T, van Dingenen R, et al. Satellite-based estimates of ambient air pollution and global variations in childhood asthma prevalence. *Environ Health Perspect.* 2012;120(9):1333–1339.

19. Islam T, McConnell R, Gauderman WJ, Avol E, Peters JM, Gilliland FD. Ozone, oxidant defense genes, and risk of asthma during adolescence. *Am J Respir Crit Care Med.* 2008;177(4):388–395.

20. Jerrett M, Shankardass K, Berhane K, Gauderman WJ, Künzli N, Avol E, Gilliland F, et al. Traffic-related air pollution and asthma on set in children: A prospective cohort study with individual exposure measurement. *Environ Health Perspect.* 2008;116(10):1433–1438.

21. McConnell R, Islam T, Shankardass K, Jerrett M, Lurmann F, Gilliland F, Gauderman J, et al. Childhood incident asthma and traffic-related air pollution at home and school. *Environ Health Perspect.* 2010;118(7):1021–1026.

22. Anderson HR, Favarato G, Atkinson RW. Long-term exposure to air pollution and the incidence of asthma: Meta-analysis of cohort studies. *Air Qual Atmos Health* 2013;6:47–56.

23. Anderson HR, Favarato G, Atkinson RW. Long-term exposure to outdoor air pollution and the prevalence of asthma: Meta-analysis of multi-community prevalence studies. *Air Qual Atmos Health* 2013;6:57–68.

24. Bernstein DI. Diesel exhaust exposure, wheezing and sneezing. *Allergy Asthma Immunol Res.* 2012;4(4):178–183.

25. Prahalad AK, Soukup JM, Inmon J, Willis R, Ghio AJ, Becker S, Gallagher JE. Ambient air particles: Effects on cellular oxidant radical gene ration in relation to particulate elemental chemistry. *Toxicol Appl Pharmacol.* 1999;158(2):81–91.

26. Becker S, Soukup JM, Gilmour MI, Devlin RB. Stimulation of human and rat alveolar macrophages by urban air particulates: Effects on oxidant radical generation and cytokine production. *Toxicol Appl Pharmacol.* 1996;141(2):637–648.

27. Poole JA, Alexis NE, Parks C, MacInnes AK, Gentry-Nielsen MJ, Fey PD, Larsson L, Allen-Gipson D, Von Essen SG, Romberger DJ. Repetitive organic dust exposure in vitro impairs macrophage differentiation and function. *J Allergy Clin Immunol.* 2008;122(2):375–382.

28. Wang F, He XY, Baines KJ, Gunawardhana LP, Simpson JL, Li F, Gibson PG. Different inflammatory phenotypes in adults and children with acute asthma. *Eur Respir J.* 2011;38(3):567–574.

29. Ordoñez CL, Shaughnessy TE, Matthay MA, Fahy JV. Increased neutrophil numbers and IL-8 levels in airway secretions in acute severe asthma: Clinical and biologic significance. *Am J Respir Crit Care Med.* 2000;161(4 Pt 1):1185–1190.

30. Goleva E, Hauk PJ, Hall CF, Liu AH, Riches DW, Martin RJ, Leung DY. Corticosteroid-resistant asthma is associated with classical antimicrobial activation of airway macrophages. *J Allergy Clin Immunol.* 2008;122(3):550–559.

31. Huang YJ, Lynch SV. The emerging relationship between the airway microbiota and chronic respiratory disease: Clinical implications. *Expert Rev Respir Med.* 2011;5(6):809–821.

32. Juhn YJ, Kita H, Yawn BP, Boyce TG, Yoo KH, McGree ME, Weaver AL, Wollan P, Jacobson RM. Increased risk of serious pneumococcal disease in patients with asthma. *J Allergy Clin Immunol.* 2008;122(4):719–723.

33. Talbot TR, Hartert TV, Mitchel E, Halasa NB, Arbogast PG, Poehling KA, Schaffner W, Craig AS, Griffin MR. Asthma as a risk factor for invasive pneumococcal disease. *N Engl J Med.* 2005;352(20):2082–2090.

34. Vieira SE, Stein RT, Ferraro AA, Pastro LD, Pedro SS, Lemos M, da Silva ER, Sly PD, Saldiva PH. Urban air pollutants are significant risk factors for asthma and pneumonia in children: The influence of location on the measurement of pollutants. *Arch Bronconeumol.* 2012;48(11):389–395.

35. Alexis NE, Soukup J, Nierkens S, Becker S. Association between airway hyperreactivity and bronchial macrophage dysfunction in individuals with mild asthma. *Am J Physiol Lung Cell Mol Physiol.* 2001;280(2):L369–L375.

36. Kongerud J, Crissman K, Hatch G, Alexis N. Ascorbic acid is decreased in induced sputum of mild asthmatics. *Inhal Toxicol.* 2003;15(2):101–109.

37. Newcomb DC, Peebles Jr RS. Bugs and asthma: A different disease? *Proc Am Thorac Soc.* 2009;6(3):266–271.

38. Brickey WJ, Alexis NE, Hernandez ML, Reed W, Ting JP, Peden DB. Sputum inflammatory cells from patients with allergic rhinitis and asthma have decreased inflammasome gene expression. *J Allergy Clin Immunol.* 2011;128(4):900–903.

39. Hernandez ML, Lay JC, Harris B, Esther Jr CR, Brickey WJ, Bromberg PA, Diaz-Sanchez D, et al. Atopic asthmatic subjects but not atopic subjects without asthma have enhanced inflammatory response to ozone. *J Allergy Clin Immunol.* 2010;126(3):537–544.

40. Hernandez M, Brickey WJ, Alexis NE, Fry RC, Rager JE, Zhou B, Ting JP, Zhou H, Peden DB. Airway cells from atopic asthmatic patients exposed to ozone display an enhanced innate immunegene profile. *J Allergy Clin Immunol.* 2012;129(1):259–261.

41. Alexis NE, Eldridge MW, Peden DB. Effect of inhaled endotoxin on airway and circulating inflammatory cell phagocytosis and CD11b expression in atopic asthmatic subjects. *J Allergy Clin Immunol.* 2003;112(2):353–361.

42. Svendsen ER, Yeatts KB, Peden D, Orton S, Alexis NE, Creason J, Williams R, Neas L. Circulating neutrophil CD14 expression and the inverse association of ambient particulate matter on lung function in asthmatic children. *Ann Allergy Asthma Immunol.* 2007;99(3):244–253.

43. Soukup JM, Becker S. Human alveolar macrophage responses to air pollution particulates are associated within soluble components of coarse material, including particulate endotoxin. *Toxicol Appl Pharmacol.* 2001;171(1):20–26.

44. Rylander R, Michel O. Organic dust induced inflammation— Role of atopy and TLR-4 and CD14 gene polymorphisms. *Am J Ind Med.* 2005;48(4):302–307.

45. Larsson KA, Eklund AG, Hansson LO, Isaksson BM, Malmberg PO. Swine dust causes intense airways inflammation in healthy subjects. *Am J Respir Crit Care Med.* 1994;150(4):973–977.

46. Clapp WD, Becker S, Quay J, Watt JL, Thorne PS, Frees KL, Zhang X, Koren HS, Lux CR, Schwartz DA. Grain dust-induced airflow obstruction and inflammation of the lower respiratory tract. *Am J Respir Crit Care Med.* 1994;150(3):611–617.

47. Michel O. Role of lipopolysaccharide (LPS) in asthma and other pulmonary conditions. *J Endotoxin Res.* 2003;9(5):293–300.

48. Eldridge MW, Peden DB. Airway response to concomitant exposure with endotoxin and allergen in atopic asthmatics. *J Toxicol Environ Health A.* 2000;61(1):27–37.

49. Boehlecke B, Hazucha M, Alexis NE, Jacobs R, Reist P, Bromberg PA, Peden DB. Low-dose airborne endotoxin exposure enhances bronchial responsiveness to inhaled allergen in atopic asthmatics. *J Allergy Clin Immunol.* 2003;112(6):1241–1243.

50. Alexis N, Eldridge M, Reed W, Bromberg P, Peden DB. CD14-dependent airway neutrophil response to inhaled LPS: Role of atopy. *J Allergy Clin Immunol.* 2001;107(1):31–35.

51. Alexis NE, Peden DB. Blunting airway eosinophilic inflammation results in a decreased airway neutrophil response to inhaled LPS in patients with atopic asthma: A role for CD14. *J Allergy Clin Immunol.* 2001;108(4):577–580.

52. Rylander R, Bake B, Fischer JJ, Helander IM. Pulmonary function and symptoms after inhalation of endotoxin. *Am Rev Respir Dis.* 1989;140(4):981–986.

53. Michel O, Ginanni R, Le Bon B, Content J, Duchateau J, Sergysels R. Inflammatory response to acute inhalation of endotoxin in asthmatic patients. *Am Rev Respir Dis.* 1992;146(2):352–357.

54. Michel O, Nagy AM, Schroeven M, Duchateau J, Nève J, Fondu P, Sergysels R. Dose–response relationship to inhaled endotoxin in normal subjects. *Am J Respir Crit Care Med.* 1997;156(4 Pt 1):1157–1164.

55. Michel O. Role of house-dusten dotoxin exposure in aetiology of allergy and asthma. *Mediators Inflamm.* 2001;10(6):301–304.

56. Alexis NE, Brickey WJ, Lay JC, Wang Y, Roubey RA, Ting JP, Peden DB. Development of an inhaled endotoxin challenge protocol for characterizing evoked cell surface phenotype and genomicresponses of airway cells in allergic individuals. *Ann Allergy Asthma Immunol.* 2008;100(3):206–215.

57. Dubin W, Martin TR, Swoveland P, Leturcq DJ, Moriarty AM, Tobias PS, Bleecker ER, Goldblum SE, Hasday JD. Asthma and endotoxin: Lipopolysaccharide-binding protein and soluble CD14 in broncho alveolar compartment. *Am J Physiol.* 1996;270(5 Pt 1):L736–L744.

58. Kline JN, Cowden JD, Hunninghake GW, Schutte BC, Watt JL, Wohlford-Lenane CL, Powers LS, Jones MP, Schwartz DA. Variable airway responsiveness to inhaled lipopolysaccharide. *Am J Respir Crit Care Med.* 1999;160(1):297–303.

59. Wagner JG, Morishita M, Keeler GJ, Harkema JR. Divergent effects of urban particulate air pollution on allergic airway responses in experimental asthma: A comparison of field exposure studies. *Environ Health.* 2012;11(1):45.

60. Mar TF, Larson TV, Stier RA, Claiborn C, Koenig JQ. An analysis of the association between respiratory symptoms in subjects with asthma and daily air pollution in Spokane, Washington. *Inhal Toxicol.* 2004;16(13):809–815.

61. Diaz-Sanchez D, Tsien A, Fleming J, Saxon A. Combined diesel exhaust particulate and ragweed allergen challenge markedly enhances human in vivo nasal ragweed-specific IgE and skews cytokine production to a T helper cell 2-type pattern. *J Immunol.* 1997;158(5):2406–2413.

62. Diaz-Sanchez D, Garcia MP, Wang M, Jyrala M, Saxon A. Nasal challenge with diesel exhaust particles can induce sensitization to a neoallergen in the human mucosa. *J Allergy Clin Immunol.* 1999;104(6):1183–1188.

63. Diaz-Sanchez D, Penichet-Garcia M, Saxon A. Diesel exhaust particles directly induce activated mast cells to degranulate and increase histamine levels and symptom severity. *J Allergy Clin Immunol.* 2000;106(6):1140–1146.

64. Nordenhäll C, Pourazar J, Ledin MC, Levin JO, Sandström T, Adelroth E. Diesel exhaust enhances airway responsiveness in asthmatic subjects. *Eur Respir J.* 2001;17(5):909–915.

65. Stenfors N, Nordenhäll C, Salvi SS, Mudway I, Söderberg M, Blomberg A, Helleday R, et al. Different airway inflammatory responses in asthmatic and healthy humans exposed to diesel. *Eur Respir J.* 2004;23(1):82–86.

66. Behndig AF, Larsson N, Brown JL, Stenfors N, Helleday R, Duggan ST, Dove RE, et al. Proinflammatory doses of diesel exhaust in healthy subjects fail to elicit equivalent or augmented airway inflammation in subjects with asthma. *Thorax.* 2011;66(1):12–19.

67. Noonan CW, Balmes JR. Biomass smoke exposures: Health outcomes measures and study design. *Inhal Toxicol.* 2010;22(2):108–112.

68. Reddy A (ed.). *Energy after Rio: Prospects and Challenges.* New York: United Nations Development Programme, 1996.

69. Prüss-Ustün A, Bonjour S, Corvalán C. The impact of the environment on health by country: A meta-synthesis. *Environ Health.* 2008;7:7.

70. Po JY, FitzGerald JM, Carlsten C. Respiratory disease associated with solid biomass fuel exposure in rural women and children: Systematic review and meta-analysis. *Thorax.* 2011;66(3):232–239.

71. Barry AC, Mannino DM, Hopenhayn C, Bush H. Exposure to indoor biomass fuel pollutants and asthma prevalence in Southeastern Kentucky: Results from the Burden of Lung Disease (BOLD) study. *J Asthma.* 2010;47(7):735–741.

72. Behera D, Chakrabarti T, Khanduja KL. Effect of exposure to domestic cooking fuels on bronchial asthma. *Indian J Chest Dis Allied Sci.* 2001;43(1):27–31.

73. Romieu I, Riojas-Rodríguez H, Marrón-Mares AT, Schilmann A, Perez-Padilla R, Masera O. Improved biomasss to intervention in rural Mexico: Impact on the respiratory health of women. *Am J Respir Crit Care Med.* 2009;180(7):649–656.

74. Smith KR, McCracken JP, Weber MW, Hubbard A, Jenny A, Thompson LM, Balmes J, Diaz A, Arana B, Bruce N. Effect of reduction in household air pollution on childhood pneumoniain Guatemala (RESPIRE): A randomised controlled trial. *Lancet.* 2011;378(9804):1717–1726.

12 Exercise-Induced Bronchoconstriction

Christopher Randolph and John M. Weiler

CONTENTS

CASE PRESENTATION

A 12-year-old white male who was diagnosed with asthma after being hospitalized for an acute exacerbation in 2002 presents with cough and wheezing after running in cross-country meets. The patient also noted increased nasal congestion, postnasal drainage, sneezing, and rhinorrhea during the spring, summer, and fall months. Pulmonary function testing revealed a forced vital capacity (FVC) of 1.75 (119% predicted), a forced expiratory volume in 1 sec (FEV$_1$) of 1.47 (113%), and a forced expiratory flow at 25%–75% (FEF$_{25-75}$) of 1.65 (100%) without response to a beta$_2$-agonist bronchodilator. A mannitol challenge, which is a surrogate indirect provocation method that is used to diagnose exercise-induced bronchoconstriction (EIB), was positive, revealing a decline in FEV$_1$ of 30% at the 5 mg dose (normal <15% fall in FEV$_1$ postchallenge). Skin prick testing (SPT) to inhalants indicated sensitization to cockroaches, dust mites, trees, grass, ragweed pollens, and Alternaria mold spores. An exhaled nitric oxide (eNO) test was negative (value of 12) indicating no evidence of airway inflammation. Based on the patient's tests, avoidance measures to dust mites and cockroaches were provided, and he was started on a nasal corticosteroid to reduce his nasal congestion during exercise, and control his underlying seasonal allergic rhinitis. He was also instructed to use a short-acting beta$_2$-adrenergic agonist 15 min before all exercise activity. A follow-up visit 4 weeks later revealed that he was now able to complete all of his training workouts and his times during cross-country meets had significantly improved. His nasal congestion was also dramatically improved, as he was now able to breathe through his nose while running. A 6-month follow-up evaluation was recommended.

INTRODUCTION

EIB is defined as a transient narrowing of the lower airway with an associated increase in airway resistance, during or following exercise.[1–3] EIB is a more accurate descriptor of this condition than is exercise-induced asthma (EIA), because exercise induces bronchoconstriction, not asthma, and not all EIB is associated with chronic asthma.[4] Indeed, the term *exercise-induced asthma* should be abandoned.[3]

This chapter addresses the two forms of EIB: EIB in patients who do not have evidence of chronic asthma (called EIB alone); and EIB in patients who also have chronic asthma (called EIB with asthma). EIB alone, which is less common, occurs with strenuous exercise, and it has been studied in schoolchildren, armed-forces recruits, and highly competitive and elite athletes.[1,5–8] EIB alone may be considered a form of injury-related lung disease. The more common condition, EIB with asthma, is seen in as many as 90% of asthmatic patients.[1–3] In contrast, EIB alone without known asthma is seen in 40%–50% of patients who have allergic rhinitis, 10% of the general population, and as many as 60% of elite or highly competitive athletes.[1–3] The prevalence of EIB in athletes who do not otherwise have asthma depends on the intensity and the duration of exercise and is particularly prevalent in the most strenuous endurance sports, with the highest degree of ventilation injuring the airway in conjunction with environmental irritants such as cold air. Thus, ice hockey, cross-country skiing, skating, cycling, mountain biking, swimming, rowing, and track and field ("athletics") have the highest prevalence of EIB alone without known asthma (ranging to about 60%). Less strenuous sports, such as badminton, baseball, and diving, have a lesser prevalence of EIB.[9,10]

EIB with asthma may represent the earliest sign of asthma in childhood and may be the last sign to resolve after an exacerbation.[1] The prevalence of EIB in patients who have underlying chronic asthma depends on the sport or activity, the environment, and the degree of control of the underlying asthma.[1-4] EIB reflects the control (or lack of control) of asthma and the evidence of airway bronchial hyperreactivity. The more severe the EIB is, the more poorly controlled the chronic asthma will be.[2,4] In the latest Expert Panel Report (EPR) of the National Asthma Education and Prevention Program (NAEPP-3), EIB is listed as an important indicator of the impairment of pulmonary function.[11] EIB exacerbations suggest the need to increase controller therapy for underlying asthma.[1-4]

A history of respiratory symptoms alone, during or following exercise, is not reliable for the diagnosis of EIB.[1-4,12,13] EIB is identified by establishing objective evidence for a fall in postexercise FEV_1 of at least 10% from its preexercise value, after 8 min of strenuous aerobic exercise. Exercise is conducted to achieve at least 80%–95% of the maximum heart rate as a surrogate for a maximum voluntary ventilation (MVV) of 40%–80% of the predicted maximum.[1-3,14] In children aged 3–6 years, a fall in FEV in one-half second (FEV0.5) may be used to define EIB.[15] The fall in FEV_1 may begin during exercise; in 80% of patients, the fall in FEV_1 occurs between 5 and 12 min and rarely as late as 30 min postexercise.[16] Recovery from the bronchoconstriction occurs within 30–60 min after exercise is completed.[17] Repeated exercise within 2–4 h may lead to a refractory period in 50% of individuals, in which exercise does not induce additional bronchoconstriction.[17]

This chapter describes the epidemiology, pathogenesis, presentation, diagnosis, and management (both pharmaceutical and nonpharmaceutical) of EIB alone and EIB with asthma. The appropriate management of EIB should allow patients, whether recreational or elite athletes or nonathletic patients with activity-induced symptoms, to have a healthy lifestyle, with the ability to participate in physical activity, including their selected sports activities.[1-4]

EPIDEMIOLOGY

The prevalence of EIB varies with the population being studied, including age, sex, ethnicity, urbanization, exercise level of intensity, type of exercise challenge, criteria for a positive test, the presence or absence of chronic asthma, and environmental conditions, including the season in which the challenge is being performed.[3,18] EIB may be suggested when a patient has a fall in FEV_1 or peak expiratory flow

(PEF) from prechallenge to postexercise. Some authors have considered a fall in peak flow of 15% following a 6-min free-running test to be diagnostic of the condition. Such falls in PEF are common in children. In one study in a South Wales population of children aged 12 years, the prevalence was 6.7% in 1973, 7.7% in 1988, and 4.7% in 2003. The lower prevalence in 2003 was attributed to an increased use of inhaled corticosteroids (ICS).[19,20] In a study of adolescent athletes participating in a variety of sports, who were examined prior to their participation, 9.4% had a positive challenge after a free-running exercise, with a positive challenge defined as a fall of at least 10% in FEV_1 by 15 min postchallenge.[21] In a second study, high-school athletes were examined on a treadmill prior to their participation, with a positive test defined as a fall of at least 10% in FEV_1, and 28% had a positive challenge.[22]

In a third study, eucapneic voluntary hyperventilation (EVH) was used to screen athletes in a Midwestern high school.[23] A positive challenge was defined as a fall of at least 10% in FEV_1 or a fall of at least 20% in FEF_{25-75} or a fall of at least 10% in PEF at 1, 5, and 10 min postchallenge.[23] Of the athletes, 38% had a positive challenge. A follow-up study by the same authors using a similar protocol in adults who had no history of asthma showed that 19% had a positive challenge.[24]

The socioeconomic impact of EIB was demonstrated in two surveys in Ghana performed 10 years apart (1993 and 2003) using a 6-min free-running test among children aged 9–13 years. The urban rich children demonstrated an increased prevalence of EIB from 4.2% to 8.3%, whereas the urban poor children had an increased prevalence from 1.4% to 3.0% and the rural poor prevalence increased from 2.2% to 3.9%.[25,26]

In Algeria, a 6-min free-running test was used to screen schoolchildren, with a positive result defined as at least a 15% fall in PEF within 10 min of the challenge. The prevalence of EIB was 47% for children with known asthma versus 13.9% for nonasthmatic children.[27] This is consistent with the prevalence of EIB in another large study by Cabral et al., who noted a higher prevalence of EIB in a population of children with moderate to severe asthma when studied using cycle ergonometry.[28] In Australian schoolchildren, 19.6% had EIB defined by a FEV_1 fall of at least 15%, and 40% of these children had no history of asthma.[29] Prevalence is affected by gender and urbanization, with girls (8.5%) more likely than boys (6.4%), and an urban setting (8.9%) more likely than a rural setting (7%) to have a positive challenge with a 6-min run using a 15% fall in PEF.[30] Ethnic and racial differences are also noted, with African Americans having a higher prevalence of EIB (13%) than European Americans (2%) using a free-running test with PEF monitoring.[31]

A British study used cycle ergometry in 9-year-old Asian children from the Indian subcontinent and found a 3.6 times higher prevalence of EIB than in white urban children when EIB was defined as at least a 15% fall in PEF within 10 min of the end of the exercise.[32]

In elite athletes, the prevalence of EIB has been reported to be 18%–50% in winter Olympians following an exercise challenge; the prevalence was 50% in skiers with a field exercise and 30%–35% in figure skaters with an exercise challenge.[33,34] In summer athletes, EVH prevalence was 50%; with the same technique in winter Olympians, the prevalence was 45%.[35,36] In asymptomatic individuals with a history of EIB only but no history of asthma, the prevalence of EIB was 12% and EIB was predictive of adult asthma.[37]

In Olympic athletes, the prevalence of EIB was highest in athletes participating in the most strenuous endurance sports, ranging from winter sports with 17.6% in cross-country skiing and 16.2% in speed skating, to summer sports with 15.3% in cycling, 11.3% in swimming, and 10.1% in the modern pentathlon.[38] In another study, scuba divers had a 17% prevalence of EIB defined as a 15% fall in FEV_1 from baseline secondary to the use of inhaled saline (4.5%), a surrogate for an exercise challenge.[39]

Elite athletes have a higher prevalence of EIB related to certain atmospheric conditions such as high pollen levels, high pollution, chemical exposure, and cold air.[3] EIB can be present with or without symptoms, but symptoms alone are not a sensitive index for the diagnosis of EIB. Thus, the prevalence not only varies with the form of the exercise but also with the type of challenge that is used to elicit EIB (surrogate or exercise).[3] Other factors related to the presence of EIB include environmental factors such as chlorinated pools, ice hockey rinks surfaced with fossil fuel, a family history of atopy, uncontrolled asthma, lower respiratory illness, a personal history of atopy, and urbanization.[4]

EIB has an impact on physical functioning including school activities and emotional functioning in quality of life. This impact was demonstrated in studies in high-school athletes and in children in Tokyo with EIB with and without asthma, and in telephone surveys of parents of 4- to 17-year-old children with current asthma and adults aged 18 years and older.[40–43]

Children with EIB were profoundly impacted with lower scores in the areas of physical functioning, emotional functioning, and school activities compared with those without EIB.[42] In the telephone survey, the most frequently reported symptoms of EIB were cough, wheezing, and shortness of breath. In a large survey of EIB, more than 1 in 5 (22.2%) of 4- to 12-year-old children with EIB avoided selected activities and almost 1 in 3 (31.8%) of 13- to 18-year-old adolescents with EIB reported avoidance of activities related to EIB.[41,43] Parents reported that asthma impacted their children "a lot or some" in 30% of sports or recreation activities, in 30.9% of normal nonsports-related activities, and in 26% of other outdoor activities. Despite the frequency of EIB, only 23% stated that they used bronchodilators always or most of the time and 43.4% reported that they "never" used bronchodilators.[41] Parents frequently express worries that asthma may limit exercise in their children; however, if they were properly educated and their children's EIB was better managed, these concerns could be resolved in most cases.[44]

PATHOGENESIS (TABLE 12.1)

The physiological determinant for EIB is the transfer or loss of water from the airway surface in response to the inspiration and conditioning of large amounts of dry air in a short period of time.[1–3] There are two theories for the evolution of EIB; the more widely accepted osmolar theory and the possibly contributory thermal theory. The osmolar theory postulates that mediator release follows degranulation of the mast cells caused by a hyperosmolar environment created by dehydration.[1–3,25,45] The thermal theory suggests that EIB is a vascular event with vasoconstriction as a result of airway cooling and reactive hyperemia following rewarming[1–3] (Table 12.1).

The evaporation of water results in the cooling and dehydration of the airway. Dehydration creates a hyperosmolar environment that leads to degranulation of the mast cells with a mediator release, including histamine, tryptase, leukotrienes, and prostaglandins, as well as chemotactic factors leading to the recruitment of inflammatory cells, most notably eosinophils but also lymphocytes and neutrophils. This response is also associated with reverse axonal sensory nerve mediator release. This orchestrated release of mediators, cytokines, and chemokines contributes to bronchial smooth muscle constriction, airway inflammation characterized by dense infiltrates of inflammatory cells (lymphocytes and eosinophils), and increased inspissated mucus secretions and cellular debris due to the denudation of the bronchial epithelial cells. Epithelial cell injury leads to an increase in transglutaminase 2, which regulates phospholipases and the leukotriene pathway. Leukotrienes are more predominant than prostaglandins in the airways of patients with EIB and they play a significant role in inducing bronchoconstriction mediated by the sensory nerves and the release of mucus from goblet cells (MUCSAC).[25] Thus, EIB is the outcome of the dehydration of the airway leading to a hyperosmolar environment. Extensive studies of the airway cells, mucosa, epithelium, exhaled breath condensate, proteomics, the genetics of the airway mucosa, sputum, and bronchoalveolar lavage support the osmolar mechanism of action for EIB.[25]

EIB alone without known asthma in the competitive or elite athlete is postulated to be due to an overuse injury to the airway. Hyperventilation, often of cold and dry air, results in compensation by the airway down to the smaller airways, where there is an enhanced risk of injury to the epithelium.[1–3,25,46] Plasma exudation occurs in the repair

TABLE 12.1
Pathogenesis[1–3,25]

EIB alone	Syndrome of overuse injury in competitive or elite athletes
EIB with asthma	Osmolar theory with contributory thermal theory peripherally with cold air

Note: Pronounced leukotriene production is regulated by epithelial injury via transglutaminase (TGM2) and phospholipase A2.

process so that repeated exposure leads to smooth muscle hyperresponsiveness and EIB.[45,46] This is seen in endurance athletes, particularly those exercising in cold climates, and swimmers.[45,47–50]

CLINICAL PRESENTATION OF EIB

The symptoms of EIB include cough, wheeze, chest tightness (or chest pain in children), shortness of breath, dyspnea, excessive mucus production, and "feeling out of shape" even though the individual is really in an acceptable physical condition.[3,13,51–57] The signs and symptoms may also be vague, including poor performance, heavy legs, muscle cramps, sore throat, and stomachache.[3,13,36,51,52] Post-race cough is the most commonly reported symptom in elite athletes. Nevertheless, a sensitivity/specificity analysis did not demonstrate the effectiveness of self-reported symptoms as a negative or positive predictor of changes in the pulmonary function after exercise.[3,13,52]

Rundell noted that in elite cold-weather athletes, 91% of EIB-positive athletes had at least one symptom whereas 48% of EIB-negative athletes also had at least one symptom.[3,13] Parsons et al. reported similar findings in collegiate athletes, with both EIB-positive and EIB-negative athletes having a similar prevalence of symptoms.[54] This is consistent with other studies that show that the percentage change in FEV_1 from pre- to postchallenge follows a normal distribution, suggesting that there is no specific cut point for a fall in FEV_1 that distinguishes between those individuals with or without EIB.[51]

Additionally, exercise-induced dyspnea is one of the most common symptoms of EIB. It has been demonstrated that many individuals who are thought to have EIB have other conditions that contribute to or precipitate their symptoms, including exercise-induced hyperventilation, exercise-related laryngomalacia, exercise-precipitated vocal cord dysfunction, nasal congestion, gastroesophageal reflux disease (GERD), cardiac abnormalities, and poor conditioning.[58,59] In one study, only 8% of children presenting with exercise-induced dyspnea had EIB; the remaining 92% had another diagnosis that manifested as EIB.[59]

DIAGNOSIS OF EIB (TABLE 12.2)

A self-reported history alone does not predict who will have a positive exercise challenge and therefore it is not reliable for the diagnosis of EIB. The outcome of a challenge may also be modified by the training environmental conditions and the level of competition, particularly in competitive or elite athletes.[3,12–14,30,55,60–65] Therefore, an evaluation of EIB mandates objective pulmonary function monitoring with exercise at 85%–90% of the maximum heart rate (40%–80% of MVV). This level of exercise may be achieved by exercising for 6 min (in children) and 8 min (in adults) at a minute ventilation of at least 17.5–21 times FEV_1 and up to 30 times FEV_1 for EVH. The latter two ventilation rates equal 60%–85% of MVV.[3,14,55,65] Interestingly, when exercise is performed in

a laboratory (e.g., on a treadmill) rather than in the venue in which an athlete participates, there may be a high rate of false-negative results for EIB. This may be due to the natural variability of EIB, but it is likely to be impacted more by factors that affect the airway response, including type, duration, and intensity of exercise, temperature and humidity of the inspired air, pollutants in the air, time since the last episode of EIB, and the duration of medication withholding[14,55] (Table 12.2).

The most commonly used and effective procedure for the diagnosis of EIB is a laboratory exercise treadmill challenge, which uses a protocol that incrementally increases the exercise intensity rapidly over 2–4 min followed by 6–8 min of strenuous exercise for a total of 10 min. The ventilation for athletes should be more than 21 times the FEV_1 during the final 8 min. Protocols generally encourage that patients breathe medical-grade dry air with a nose clip, while running or cycling at a level sufficient to increase the heart rate to 80%–95% of the maximum heart rate (max HR = 220 – age in years).[14,55]

Free running or running on a treadmill may be preferable to cycling because ventilation increases more rapidly when running. Again, as noted above, the patient should breathe dry air to ensure a low water content of inspired air. The apparatus to produce cool air is considerably more complex and few laboratories provide both dry and cool air. If available, cool air may be preferable in skiers to simulate the natural environment in which they participate.[1–3]

There is a natural variation in the airway reactivity to exercise so that a single negative test may not be sufficient to rule out EIB.[14,55] As many as 25% of individuals without known asthma but with exercise-induced symptoms may have one positive test and one negative test when an exercise is repeated under the same conditions over a short span of days.[14] A natural variation can also occur with known asthmatic patients in whom exposure to allergens or irritants can temporarily increase the severity of EIB and the elimination of these factors will diminish the severity of EIB.[65]

Generally, elite athletes should be evaluated using a sports-specific exercise that reproduces the symptoms in the laboratory that occur "on the field".[3,30,35] The environmental conditions, including temperature, humidity, pollen level, and pollution index, may impact the response on the field and are difficult to replicate in the laboratory.

Measurements of FEV_1 are made in duplicate at 0, 3, 5, 10, 15, 20, and 30 min after exercise and the highest (best) value at each postexercise stage is used in the calculations. Full FVC maneuvers should not be performed postexercise; an FEV_1 lasting at least 2 sec but no more than 3 sec leads to less fatigue than a full FVC maneuver.[1–3,55]

The percentage fall in FEV_1 is:

$$100 \times \frac{\left(\text{Best prechallenge } FEV_1 - \text{lowest best postchallenge } FEV_1\right)}{\text{Best prechallenge } FEV_1}$$

TABLE 12.2

Diagnostic Tests (1–3): Challenges to Perform When Response to Bronchodilator Shows <12% and 200 mL Increase in FEV$_1$[3]

	Advantage	Disadvantage	Diagnostic Cutoff
Indirect challenge	Specificity	Sensitivity less than with methacholine	At least a 10% fall in FEV$_1$ from baseline
Exercise: cycle, treadmill, run, sport	Specificity	Requires facilities to perform challenge (e.g., laboratory equipped with treadmill and crash cart)	At least a 10% fall in FEV$_1$ from baseline
Surrogate challenges	Specificity; requires no exercise equipment	Sensitivity less than with methacholine	At least a 10% fall in FEV$_1$ from baseline
Mannitol	Specificity; requires no exercise equipment; commercially available; relatively inexpensive; produces a response–dose ratio	May not diagnose mild asthma	PD$_{15}$: at least a 15% fall in FEV$_1$ from baseline or 10% fall in FEV$_1$ between stages
EVH	Standard for evaluating Olympic athletes to confirm EIB	May be more sensitive than mannitol for EIB	At least a 10% fall in FEV$_1$ from baseline
Hypertonic saline	Specificity (88%)	Sensitivity (46%); not standardized	At least a 15% fall in FEV$_1$ from baseline
Adenosine monophosphate[151]	Sensitivity (70%); specificity (94%)	Sputum eosinophilia; not approved by the FDA; limited publications support its use in this setting	At least a 10% fall in FEV$_1$ from baseline
Direct challenge	Sensitivity	May lack specificity	PC$_{20}$: at least a 20% fall in FEV$_1$ from baseline
Methacholine	Sensitivity	May lack specificity	PC$_{20}$: at least a 20% fall in FEV$_1$ from baseline

where the lowest FEV$_1$ postchallenge is the best (highest) FEV$_1$ at the stage with the largest fall in FEV$_1$.

The diagnosis of EIB requires at least a 10% fall in FEV$_1$, preferably at two or more time points postchallenge. The severity of EIB may be rated based on the fall in FEV$_1$ as mild (>10% but <25%), moderate (>25% but <50%), and severe (>50%), from prechallenge.[1–3]

Other end points are time to recovery to 95% of baseline FEV$_1$ and area under the curve (AUC) until 30 min postexercise. Flow rates (FEF$_{25-75}$) and PEF are rarely useful.

Given the variability in the performance of exercise challenges, surrogate challenges have been developed to assess EIB.[35] These include inhaling dry powder mannitol (Aridol) and EVH. EVH is the recommended test for Olympic athletes. Mannitol is a graduated dose–response test, which has intrinsic safety and may provide the level of sensitivity (e.g., using the response–dose ratio [RDR]). In contrast to other challenges, patients undergoing EVH may be more susceptible to severe reactions with extreme falls in FEV$_1$.[1–3]

EVH was developed in the 1980s to evaluate armed-forces personnel for EIB. The EVH test requires inhalation of a fixed dry gas mixture containing 4.9%–5% carbon dioxide, 21% oxygen, and the remaining balance of nitrogen.[66] The procedure necessitates hyperventilation of the dry gas mixture for 6 min at 30 times FEV$_1$ to reach about 85% of MVV. The higher ventilation achieved (vs. 17–21 times FEV$_1$ with exercise) and the use of dry air result in a low rate of false-negative outcomes for EIB. However, EVH is a challenge without a standardized dose response and is very potent with the potential for a larger fall in FEV$_1$ than that with a graduated test such as the inhalation of mannitol (or methacholine).

EVH should probably not be the first challenge performed for individuals with a documented diagnosis of asthma.[66] However, EVH has been useful in the diagnosis of previously undiagnosed elite athletes and in excluding asthma in others previously clinically diagnosed as having EIB.[67–69] The disadvantages of EVH are a sore throat from breathing dry air, the need for a very low-resistance breathing circuit, and, as noted, severe falls in FEV$_1$.[1–3] Following the EVH challenge, FEV$_1$ is evaluated for about 30 min. A sustained fall in FEV$_1$ of at least 10% following EVH is consistent with EIB[68,70,71]; EVH is considered the gold standard for the diagnosis of asthma in Olympic athletes who are being screened for EIB. Nevertheless, general screening of all elite athletes for EIB with EVH is not recommended, as there is a relatively low prevalence of EIB among these athletes, suggesting that a history of EIB is unreliable.[12]

For individuals with known asthma, a mannitol dry powder challenge could be the initial procedure to evaluate the potential for EIB. This challenge test is standardized and patients rarely have large falls in FEV$_1$ as may be seen with the exercise challenge or EVH; moreover, exercise and EVH do not provide a RDR.[1–3]

Mannitol creates a hyperosmolar environment, which causes a mediator release similar to exercise and EVH. The challenge involves the inhalation of progressively increasing doses of mannitol powder to a cumulative dose of 635 mg, with determinations of FEV$_1$ 60 sec after each dose. The mannitol kit is commercially available in many countries with prepackaged capsules containing 5, 10, 30, or 40 mg of mannitol and an Osmohaler device to deliver the drug.[72,73] The FEV$_1$ is determined in duplicate. A fall of 15% from baseline in FEV_1 (or a fall of 10% between doses) at a cumulative dose of no more than 635 mg is considered a positive test. The test has a repeatability of about one doubling dose. Spontaneous recovery usually occurs rapidly after a mannitol challenge[72–74] in those with known asthma who are not receiving ICS, there is a consistent relationship between mannitol PD_{15} and the percentage fall in FEV_1 after exercise and EVH. This relationship is not as consistent in patients using ICS or in those without a defined asthma diagnosis.[75] A mannitol challenge completed in less than 35 min demonstrated sensitivities of 64%, 75%, and 83% to characterize exercise-associated FEV_1 falls of 10%, 15%, and 20%, respectively.[73]

Hypertonic saline (4.5%) is not commercially available for challenge testing but it has been used for the diagnosis of EIB and airway hyperresponsiveness in individuals with known asthma.[29,76] During a saline challenge, the nebulizer output is kept unchanged and the dose of saline is increased consecutively by doubling the inhalation time beginning with 0.5 min, then 1, 2, 4, and 8 min with subjects inhaling at tidal volumes. FEV_1 is determined in duplicate 1 min after each challenge step and the best (highest) of the duplicate readings at each stage is used. The challenge is terminated when FEV_1 falls ≥15% or more from baseline or the cumulative inhalation time of 15.5 min is achieved.[77] The level of aerosol delivered is determined by the alteration in the weight of the nebulizer. A 15% fall in FEV_1 in response to an inhalation of 23 g of saline or less is considered a positive result.[77] The sensitivity of a 4.5% saline provocative dose to diagnose EIB (with a fall in FEV_1 of at least 10%) was 53.9% with a specificity of 84.7% in a pediatric population.[78] Adenosine monophosphate is another investigational surrogate diagnostic test that creates a hyperosmolar environment.[3,76]

In a review of 20 relevant studies of diagnostic tests versus exercise challenge tests, the sensitivity and specificity for each test were as follows[79]:

- Self-report of symptoms to detect EIB (two studies): sensitivity 36.8%, specificity 85%–86%
- Sports-specific challenge for exercise bronchoprovocation to detect EIB (five studies): sensitivity 0%–100%, specificity 0%–100%
- EVH (seven studies) to detect EIB: sensitivity 25%–90%, specificity 0%–71%
- Free-running test (three studies) to detect EIB: sensitivity 60%–67%, specificity 47%–67%
- Mannitol (three studies) to detect EIB: sensitivity 58%–96%, specificity 65%–78%

These studies reflect small numbers and heterogeneity, with different study populations of adult and pediatric patients, elite and professional athletes, and different methods to induce EIB. This demonstrates that there is no consensus on a gold standard that replaces the standard exercise challenge to diagnose EIB.[79]

Direct challenges with pharmaceutical agents such as methacholine (which is available commercially) and histamine (which is investigational) are not recommended for

the diagnosis of EIB because they are not specific for EIB. Although methacholine may be used to exclude reactive airway disease, winter athletes who had a positive methacholine challenge did not demonstrate bronchoconstriction when evaluated with exercise, EVH, or mannitol.[8] A positive methacholine challenge in cold-weather athletes may reflect airway injury with bronchial hyperresponsiveness secondary to the hyperventilation of cold and dry air. Athletes performing in cold and dry environments, in swimming pools, or on ice rinks with air polluted with irritants may have airway hyperresponsiveness secondary to injury. In these patients, a methacholine challenge is not recommended for the diagnosis of EIB because a positive methacholine challenge merely reflects nonspecific airway injury. Individuals with "ski asthma," with airway hyperresponsiveness to methacholine and symptoms simulating asthma, fail to respond to ICS. This finding corroborates the contention that ski asthma with a positive methacholine challenge represents nonspecific airway injury with hyperresponsiveness and not the characteristic airway inflammation seen with chronic asthma.[80]

Comparative studies of EVH and methacholine in swimmers showed that the majority of swimmers who have positive EVH challenges also have positive methacholine challenges.[48] However, discrepancies exist because it is not uncommon to see a patient who has a positive EVH challenge and a negative methacholine challenge.[4,81]

The differential diagnosis of EIB should include vocal cord dysfunction, nasal congestion, cardiac and/or pulmonary abnormalities, and poor exercise conditioning, which all mimic EIB. Vocal cord dysfunction usually presents with inspiratory stridor with flattening and/or premature closure of the inspiratory loop on pulmonary function testing.[3] Dyspnea alone usually suggests poor physical conditioning and, less frequently, exercise-induced hyperventilation or other pulmonary conditions such as chronic obstructive pulmonary disease (COPD).[59] Patients with dyspnea may rarely have cardiac disorders (including arrhythmias, congestive heart failure, structural disease such as myopathies or idiopathic hypertrophic subaortic stenosis, or mitochondrial defects), gastrointestinal diseases (such as GERD), or skeletal abnormalities such as scoliosis. Rarely, if pruritus and urticaria are coexistent with symptoms suggesting EIB, then exercise-induced anaphylaxis syndromes with or without food dependence should be considered. With the proper use of diagnostic exercise challenge testing and rhinolaryngoscopy to visualize vocal cord adduction for vocal cord dysfunction, these other conditions can be ruled in or out.[1–3,58,59]

MANAGEMENT; PHARMACEUTICAL AND NONPHARMACEUTICAL AGENTS (TABLES 12.3 AND 12.4)

The treatment of individuals who have EIB requires an awareness of the variability of patient responses. The environmental conditions, the type of activity, and the underlying asthma must all be carefully evaluated when initiating and adjusting therapies.[82]

As noted earlier, EIB is triggered by inhaling dry air, leading to a hyperosmolar airway, resulting in airway inflammation and bronchoconstriction. The severity of EIB may be diminished in some patients by inspiring warm and humid air during exercise.[83] Nevertheless, severe EIB can still develop in patients inhaling hot dry air.[84] Thus, it is important to recognize that the principal stimulus for EIB is loss of water rather than airway rewarming. Medications that are effective in blocking the physiological effects of the bioactive mediators released from inflammatory cells as a result of this hyperosmolar state in the airway are useful in preventing EIB.[85-90]

BETA-AGONISTS

To prevent EIB, either inhaled short-acting beta-agonists (SABAs) or long-acting beta-agonists (LABAs) can be administered 15–30 min prior to exercise on an intermittent basis in the majority of individuals.[91-93] SABAs have an onset of action within 5–20 min with a duration of activity of about 2–4 h.[91,94,95] Inhaled beta-agonists inhibit EIB by activating two sites of beta$_2$-receptors on the mast cells to inhibit mediator release and on the bronchial smooth muscle to block contraction in response to mediators including histamine, leukotrienes, and prostaglandin D2.[1]

Beta-agonists alone are able to treat the bronchoconstrictive component of EIB, but they have no impact on inflammation.[95,96] A tolerance to beta-agonist therapy develops with daily administration at the level of both the mast cell and the airway smooth muscle within a week of regular use and this tachyphylaxis is not impacted by simultaneous therapy with ICS.[1-3]

Tolerance is reflected first by shortening the duration of protection to 2 h with SABAs and to 4–6 h with LABAs.[95,97-102] Additionally, the time to recovery to baseline FEV$_1$ following exercise may be extended after prolonged use of beta-agonists. The dose of inhaled beta-agonists needed to achieve protection may be higher if a daily beta-agonist is administered.[103,104] The EIB episode may be more severe with daily administration of a beta-agonist.[104] The likely mechanism of tolerance is a decreased number or a downregulation of beta$_2$-adrenergic receptors on the mast cells.[97,105] Tachyphylaxis is often managed by increasing the dose of the beta-agonist prior to exercise, making the problem even worse. Intermittent use of a beta-agonist, no more than three times a week, for prophylaxis or treatment, is most effective in preventing tachyphylaxis.[106] The discontinuation of a beta-agonist for 3 days will generally lead to a return of responsiveness to beta-agonists.[101]

ANTICHOLINERGIC AGENTS

Anticholinergic agents, such as ipratropium bromide, have been inconsistent in attenuating EIB; however, it is clear that some patients do respond to this therapy. This agent has bronchodilator activity by inhibiting vagally mediated bronchomotor tone. Ipratropium has been used alone and in conjunction with SABAs for acute exacerbations of asthma, but it has not been consistent in double-blind, placebo-controlled investigations and intrapatient variability has been reported.[107-110]

CHROMONES AND NONSTEROIDAL ANTI-INFLAMMATORY AGENTS

Chromones are mast cell stabilizing medications that block EIB.[111] These agents, including sodium cromoglycate and nedocromol sodium, are administered by inhalation, immediately prior to exercise, to provide up to 60% inhibition of EIB; but they are no longer available in the United States.[111] Complete inhibition of EIB is defined as a fall in FEV$_1$ postexercise of no more than 10%.[1,2] The duration of these agents' protection is usually less than 4 h, but their onset of action is immediate so they can be inhaled just prior to exercise on an as-needed basis.[2,112] Tolerance has not been reported to the recurrent administration of these drugs. These agents reportedly work by inhibiting the release of prostaglandin D2 and leukotrienes.[112] Unfortunately, the armamentarium of medications to treat EIB has been significantly weakened since these agents are no longer available.

LEUKOTRIENE ANTAGONISTS

Leukotriene receptor antagonists (LTRAs) such as montelukast and zafirlukast and 5-lipoxygenase inhibitors such as zileuton provide approximately 60% protection against EIB. Montelukast is the most commonly used agent. It is administered as a tablet and should be taken about 2 h prior to the activity so that it can be fully effective.[113] Although it is not effective for all asthmatic patients, it can provide protection for as long as 24 h.[114,115] Unlike beta-agonists, montelukast can be taken continuously, daily, prophylactically, and without tolerance developing.[115] Montelukast promotes the recovery of FEV$_1$ to baseline by decreasing the time to recovery and it diminishes the duration and severity of the asthma episode following exercise.[1-3] Combination therapy with loratidine may provide effective attenuation of EIB with a decreased mediator release.[116-118] Zafirlukast, a second leukotriene antagonist, has a duration of action of about 8 h.[117,118] Zileuton, a 5-lipoxygenase inhibitor, has a duration of prophylaxis for EIB of 4 h, equivalent to zafirlukast, but it is less efficacious by 8 h than zafirlukast, montelukast, and salmeterol and there is no difference between it and placebo by 12 h.[118-120]

NONPHARMACEUTICAL MANEUVERS

Nonpharmaceutical maneuvers that can attenuate or provide prophylaxis against EIB include hydration and inspiring air conditioned to the physiological temperature and humidity, which may provide 80% or more protection, similar to medications[113,117,118,121-125] (Table 12.3). The use of a face mask or instruments for heat exchange permits the retention of water

TABLE 12.3

Nonpharmacological

Therapy[1–3,127–132,147–150]

Breathing through mouth/face mask

Warm-up refractory period

Vitamin C

Fish oil

Low-salt diet

Aerobic conditioning

vapor allowing rebreathing. This may decrease the number of airway generations required for adjusting the inspired air to the physiological conditions.[1–3] Finally, recurrent exercise repeated within a limited period of time from the first exercise (e.g., about 2 h) will lead to a refractory period of tolerance to further bronchoconstriction.[122] Warming up with aerobic exercises, such as short sprints with the achievement of 40%–60% of the maximum heart rate, may attenuate EIB, particularly in conjunction with SABAs.[126–129] Agents such as ascorbic acid, fish oil, and dietary sodium restriction have been demonstrated to attenuate EIB in small, placebo-controlled trials.[130–132]

APPROACH TO TREATMENT OF EIB WITH ASTHMA

As described earlier, SABA or LABA may be administered up to 30 min prior to exercise, as many as three times a week, to prevent mild intermittent episodes of EIB. Tolerance to SABA and LABA occurs after only a few doses and is indicated by decreased bronchodilation when these drugs are given for an asthma exacerbation, even with concomitant ICS therapy.[101,104,133–135] This tolerance may lead the patient or health-care provider to further increase the use of beta-agonists with a greater chance of adverse events and no increase in efficacy. However, despite the concern regarding the daily use of beta-agonists leading to tolerance and impairing the response to emergency therapy for asthma, there are limited data to support that this tolerance is clinically important in the elite athlete.[62] With competitive and elite athletes who exercise daily or even more frequently, the use of beta-agonists for prophylaxis during or following exercise could theoretically lead to exceeding the optimal guidelines for beta-agonist monotherapy stated in the National Heart, Lung, and Blood Institute (NHLBI) and the Global Initiative for Asthma (GINA) guidelines and tolerance could then potentially be of clinical importance.[1–3,62]

If asthma is more persistent and not well controlled, then either montelukast or ICS may be started. Montelukast is administered once a day at night, with onset within about 2 h and a duration of about 24 h. Montelukast is effective in at least one-half of asthmatic patients but the other half will have no improvement with this drug. No tolerance develops to montelukast, as occurs with beta-agonists. ICS therapy is indicated for persistent asthma that is mild to severe and that does not respond to beta-agonists or montelukast[1,2]: (Table 12.4).

Nonsteroidal medications, such as the mast cell stabilizers (MCS), cromolyn (cromoglycate), or nedocromil, are also deemed effective for chronic mild persistent asthma as stated in previous NHLBI guidelines. Cromolyn has been demonstrated to be effective versus a placebo in decreasing the fall in FEV_1 after a EVH challenge in the most competitive or elite athletes with EIB.[112] These findings support the importance of the mast cell mediator release in EIB severity. The limitation of the study is that cromoglycate was compared in a single dose with a placebo, and not with an active comparator.[62,112] In a Cochrane analysis of 20 randomized, controlled trials, nedocromil (4 mg inhaled 15–60 min prior to exercise) significantly diminished the severity and the duration of EIB in both adults and children.[111] A Cochrane analysis of eight studies demonstrated no significant difference between cromolyn and nedocromil in the maximum decrease in FEV_1, complete protection (defined as the maximum percentage fall in FEV_1 less than 10% from baseline), clinical protection (defined as 50% improvement over a placebo), or side effects.[136] Unfortunately, as noted earlier, neither agent is marketed or sold in the United States, the United Kingdom, or Europe.

ICS therapy is indicated in both adults and children who have chronic persistent asthma not responsive to beta-agonist and montelukast. When administered on a daily basis, these agents have been demonstrated to be effective in decreasing the severity of EIB.[1–3] The dose and the duration of the therapy are dependent on the various preparations.[1–3,121] ICS therapy is the most widely utilized and the most effective inhaled anti-inflammatory therapy preferred in both the NHLBI and GINA guidelines.[1–3] ICS therapy prevents asthma episodes and enhances quality of life and pulmonary functions, while diminishing airway inflammation and hyperresponsiveness as well as the severity and frequency of exacerbations and mortality.[137,138] Used in the recommended doses, ICS therapy requires days to weeks to become fully effective. The onset of the effects of ICS therapy usually requires 7–14 days, and is most efficacious after 8 weeks of treatment.[64] ICS may be administered in very high doses a few hours prior to exercise for EIB alone in competitive athletes, but this is not recommended as an ongoing clinical practice.[139]

Our understanding of the efficacy of ICS therapy is derived from similar studies lasting from 3 weeks to 2 years in children and adults. In a study with budesonide (800 µg

TABLE 12.4

Pharmacological Therapy[109,111,112,121,124]

Beta-agonists: long acting and short acting (LABA, SABA)

Anticholinergic agents

Montelukast

Nonsteroidal agents

Inhaled steroids (ICS)

Combination therapy (such as ICS plus LABA)

bid) versus a placebo, in which adults were randomized to treatment for 6 weeks of therapy, there was a postexercise fall in FEV_1 of 7% in the budesonide cohort and 22% in the placebo cohort with similar outcomes in pediatric studies.[62,140] When combination therapy was examined, the ICS component remained effective in controlling the severity of EIB when the beta-agonist was withdrawn from the combination therapy.[141] ICS, including budesonide, ciclesonide, and fluticasone, have been demonstrated to be efficacious in decreasing the severity of EIB within 3–12 weeks of the initiation of ICS therapy.[123,124,142,143] The time to onset of protection is quicker with higher doses of ICS than with lower doses.[121] ICS alone, used daily, are effective, as the majority of individuals with EIB have normal spirometry and require a beta-agonist only prior to exercise. However, in individuals with an abnormal baseline spirometry, the combination of ICS with LABAs has been demonstrated to be effective in decreasing the severity of EIB.[142,143] Combination therapy with LABAs, including salmeterol and formoterol, is often used in the management of asthma that is not controlled with ICS therapy alone. The combinations (of ICS with LABA) are usually prescribed in fixed combinations, but may be administered as separate inhalers. The use of monotherapy with LABAs for chronic or persistent asthma is never recommended on a continuous basis because of the danger of adverse outcomes with therapeutic failure and the danger of asthma exacerbation.[144] However, a review of the literature indicates that combined fluticasone and salmeterol was more effective than fluticasone alone for the prophylaxis of EIB with asthma.[145] Similarly, in a randomized, double-blind investigation, combination therapy with budesonide and formoterol was more effective in improving asthma control and symptoms compared with budesonide alone.[146] As noted above, a pilot study in children with clinically stable asthma, who were being treated with a combination therapy (ICS and LABA), demonstrated that the removal of the LABA reduced the severity of EIB and may even have eliminated EIB.[141] This observation suggests that ICS alone may be more effective over time than the combination of ICS and LABA for EIB. Indeed, patients should attempt to discontinue the inhaled beta-agonist prior to exercise to determine if EIB is still present. This policy will avoid administering inhaled beta-agonists when these agents are unnecessary.[1]

An evidence-based review of the literature reveals that SABA provided greater protection than MCS in 12 studies.[79] However, combining SABAs and MCS provided no further benefits in five studies. LTRAs, MCS, ipratropium bromide, and interval warm-up routines demonstrated a statistically significant reduction in EIB with asthma, measured as the mean difference in the percentage fall in FEV_1 and 95% confidence intervals when compared with a placebo. Nine studies demonstrated the efficacy of single-dose interventions with LTRA (8.9% mean difference); 17 studies with nedocromil sodium (15.6% mean difference); 4 studies with interval warm-up (10.6% mean difference); 4 studies with ICS (5% mean difference); 2 studies with

continuous high-intensity warm-up (9.8% mean difference); and 3 studies with continuous low-intensity warm-up versus no warm-up (12.6% mean difference).[79] Notably, after daily LABA use for 3–4 weeks in four studies, the percentage fall in FEV_1 following an exercise challenge at 2 and 4 weeks was greater than at day 1, presumably related to tachyphylaxis. Interestingly, both SABA and LABA continue to lessen EIB in patients with known asthma when given prophylactically even though the effect of these drugs is diminished by tachyphylaxis with a prolonged time to recovery.[79,95,97–103]

Supplements to the diet such as fish oil and vitamin C as well as a low-salt diet have been demonstrated to be effective for protection against EIB.[147,148] However, these studies, while often placebo controlled, were performed in individuals with mild EIB and do not apply to the more severe forms of EIB.[147,148] Agents such as heparin, theophylline, furosemide, and calcium channel blockers have also been evaluated as therapy for EIB, but there is insufficient evidence to recommend their routine use.[1–3]

Maintaining physical conditioning may raise the threshold for EIB.[149,150] For the elite athlete, national and global guidelines and standards as well as regulations must be followed. For the elite athlete with EIB alone, the use of ICS in large doses (i.e., beclomethasone at 1500 µg given 4 h prior to exercise) or cromolyn sodium or beta-agonists given prior to exercise have some demonstrated efficacy[112,139]; but a reduction in prolonged training and the avoidance of triggers in the environment may be the only effective management of EIB.[1–3] Chronic use of ICS is less effective in the setting of neutrophil predominance with EIB alone.[1,2,62,82]

CONCLUSION

EIB is the most specific and earliest presentation of asthma and the last to resolve with an asthma exacerbation. This condition generally reflects underlying asthma control (or lack of control) but it may present alone in highly competitive or elite athletes. EIB has bronchoconstrictive and inflammatory components. The diagnosis of EIB requires pulmonary function evaluation with an exercise or surrogate challenge. A differential diagnosis includes poor conditioning, vocal cord dysfunction, nasal congestion, and, rarely, cardiac or other pulmonary conditions. The management of EIB should follow the general guidelines that the NHLBI has developed or the more recently published practice parameter on EIB so that the exercising individual may pursue a healthy lifestyle with the ability to participate in the exercise of choice.[3]

DECLARATION OF INTEREST

The authors have no conflicts of interest to report. Both authors are members of the workgroup for the Joint Task Force Practice Parameter on Exercise-Induced Asthma. The authors alone are responsible for the content, preparation, and writing of this chapter.

REFERENCES

1. Anderson, S.D., Exercise-induced bronchoconstriction in the 21st century. *J Am Osteopath Assoc*, 2011. **111**(11 Suppl 7): S3–S10.

2. Anderson, S.D. and P. Kippelen, Assessment and prevention of exercise-induced bronchoconstriction. *Br J Sports Med*, 2012. **46**(6): 391–396.

3. Weiler, J.M., S.D. Anderson, and C.C. Randolph, Pathogenesis, prevalence, diagnosis, and management of exercise-induced bronchoconstriction: A practice parameter. *Ann Allergy Asthma Immunol*, 2010. **105**(6 Suppl): S1–S47.

4. Khan, D.A., Exercise-induced bronchoconstriction: Burden and prevalence. *Allergy Asthma Proc*, 2012. **33**(1): 1–6.

5. Bougault, V., J. Turmel, and L.P. Boulet, Bronchial challenges and respiratory symptoms in elite swimmers and winter sport athletes: Airway hyperresponsiveness in asthma—Its measurement and clinical significance. *Chest*, 2010. **138**(2 Suppl): 31S–37S.

6. Langdeau, J.B. and L.P. Boulet, Is asthma over- or under-diagnosed in athletes? *Respir Med*, 2003. **97**(2): 109–114.

7. Lund, T.K., Are asthma-like symptoms in elite athletes associated with classical features of asthma? *Br J Sports Med*, 2009. **43**(14): 1131–1135.

8. Sue-Chu, M., J.D. Brannan, S.D. Anderson, et al., Airway hyperresponsiveness to methacholine, adenosine 5-monophosphate, mannitol, eucapnic voluntary hyperpnoea and field exercise challenge in elite cross-country skiers. *Br J Sports Med*, 2010. **44**(11): 827–832.

9. Weiler, J.M., T. Layton, and M. Hunt, Asthma in United States Olympic athletes who participated in the 1996 Summer Games. *J Allergy Clin Immunol*, 1998. **102**(5): 722–726.

10. Weiler, J.M. and E.J. Ryan, 3rd, Asthma in United States olympic athletes who participated in the 1998 olympic winter games. *J Allergy Clin Immunol*, 2000. **106**(2): 267–271.

11. National Asthma, E. and P. Prevention, Expert Panel Report 3 (EPR-3): Guidelines for the Diagnosis and Management of Asthma-Summary Report 2007. *J Allergy Clin Immunol*, 2007. **120**(5 Suppl): S94–S138.

12. Parsons, J.P., D. Cosmar, G. Phillips, et al., Screening for exercise-induced bronchoconstriction in college athletes. *J Asthma*, 2012. **49**(2): 153–157.

13. Rundell, K.W., J. Im, L.B. Mayers, et al., Self-reported symptoms and exercise-induced asthma in the elite athlete. *Med Sci Sports Exerc*, 2001. **33**(2): 208–213.

14. Anderson, S.D., D.S. Pearlman, K.W. Rundell, et al., Reproducibility of the airway response to an exercise protocol standardized for intensity, duration, and inspired air conditions, in subjects with symptoms suggestive of asthma. *Respir Res*, 2010. **11**: 120.

15. Vilozni, D., Exercise challenge test in 3- to 6-year-old asthmatic children. *Chest*, 2007. **132**(2): 497–503.

16. van Leeuwen, J.C., J.M. Diessen, F.H. deJongh, et al., Monitoring pulmonary function during exercise in children with asthma. *Arch Dis Child*, 2011. **96**(7): 664–668.

17. Freed, A.N. and S.D. Anderson, Exercise induced bronchoconstriction: Human models. In: Kay, A.B., J. Bousquet, P.G. Holt, and A.P. Daplan (eds.), *Allergy and Allergic Diseases*, pp. 808–822, 2009. Oxford: Blackwell Scientific Publications.

18. Goldberg, S., F. Mimouni, L. Joseph, et al., Seasonal effect on exercise challenge tests for the diagnosis of exercise-induced bronchoconstriction. *Allergy Asthma Proc*, 2012. **33**(5): 416–420.

19. Burr, M.L., B.A. Eldridge, and L.K. Borysiewicz, Peak expiratory flow rates before and after exercise in schoolchildren. *Arch Dis Child*, 1974. **49**(12): 923–926.

20. Burr, M.L., B.K. Butland, S. King, et al., Changes in asthma prevalence: Two surveys 15 years apart. *Arch Dis Child*, 1989. **64**(10): 1452–1456.

21. Hallstrand, T.S., Effectiveness of screening examinations to detect unrecognized exercise-induced bronchoconstriction. *J Pediatr*, 2002. **141**(3): 343–348.

22. Rupp, N.T., M.F. Guill, and D.S. Brudno, Unrecognized exercise-induced bronchospasm in adolescent athletes. *Am J Dis Child*, 1992. **146**(8): 941–944.

23. Mannix, E.T., M.A. Roberts, H.J. Dukes, et al., Airways hyperresponsiveness in high school athletes. *J Asthma*, 2004. **41**(5): 567–574.

24. Mannix, E.T., M. Roberts, D.P. Fagin, et al., The prevalence of airways hyperresponsiveness in members of an exercise training facility. *J Asthma*, 2003. **40**(4): 349–355.

25. Hallstrand, T.S., New insights into pathogenesis of exercise-induced bronchoconstriction. *Curr Opin Allergy Clin Immunol*, 2012. **12**(1): 42–48.

26. Addo-yobo, E.O., A. Woolcock, A. Allotey, et al., Exercise-induced bronchospasm and atopy in Ghana: Two surveys ten years apart. *PLoS Med*, 2007. **4**(2): e70.

27. Benarab-Boucherit, Y., H. Mehliouni, F. Nediar, et al., Prevalence rate of exercise-induced bronchoconstriction in Annaba (Algeria) schoolchildren. *J Asthma*, 2011. **48**(5): 511–516.

28. Cabral, A.L., G.M. Conceicao, C.H. Fonseca-Guedes, et al., Exercise-induced bronchospasm in children: Effects of asthma severity. *Am J Respir Crit Care Med*, 1999. **159**(6): 1819–1823.

29. Haby, M.M., J.K. Peat, C.M. Mellis, et al., An exercise challenge for epidemiological studies of childhood asthma: Validity and repeatability. *Eur Respir J*, 1995. **8**(5): 729–736.

30. DeBaets, F., E. Bodart, M. Dramaix-Wilmet, et al., Exercise-induced respiratory symptoms are poor predictors of bronchoconstriction. *Pediatr Pulmonol*, 2005. **39**(4): 301–305.

31. Kufkafka, D.S., D.M. Lang, S. Porter, et al., Exercise-induced bronchospasm in high school athletes via a free running test: Incidence and epidemiology. *Chest*, 1998. **114**(6): 1613–1622.

32. Jones, C.O., S. Quereshi, R.J. Rona, et al., Exercise-induced bronchoconstriction by ethnicity and presence of asthma in British nine year olds. *Thorax*, 1996. **51**(11): 1134–1136.

33. Wilber, R.I., K.W. Rundell, E. Szmedra, et al., Incidence of exercise-induced bronchospasm in Olympic winter sport athletes. *Med Sci Sports Exerc*, 2000. **32**(4): 732–737.

34. Mannix, E.T., M.O. Farbre, P. Palange, et al., Exercise-induced asthma in figure skaters. *Chest*, 1996. **109**(2): 312–315.

35. Rundell, K.W., S.D. Anderson, B.A. Spierling, et al., Field exercise vs laboratory eucapnic voluntary hyperventilation to identify airway hyperresponsiveness in elite cold weather athletes. *Chest*, 2004. **125**(3): 909–915.

36. Holzer, K., S.D. Anderson, and J. Douglass, Exercise in elite summer athletes: Challenges for diagnosis. *J Allergy Clin Immunol*, 2002. **110**(3): 374–380.

37. Porsbjerg, C., M.L. vonLinstow, C.S. Ulrik, et al., Outcome in adulthood of asymptomatic airway hyperresponsiveness to histamine and exercise-induced bronchospasm in childhood. *Ann Allergy Asthma Immunol*, 2005. **95**(2): 137–142.

38. Carlsen, K.M., S.D. Anderson, and L. Bjermer, Exercise-induced asthma, respiratory and allergic disorders in elite athletes: Epidemiology, mechanisms and diagnosis: Part I of the report from the Joint Task Force of the European Respiratory Society (ERS) and the European Academy of Allergy and Clinical Immunology (EAACI) in cooperation with GA2LEN. *Allergy*, 2008. **63**(4): 387–403.

39. Anderson, S.D., R. Wong, M. Bennett, et al., Summary of the knowledge and thinking about asthma and diving since 1993. *Diving Hyperb Med*, 1993. **36**: 12–22.

40. Parsons, J.P., T.J. Craig, S.W. Stoloff, et al., Impact of exercise-related respiratory symptoms in adults with asthma: Exercise-Induced Bronchospasm Landmark National Survey. *Allergy Asthma Proc*, 2011. **32**(6): 431–437.

41. Ostrom, N., N. Eid, T.J. Craig, et al., Exercise-induced bronchospasm in children with asthma in the United States: Results from the Exercise-Induced Bronchospasm Landmark Survey. *Allergy Asthma Proc*, 2011. **32**(6): 425–430.

42. Kojima, N., Y. Ohya, M. Futamura, et al., Exercise-induced asthma is associated with impaired quality of life among children with asthma in Japan. *Allergol Int*, 2009. **58**(2): 187–192.

43. Hallstrand, T.S., Quality of life in adolescents with mild asthma. *Pediatr Pulmonol*, 2003. **36**(6): 536–543.

44. Correia, M.A. Jr., Effect of exercise-induced bronchospasm and parental beliefs on physical activity of asthmatic adolescents from a tropical region. *Ann Allergy Asthma Immunol*, 2012. **108**(4): 249–253.

45. Anderson, S.D. and P. Kippelen, Airway injury as a mechanism for exercise-induced bronchoconstriction in elite athletes. *J Allergy Clin Immunol*, 2008. **122**(2): 225–235; quiz 236–237.

46. Anderson, S.D. and P. Kippelen, Exercise-induced bronchoconstriction: Pathogenesis. *Curr Allergy Asthma Rep*, 2005. **5**(2): 116–122.

47. Stensrud, T., K.V. Myland, K. Gabrielsen, et al., Bronchial hyperresponsiveness in skiers: Field test versus methacholine provocation? *Med Sci Sports Exerc*, 2007. **39**(10): 1681–1686.

48. Stadelmann, K., T. Stensrud, and K.H. Carlsen, Respiratory symptoms and bronchial responsiveness in competitive swimmers. *Med Sci Sports Exerc*, 2011. **43**(3): 375–381.

49. Bougault, V., J. Turmel, J. St-Laurent, et al., Asthma, airway inflammation and epithelial damage in swimmers and cold-air athletes. *Eur Respir J*, 2009. **33**(4): 740–746.

50. Rundell, K.W., B.A. Spierling, T.M. Evans, et al., Baseline lung function, exercise-induced bronchoconstriction, and asthma-like symptoms in elite women ice hockey players. *Med Sci Sports Exerc*, 2004. **36**(3): 405–410.

51. Weiler, J.M., S. Bonini, R. Coifman, et al., American Academy of Allergy, Asthma & Immunology Work Group report: Exercise-induced asthma. *J Allergy Clin Immunol*, 2007. **119**(6): 1349–1358.

52. Rundell, K.W., R.L. Wilber, L. Szmedra, et al., Exercise-induced asthma screening of elite athletes: Field versus laboratory exercise challenge. *Med Sci Sports Exerc*, 2000. **32**(2): 309–316.

53. Rundell, K.W. and J.B. Slee, Exercise and other indirect challenges to demonstrate asthma or exercise-induced bronchoconstriction in athletes. *J Allergy Clin Immunol*, 2008. **122**(2): 238–246; quiz 247–248.

54. Parsons, J.P., C. Kaeding, and G. Phillips, Prevalence of exercise-induced bronchospasm in a cohort of varsity college athletes. *Med Sci Sports Exerc*, 2007. **39**(9): 1487–1492.

55. Crapo, R.O., R. Casaburi, A.L. Coates, et al., Guidelines for methacholine and exercise challenge testing-1999. This official statement of the American Thoracic Society was adopted by the ATS Board of Directors, July 1999. *Am J Respir Crit Care Med*, 2000. **161**(1): 309–329.

56. Cockcroft, D. and B. Davis, Direct and indirect challenges in the clinical assessment of asthma. *Ann Allergy Asthma Immunol*, 2009. **103**(5): 363–369; quiz 369–372, 400.

57. Carlsen, K.H., G. Engh, and M. Mork, Exercise-induced bronchoconstriction depends on exercise load. *Respir Med*, 2000. **94**(8): 750–755.

58. Vasudev, M., Evaluation of paradoxical vocal fold motion. *Ann Allergy Asthma Immunol*, 2012. **109**(4): 233–236.

59. Abu-Hasan, M., B. Tannous, and M. Weinberger, Exercise-induced dyspnea in children and adolescents: If not asthma then what? *Ann Allergy Asthma Immunol*, 2005. **94**(3): 366–371.

60. Rundell, K.W., Pulmonary function decay in women ice hockey players: Is there a relationship to ice rink air quality? *Inhal Toxicol*, 2004. **16**(3): 117–123.

61. Rundell, K.W., High levels of airborne ultrafine and fine particulate matter in indoor ice arenas. *Inhal Toxicol*, 2003. **15**(3): 237–250.

62. Pedersen, L., J. Elers, and V. Backer, Asthma in elite athletes: Pathogenesis, diagnosis, differential diagnoses, and treatment. *Phys Sportsmed*, 2011. **39**(3): 163–171.

63. McKenzie, D.C. and L.P. Boulet, Asthma, outdoor air quality and the Olympic Games. *CMAJ*, 2008. **179**(6): 543–548.

64. Fitch, K.D., M. Sue-Chu, S.D. Anderson, et al., Asthma and the elite athlete: Summary of the International Olympic Committee's consensus conference, Lausanne, Switzerland, January 22–24, 2008. *J Allergy Clin Immunol*, 2008. **122**(2): 254–260, 260 e1–7.

65. Anderson, S.D., S. Lambert, J.D. Brannan, et al., Laboratory protocol for exercise asthma to evaluate salbutamol given by two devices. *Med Sci Sports Exerc*, 2001. **33**(6): 893–900.

66. Anderson, S.D., G.J. Argyros, H. Magnussen, et al., Provocation by eucapnic voluntary hyperpnoea to identify exercise induced bronchoconstriction. *Br J Sports Med*, 2001. **35**(5): 344–347.

67. Dickinson, J., A. McConnell, and G. Whyte, Diagnosis of exercise-induced bronchoconstriction: Eucapnic voluntary hyperpnoea challenges identify previously undiagnosed elite athletes with exercise-induced bronchoconstriction. *Br J Sports Med*, 2011. **45**(14): 1126–1131.

68. Arygros, G.J., J.M. Roach, K.M. Hurowitz, et al., Eucapnic voluntary hyperventilation as a bronchoprovocation technique: Development of a standarized dosing schedule in asthmatics. *Chest*, 1996. **109**(6): 1520–1524.

69. Ansley, L., P. Kippelen, J. Dickinson, et al., Misdiagnosis of exercise-induced bronchoconstriction in professional soccer players. *Allergy*, 2012. **67**(3): 390–395.

70. Spiering, B.A., D.A. Judelson, and K.W. Rundell, An evaluation of standardizing target ventilation for eucapnic voluntary hyperventilation using FEV_1. *J Asthma*, 2004. **41**(7): 745–749.

71. Brummel, N.E., J.G. Mastronarde, D. Rittinger, et al., The clinical utility of eucapnic voluntary hyperventilation testing for the diagnosis of exercise-induced bronchospasm. *J Asthma*, 2009. **46**(7): 683–686.

72. Brannan, J.D., S.D. Anderson, C.P. Perry, et al., The safety and efficacy of inhaled dry powder mannitol as a bronchial provocation test for airway hyperresponsiveness: A phase 3 comparison study with hypertonic (4.5%) saline. *Respir Res*, 2005. **6**: 144.

73. Anderson, S.D., B. Charlton, J.M. Weiler, et al., Comparison of mannitol and methacholine to predict exercise-induced bronchoconstriction and a clinical diagnosis of asthma. *Respir Res*, 2009. **10**: 4.

74. Holzer, K., S.D. Anderson, H.K. Chan, et al., Mannitol as a challenge test to identify exercise-induced bronchoconstriction in elite athletes. *Am J Respir Crit Care Med*, 2003. **167**(4): 534–537.

75. Brannan, J.D., H. Koskela, S.D. Anderson, et al., Responsiveness to mannitol in asthmatic subjects with exercise- and hyperventilation-induced asthma. *Am J Respir Crit Care Med*, 1998. **158**(4): 1120–1126.

76. Anderson, S.D., Indirect challenge tests: Airway hyperresponsiveness in asthma—Its measurement and clinical significance. *Chest*, 2010. **138**(2 Suppl): 25S–30S.

77. Anderson, S.D. and J.D. Brannan, Methods for "indirect" challenge tests including exercise, eucapnic voluntary hyperpnea, and hypertonic aerosols. *Clin Rev Allergy Immunol*, 2003. **24**(1): 27–54.

78. Riedler, J., T. Reade, M. Dalton, et al., Hypertonic saline challenge in an epidemiologic survey of asthma in children. *Am J Respir Crit Care Med*, 1994. **150**(6 Pt 1): 1632–1639.

79. Dryden, D.M., C.H. Spooner, D.M. Srickland, et al., Exercise-induced bronchoconstriction and asthma. *Evidence Reports/Technology Assessments, No. 189*, 2010.

80. Sue-Chu, M., E.M. Karljalainen, A. Laitinen, et al., Placebo-controlled study of inhaled budesonide on indices of airway inflammation in bronchoalveolar lavage fluid and bronchial biopsies in cross-country skiers. *Respiration*, 2000. **67**(4): 417–425.

81. Pederson, L., S. Winther, V. Backer, et al., Airway responses to eucapnic hyperpnea, exercise, and methacholine in elite swimmers. *Med Sci Sports Exerc*, 2008. **40**(9): 1567–1572.

82. Spector, S. and R. Tan, Exercise-induced bronchoconstriction update: Therapeutic management. *Allergy Asthma Proc*, 2012. **33**(1): 7–12.

83. Anderson, S.D., R.E. Schoeffel, R. Follett, et al., Sensitivity to heat and water loss at rest and during exercise in asthmatic patients. *Eur J Respir Dis*, 1982. **63**(5): 459–471.

84. Anderson, S.D., R.E. Schoeffel, J.L. Black, et al., Airway cooling as the stimulus to exercise-induced asthma—A re-evaluation. *Eur J Respir Dis*, 1985. **67**(1): 20–30.

85. Reiss, T.F., J.B. Hill, E. Harman, et al., Increased urinary excretion of LTE4 after exercise and attenuation of exercise-induced bronchospasm by montelukast, a cysteinyl leukotriene receptor antagonist. *Thorax*, 1997. **52**(12): 1030–1035.

86. O'Sullivan, S., A. Roquet, B. Dahlen, et al., Evidence for mast cell activation during exercise-induced bronchoconstriction. *Eur Respir J*, 1998. **12**(2): 345–350.

87. Leff, J.A., W.W. Busse, D. Pearlman, et al., Montelukast, a leukotriene-receptor antagonist, for the treatment of mild asthma and exercise-induced bronchoconstriction. *N Engl J Med*, 1998. **339**(3): 147–152.

88. Brannan, J.D., M. Gulliksson, S.D. Anderson, et al., Inhibition of mast cell PGD2 release protects against mannitol-induced airway narrowing. *Eur Respir J*, 2006. **27**(5): 944–950.

89. Brannan, J.D., M. Gulliksson, S.D. Anderson, et al., Evidence of mast cell activation and leukotriene release after mannitol inhalation. *Eur Respir J*, 2003. **22**(3): 491–496.

90. Brannan, J.D., S.D. Anderson, K. Gomas, et al., Fexofenadine decreases sensitivity to and montelukast improves recovery from inhaled mannitol. *Am J Respir Crit Care Med*, 2001. **163**(6): 1420–1425.

91. Pearlman, D.S., W. Rees, K. Schaefer, et al., An evaluation of levalbuterol HFA in the prevention of exercise-induced bronchospasm. *J Asthma*, 2007. **44**(9): 729–733.

92. Larsson, K., K.H. Carlsen, and S. Bonini, Ani-asthmatic drugs: Treatment of athletes and exercise induced bronchoconstriction. *Eur Respir Mon*, 2005. **33**: 73–88.

93. Anderson, S.D., Single-dose agents in the prevention of exercise-induced asthma: A descriptive review. *Treat Respir Med*, 2004. **3**(6): 365–379.

94. Anderson, S.D., J.P. Seale, P. Rozea, et al., Inhaled and oral salbutamol in exercise-induced asthma. *Am Rev Respir Dis*, 1976. **114**(3): 493–500.

95. Anderson, S.D., C. Caillaud, and J.D. Brannan, Beta2-agonists and exercise-induced asthma. *Clin Rev Allergy Immunol*, 2006. **31**(2–3): 163–180.

96. Bisgaard, H., Long-acting beta(2)-agonists in management of childhood asthma: A critical review of the literature. *Pediatr Pulmonol*, 2000. **29**(3): 221–234.

97. Scola, A.M., L.K. Chong, S.K. Suvarna, et al., Desensitisation of mast cell beta2-adrenoceptor-mediated responses by salmeterol and formoterol. *Br J Pharmacol*, 2004. **141**(1): 163–171.

98. Nelson, J.A., L. Strauss, M. Skowronski, et al., Effect of long-term salmeterol treatment on exercise-induced asthma. *N Engl J Med*, 1998. **339**(3): 141–146.

99. Johnson, M., Molecular mechanisms of beta(2)-adrenergic receptor function, response, and regulation. *J Allergy Clin Immunol*, 2006. **117**(1): 18–24; quiz 25.

100. Haney, S. and R.J. Hancox, Recovery from bronchoconstriction and bronchodilator tolerance. *Clin Rev Allergy Immunol*, 2006. **31**(2–3): 181–196.

101. Haney, S. and R.J. Hancox, Rapid onset of tolerance to beta-agonist bronchodilation. *Respir Med*, 2005. **99**(5): 566–571.

102. Drotar, D.E., E.E. Davis, and D.W. Cockcroft, Tolerance to the bronchoprotective effect of salmeterol 12 hours after starting twice daily treatment. *Ann Allergy Asthma Immunol*, 1998. **80**(1): 31–34.

103. Storms, W.W., P. Chervinsky, A.F. Ghannam, et al., A comparison of the effects of oral montelukast and inhaled salmeterol on response to rescue bronchodilation after challenge. *Respir Med*, 2004. **98**(11): 1051–1062.

104. Hancox, R.J., P. Subbarao, D. Kamada, et al., Beta2-agonist tolerance and exercise-induced bronchospasm. *Am J Respir Crit Care Med*, 2002. **165**(8): 1068–1070.

105. Peachell, P., Regulation of mast cells by beta-agonists. *Clin Rev Allergy Immunol*, 2006. **31**(2–3): 131–142.

106. Davis, B.E., J.K. Reid, and D.W. Cockcroft, Formoterol thrice weekly does not result in the development of tolerance to bronchoprotection. *Can Respir J*, 2003. **10**(1): 23–26.

107. Knopfli, B.H., O. Bar-Or, and C.G. Araujo, Effect of ipratropium bromide on EIB in children depends on vagal activity. *Med Sci Sports Exerc*, 2005. **37**(3): 354–359.

108. Boulet, L.P., H. Turcotte, and S. Tennina, Comparative efficacy of salbutamol, ipratropium, and cromoglycate in the prevention of bronchospasm induced by exercise and hyperosmolar challenges. *J Allergy Clin Immunol*, 1989. **83**(5): 882–887.

109. Boner, A.L., G. Vallone, and G. De Stefano, Effect of inhaled ipratropium bromide on methacholine and exercise provocation in asthmatic children. *Pediatr Pulmonol*, 1989. **6**(2): 81–85.

110. Blake, K., Review of guidelines and the literature in the treatment of acute bronchospasm in asthma. *Pharmacotherapy*, 2006. **26**(9 Pt 2): 148S–155S.

111. Spooner, C.H., G.R. Spooner, and B.H. Rowe, Mast-cell stabilising agents to prevent exercise-induced bronchoconstriction. *Cochrane Database Syst Rev*, 2003. (4): CD002307.

112. Kippelen, P., J. Larsson, S.D. Anderson, et al., Effect of sodium cromoglycate on mast cell mediators during hyperpnea in athletes. *Med Sci Sports Exerc*, 2010. **42**(10): 1853–1860.

113. Pearlman, D.S., J. vanAdelsberg, G. Phillip, et al., Onset and duration of protection against exercise-induced bronchoconstriction by a single oral dose of montelukast. *Ann Allergy Asthma Immunol*, 2006. **97**(1): 98–104.

114. Philip, G., D.S. Pearlman, C. Villaran, et al., Single-dose montelukast or salmeterol as protection against exercise-induced bronchoconstriction. *Chest*, 2007. **132**(3): 875–883.

115. Edelman, J.M., J.A. Turpin, E.A. Bronsky, et al., Oral montelukast compared with inhaled salmeterol to prevent exercise-induced bronchoconstriction. A randomized, double-blind trial. Exercise Study Group. *Ann Intern Med*, 2000. **132**(2): 97–104.

116. Hallstrand, T.S., M.W. Moody, M.M. Wurtel, et al., Inflammatory basis of exercise-induced bronchoconstriction. *Am J Respir Crit Care Med*, 2005. **172**(6): 679–686.

117. Dahlen, B., A. Roquet, M.D. Inman, et al., Influence of zafirlukast and loratadine on exercise-induced bronchoconstriction. *J Allergy Clin Immunol*, 2002. **109**(5): 789–793.

118. Coreno, A., M. Skowronski, C. Kotaru, et al., Comparative effects of long-acting beta2-agonists, leukotriene receptor antagonists, and a 5-lipoxygenase inhibitor on exercise-induced asthma. *J Allergy Clin Immunol*, 2000. **106**(3): 500–506.

119. Krawiec, M.E. and S.E. Wenzel, Leukotriene inhibitors and non-steroidal therapies in the treatment of asthma. *Expert Opin Pharmacother*, 2001. **2**(1): 47–65.

120. Kraft, M., LTRA inhibition of exercise-induced bronchoconstriction. *Postgrad Med*, 2000. **108**(4 Suppl): 32–39.

121. Subbarao, P., M. Duong, E. Adelroth, et al., Effect of ciclesonide dose and duration of therapy on exercise-induced bronchoconstriction in patients with asthma. *J Allergy Clin Immunol*, 2006. **117**(5): 1008–1013.

122. Larsson, J., C.P. Perry, S.D. Anderson, et al., The occurrence of refractoriness and mast cell mediator release following mannitol-induced bronchoconstriction. *J Appl Physiol*, 2011. **110**(4): 1029–1035.

123. Jonasson, G., K.H. Carlsen, and C. Hultquist, Low-dose budesonide improves exercise-induced bronchospasm in schoolchildren. *Pediatr Allergy Immunol*, 2000. **11**(2): 120–125.

124. Hofstra, W.B., H.J. Neijens, E.J. Duiverman, et al., Dose-responses over time to inhaled fluticasone propionate treatment of exercise- and methacholine-induced bronchoconstriction in children with asthma. *Pediatr Pulmonol*, 2000. **29**(6): 415–423.

125. Hermansen, M.N., K.G. Nielson, F. Buchvald, et al., Acute relief of exercise-induced bronchoconstriction by inhaled formoterol in children with persistent asthma. *Chest*, 2006. **129**(5): 1203–1209.

126. Svenonius, E., R. Kautto, and M. Arborelius Jr., Improvement after training of children with exercise-induced asthma. *Acta Paediatr Scand*, 1983. **72**(1): 23–30.

127. Mickleborough, T.D., M.R. Lindley, and L.A. Turner, Comparative effects of a high-intensity interval warm-up and salbutamol on the bronchoconstrictor response to exercise in asthmatic athletes. *Int J Sports Med*, 2007. **28**(6): 456–462.

128. Henriksen, J.M. and T.T. Nielsen, Effect of physical training on exercise-induced bronchoconstriction. *Acta Paediatr Scand*, 1983. **72**(1): 31–36.

129. Haas, F., Effect of aerobic training on forced expiratory airflow in exercising asthmatic humans. *J Appl Physiol*, 1987. **63**(3): 1230–1235.

130. Tecklenburg, S.L., Ascorbic acid supplementation attenuates exercise-induced bronchoconstriction in patients with asthma. *Respir Med*, 2007. **101**(8): 1770–1778.

131. Mickleborough, T.D., M.R. Lindley, and G.S. Montgomery, Effect of fish oil-derived omega-3 polyunsaturated fatty acid supplementation on exercise-induced bronchoconstriction and immune function in athletes. *Phys Sportsmed*, 2008. **36**(1): 11–17.

132. Mickleborough, T.D. and A. Fogarty, Dietary sodium intake and asthma: An epidemiological and clinical review. *Int J Clin Pract*, 2006. **60**(12): 1616–1624.

133. Pauwels, R.A., C.G. Lofdahl, D.S. Postma, et al., Effect of inhaled formoterol and budesonide on exacerbations of asthma. Formoterol and Corticosteroids Establishing Therapy (FACET) International Study Group. *N Engl J Med*, 1997. **337**(20): 1405–1411.

134. Hancox, R.J. and D.R. Taylor, Long-acting beta-agonist treatment in patients with persistent asthma already receiving inhaled corticosteroids. *BioDrugs*, 2001. **15**(1): 11–24.

135. Elers, J., U. Strandbygaard, L. Pederson, et al., Daily use of salmeterol causes tolerance to bronchodilation with terbutaline in asthmatic subjects. *Open Respir Med J*, 2010. **4**: 48–50.

136. Kelly, K.D., C.H. Spooner, and B.H. Rowe, Nedocromil sodium versus cromoglycate for the pre-treatment of exercise induced bronchoconstriction in asthma. *Cochrane Database Syst Rev*, 2000. (2): CD002169.

137. Suissa, S., P. Ernst, S. Benayoun, et al., Low-dose inhaled corticosteroids and the prevention of death from asthma. *N Engl J Med*, 2000. **343**(5): 332–336.

138. Jeffrey, P.K., R.W. Godfrey, E. Adelroth, et al., Effects of treatment on airway inflammation and thickening of basement membrane reticular collagen in asthma. A quantitative light and electron microscopic study. *Am Rev Respir Dis*, 1992. **145**(4 Pt 1): 890–899.

139. Kippelen, P., J. Larsson, S.D. Anderson, et al., Acute effects of beclomethasone on hyperpnea-induced bronchoconstriction. *Med Sci Sports Exerc*, 2010. **42**(2): 273–280.

140. Valthenen, A.S., A.J. Knox, A. Wisniewski, et al., Effect of inhaled budesonide on bronchial reactivity to histamine, exercise, and eucapnic dry air hyperventilation in patients with asthma. *Thorax*, 1991. **46**(11): 811–816.

141. Kersten, E.T., J.M. Driessen, J.C. van Leeuwen, et al., Pilot study: The effect of reducing treatment on exercise induced bronchoconstriction. *Pediatr Pulmonol*, 2010. **45**(9): 927–933.

142. Weiler, J.M., R.A. Nathan, N.T. Rupp, et al., Effect of fluticasone/salmeterol administered via a single device on exercise-induced bronchospasm in patients with persistent asthma. *Ann Allergy Asthma Immunol*, 2005. **94**(1): 65–72.

143. Pearlman, D.S., P. Qaqundah, J. Matz, et al., Fluticasone propionate/salmeterol and exercise-induced asthma in children with persistent asthma. *Pediatr Pulmonol*, 2009. **44**(5): 429–435.

144. Lazarus, S.C., H.A. Boushey, J.V. Fahy, et al., Long-acting beta2-agonist monotherapy vs continued therapy with inhaled corticosteroids in patients with persistent asthma: A randomized controlled trial. *JAMA*, 2001. **285**(20): 2583–2593.

145. Reynolds, N.A., K.A. Lyseng-Williamson, and L.R. Wiseman, Inhaled salmeterol/fluticasone propionate: A review of its use in asthma. *Drugs*, 2005. **65**(12): 1715–1734.

146. Noonan, M., L.J. Rosenwasser, P. Martin, et al., Efficacy and safety of budesonide and formoterol in one pressurised metered-dose inhaler in adults and adolescents with moderate to severe asthma: A randomised clinical trial. *Drugs*, 2006. **66**(17): 2235–2254.

147. Mickleborough, T.D., R.L. Murray, A.A. Ionescu, et al., Fish oil supplementation reduces severity of exercise-induced bronchoconstriction in elite athletes. *Am J Respir Crit Care Med*, 2003. **168**(10): 1181–1189.

148. Mickleborough, T.D., M.R. Lindley, A.A. Ionescu, et al., Protective effect of fish oil supplementation on exercise-induced bronchoconstriction in asthma. *Chest*, 2006. **129**(1): 39–49.

149. Ram, F.S., S.M. Robinson, P.N. Black, et al., Physical training for asthma. *Cochrane Database Syst Rev*, 2005. (4): CD001116.

150. Hallstrand, T.S., P.W. Bates, and R.B. Schoene, Aerobic conditioning in mild asthma decreases the hyperpnea of exercise and improves exercise and ventilatory capacity. *Chest*, 2000. **118**(5): 1460–1469.

151. Hildebrand, K., Usefulness of selected tests in the diagnosis of exercise induced bronchoconstriction. *Pneumonol Alergol Pol*, 2011. **79**(6): 397–406.

Section IV

Asthma Education and Outcomes

13 Asthma Education

Vanessa M. McDonald and Peter G. Gibson

CONTENTS

CASE PRESENTATION

Lucy is a 42-year-old female who presented to the ambulatory care asthma clinic of a tertiary care hospital for clinical review following her first admission to hospital since childhood with an acute exacerbation of her asthma. She is a nonsmoker with a history of asthma since childhood. Her main exacerbation trigger is respiratory tract infections. Her body mass index (BMI) is 31.6 kg/m² and she is atopic.

ASTHMA CONTROL

Lucy stated that she felt fine. When asked specifically about her asthma symptoms, she said that she had woken from her sleep with a cough and wheeze every night over the past week, she had symptoms of asthma each morning on waking, and, when probed, she stated that her activity was somewhat limited during intensive exercise but that this was normal. She was using short-acting beta₂-adrenergic agonists three times per day for the relief of her symptoms. Her forced expiratory volume in 1 sec (FEV₁) was 2.10 L (72% predicted), her forced vital capacity (FVC) was 3.25 L (90% predicted), and her FEV₁/FVC (forced expiratory ratio [FER]) was 0.65. Her best peak flow reading was 400 L/min. Her assessment indicated that her asthma was uncontrolled.

CURRENT PRESCRIBED TREATMENT

- *Fluticasone propionate/salmeterol xinafoate 250/25 μg, two inhalations bid via a pressurized metered-dose inhaler (pMDI) and a valved holding chamber (spacer).*
- *Terbutaline 500 μg via a Turbuhaler as needed.*

ASTHMA MANAGEMENT SKILLS AND KNOWLEDGE

Adherence

Lucy said that she was adherent to her prescribed treatment. However, she said that she had missed two doses of her combination inhaled corticosteroid/long-acting beta₂-adrenergic agonist (ICS/LABA) in the past week.

Asthma Knowledge and Symptom Perception

Lucy had a lifelong history of asthma. While she was aware of the role of her inhaled therapies, she had never undergone an asthma education and self-management program. Her symptom perception was poor.

Inhaler Technique

Lucy's inhaler technique with both her pMDI and spacer was optimal. Her technique using the Turbuhaler was inadequate; she held it to the side during activation and did not inhale deeply enough. Inhaler device polypharmacy was evident with this regime.

Self-Monitoring

Lucy was not monitoring her symptoms or her peak flow readings. She did not own a peak flow meter and was not familiar with self-monitoring diaries.

Exacerbation Management

Lucy had a written action plan that was prescribed by her general practitioner (GP) in 2004. The maintenance therapy and escalation plan were not reflective of her current treatment regime.

CASE SUMMARY

Lucy has uncontrolled asthma with poor symptom perception. Her treatment knowledge is adequate but she is not aware of the severity of her asthma, the level of poor control, how to recognize exacerbations, or how to escalate treatment. The number of devices she uses could be minimized. While she reports an adherence to her treatment of greater than 80%, this may not be an accurate reflection of what is actually occurring.

Lucy would benefit from education to improve her knowledge of the desired level of asthma control and symptom recognition. She will start self-monitoring her symptoms and/or her peak flow and she will need a personalized written action plan for exacerbation management. Regular follow-up will be required.

INTRODUCTION

We have presented Lucy, a 42-year-old female with asthma, who was recently admitted to hospital with an acute exacerbation of her asthma. Currently, she has ongoing poor symptom control despite being prescribed a combination high-dose ICS/LABA. An assessment of her asthma management skills and knowledge indicates that there are a number of areas that require addressing. Asthma education will be integral to Lucy's management of her asthma.

Asthma education not only involves the transfer of information and knowledge, but it also incorporates strategies to improve skills and change attitudes, ultimately leading to behavioral change.[1] This approach is termed *asthma self-management education.*

In this chapter, we will describe the essential components of effective education and discuss best-practice recommendations. We will also present evidence supporting asthma self-management education in a number of different patient populations.

ASTHMA EDUCATION

There is unequivocal evidence to support asthma self-management education and its ability to improve the morbidity of this disease in both children and adults[2–6]; as such, asthma self-management education is fundamental to optimal asthma management.

Self-management support is defined as "the systematic provision of education and supportive interventions by health care staff to increase patients' skills and confidence in managing their health problems, including regular assessment of progress and problems, goal setting, and problem-solving support. Self-management is defined as the tasks that individuals must undertake to live well with one or more chronic conditions. These tasks include having the confidence to deal with medical management, role management, and emotional management of their conditions."[7]

Meta-analyses of randomized controlled trials (RCT) have identified the essential components of asthma self-management education.[3,6,8,9] The most effective programs include the transfer of information, skills training, regular medical follow-up, the delivery of written asthma action plans (WAAPs), and regular monitoring of symptoms or lung function by the patient. These are achieved through effective therapeutic patient–clinician partnerships using a person-centered approach (Figure 13.1). While successful asthma self-management programs have considerable variability, they remain a multifaceted intervention and are most effective when their components are delivered in combination rather than as individual aspects.[3,10]

Asthma self-management education can be delivered in a variety of settings. Improvements in asthma knowledge and control have been demonstrated in programs delivered in the primary care outpatient, hospital, and emergency department settings as well as through the internet and mobile phone technologies.[11] The programs that have reported the best outcomes are those that are implemented in secondary care settings in patients with moderate to severe asthma.[12]

ESSENTIAL COMPONENTS OF ASTHMA EDUCATION

DEVELOPING EFFECTIVE PATIENT–CLINICIAN PARTNERSHIPS

The development of effective patient–clinician partnerships is an important aspect of asthma self-management. One

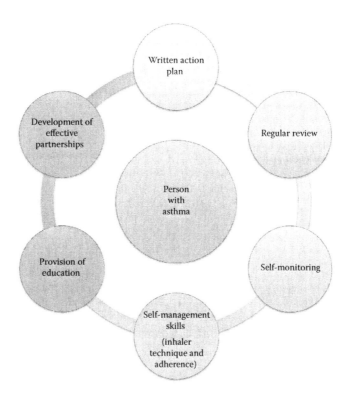

FIGURE 13.1 The key components of effective asthma education, placing the patient at the center of the educative process.

model that facilitates these effective partnerships is person-centered or patient-centered care. The concept of "patient centeredness" was first presented in the medical literature in the mid-1950s by Balint,[13] who contrasted this concept with illness-centered medicine. Since then, several definitions of person-centered and patient–client-centered care have emerged in the literature. The paradigm of person-centered care relates to holism, suggesting that patients be treated from a biopsychosocial perspective.[14] Person-centered care is, therefore, the treatment and care provided by health services that place the person at the center of his or her own care.[15] This is necessary to deliver effective asthma self-management education (Figure 13.1). A definition of this concept of care is as follows:

> A collaborative effort consisting of patients, patients' families, friends, the doctors and other health professional achieved through a comprehensive system of patient education where patients and health professionals collaborate as a team, share knowledge and work towards the common goals of optimum healing and recovery.[15]

The hallmark features of person centeredness concern the creation and maintenance of respectful and collaborative relationships between patients, their families, and health-care staff, and the recognition of individuality. Practicing person-centered care involves treating patients as partners, involving them in decision making, improving their autonomy, and respecting their beliefs and concerns. Health-care providers should respect and establish the contribution that the patients or their families make to their own health, such as their values, goals, past experience, and knowledge of their own health needs, and the patients and their families should respect the contribution that health-care providers can make, including their professional expertise and their knowledge and information about the options available. Both the health-care provider and the service user are important within the partnership; neither is interchangeable.[15] Person-centered care is particularly well suited to the needs of people with asthma during the educative process.

Person-centered care requires the clinician to have an appreciation of the patient's expectations, beliefs, and concerns; an understanding of the patient's personal circumstances; a willingness and motivation to provide information surrounding the diagnosis, pathology, treatment, and prognosis; and the knowledge to inform evidence-based treatment decisions.[16–18]

Poor patient–clinician partnerships have negative effects on health outcomes. By including patients in the decision-making process, outcomes such as adherence can be improved. A recent study in an asthma population by Wilson et al.[19] examined the effect of shared decision making compared with clinician decision making among patients with asthma, using adherence to controller therapy as the outcome. In the shared-decision group, treatment was negotiated with the participants who had the opportunity to summarize their treatment goals, were provided with information about the necessary treatments for disease control, and were presented with a range of treatment options, which enabled them to make a shared decision with the clinician. This approach resulted in statistically significant improvements in adherence to medical advice and clinically significant improvements in outcomes such as asthma-related quality of life, health-care use, rescue medication use, asthma control, and lung function.

ASSESSMENT OF KNOWLEDGE AND SKILLS AND PROVISION OF INFORMATION

The content and style of the information transfer and skills training will depend somewhat on the specific needs of the patient, taking into consideration the patient's age, level of education, and disease severity, and environmental factors such as the patient's social and emotional status and family support.[12] There are, however, core information and skills that should be included, and these are illustrated in the suggested content checklist for asthma education consultations (Table 13.1). These content areas can be addressed during the initial consultation, and they can be reinforced and reviewed during follow-up consultations.

With respect to the transfer of information, asthma education should include:

- The provision of information relating to the nature of asthma and its mechanisms
- Asthma treatment, including the concept of different classes of asthma medication, when to use medications, possible side effects, and ways to minimize these side effects
- The concept that asthma is a long-term condition and, as such, the requirements for treatment are also long term
- Practical information about how to use the inhaled therapy, inhaler cleaning instructions, and information about knowing when the device is empty
- Recognizing the signs and symptoms of worsening asthma and what to do if they occur
- Ways of preventing exacerbations
- Trigger identification, avoidance, and management
- An assessment of adherence and discussions focusing on adherence-aiding strategies
- The importance and benefits of self-monitoring
- WAAPs
- The need for regular follow-up

In terms of asthma management skills, inhaler technique assessment and correction are vital as are the initiation of self-monitoring of the symptoms and/or peak flows, the prescription, and an agreement on a written action plan that includes the course of action to take following an increase in asthma signs and symptoms.[1,4]

INHALER TECHNIQUE

Adequate skill in the use of inhaler devices is integral to achieving good asthma outcomes. The majority of asthma medications are delivered via the inhaled route, as this offers the best balance between efficacy and safety.[20,21] Unfortunately, as many as 90% of patients have poor inhalation technique.[22]

The assessment and correction of inhaler technique are essential features of asthma education, and can effectively overcome errors and improve outcomes.[23] A number of known factors can increase the error rate for inhalation devices and these factors need to be considered when educating patients and choosing the inhaled therapy. Both older people and people with more severe airflow obstruction are at greatest risk of poor inhaler technique, which is related to decreased cognitive function and manual dexterity in older people and reduced peak inspiratory flow rates in both older people and those with severe airflow obstruction.[20,24] Furthermore, data suggest that there is a lack of education and instruction on inhalation technique among patients who are prescribed treatment; as many as 25% of asthma or chronic obstructive pulmonary disease (COPD) patients have never been provided with inhaler device instruction.[25] This may be related to clinicians' confidence to educate patients, as other data suggest that the proportion of health professionals who are unable to demonstrate adequate inhaler technique is between 31% and 85%.[26] The document "Inhaler Technique in Adults with Asthma or COPD" (http://www.nationalasthma.org. au/uploads/content/237-Inhaler_technique_in_adults_with_ asthma_or_COPD.pdf) details the essential steps that are required to develop an adequate technique for each of the most common inhaler devices used in asthma treatment. The following is a TEACHER mnemonic to aid in the vital steps for inhaler technique education.

Tailor: Individualize the device to the patient's needs.
Educate: Educate and demonstrate the correct technique.
Assess: Assess the patient's ability for using the device.
Correct: Correct the technique.
Have Another Go: After correction, reassess.
Evaluate: Is this the correct device for this patient?
Reduce: Minimize the number of devices prescribed.

These include the need to individualize the choice of inhaler to the individual patient's skill and preference; the need to explain and demonstrate to the patient how to use the device, and why an effective technique is important; the need to assess the patient's technique and to correct the essential steps when necessary; and the continued evaluation of the patient's technique as his or her proficiency may decrease over time. Finally, we recommend minimizing the number of different devices prescribed to avoid inhaler device polypharmacy.[21]

Over time, there has been a progressive increase in the types of inhalation devices used in the management of asthma and other obstructive airway diseases; this has led to the frequent problem of inhaler device polypharmacy, which is the use of multiple types of inhalation devices by one individual.[21] We have previously demonstrated that this is a common problem among adults with asthma and that an inadequate inhalation device technique is most common among patients using three or more delivery devices.[21] As the array of devices continues to increase, this is becoming a very important issue to address.

TABLE 13.1
Content of Asthma Education Consultations

	Case Study "Lucy"
Nature of Disease	●
Provide basic patient-centered review of respiratory anatomy and asthma physiology, including the concept of asthma as an inflammatory disease and the concept of airway narrowing	
Asthma Treatment	●
Concept of asthma medication classes	
Actions—relievers for bronchoconstriction; preventers for airway inflammation	
When to use medication	
Possible side effects and ways to minimize	
Inhaler Technique	✹
Assess inhaler technique	Needs correction
Correct inhaler technique	Minimize the number
Continually reassess and correct inhaler technique at follow-up	
Assess and, when possible, correct inhaler device poly-pharmacy	
Self-Monitoring	✹
Establish patient preference for self-monitoring	Commenced on peak flow and symptom monitoring
Have the patient understand the rationale for self-monitoring	
Commence either peak flow or symptom monitoring based on the patient's ability and preference	
Continually review self-monitoring at follow-up	
Asthma Control	✹
Ensure the patient understands the concept of good asthma control	Poor control
Ensure the patient is able to recognize the signs and symptoms of worsening asthma and knows the actions to take	Poor recognition Given WAP
Written Action Plan	✹
Prescribe a written action plan	Plan developed
Include the patient in the decision-making process	Scripts given
Ensure the patient understands and accepts the treatment recommendations	Knowledge and agreement of plan assessed
Provide the patient with prescriptions for the recommended treatments	
Reinforce the plan at follow-up	
Review the plan following each exacerbation or every 6 months	
Adherence	●
Assess adherence to treatment	Requires ongoing assessment and review
Establish reason for nonadherence in a supportive and nonjudgmental way	
Discuss ways to implement adherence-aiding strategies	
Triggers	●
Identify relevant trigger factor with the patient	
Provide advice on trigger factor management	
Review regularly	
Smoking	N/A
Establish smoking status	
Engage in discussions about smoking cessation	
Individual Patients' Needs	●
Establish what is important to each patient	
Ensure patients' needs are addressed	
Allow time to explore patients' questions and concerns	
Follow-up/review	●

●, assessed and adequate; ✹, assessed and inadequate; N/A, not applicable.

Source: Adapted from McDonald, V.M. and Gibson, P.G., *Allergy Frontiers: Diagnosis and Health Economics,* Springer Publishing, Japan, 2009. With permission.

Figure 13.2 provides guidance for the selection of inhaler devices taking into consideration the potential errors. Regardless of the device selected, the practitioner must demonstrate the technique, and provide regular reassessment and instruction.[20]

SELF-MONITORING

Self-monitoring is the regular self-recording of symptoms and/or peak expiratory flow (PEF) measurements that patients perform in their home and work or school environment. Self-monitoring is useful as it provides patients with a tool for assessing their level of asthma control and aids in the recognition of the early signs of an exacerbation. Self-monitoring also assists clinicians in reviewing the level of asthma control over time and the results provide clinicians with data to determine the action to be taken at certain points of the early exacerbation written action plan.

In children, it appears that symptom-based action plans are superior to peak flow-based plans, but it is not known if this is related to differences in adherence for either option.[9] In adult patients, a number of studies have compared the two forms of monitoring and a meta-analysis concluded

that when self-monitoring is coupled with a written action plan, the results from symptom or peak flow monitoring are equivalent.[27] One study did, however, show that patients preferred symptom monitoring over the use of peak flow[28] and while adherence to self-monitoring can be poor, the notion of establishing individual patient preferences is important in determining the approach each patient might take.

While the effects of peak flow or symptom monitoring are equivalent, each has its pros and cons. Peak flows provide more objective data and may be more useful in patients (such as in the earlier "Lucy" case study) who have a poor perception of their symptoms[29]; however, they may be considered by patients as less practical and an unnecessary financial burden. Conversely, symptom monitoring provides less objective data, but it is less costly and more practical. In some patients, symptoms may deteriorate before a fall in the peak flow is evident; in this group of patients, symptom monitoring is preferred.[29]

A number of other factors should also be considered when establishing and reviewing self-monitoring practices with patients. Factors such as literacy, cognition, and the ability to record symptoms or peak flow are important. Additionally, patients should be provided with information

Potential problems with technique	pMDI	pMDI + holding chamber	DPI
Decreased PIF	✔	✔	🚫
Impaired cognition	?	?	?
Decreased manual dexterity	🚫	?	?
Decreased press and breathe coordination	🚫	✔	✔

Key: pMDI, pressurized-metered dose inhaler; DPI, dry powder inhaler; PIF, peak inspiratory flow.

✔ The patient should be able to master the technique in the presence of the impairment.

? The patient may possibly master the technique in the presence of the impairment.

🚫 The device is not recommended when the impairment is present.

Regardless of the device selection, the practitioner must demonstrate the technique, and provide regular reassessment and instruction. Minimization of inhaler device polypharmacy is recommended.

FIGURE 13.2 **(See color insert)** A guide to inhaler device selection recognizing the potential problems associated with the optimal technique. (Reprinted from *The Lancet*, 374, Gibson, P.G., McDonald, V.M., and Marks, G.B., Asthma in the older adult, 803–813, ©2010, with permission from Elsevier.)

or examples about the rationale and the benefits of self-monitoring, including the interpretation and the relevance of the results on asthma control. A chart display also influences the ability to recognize deteriorating asthma.[30]

REGULAR REVIEW

A regular medical review is another key element contributing to the success of asthma self-management education.[3] The review provides practitioners with the opportunity to assess asthma control, measure lung function, review treatment response, and reinforce asthma knowledge and skills.

The key questions to assess during the review are the frequency of symptoms, including nocturnal awakening and symptoms on waking up in the morning. The degree of activity limitation and the frequency of short-acting beta$_2$-adrenergic agonist use should also be elicited, as should the exacerbation history.

Due to the time pressures faced by medical practitioners, asthma education opportunities may be limited during both the initial consultation and at follow-up review. Working in partnership with asthma educators, specialist nurses, and allied health professionals will increase the asthma education opportunities for patients.

WRITTEN ASTHMA ACTION PLANS

Exacerbations are a common feature in asthma, putting the patient at immediate risk for distress, hospitalization, and even death. Acute exacerbations represent a significant contribution to health-care costs.[24] Exacerbations may occur over days or weeks and, as such, patients frequently have an opportunity to recognize their deterioration and escalate their treatment to reduce both the severity of the exacerbation and the recovery time. WAAPs are used to facilitate asthma management, particularly exacerbation management.[1,31]

WAAPs are developed by a medical practitioner or an accredited nurse practitioner to provide patients with written instructions, either in the form of text[31] or as pictorial information,[32] about their maintenance treatment and instructions for the escalation of treatment during both moderate and severe asthma exacerbations. WAAPs allow people with asthma to detect the early signs and symptoms of exacerbations in addition to providing instructions about how to manage these exacerbations.[1] They are an essential component in the effective self-management of asthma,[3] and are a key recommendation of international clinical practice asthma guidelines.[12,33]

When written action plans are coupled with self-management education there is irrefutable evidence to support their effect on reducing asthma morbidity.[3] Unfortunately, the uptake of WAAPs in practice remains poor.[34] A population survey in South Australia demonstrated that the proportion of people who stated that they had a WAAP was 42% in 1995, which fell to 20.8% in 2003.[34] The reasons for the low-level uptake of WAAPs by health-care professionals are likely to be multifactorial; it may reflect the poor training of doctors and other health professionals in creating and delivering negotiated action plans in partnership with people with asthma,[35] suggesting a need for additional training in self-management plans among health professionals. It may also be related to the time required for medical practitioners to develop and effectively convey the plan to the patient. This can be overcome by developing asthma management programs in partnership with asthma educators, specialist nurses, and other allied health-care professionals. Finally, the poor uptake could be related to the attitudes of clinicians and patients regarding the importance of such plans. In a recent study published by the present authors, the importance of the clinical problems experienced by older people with asthma and COPD was rated by both patients and their physicians. The problems related to self-management, including WAAPs,[18] received the lowest rating of importance from patients and doctors. This suggests a need to improve clinicians' and patients' knowledge of the efficacy and benefits of written action plans.

Many different written action plan templates are available to aid both clinicians and patients in completing these agreed treatment plans. Examples may be found at the following websites: http://www.nationalasthma.org.au/health-professionals/tools-for-primary-care/asthma-action-plans/asthma-action-plan-library (accessed 11/08/12), http://www.aaaai.org/Aaaai/media/MediaLibrary/PDF%20Documents/Libraries/NEW-WEBSITE-LOGO-asthma-action-plan_HI.pdf (accessed 11/08/12), and http://asthma.ca/adults/control/pdf/AsthmaActionPlan_ENG.pdf (accessed 11/08/12).

Gibson and Powell[31] undertook a study to review the evidence supporting WAAPs and they recommended that the key components of WAAPs include detail describing:

- When to increase treatment (action point)
- How to increase treatment
- For how long
- When to seek medical help

An example of a WAAP incorporating these components for the "Lucy" case study is presented in Figure 13.3. In addition to the written component, engagement with the patient is also essential to ensure that he or she understands the plan, agrees to the treatment recommendations, and has the capacity to implement all elements of the plan.

ADHERENCE

Adherence to medical advice is a well-known problem in people with asthma,[36] and as health professionals, we need to recognize and expect nonadherence. The reality that patients do not always follow the prescribed treatment advice has been evident for thousands of years. As Hippocrates said

> ... to be alert to the faults of the patients which make them lie about their taking of the medicines prescribed and when things go wrong, refuse to confess that they have not been taking their medicine.[37]

Case Study: Lucy's Written Asthma Action Plan

When Well
Seretide 250/25 mcg _____   Dose: Two puffs via your spacer morning and night
Ventolin* 100 mcg _____   Dose: Two puffs as needed
Take Ventolin two puffs 10 minutes before exercise

When Not Well

- If your peak flow reading does not reach 80% of your best value, which is **320 L/m** following your medication for a 24 hour period.

or

- If you are waking at night due to your asthma or have symptoms when you wake in the morning.

or

- If you require your Ventolin more frequently than usual and are not getting the same effect.

or

- You are getting a cold.

Then

- Increase your Ventolin: Take two extra puffs as needed.
- Start prednisone 37.5 mg a day for 14 days.
- See your doctor if you are no better in 2–3 days of increased treatment.

For a Severe Attack

- If your peak flow does not reach 50% of best value, which is **200 L/m**.

or

- If you have a severe shortness of breath and can only speak in short sentences.

or

- If you are having a severe attack of asthma and are frightened.

or

- If you need to take your Ventolin more than 4 hourly and do not gain an effect.

Then

- Take Ventolin four puffs in your spacer: repeat if you do not improve.
- Take 50 mg of prednisone.
- Seek medical attention immediately by calling an ambulance on 000.
- Continue to use your Ventolin in your spacer four puffs every 4 minutes until help arrives.

Signature_____   Date_____

*Changed from terbutaline due to poor technique and inhaler poly device pharmacy.

FIGURE 13.3   (See color insert) An example of a written asthma action plan. (©Department of Respiratory and Sleep Medicine, John Hunter Hospital, used with permission. Adapted from McDonald, V.M. and Gibson, P.G., Asthma patient education, In: Pawankar, R., Holgate, S., and Rosenwaser, L. (eds), *Allergy Frontiers: Diagnosis and Health Economics*, Springer, Japan, 2009. With permission.) *Note:* Trade names have been used to represent the language used in patient communication.

He was referring to health behavior that is now referred to as nonadherence. There are now several terms used in the medical literature to describe a patient's health behavior regarding treatment. These include *compliance*, *adherence*, and *concordance*. While these terms are frequently used interchangeably, they have different meanings that must be recognized.

The now largely outmoded term compliance refers to the extent to which the patient's behavior matches the prescriber's advice.[36] Compliance is associated with negative connotations as it infers that a paternal relationship exists between the patient and the prescriber in which the role of the prescriber is to issue treatment and the role of the patient is to follow orders.[36,38]

The preferred term 'adherence' refers to the extent to which a patient's behavior with respect to their medication, diet or lifestyle is consistent or matches the recommendations of the prescriber.[36,38]

In contrast with the term compliance, adherence is intended to be nonjudgmental rather than attributing blame to the patient, prescriber, or treatment.[38,39] Moreover, adherence refers to both the underuse and overuse of medications and therapies.[38] However, in asthma the most frequent form of nonadherence is the underuse of treatment.[12]

The term concordance is a more complex notion that relates to the relationship between the patient and the prescriber, which is based on equality and respect and considers the patient's beliefs and preferences.[36] Concordance fits the model of person-centered care as it recognizes the need for patients and clinicians to work in partnership to reach agreement around treatment decisions and further recognizes that patients and clinicians may have opposing views.[36] Concordance can be thought of as the process required for achieving adherence.

It is well known that adherence in chronic disease can be poor, and this is particularly true in chronic respiratory conditions. In a meta-analysis of 569 studies, adherence to therapy in respiratory diseases ranked poorly, with a mean adherence rate of 68.8%, which was fifteenth out of seventeen different diseases.[40] A prospective study of asthma found that 24% of severe exacerbations were attributable to nonadherence.[41]

There are two distinct patterns of behavior associated with nonadherence, which are referred to as intentional and unintentional nonadherence.[36,38,42] Understanding the behavior pattern of nonadherence in individuals will guide their education and help develop adherence-aiding strategies.

Intentional nonadherence occurs when patients make purposeful decisions to take and perform treatments in a way other than that prescribed. This often refers to the self-adjustment or titration of treatment according to the patient's symptoms or beliefs, or the cessation of treatment earlier than prescribed.[36] Intentional nonadherence usually results when the patient weighs the risks against the benefits of taking medication and makes a decision based on his or her reasoning.[38] While intentional nonadherence may result from a balance of reasoning, the decision could result from poor knowledge about the treatment, or an erroneous understanding regarding the nature or consequence of the problem, the prescribed therapy, and the potential benefit of treatment. Therefore, this form of nonadherence can often be addressed through strategies that improve patients' knowledge and influence their health beliefs and concerns.[38]

Unintentional nonadherence occurs when patients do not adhere to treatment advice due to reasons out of their control.[36] These are often related to cognitive impairments, language barriers, and physical disabilities. In the case of an older person with asthma, this could relate to impaired vision or musculoskeletal problems affecting his or her ability to use inhaled medications. Further unintentional nonadherence could also result from ineffective communication or inaccurate recollection of the prescribed treatment prescription.[36] Studies of how well patients retain health information suggest that less than 50% of the information conveyed by the physician is recalled immediately after an office visit.[40]

Recognizing nonadherence, establishing the reasons for nonadherence, and working with patients to improve their adherence are essential elements of asthma education.

ASTHMA EDUCATION IN DIFFERENT POPULATIONS

Asthma self-management education has been tested in many different patient groups, including adults, children and adolescents, elderly people, pregnant women, and culturally and linguistically diverse populations. Evidence supports asthma self-management education in these populations and recognizes that the education should be tailored to the specific needs of the population.[12]

ADULTS

Many RCTs of asthma education have been conducted in adults with asthma and the results of these trials have been summarized in Cochrane systematic reviews.[3,10] One review examined limited education that included the provision of information only. The review included 12 RCTs, and the results indicated that the provision of information alone was effective in terms of improving knowledge but it did not reduce asthma morbidity, hospital admissions, or unscheduled doctors' visits for asthma. Furthermore, these studies showed that the provision of information alone did not improve lung function or reduce medication use. From this analysis, it can be concluded that limited education involving the transfer of information alone improves knowledge but not asthma health outcomes.[10] A second systematic review evaluated 36 RCTs comparing self-management education with usual medical care. This analysis demonstrated that self-management education is effective in reducing hospitalizations, emergency department and unscheduled physician office visits, as well as reducing days off work or school, reducing nocturnal asthma, and improving patients' quality of life. The estimated number needed to treat (NNT) with asthma self-management education in order to prevent 1 asthma hospitalization is 20 and to prevent one emergency department visit the NNT is 8.[11] The authors conclude that asthma self-management education that includes the provision of information, self-monitoring by either PEF or symptoms, regular medical review, and a WAAP improves the health outcomes for adults with asthma.[3]

OLDER PEOPLE

Older people with asthma are an important population as the morbidity and mortality from asthma in this population is high.[43] The optimal self-management education for older people with asthma is still unclear. In the majority of the studies included in the previously described systematic review,[3] the participants were a mean age of less than 52 years and older people were excluded in some of the trials.[3] While asthma deaths have fallen in younger populations over the last few decades, Australia, for example, has witnessed a rise in mortality in older adults.[44] While advances in pharmacotherapy and self-management education policy initiatives have led to positive outcomes in younger people with asthma, the same has not been seen in older people, suggesting that the results of these RCTs cannot be extrapolated or applied to older populations who remain at risk.[20]

While less data exist related to self-management techniques in older people, a small number of recent trials have examined interventions in this population. Patel et al. showed that a telephone interview intervention could improve outcomes in older people with asthma. This intervention improved the use of ICS use, decreased emergency department attendance, and increased the uptake of WAAPs in older participants with asthma compared with a control group.[45]

Huang et al. also conducted a RCT in older people with moderate to severe asthma involving telephone interventions. This trial had three arms: usual care, individualized education with weekly telephone consults, and the former plus peak flow monitoring. Written information was provided in large fonts and used pictures with few words. Participants in the two intervention arms demonstrated significant improvements in their asthma knowledge and skills, self-care behaviors and self-efficacy, and prebronchodilator FEV_1 compared with a control group.[46] In another RCT, Goeman et al. evaluated the effectiveness of a multifaceted educational intervention for GPs aimed at improving the outcomes of older people with asthma. In this study, GPs received an educational intervention that was designed to improve the care of older people with asthma. This educational intervention was associated with improved content and style in communication, but it did not improve patient outcomes. It should be noted that the baseline characteristics of the patient population in this study did indicate good baseline asthma control, which may have limited the room for improvement.[47]

These studies suggest that older people with asthma can be instructed in an effective self-management program and achieve improvements in self-management efficacy,[46] quality of life,[48] and lung function.[46] The benefits of asthma self-management education come from integrated programs with active involvement by the participant.

Pregnant Women

Irrespective of the level of asthma severity, exacerbations of asthma in pregnant women are common. Achieving good control in this population is vital, as uncontrolled asthma during pregnancy is associated with adverse maternal and fetal outcomes.[49] Asthma self-management education in this population has been shown to improve asthma knowledge and skills. Murphy et al.[50] conducted a study in which pregnant women were recruited from the antenatal clinic of a tertiary hospital. The women were interviewed by an asthma educator at 20 and 33 weeks gestation. Their asthma knowledge and skills were poor at the baseline visit but improved significantly following education by the asthma educator, suggesting that asthma self-management education should be integrated into standard antenatal care.[50]

An important aspect of asthma education for pregnant women is to ensure that they understand the importance of good asthma control in order to avoid poor maternal and fetal outcomes. The safety of asthma treatment during pregnancy must also be stressed, as pregnant women may have concerns about using their treatment and a misconstrued understanding of the risk of taking medications during pregnancy may lead to poor adherence and adverse outcomes.

Children

There is good evidence of the benefits of self-management education for children with asthma.[8] A number of systematic reviews have evaluated the value of asthma self-management education in pediatric and adolescent populations.[2,6,8,9] While the setting and the type of intervention vary, the reviews are supportive of educational intervention for children with asthma. In the most comprehensive review by Wolf et al., the effects of self-management education in children were evaluated. Thirty-two RCTs were included, and the results of the analysis indicated that self-management education of children was associated with improvements in airflow obstruction and self-efficacy. Furthermore, education was also associated with a reduction in emergency department presentations and reduced absenteeism from school.[6] Asthma self-management education is recognized as standard practice in children and adolescents with asthma.[11,12]

SUMMARY

Asthma self-management education is an effective and integral part of asthma management in both adults and children. It can be successfully delivered in a variety of settings. The key components of asthma self-management education involve the transfer of information to improve knowledge, skills training, self-monitoring, the prescription of WAAPs, and regular medical review. These components of asthma education are best delivered in a model of person-centered care where the needs of the individual patient are understood and effective clinician–patient partnerships are developed.

REFERENCES

1. McDonald VM, Gibson PG. Asthma patient education. In: Pawankar R, Holgate S, Rosenwaser L (eds). *Allergy Frontiers: Diagnosis and Health Economics*. Japan: Springer, 2009.
2. Coffman JM, Cabana MD, Yelin EH. Do school-based asthma education programs improve self-management and health outcomes? *Pediatrics*. 2009;124(2):729–742.
3. Gibson PG, Powell H, Coughlin J, Wilson AJ, Abramson M, Haywood P, et al. Self-management education and regular practitioner review for adults with asthma. *Cochrane Database Syst Rev*. 2003(Issue 3. Art. No.: CD001117. DOI: 10.1002/14651858.CD001117).
4. McDonald VM, Gibson PG. Asthma self-management education. *Chron Respir Dis*. 2006;3(1):29–37.
5. Shah S, Roydhouse JK, Sawyer SM. Asthma education in primary healthcare settings. *Curr Opin Pediatr*. 2008;20(6):705–710.
6. Wolf FM, Guevara JP, Grum CM, Clark NM, Cates CJ. Educational interventions for asthma in children. *Cochrane Database Syst Rev*. 2002(Issue 4. Art. No.: CD000326. DOI: 10.1002/14651858.CD000326).
7. Adams K, Greiner SC, Corrigan JM. *The 1st Annual Crossing the Quality Chasm Summit—A Focus on Communities*. Washington, DC: Institute of Medicine of the National Academies, The National Academic Press, 2004.
8. Boyd M, Lasserson TJ, McKean MC, Gibson PG, Ducharme FM, Haby M. Interventions for educating children who are at risk of asthma-related emergency department attendance. *Cochrane Database Syst Rev*. 2009;15(2):CD001290.

9. Bhogal S, Zemek R, Ducharme FM. Written action plans for asthma in children. *Cochrane Database Syst Rev*. 2006;19(3).

10. Gibson PG, Powell H, Coughlan J, Wilson AJ, Hensley MJ, Abramson M, et al. Limited (information only) patient education programs for adults with asthma. *Cochrane Database Syst Rev*. 2002(Issue 2. CD001005).

11. Global Initiative for Asthma (GINA). Global Strategy for Asthma Management and Prevention, 2011.

12. British Thoracic Society (BTS/SIGN). British Guideline on the Management of Asthma, 2012.

13. Balint M. The doctor, his patient, and the illness. *Lancet*. 1955;268(6866):683–688.

14. Mead N, Bower P. Patient-centred consultations and outcomes in primary care: A review of the literature. *Patient Educ Couns*. 2002;48(1):51–61.

15. National Ageing Research Institute. What is person-centred health care? A literature review. Melbourne, Australia, 2006.

16. Bauman AE, Fardy HJ, Harris PG. Getting it right: Why bother with patient-centered care? *Med J Aust*. 2003;179(5):253–256.

17. Irwin RS, Richardson ND. Patient-focused care: using the right tools. *Chest*. 2006;130:73S–82S.

18. McDonald VM, Higgins I, Simpson JL, Gibson PG. The importance of clinical management problems in older people with COPD and asthma: do patients and physicians agree? *Prim Care Respir J*. 2011;20(4):389–395.

19. Wilson SR, Strub P, Buist AS, Knowles SB, Lavori PW, Lapidus J, et al. Shared treatment decision making improves adherence and outcomes in poorly controlled asthma. *Am J Respir Crit Care Med*. 2010;181(6):566–577.

20. Gibson PG, McDonald VM, Marks GB. Asthma in the older adult. *Lancet*. 2010;374(9743):803–813.

21. McDonald VM, Gibson PG. Inhalation device polypharmacy in asthma. *Med J Aust*. 2005;182(5):250–251.

22. Plaza V, Sanchis J. Medical personnel and patient skill in the use of metered dose inhalers: A multicentric study. CESEA Group. *Respiration*. 1998;65(3):195–198.

23. Basheti IA, Reddel HK, Armour CL, Bosnic-Anticevich SZ. Improved asthma outcomes with a simple inhaler technique intervention by community pharmacists. *J Allergy Clin Immunol*. 2007;119(6):1537–1538.

24. McDonald VM, Gibson PG. Exacerbations of severe asthma. *Clin Exp Allergy*. 2012;42(5):670–677.

25. Lavorini F, Magnan A, Dubus JC, Voshaar T, Corbetta L, Broeders M, et al. Effect of incorrect use of dry powder inhalers on management of patients with asthma and COPD. *Respir Med*. 2008;102(4):593–604.

26. Basheti IA, Armour CL, Bosnic-Anticevich SZ, Reddel HK. Evaluation of a novel educational strategy, including inhaler-based reminder labels, to improve asthma inhaler technique. *Patient Educ Couns*. 2008;72(1):26–33.

27. Powell H, Gibson PG. Options for self-management education for adults with asthma. *Cochrane Database Syst Rev*. 2003 (Issue 3. Art. No.: CD004107. DOI: 10.1002/14651858.CD004107).

28. Harver A, Humphries CT, Kotses H. Do asthma patients prefer to monitor symptoms or peak flow? *J Asthma*. 2009;46(9):940–943.

29. Gibson PG. Monitoring the patient with asthma: An evidenced-based approach. *J Allergy Clin Immunol*. 2000;106:17–26.

30. Turner RM, Hayen A, Macaskill P, Irwig L, Reddel HK. Control charts demonstrated limited utility for the monitoring of lung function in asthma. *J Clin Epidemiol*. 2012;65(1):53–61.

31. Gibson PG, Powell H. Written action plans for asthma: An evidence-based review of the key components. *Thorax*. 2004;59:94–99.

32. Roberts NJ, Evans G, Blenkhorn P, Partridge MR. Development of an electronic pictorial asthma action plan and its use in primary care. *Patient Educ Couns*. 2010;80(1):141–146.

33. Global Initiative for Asthma (GINA). Global Strategy for Asthma Management and Prevention. NHLBI/WHO Workshop Report 2006.

34. Wilson DH, Adams RJ, Tucker G, Appleton S, Taylor AW, Ruffin RE. Trends in asthma prevalence and population changes in South Australia, 1990–2003. *Med J Aust*. 2006;184(5):226–229.

35. Walters EH, Walters JAE, Wood-Baker R. Why have asthma action plans failed the consumer test? *Med J Aust*. 2003;178:477–478.

36. Horne R. Compliance, adherence, and concordance—Implications for asthma treatment. *Chest*. 2006;130(1 Suppl.):65S–72S.

37. Hippocrates. *Decorum*, c 200 BC.

38. Goeman DP, Douglass JA. Optimal management of asthma in elderly patients: Strategies to improve adherence to recommended interventions. *Drugs Aging*. 2007;24(5):381–394.

39. MacLaughlin EJ, Raehl CL, Treadway AK, Sterling TL, Zoller DP, Bond CA. Assessing medication adherence in the elderly: Which tools to use in clinical practice? *Drugs Aging*. 2005;22(3):231–255.

40. DiMatteo MR. Variations in patients' adherence to medical recommendations: A quantitative review of 50 years of research. *Med Care*. 2004;42(3):200–209.

41. Williams LK, Peterson EL, Wells K, Ahmedani BK, Kumar R, Burchard EG, et al. Quantifying the proportion of severe asthma exacerbations attributable to inhaled corticosteroid nonadherence. *J Allergy Clin Immunol*. 2011;128(6):1185–1191.

42. Banning M. Older people and adherence with medication: A review of the literature. *Int J Nurs Stud*. 2008;45(10):1550–1561.

43. Australian Centre for Asthma Monitoring. Asthma in Australia 2011. AIHW Asthma Series no. 4. Cat. no. ACM 22. Canberra: Australian Institute of Health and Welfare, 2011.

44. McDonald VM, Gibson PG. Asthma mortality and management in older Australians: Time for a new approach? *Australas J Ageing*. 2008;27:215.

45. Patel RR, Saltoun CA, Grammer LC. Improving asthma care for the elderly: A randomized controlled trial using a simple telephone intervention. *J Asthma*. 2009;46(1):30–35.

46. Huang TT, Li YT, Wang CH. Individualized programme to promote self-care among older adults with asthma: Randomized controlled trial. *J Adv Nurs*. 2009;65(2):348–358.

47. Goeman DP, Sanci LA, Scharf SL, Bailey M, O'Hehir RE, Jenkins CR, et al. Improving general practice consultations for older people with asthma: A cluster randomised control trial. *Med J Aust*. 2009;191(2):113–117.

48. Buist AS, Vollmer WM, Wilson SR, Frazier EA, Hayward AD. A randomized clinical trial of peak flow versus symptom monitoring in older adults with asthma. *Am J Respir Crit Care Med*. 2006;174(10):1077–1087.

49. Powell H, Murphy VE, Taylor DR, Hensley MJ, McCaffery K, Giles W, et al. Management of asthma in pregnancy guided by measurement of fraction of exhaled nitric oxide: A double-blind, randomised controlled trial. *Lancet*. 2011;378(9795):983–990.

50. Murphy VE, Gibson PG, Talbot PI, Kessell CG, Clifton VL. Asthma self-management skills and the use of asthma education during pregnancy. *Eur Respir J*. 2005;26:435–441.

14 Adherence and Outcomes

Andrew G. Weinstein

CONTENTS

CASE PRESENTATION

A 40-year-old female was referred after a recent 3-day hospital admission for asthma, her second in the past year. An evaluation of the causes of the factors precipitating her asthma (gastroesophageal reflux disease [GERD], nonsteroidal anti-inflammatory drug [NSAID] sensitivity, atopy, and sinusitis) was negative. A chest x-ray and alpha-1-antitrypsin were negative. The patient stated that she had been receiving the following medications: fluticasone 110 µg two inhalations bid; theophylline 400 mg bid; and albuterol two inhalations Q 4 h prn. Her spirometry revealed a forced vital capacity (FVC) of 87%, a forced expiratory volume in 1 sec (FEV$_1$) of 62%, and a forced expiratory flow (FEF$_{25-75}$) of 37% predicted. The patient is currently employed in an office setting with no exposure to irritant fumes or mold. The possible factors that precipitated her asthma flare were cheering her daughter at a softball game and playing in a softball game in which she did more running than usual. An adherence evaluation revealed a theophylline level of <2.0 µg/dL and one refill of fluticasone 110 (after her recent admission) from a local pharmacy in the previous 6 months. She completed an asthma adherence survey, which identified concerns about the cost of medicine; corticosteroids side

effects; the need for daily preventative inhaled corticosteroid (ICS) treatment; spouse disagreement about medication use; and forgetting to take the medication. An asthma information assessment identified poor comprehension of the action, side effects, and rationale for the daily use of inhaled steroids; no prior use of a peak flow meter; and no written asthma action plan. The physician had recommended discontinuing Theo-24 and QVAR and starting mometasone/fomoterol 200/5 two inhalations bid to improve her asthma control and decrease the number of insurance medication payments.

The patient received an asthma education program from a nurse practitioner (NP) to evaluate the aforementioned problems/concerns with care. At the outset, the NP asked the patient what area she would like to discuss and the response was the need for daily asthma treatment. The NP responded that she would address that issue but explained that she would need to review information with the patient about asthma and the use of a peak flow meter, which would help answer the patient's primary concern. The NP suggested using the peak flow meter as a way to determine the patient's need for daily ICSs. In consultation with the physician, they both recommended not using the mometasone/fomoterol 200/5 for 2 weeks and measure peak flow twice daily. At the end of 2 weeks, the patient was to start using the mometa-sone/fomoterol 200/5 two inhalations bid and continue peak flow measurements until the next visit 2 weeks later. In the meantime, she was to use the Proventil HFA prn if she had symptoms; however, should the symptoms persist, she was to start the mometasone/fomoterol 200/5 two inhalations and contact the office. The physician recommended an electronic adherence monitoring device for the mometasone/fomoterol 200/5. The patient agreed to medication monitoring.

At follow-up 4 weeks later, the patient recognized the benefit of daily mometasone/fomoterol 200/5. She had less symptoms and higher peak flow values during the previous 2 weeks. FEV$_1$ improved to 80% predicted. A review of the patient's adherence monitoring showed that she used mometasone/fomoterol 200/5 10 days bid and 4 days qd. She agreed to continue with this new medication plan because it was effective (Figure 14.1).

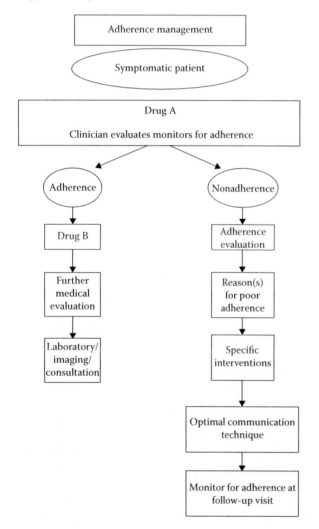

FIGURE 14.1 Adherence management is appropriate for any chronic disease that requires continuous pharmacological therapy. Once an individual is identified as nonadherent, an evaluation is performed to identify the cause(s); the specific strategy(s) to be implemented; and the appropriate communication technique. (From Weinstein, A.G., *Ann. Allergy Asthma Immunol.*, 106(4), 283–291, 2011.)

INTRODUCTION

The components of a successful clinician–patient interaction are (1) the accurate diagnosis of the patient's problem, (2) the selection of an effective treatment, and (3) the willingness of the patient and physician to develop an agreeable treatment plan. Unfortunately, many clinicians do not focus on step 3 and do not achieve the desired outcomes of symptom reduction and improved quality of life that are gained by adherence to treatment. This chapter will examine the different reasons why individuals fail to follow their clinicians' instructions and/or recommendations and various interventions that have been shown to be effective to improve patient adherence. Adherence to asthma medication will focus on ICS therapy since it is the most widely used therapy and recommended by the Expert Panel Report-3, except for mild asthma.

KEY CONCEPTS REGARDING ADHERENCE TO ASTHMA THERAPIES

- All asthma patients should be evaluated for adherence at the time of consultation with an asthma specialist.
- Providers should not rely solely on patient report for adherence history.
- Adherence is simultaneously influenced by several factors: characteristics of the disease; concomitant disorders (e.g., depression and anxiety); treatment type; socioeconomics; health-care system access; and personal. Each must be considered, preferably at the initial evaluation.
- Patient-tailored interventions are recommended since no one intervention is effective for all.
- When patients are identified as nonadherent, they should be supported and not blamed.
- When patients state that they have been nonadherent, believe them.
- Patient-centered communication skills will enhance patient adherence. Assessing the readiness of a patient to accept a medical recommendation is essential.
- Physician extenders (NPs, physician's assistant, and nurses) can work with physicians to promote adherence.
- Disease management companies should work with physicians to optimize care.

DEFINITION

The term *compliance* has been used to define "the extent to which patients follow physician instructions prescriptions and proscriptions." It implies that treatment decision making is entirely the physician's responsibility and that the patient must obey or acquiesce.[1] Adherence is defined by the World Health Organization as "the extent to which a person's behavior, such as: taking medication, following a diet, and/or executing lifestyle changes, corresponds with agreed recommendations from a healthcare provider."[2] The main difference between adherence and compliance is that adherence is consensual. It requires patients' agreement to the recommendations, that patients should be active partners with health professionals in their own care, and that good communication between patients and health professionals is a must for an effective clinical practice.[2] The WHO definition also expands the definition of regimen beyond medication. It is important to note that many organizations use the terms *adherence* and *compliance* interchangeably. Adherence to asthma therapy is essential since it is a chronic disease, requiring daily medication administration and long-term supervision by a health-care provider.

TO WHAT DEGREE ARE PATIENTS ADHERENT WITH ASTHMA TREATMENT REGIMENS?

Nonadherence with prescriptions can be classified as primary (failure to get the initial prescription refilled) and secondary (underuse of therapy or premature discontinuation of treatment). Primary nonadherence may range from 7% to 44%. An Australian study in a primary care setting found primary nonadherence with asthma medication to be 30%.[3] Secondary nonadherence in a U.S. asthma clinic, determined by prescription refill, was 21% for theophylline and 41% for ICSs over 12 months.[4] The examples of secondary nonadherence only determine that the medication was received by the patient, but do not provide information regarding its actual use. The rates of secondary ICS adherence in both children and adults are approximately 50%.[5] On examining an insurance database, Williams et al. determined that approximately 50% of adults did not refill ICSs.[6] Bender et al. examined refills of fluticasone/salmeterol over 12 months in over 5500 patients.[7] On average, patients filled enough medication to cover 22.2% of days and more than one-half of the patients filled a 30-day prescription only once over the 1-year period.[7] Using electronic adherence monitors, Onyirimba et al. found that adherence to ICSs decreased by 50% in 1 week and dropped as low as 20% after 12 weeks.[8] Krishnan also found a 50% decrease in ICS usage postdischarge from a hospital ICU.[9] Jonasson et al. reported on adherence to inhaled budesonide administered with a breath-driven asthma inhaler in 163 Swedish children.[10] Adherence was 70% after 6 months and dropped to 60% after 1 year.

Significance of Nonadherence and Clinical Outcomes

Nonadherence is related to adverse outcomes. In a review of an epidemiological database, Suissa found that subjects treated regularly with ICSs for at least 16 days and as long as 6 months were 40% less likely to be readmitted for asthma.[11] In another study, Suissa compared the deaths of a known asthma population with a control group of individuals who died from asthma.[12] The rate of death from asthma during the first 3 months after the discontinuation of ICSs was higher than the rate among patients who continued to use the drugs.

They concluded that the regular use of low-dose ICSs is associated with a decreased risk of death from asthma. Milgrom examined the adherence of 24 children aged 8–13 years with moderate to severe asthma in an outpatient setting.[13] They received ICSs with an electronic monitor over 3 months. The children with low adherence (median 11%) required oral steroid bursts while the adherent group (median 64%) did not require oral steroids. These findings support the concept that adherence enhances outcomes.

Williams et al. found that less adherent adult patients treated in a health maintenance organization (HMO) were more likely to be seen in an emergency department (ED), hospitalized, and receive more oral corticosteroids during the study period.[6] Similarly, Krishnan found that patients discharged from an intensive care unit who were subsequently nonadherent with both ICSs and oral corticosteroids had reduced asthma control as measured by the Asthma Control Test (ACT).[9] Murphy et al. examined the prescription refill data for ICSs of 115 adult asthma patients in a clinic. Suboptimal adherence (<80%) was found in 65% of patients prescribed ICSs. Patients with suboptimal ICS adherence had reduced FEV_1 and higher sputum eosinophil counts.[14]

Methods to Assess Adherence

There are a variety of methods to assess a patient's adherence, which are summarized in Table 14.1. Several methods are considered here. Self-reporting, asking patients about their medication use, or keeping a diary are not accurate measures. Patients may not want to disappoint a provider and therefore may overestimate their medication use.[15] As a result, clinicians tend to overestimate patient adherence.[15] Studies comparing patient diary with electronic adherence devices demonstrate the weakness of patient reporting.[13] Direct measures, such as blood and saliva measures of theophylline, an

TABLE 14.1
Assessing Adherence

Indirect Methods	Direct Methods
Question the patient	Observation
Ask patient to complete questionnaire	Measure levels of medicine (e.g., blood/urine)
Evaluate patient diaries for completeness	Measure biological marker attached to the medicine
Assess adherence based on response to treatment	Conduct unannounced spot checks of patients at home/clinic
Conduct pill counts	Measure clinic attendance
Use electronic monitors for physiological markers (e.g., pulmonary function)	
Determine from pharmacy whether prescriptions were filled	

Source: Weinstein, A.G., *Ann. Allergy Asthma Immunol.*, 106(4), 283–291, 2011.

oral bronchodilator, were commonly used to evaluate patient adherence in the 1970s and 1980s in the United States before anti-inflammatory medication became the standard of care. The primary advantage of a direct measure is in identifying the medication has actually been taken by the patient.[17] One disadvantage is that serum levels are affected by medication, food, and smoking behavior, which alter absorption and excretion and confound the results. Another disadvantage is that the direct measure provides data for one point in time and does not necessarily reflect overall adherence. Some individuals may take a monitored medicine immediately prior to a visit in anticipation of a direct measure. Electronic monitors for metered-dose inhalers (MDIs) have become more prevalent in research and practice. Electronic monitors are able to identify the pattern of medication use for more than a month, giving the physician the opportunity to review these results with the patient in relation to symptoms and lung function measures at home. Cochrane observed subjects who were given an electronic adherence monitor with their MDI but were unaware that they were being tracked. The medication use records of some subjects identified multiple actuations immediately before their clinic appointment, which was described as "dumping."[18] The disadvantage of the electronic monitor approach is its cost. The Doser CT is less expensive but it only records 30–45 days of data and it does not generate an electronic record for the clinician regarding the date and time of use.[19] The Smart Inhaler technology is more expensive but it provides documentation of the patient's adherence record and it can be applied to a greater variety of the MDIs (aerosol and dry powder) currently in use. It also provides audible feedback as reminders and includes wireless capability to permit remote monitoring.[20] These assays and devices permit clinicians to determine whether symptoms are secondary to treatment failure versus failure to administer treatment.

Patient questionnaires have been used to assess adherence for multiple diseases by identifying patient barriers to medication use. Recent questionnaires have been used to assess asthma adherence. Patients self-identify concerns, including the need for medication, the effectiveness of treatment, and the cost. McHorney et al.[21] developed a three-question survey, the Adherence Estimator, which identifies a patient's (a) perceived need for medications; (b) perceived concerns for medications; and (c) perceived affordability of medications, and they related these items to prescription refill data and patient self-report of medication use. The authors felt that there were some research design problems with this instrument, specifically that there was a small cohort of asthma subjects; patients received a mixture of ICSs and leukotriene modifiers; and there were inaccuracies with patient self-report of adherence. They suggested that future research with a larger sample of asthma patients treated exclusively with ICSs would be required before relying on the Adherence Estimator. Weinstein et al. have developed a web-based questionnaire with 90 items to examine the causes of patient nonadherence.[22] The questionnaire was derived from an inpatient rehabilitation program for severe asthmatic children.

This instrument was subsequently completed by 160 adult asthma patients with all levels of illness severity treated with ICSs.[23] Three factors were identified in this analysis: a symptom severity factor, a quality of life disruption factor, and an adherence factor. To build on these studies, Schatz et al.[24] enrolled 440 adult asthma patients receiving ICSs and followed them for 1 year. They identified five questions: I follow my medication plan; I do not need preventative treatment; I forget at least one dose per day; my ICS causes side effects; and I cannot afford my medication. All five questions were related to asthma control, and the specific barrier questions were related to subsequent adherence or asthma-related health-care utilization.

Pharmacy prescription refill databases have proved valuable in assessing adherence. Some local pharmacies may be helpful in giving individual patient prescription refill data. Although refill information does not answer the question of actual medication use, it does give data as to whether the medicine was obtained by the patient. One learns how "persistent" the patient is about continuing the prescription over time, as well as computing "adherence", the average daily medication dispensed from the inhaler.[8] In the past, HMOs have had pharmacy databases to assist their clinicians in determining if treatment failure may be related to nonadherence. More clinicians are getting access to these data; additionally, more local pharmacies are now more willing to provide refill data.

Clinical Method to Determine Adherence

One way to estimate adherence with the patient in the clinic is to ask a question that suggests that most patients do not follow directions fully. The question is "I wanted to find out how you are doing with the medication regimen we had discussed during the last visit. Most patients follow the plan 50% of the time. So if they were to take their ICS twice a day for 1 week (14 times), that would be seven times. How often are you using the ICS?"

By normalizing nonadherence, it offers the patient the opportunity to honestly reply to the question. One must not scold the patient if he or she is nonadherent, but start a dialogue on why the patient is having difficulties and determine a potential solution that is developed between the patient and the clinician. Choo et al. demonstrated the validity of self-reported nonadherence by comparing patient report, pill count, electronic monitoring device, and automated pharmacy records. Nonadherence reported by patients can serve as a qualitative indicator and a predictor of reduced adherence.

Types of Nonadherence

Patients may be categorized by type of behavior and nonadherence.[2] *Erratic* patients have difficulty following treatment because of the complexity of the treatment or the chaos of their lives. They tend to be forgetful, to be too busy with changing schedules, and frequently run out of medication.

Their priorities do not match the requirements to follow the regimen recommended by their provider. *Unwitting* patients misunderstand the dosing regimen or forget instructions. They fail to understand the rationale for therapy and do not distinguish acute from preventative therapies. There may be language barriers or health literacy issues or they may never have been properly informed by the physician. *Intelligent* patients frequently believe that they know more about the appropriate treatment than the provider does. They may say that they do not need treatment or it is ineffective; they are concerned about drug dependence, side effects, or addiction; or they have a different cultural belief from the provider.

FACTORS OR BARRIERS RELATED TO NONADHERENCE

Barriers can be categorized as related to the characteristics of the disease, the therapy required, the individual patient, the clinician, the practice and health system, or general societal conditions.[2] A patient's barriers may change over time and a review of these barriers should be made at each visit. In the following sections, we discuss the most common barriers affecting asthma management.

THERAPY-RELATED FACTORS

Regimen factors that may affect adherence include: *duration, frequency, complexity, cost, efficacy,* and *real or perceived concerns about side effects.* The correct use of MDIs is key, and an incorrect technique may be considered a form of poor adherence. Patients must also differentiate when to supplement daily ICS use with prn use of rescue medication. Individuals may not use ICS inhalers because they do not perceive the immediate bronchodilation effect experienced with beta$_2$-agonists.

PATIENT-RELATED FACTORS

According to the World Health Organization, "patient-related factors" represent the resources, knowledge, beliefs, perceptions, and expectations of the patient (Videos 14.1 and 14.2).[2] Poverty may lead to decreased access to medication and health-care providers. Individuals in poverty may have lower adherence since they have a greater incidence of depression and stresses that can influence their understanding of instructions, beliefs, and expectations about treatment. Age may also be a factor affecting adherence. Older individuals may forget to take their medicine. Adolescents may be reluctant to follow medication recommendations

http://goo.gl/LTxgCD

VIDEO 14.1 Health belief model.

http://goo.gl/E6Drlz

VIDEO 14.2 Adolescent nonadherence, physician with communication skills: follow-up visit.

because of body image, peer pressure, or autonomy issues (Videos 14.2 through 14.4). The comprehension of asthma care instructions may be a barrier secondary to poor literacy or poor instruction from the provider.

Health beliefs are associated with adherence. Individuals who do not believe that the treatment is effective will not follow through with the recommendations.[26] Distrust of the health-care provider leads to less adherence.[27] In asthma, low literacy has been associated with improper use of MDIs.[28] One aspect of literacy may be particularly important: the ability to understand and use numerical concepts. Poor numerical scores have been shown to be related to ED visits and hospitalizations.[29] This suggests that the comprehension of numerical concepts can affect outcomes.

Patient beliefs about ICSs directly affect their adherence and outcomes. Patients who are concerned about corticosteroid use may underdose or discontinue long-term use in an effort to be "corticosteroid sparing."[2] A survey of over 600 adult asthma patients was conducted to find out patients' perception of the role of ICSs in the treatment of asthma and the potential side effects of asthma. For example, 40% believed that ICSs were bronchodilators and only 25% were aware that ICSs reduced inflammation (Videos 14.5 and 14.6).[30] This would suggest that physicians should identify these concerns before prescribing ICSs.

PROVIDER-RELATED FACTORS

Physician communication skills are appreciated by patients and can influence their adherence and outcomes.[31] A

http://goo.gl/eSZ6N4

VIDEO 14.3 Introduction.

http://goo.gl/wxnId

VIDEO 14.4 Adolescent nonadherence, physician with communication skills: initial visit.

http://goo.gl/xUYYL

VIDEO 14.5 Steroid phobia, physician with communication skills: initial visit.

http://goo.gl/HKpTCY

VIDEO 14.6 Steroid phobia, physician with communication skills: follow-up visit.

significant body of research supports the concept that providers who are friendly and empathetic have the ability to earn the trust of patients, can relate to the patient at his or her level of comprehension, and have the sensitivity to assess and overcome patient barriers that will enhance adherence and outcomes (Videos 14.7 through 14.9).[32]

DISEASE-RELATED FACTORS

A primary role of asthma management is to achieve adherence. Unfortunately, the following characteristics of asthma are associated with poor adherence: the disease is chronic requiring continuous medication administration, there may be periods when patients are asymptomatic, and a portion

http://goo.gl/LvWtFq

VIDEO 14.7 Reflective listening.

http://goo.gl/CmiG3h

VIDEO 14.8 Open-ended questions.

http://goo.gl/WX2nJi

VIDEO 14.9 Empathy.

of patients has difficulty appreciating bronchoconstriction requiring bronchodilator therapy.[2]

PRACTICE AND SYSTEM-RELATED FACTORS

Studies have shown that the organization of the clinic affects adherence to asthma treatment. Fewer patients seen per hour, appointment length, evening hours, multilingual staff, consistency of care, ease of making appointments, ease and effectiveness of telephone communication, and use of the telephone for reminders and follow-ups all promote adherence.[33] At a system level, physicians who have more access to pharmacy refill data are more likely to identify patient adherence. Increasing co-payments for visits and medication are one of the causes of nonadherence. By reducing co-payments for ICSs, one can increase adherence by 5.88%.[34]

INTERVENTIONS TO IMPROVE ADHERENCE

Interventions should focus on the individual barriers identified by the patient. The approach to overcome these barriers can focus on the regimen, the patient, and the providers of care, and can be tailored to the individual patient.[2]

REGIMEN INTERVENTIONS

Attempts to decrease the complexity of the regimen to once daily and combining medications into one MDI to reduce the number of medicines to be taken have been reported to be helpful in increasing adherence.[35] Patients frequently report that forgetting is a common cause of nonadherence. One should carefully assess if forgetting is the "real reason" for missing medication doses. A patient may use "forgetting" as a reason when the individual may have one or more concerns about the medication prescribed. Incorrect inhaler use is a common reason for treatment failure when the patient has been "adherent" using a faulty technique. The techniques of inhaling aerosol and dry powder are significantly different. It is essential to review MDI and dry powder inhaler (DPI) use and correct the technique when needed.

PATIENT INTERVENTIONS

Gibson et al. in the Cochrane Airways Group reviewed adherence articles related to asthma interventions.[36] Most of the studies focused on self-management programs. Successful programs involved self-monitoring of peak expiratory flow rates and symptoms as well as regular medical review and written action plans. Studies of adult self-management programs demonstrated improved health outcomes such as a reduction in nocturnal asthma, hospitalizations, physician visits, and missed days at school and work. Superior outcomes were achieved for patients with written asthma action plans who had the ability to adjust their medication. Kotses et al. developed an adult self-management program conducted over 7 weeks in which the investigators were not only able to reduce symptoms and improve control but they were also able to demonstrate cost effectiveness.[37,38]

Over the short term, self-management training led to fewer asthma symptoms and physician visits and an improvement in asthma management skills and cognitive abilities. Over the long term, self-management training was related to a lower frequency of asthma attacks, reduced medication use, an improvement in cognitive measures, and an increased use of self-management skills. A cost–benefit analysis indicated that the program was beneficial, reducing the cost of asthma to each patient by $475.29. The benefits came primarily from reductions in hospital admissions (reduced from $18,488 to $1,538) and income lost as a result of asthma (reduced from $11,593 to $4,589). Thus, the program more than paid for itself.

In another Cochrane review of adherence to multiple chronic diseases, Haynes reported that the most effective interventions for patients included providing reinforcement for patients' efforts to change their health-related behaviors, giving feedback on progress, tailoring the education intervention to the specific needs of the patient, teaching self-management skills, and providing the patient with educational resources.[39] McDonald et al. evaluated adult patient-focused adherence interventions with varying medical chronic diseases.[40] Although they recognized that there have been significant gains in strategies to improve adherence, most strategies were too costly, complex, labor-intensive, and of variable effectiveness. They encouraged more innovative strategies to be developed.

Providing patients with feedback about medication use has been shown to be helpful in increasing adherence to asthma therapies. Onyirimba et al., using electronic monitors to follow adult inner-city women's use of ICSs, found that those who were given feedback about their medication use had higher (78%) adherence during the 10-week outpatient study than those in the control group who received no feedback.[8] Weinstein et al. employed theophylline monitoring in the outpatient phase of an uncontrolled trial of 59 children with severe asthma who were initially treated in a 10-day rehabilitation protocol.[41] Prior to rehabilitation, the median number of hospital days was 7, the number of emergency care visits was 4, and the asthma-related costs were $10,420. Using psychoeducational strategies to improve self-management behaviors, to assess and remove barriers to adherence, and theophylline monitoring at each outpatient visit, they were able to achieve reductions in morbidity. Hospitalizations and emergency care visits were zero for all 4 years of follow-up and the cost of care at the fourth-year follow-up was $1940. Furthermore, the median theophylline dose was 7.9 µg/mL.

Information technologies are being developed to utilize interactive Internet and mobile device platforms to improve asthma knowledge and/or asthma outcomes. Mosnaim and colleagues conducted an 8-week study in which four low-income black adolescents aged 12–18 years received 10–15 MP3 tracks with coping messages recorded by their peers as well as twice-daily telephone messages to use their ICS.[42] The researchers found that treatment adherence improved from less than 40% to more than 70%, and that asthma control scores (ACT) improved from 19 to more than 20.[42] While this technological research is in its early stages, with small studies and pilot projects, its findings suggest further study with randomized trials.

Recently, patient-centered communication strategies have been introduced to help patients be more consistent with their medication regimen. Patient-centered approaches are associated with better patient retention, adherence, and treatment outcomes, without increased time and cost (Video 14.10).[31] Motivational interviewing (MI) is a patient-centered counseling approach that can be briefly integrated into patient encounters and is specifically designed to enhance motivation to change among patients not ready to change.[32] Existing asthma management approaches (e.g., education and self-management) increase the resistance among patients not ready or willing to follow medical recommendations. MI helps patients resolve their ambivalence about behavior change and builds their intrinsic motivation before providing education (Video 14.11). Although MI overlaps with patient-centered communication, it additionally includes some concrete motivational strategies that can be briefly and easily implemented in medical settings (e.g., setting an agenda, reflective listening (Video 14.7), assessing motivation and confidence for change (Video 14.12), helping the patient weigh the costs and benefits of change (Video 14.4), and providing medical advice and health feedback (Video 14.8)). Wilson et al.[31] used a patient-centered counseling approach, shared-decision making (SDM), to determine its effectiveness in increasing adherence and asthma control in 612 adults with asthma. Practitioners in the study were nonphysicians. SDM uses many of the strategies of MI. The focus of SDM is the negotiation of a treatment regimen that accommodates patients' goals and preferences. During this 2-year study, patients exhibited increased adherence with ICSs and

http://goo.gl/t3hORf

VIDEO 14.10   Patient-centered counseling.

http://goo.gl/s6PULO

VIDEO 14.11   Ambivalence.

http://goo.gl/PkmX6

VIDEO 14.12   Motivation assessment.

long-acting beta$_2$-adrenergic agonists, improved asthma-related quality of life, reduced rescue medication use, greater asthma control and lung function, as well as decreased clinic visits. These findings support the conclusion that negotiating patients' treatment decisions significantly improves adherence to asthma pharmacotherapy and clinical outcomes.

PROVIDER INTERVENTIONS

Providers' acquisition of communication skills is related to adherence.[2] Studies have examined how to improve the communication skills of physicians caring for asthma patients. Clark et al.[43] have provided training in communication skills as well as asthma management to primary care physicians and demonstrated increased anti-inflammatory prescriptions, decreased nonemergency visits, and increased patient satisfaction persisting over 2 years. Cabana,[44] applying a similar communications asthma education program for primary care physicians, was effective in improving parent-reported provider communication skills, the number of days affected by asthma symptoms, and asthma health-care use. Patients with more frequent asthma symptoms and higher health-care utilization at baseline were more likely to benefit from their physician's participation in the program. Studies suggest that having a family member or companion accompany the patient may increase physician and patient question-asking times during the visit.[45] The Accreditation Council for Graduate Medical Education has recognized communication skills as a core area of training for residents and fellows in the United States. Skill development includes counseling patients as well as learning to communicate with health-care teams.

HEALTH-CARE SYSTEM INTERVENTIONS

In 2008, approximately 22 million Americans were determined to have asthma, 6 million under 18 years of age.[46] The annual cost of asthma care in 2007 was an estimated $19.7 billion, with 456,000 hospitalizations and 1.5 million ED visits.[47] The cost of nonadherence has been estimated to be $290 billion in 2009, leading to unavoidable medical expenses.[48] The 2003 World Health Report emphasizes the need to think beyond clinicians as the sole intervener to promote adherence to a large population.[2] Clinicians can no longer afford the time to provide personal interventions. In a response to the increasing cost of care, the United States has turned to disease management companies to improve patient outcomes. *Disease management*, *population care*, and *care management* are similar terms applied to organizations with pragmatically indistinguishable "means" in the systematic pursuit of the same "end"—improved health outcomes for a population of patients.[49] The Asheville Project, a frequently cited asthma disease management program, was successful in reducing morbidity due to asthma as well as congestive heart failure, diabetes, and hypertension.[50] A cohort of 207 adult asthma patients with duration of symptoms for greater than 5 years received one-on-one asthma

education with a pharmacist, who was also a certified asthma educator. They met for one to two sessions. Subsequently, the patients also met with a pharmacist case manager every 3 months. They discussed medication use, symptoms and triggers, inhaler technique, review of peak flow, and update of asthma action plans. The patients' spirometry was also measured. Adherence was not a main outcome measure but was assessed by patient self-report. Adherence results were determined as spending on medication for the cohort and asthma-related medical claims. The study demonstrated a significant reduction in ED visits and hospitalizations. More patients had a less severe National Asthma Education and Prevention Program (NAEPP) asthma severity classification and a higher spirometry from baseline. Although these improvements are significant, there is no way to determine how adherence interventions caused these gains. Because these patients received medication from the pharmacy in Asheville, an objective measure of adherence could have been made pre- and postintervention. By diagnosing adherence status, clinicians could have made appropriate interventions for nonadherent individuals to improve outcomes.

Two disease management outcome studies that focus on adherence, one in diabetes and the other involving both diabetes and cardiovascular disease, are instructive on how adherence measures and interventions can improve the health of a population. Thiebaud et al. prospectively evaluated the effect of telephonic care management within a diabetes management program on adherence to treatment with multiple medications (hypoglycemic agents, angiotensin converting enzyme [ACE] inhibitors, angiotensin receptor blockers, and statins) and recommended laboratory tests in a Medicaid population.[51] The entire intervention population was the focus of the intervention. The comprehensive telephonic care management model used was delivered by nurse care managers who were responsible for tailoring treatment plans to each patient. The care managers influenced adherence in at least four ways. They encouraged patients to follow through on the provider's orders and helped patients to problem-solve adherence issues. They contacted the provider's office directly with information that might result in a new medication or test order. They sent laboratory kits directly to the patients to ensure that the results were available. The care managers also had an indirect influence on adherence to guidelines by educating and empowering patients to partner with their providers. Care-managed patients increased their scripts for hypoglycemic use by 1.5 scripts ($P < .001$) and insulin use by 0.9 script ($P < .001$) relative to controls. Care-managed patients with no tests at baseline, experienced a significant increase in the number of A1C, lipid, and microalbuminuria tests and retinal examinations performed.

The second study by Lawrence et al. focused on a nonadherent population of patients with diabetes and cardiovascular disease.[52] The objectives of this study were to (1) assess the effectiveness of telephonic intervention in influencing the re-initiation of medication therapy and (2) evaluate the rate and timing of medication re-initiation. Care managers received focused training on techniques for medication behavior

TABLE 14.2
Factors Affecting Adherence to Asthma Treatment and Interventions to Improve Adherence*

Drug-Related Factors

Difficulties with inhaler devices

Identify appropriate device for patient. Demonstrate use and have patient demonstrate technique in turn.[59]

Awkward regimens—e.g., four times daily—or multiple drugs

Simplify regimen or tailor it to patient preference.[59]

Fears about side effects

Determine whether concern is theoretical or specific. If specific, relate the persistence of the symptoms versus the likelihood of side effects. Use motivational interviewing to assess the pros and cons and reduce ambivalence. Consider referral to a support group.[60]

Cost of medication

If patient has a prescription plan, select least expensive drug. If not, refer to discount pharmacy plans or pharmaceutical programs.[61]

Dislike of medication

Reduce allergic or irritant exposure to decrease symptoms or medication.[62]

Use motivational interviewing to discuss the "pros and cons" and reduce ambivalence.[60]

Distant pharmacies

Identify capability of receiving prescription by mail.[61]

Non-Drug-Related Factors

Misunderstanding or lack of instruction

If lack of instruction, provide instruction. Assess level of literacy. If low, provide a suitable education strategy. Review pathophysiology and rationale for treatment as well as the consequences of no treatment. Provide instruction and have patient demonstrate technique.[63]

Dissatisfaction with health-care professionals

Have patient speak to administrator regarding issue. May require patient to see another provider if interactions do not improve.[61]

Unexpressed/undisclosed fears or concerns

Identify concerns and address each concern. Determine whether they are theoretical or actual. Consider referral to a support group. May require psychological intervention if fears or concerns persist.[60,61]

Inappropriate expectations

Clarify expectations from a medical perspective. If patient expects greater or quicker improvement, attempt to reset expectations. Review role of allergen/irritant exposure as a factor.[63]

Poor supervision, training, or follow-up

Encourage supervision for children/elderly. Review use of medication in office. Schedule appropriate follow-up.[63]

Anger about condition or its treatment

Identify reason for anger. Express that treatment may improve condition. Assess ambivalence about treatment and review possible alternatives.[60]

Underestimation of severity

Relate symptoms with pulmonary function or use exercise challenge to demonstrate severity of condition.[62]

Cultural issues

Appreciate that varying cultures have different concepts of the development of asthma, factors that exacerbate it, and treatment choices. Take advantage of community health workers to clarify issues.[63]

Concerns about stigmatization

Assess patient reaction to diagnosis. Understand the patient's concerns and refer to support group if the concerns persist.[60]

Forgetfulness or complacency

Determine whether the problem is forgetting to follow treatment versus other reasons. Consider tailoring medication use to patient's daily activities.[63] *Address complacency by withdrawing treatment to determine actual need for treatment.*[62]

Attitudes toward ill health

Assess patient's health beliefs about asthma and treatment. For patients who question the diagnosis or efficacy of treatment, consider stopping treatment and having patient monitor lung function at home.[62]

Religious issues

Clarify how patient's religious beliefs may affect attitudes about diagnosis and treatment. Discussing this with patient's religious leader may give insight and source of support for the patient.[63,64]

Source: Weinstein, A.G., *Ann. Allergy Asthma Immunol.*, 106(4), 283–291, 2011.

* Global Strategy for Asthma Management and Prevention, Global Initiative for Asthma (GINA) 2012 Framework. Available at http://www.ginasthma.org.

change, readiness to change, MI, and active listening. The training also addressed common barriers to adherence and available resources, including side effect management, mail order benefits, drug assistance programs, medication organizers, and reminder systems. The intervention group had a significantly higher rate of medication re-initiation (59.3%) than the control group (42.1%; $P < .05$). Time to re-initiation was significantly shorter in the intervention group than in the control group (59.5 [±69.0] days vs. 107.4 [±109] days; $P < .05$). This initiative demonstrated that a targeted disease management intervention promoting patient behavior change increased the number of patients who re-initiated therapy after a period of nonadherence and decreased the time from nonadherence to adherence. In both studies, nonphysicians were the agents of change using behavioral techniques and adherence to treatment as the guideline.

Because of its low cost and its ability to reach large populations, disease management and population health studies are utilizing interactive voice recognition (IVR). IVR has been used to collect adherence and other health data.[53] The system uses voice-processing technology to link individuals with a computer database. Prerecorded voice files generally prompt the caller to press telephone buttons to answer questions or request information. The IVR system can then retrieve the appropriate health or resource information by accessing the host computer's database and provide it to the patient.

A recent study from a HMO evaluated IVR in a poorly controlled adult asthma population ($n = 50$), all of whom had been prescribed an ICS.[54] Calls were completed in less than 5 min and included content that was designed to inquire about asthma symptoms, deliver core educational messages, encourage refilling of ICS prescriptions, and increase communication with providers. Adherence was tracked during 10 weeks using objective measures that included either electronic monitors or the calculation of canister weight. Subjects completed both quality of life and asthma control surveys. Adherence was 32% higher in the IVR group but there was no difference in quality of life or asthma control.

Weinstein and colleagues have designed an asthma adherence disease management model that was developed while caring for children with severe asthma.[55] It consists of four sequential steps when evaluating symptomatic patients: (1) objective measure of medication use, (2) increase medication if adherent and identify patient barriers if nonadherent, (3) select appropriate interventions for specific barriers, and (4) use appropriate patient-centered communication techniques (Figure 14.1). The same investigators have developed a web-based asthma adherence clinical decision support system to promote adherence to asthma treatments.[56] Patients identify barriers to treatment and receive written and video responses to each barrier. Providers review the barriers and are given specific recommendations for these patients as well as patient-centered counseling techniques to achieve optimal adherence (Table 14.2). This system is being tested telephonically by clinicians trained in the MI technique who provide interventions to subjects with remote electronic adherence monitors and pulmonary function devices.[57]

SUMMARY

The case report presented demonstrates how the adherence information presented in the chapter should be used clinically. The patient reports that she is following the treatment plan, but both biological assay and pharmacy data reveal otherwise. The principal barriers and health beliefs identified include cost of medications, concern about medication side effects, and questions about whether treatment is really necessary. The secondary barriers identified include disagreement with spouse about treatment and forgetting to take treatment. The Asthma Information Test revealed that the patient questions the need for an ICS and does not understand the rationale for treatment. The physician increases the strength of the asthma treatment thereby decreasing the total number of medications (complexity of care) and the number of co-payments.

The NP uses patient-centered communication skills by asking the patient what she would like to learn from the asthma education class. She addresses the patient's concern by developing a strategy to test her health belief about the need for asthma medication and determine whether she needs a daily anti-inflammatory treatment. A strategy to help the patient answer this question is developed. Electronic adherence monitoring gives clinicians information to review with patients and come to an agreement regarding the need for medication and its short-term and long-term efficacy.

REFERENCES

1. Haynes RB, Taylor DW, Sackett DL. *Compliance in Health Care.* Baltimore: Johns Hopkins University Press, 1979.
2. Sabate E. Adherence to long-term therapies: Evidence for action, noncommunicable diseases and mental health adherence to long term therapies project. World Health Organization, Geneva, 2003.
3. Watts RW, McLennan G, Bassham I, et al. Do patients with asthma fill their prescriptions? A primary compliance study. *Aust Fam Physician* 1997;26(Suppl. 1):S4–S6.
4. Kelloway JS, Wyatt RA, Adlis SA. Comparison of patients' compliance with prescribed oral and inhaled asthma medications. *Arch Intern Med* 1994;154;1349–1352.
5. Rand CS, Nides M, Cowles MK, et al. Long-term metered-dose inhaler adherence in a clinical trial. The Lung Health Study Research Group. *Am J Respir Crit Care Med* 1995;152;580–588.
6. Williams LK, Peterson EL, Wells K, et al. A cluster-randomized trial to provide clinicians inhaled corticosteroid adherence information for their patients with asthma. *J Allergy Clin Immunol* 2010;126:225–231.
7. Bender BG, Pedan A, Varasteh LT. Adherence and persistence with fluticasone propionate/salmeterol combination therapy. *J Allergy Clin Immunol* 2006;118:899–904.
8. Onyirimba F, Apter AJ, Reisine ST. Direct clinician-to-patient feedback of inhaled steroid use: Its effect on adherence and asthma outcome. *Ann Allergy Asthma Immunol* 2003;90:411–415.
9. Krishnan JA, Riekert KA, McCoy JV, et al. Corticosteroid use after hospital discharge among high-risk adults with asthma. *Am J Respir Crit Care Med* 2004;170:1281–1285.
10. Jonasson G, Carlsen K, Mowinckel P. Asthma drug adherence in a long term clinical trial. *Arch Dis Child* 2000;83:330–331.

11. Suissa S, Ernst P, Kezouh A. Regular use of inhaled corticosteroids and the long term prevention of hospitalisation for asthma *Thorax* 2002;57(10):880–884.

12. Suissa S, Ernst P, Benayoun S, et al. Low-dose inhaled corticosteroids and the prevention of death from asthma. *N Engl J Med* 2000;343(5):332–336.

13. Milgrom H, Bender B, Ackerson L, et al. Noncompliance and treatment failure in children with asthma. *J Allerg Clin Immunol* 1996;98:1051–1057.

14. Murphy A, Proeschal A, Brightling C, et al. The relationship between clinical outcomes and medication adherence in difficult-to-control asthma *Clinical Pharmacist* 2012;4(Suppl. 2):S2.

15. Adams SA, Matthews CE, Ebbeling CB, et al. The effect of social desirability and social approval on self-reports of physical activity. *Am J Epidemiol* 2005;161:389–398.

16. Bender B, Wamboldt FS, O'Connor SL, et al. Measurement of children's asthma medication adherence by self report, mother report, canister weight, and Doser CT. *Ann Allergy Asthma Immunol* 2000;85:416–421.

17. Weinstein, AG, Cusky, W. Theophylline compliance in asthmatic children. *Ann Allergy* 1985;54:19.

18. Cochrane, GM. Compliance in asthma: A European perspective. *Eur Respir Rev* 1995;5(26):116–119.

19. O'Connor SL, Bender BG, Gavin-Devitt LA, et al. Measuring adherence with the Doser CT in children with asthma. *J Asthma* 2004;41(6):663–670.

20. Burgess SW, Sly PD, Devadason SG. Providing feedback on adherence increases use of preventive medication by asthmatic children. *J Asthma* 2010;47(2):198–201.

21. McHorney CA, Spain CV, Charles M, et al. Validity of the adherence estimator in the prediction of 9 month persistence with medications prescribed for chronic diseases: A prospective analysis of data from pharmacy claims. *Clin Ther* 2009;31:2584–2607.

22. www.AsthmaPACT.org Hosted on the Asthma and Allergy of Foundation website www.aafa.org. Reviewed August 2012.

23. Weinstein, AG, Schatz M, Laurenceau. Preliminary analysis of an adherence survey for adult asthma patients. *J Allergy Clin Immunol* 2009;123:S72.

24. Schatz M, Zeiger RS, Yang S-J, Weinstein AG, Chen W, Saris-Baglama RN, Turner-Bowker DM. Development and preliminary validation of the adult asthma adherence questionnaire. *J Allergy Clin Immunol* 2013;1:280–288.

25. Choo P, Rand C, Inui T, et al. Validation of patient reports, automated pharmacy records, and pill counts with electronic monitoring of adherence to antihypertensive therapy validation of patient reports. *Med Care* 1999;37;846–857.

26. Osman LM, Russell IT, Friend JA, et al. Predicting patient attitudes to asthma medication. *Thorax* 1993;48:827–830.

27. George M, Freedman TG, Norfleet AL, et al. Qualitative research enhanced understanding of patients' beliefs: Results of focus groups with low-income urban African-American adults with asthma. *J Allergy Clin Immunol* 2003;111:967–973.

28. Williams MV, Baker DW, Honig EG, et al. Inadequate literacy is a barrier to asthma knowledge and self-care. *Chest J* 1998;114:1008–1015.

29. Apter AJ, Cheng J, Small D, et al. Asthma numeracy skill and health literacy. *J Asthma* 2006;43:705–710.

30. Boulet LP. Perception of the role and potential side effects of inhaled corticosteroids among asthmatic patients *Chest J* 1998;113(3):587–592.

31. Wilson S, Strub P, Buist A, et al. and the Better Outcomes of Asthma Treatment (BOAT) Study Group. Shared treatment decision making improves adherence and outcomes in poorly controlled asthma. *Am J Respir Crit Care Med* 2010;181(6):566–577.

32. Borrelli B Riekert K, Weinstein A, et al. Brief motivational interviewing as a clinical strategy to promote asthma medication adherence. *J Allergy Clin Immunol* 2007;120:1023–1030.

33. Lowe RA, Localio AR, Schwarz DF, et al. Association between primary care practice characteristics and emergency department use in a Medicaid managed care organization. *Med Care* 2005;43:792–800.

34. Chernew M, Shah M, Wegh A, et al. Impact of decreasing copayments on medication adherence within a disease management environment. *Health Aff* 2008;27(1):103–112.

35. Stoloff SW, Stempel DA, Meyer J, et al. Improved refill persistence with fluticasone propionate and salmeterol in a single inhaler compared with other controller therapies. *J Allergy Clin Immunol* 2004;113:245–251.

36. Gibson PG, Powell H, Wilson A, et al. Self-management education and regular practitioner review for adults with asthma (Review). *Cochrane Airways Group*. Update 2002.

37. Kotses H, Bernstein IL, Bernstein DI, et al. A self-management program for adult asthma. Part I: Development and evaluation. *J Allergy Clin Immunol* 1995;95(2):529–540.

38. Taitel MS, Kotses H, Bernstein IL, et al. A self-management program for adult asthma. Part II: Cost–benefit analysis. *J Allergy Clin Immunol* 1995;95(3):672–676.

39. Haynes RB, Yao X, Degani A, et al. Interventions to enhance medication adherence. *Cochrane Database Syst Rev* 2005;CD000011.

40. McDonald HP, Garg AX, Haynes RB. Interventions to enhance patient adherence to medication prescriptions: Scientific review. *JAMA* 2002;288:2868–2879.

41. Weinstein, AG, McKee L, Stapleford J, et al. An economic evaluation of short-term inpatient rehabilitation for severe asthmatic children. *J Allergy Clin Immunol* 1996;98:264–273.

42. Mosnaim G, Powell L, Rathkopf M. A review of published studies using interactive Internet tools or mobile devices to improve asthma knowledge or health outcomes. *Pediat Allergy Immunol Pulmonol* 2012;25(2):55–63.

43. Clark NM, Gong M, Schork MA, et al. Long-term effects of asthma education for physicians on patient satisfaction and use of health services. *Eur Respir J* 2000;16:15–21.

44. Cabana MD, Slish KK, Evans D, et al. Impact of physician asthma care education on patient outcomes. *Pediatrics* 2006;117(6):2149–2157.

45. Schilling LM, Scatena L, Steiner JF, et al. The third person in the room: Frequency, role, and influence of companions during primary care medical encounters. *J Fam Pract* 2002;51:685–690.

46. Summary Health Statistics for US Adults: National Health Interview Survey, 2008 and Summary Health Statistics for US Children: National Health Interview Survey, 2008.

47. American Lung Association. Epidemiology & statistics unit, research and program services. *Trends in Asthma Morbidity and Mortality*. November 2007.

48. New England Health Institute. Thinking outside the pillbox: A system-wide approach to improving patient medication adherence for chronic disease, 2009.

49. Kindig D, Stoddart G. What is population health? *Am J Public Health* 2003;93(3):380–383.

50. Bunting BA, Cranor CW. The Asheville Project: Long-term clinical, humanistic, and economic outcomes of a community-based medication therapy management program for asthma. *J Am Pharm Assoc (2003)* 2006;46:133–147.

51. Thiebaud P, Demand M, Wolf S, et al. Impact of disease management on utilization and adherence with drugs and tests: The case of diabetes treatment in the Florida: A Healthy State (FAHS) program. *Diabetes Care* 2008;31(9):1717–1722.

52. Lawrence DB, Allison W, Chen JC, et al. Improving medication adherence with a targeted, technology-driven disease management intervention. *Dis Manag* 2008;11(3):141–144.

53. Kaplan B, Farzanfar R, Friedman RH. Personal relationships with an intelligent interactive telephone health behavior advisor system: A multimethod study using surveys and ethnographic interviews. *Int J Med Inform* 2003;71:33–41.

54. Bender BG, Apter A, Bogen DK, et al. Test of an interactive voice response intervention to improve adherence to controller medications in adults with asthma. *J Am Board Fam Med* 2010;23(2):159–165.

55. Weinstein AG. Asthma adherence management for the clinician. *J Allergy Clin Immunol: In Practice* 2013;1:123–128.

56. www.AsthmaPACT.org hosted by The Asthma and Allergy Foundation of America.

57. Weinstein AG. An Asthma Adherence Telehealth System to Improve Asthma Management. NIH grant No. R43HL115846.

58. Weinstein AG. The potential of asthma adherence management to enhance asthma guidelines. *Ann Allergy Asthma Immunol* 2011;106(4):283–291.

59. Guidelines for the Diagnosis and Management of Asthma (EPR3) 2007. NIH, NHLBI. August 2007. NIH publication No. 08-4051.

60. Borelli B, Riekert K, Weinstein A, Rathier L. Brief motivational interviewing as a clinical strategy to promote asthma medication adherence. *J Allergy Clin Immunol* 2007;120:1023–1030.

61. Asthma PACT (Personalized Assessment and Control Tool). Asthma and Allergy Foundation of America, 2004–2010. Available at www.AsthmaPACT.org. Accessed Feb 19, 2010.

62. Weinstein AG. Clinical management strategies to maintain drug compliance in asthmatic children. *Ann Allergy* 1995;74:304–310.

63. Rand C, Bender B, Boulet L-P, Chaustre I, Weinstein A. Asthma, Chapter 7, *World Health Organization Report 2003: Adherence to Long-Term Therapies: Evidence for Action.* Geneva: World Health Organization, 2003.

64. Ahmedani BK, Peterson EL, Wells KE, Rand C, Williams LK. Asthma medication adherence: The role of God and other health locus control factors. *Ann Allergy Asthma Immunol* 2013;110:75–79.

15 Inhaler Devices

Federico Lavorini, Mark L. Levy, and Giovanni A. Fontana

CONTENTS

CASE PRESENTATIONS

1. A 45-year-old male with a recent diagnosis of asthma presented for lung function testing. He reported shortness of breath and the lack of effect of his therapy, and he particularly mentioned that he had no symptomatic relief after inhaling salbutamol via a pressurized metered-dose inhaler (pMDI). He said he had been given the inhaler for the first time 2 weeks earlier at an internist's clinic and he had received only a brief oral instruction to "spray the medicine to the throat." As a result, he had faithfully administered the drugs by aiming and firing the aerosol toward his anterior neck around the thyroid cartilage twice a day for 2 weeks.

2. A 45-year-old female asthma patient reported that her beta-agonist pMDI inhaler was ineffective. She had increased the dose of her beta-agonist to 20 puffs a day without any obvious benefit. She insisted that she knew how to use the inhaler correctly and had been following the verbal instructions given by her general physician some months earlier. When she was asked to demonstrate her inhaler technique, she fired the aerosol twice with the dust cap on, then quickly removed the cap, placed the mouthpiece between her lips, and inhaled.

COMMENT

These two unusual cases should remind medical personnel not to rely on quick verbal instructions to patients on inhaler technique; rather, they should first demonstrate the correct use of an inhaler and then observe the patient's technique.

Furthermore, one should not assume that patients with a long history of using MDIs are able to use inhalers correctly. The absence of any effect, therapeutic or adverse, of a beta-agonist MDI, especially in patients receiving higher doses, should alert physicians to the possibility of misuse due to inadequate instructions or demonstration.

INTRODUCTION AND CASE STUDIES

The incidence of asthma continues to rise worldwide, doubling over the last 10 years[1–3]; consequently, asthma is placing a huge economic burden on health-care resources.[4] Asthma management guidelines are now widely available in virtually every country. Their aim is to achieve control of the disease with the lowest possible dose of the medication prescribed.[1] Asthma guidelines advocate a stepwise approach to pharmacological treatment: increase the amount and frequency of medication as asthma worsens ("step up"), and decrease the amount and frequency of medication when asthma is under control ("step down"). Once the control of asthma has been achieved and maintained for at least 3 months, a gradual reduction of the maintenance therapy is recommended to identify the minimum therapy required to maintain control.[1]

Unfortunately, the current level of asthma control falls far short of the published goals for long-term asthma management,[2] with many patients reporting daytime and night-time symptoms at least once a week, continuing to require unscheduled GP visits and hospitalizations.[2] One of the reasons why asthma remains poorly controlled is that patients are deriving incomplete benefit from their inhaled medication, primarily because they are unable to use their inhalers correctly.[5] Although inhaler misuse for pMDIs is commonly related to poor coordination between actuation and inhalation or, for dry powder inhalers (DPIs) to exhalation into the inhaler thus blowing the powder out of the device, patients occasionally misuse their inhalers in other unusual ways. The case histories described demonstrate some of these issues.

Several inhaler devices are currently available on the market, and these are classified as pMDIs, breath-actuated (BA) pMDIs, DPIs, soft mist inhalers (SMI), and nebulized or "wet" aerosols. Each class of inhaler device has pros as well as cons (Table 15.1). Inhalers differ in their efficiency of drug delivery to the lower respiratory tract, depending on the form of the device, its internal resistance, the formulation of the medication, its particle size, the velocity of the produced aerosol plume, and the ease with which patients can use the device.[6] The efficiency of drug delivery may also be influenced by patients' preference, which, in turn, affects patients' adherence to treatment and, indeed, the subsequent

long-term control of the disease.[7] There seems little point in prescribing an effective medication in an inhaler device that patients cannot use correctly. Thus, the choice of the right inhaler for the patient is just as important as choosing the most effective medication.

In this chapter, we will focus on the handheld inhalers (i.e., pMDI, DPI, BA pMDI, and SMI), together with the current understanding of the correct inhalation techniques for each device. We will also provide a general description of nebulizers, which are frequently used to deliver asthma medications.[8] However, since most of the current nebulizer designs are bulky and inconvenient, and drug administration is prolonged, they are better categorized as second-line devices for most asthma patients. We will also assess the problems that can lead to poor inhaler technique, which could contribute to poor asthma control. Finally, we will summarize some of the recommendations by the Aerosol Drug Management

TABLE 15.1

Advantages and Disadvantages of Different Inhaler Devices

Device	Advantages	Disadvantages
pMDI	• Portable and compact • Multidose device • Quick to use • Relatively cheap • Cannot contaminate contents • Available for most inhaled medications	• Contains propellants • Not breath actuated • Many patients cannot use it correctly (e.g., coordination difficulties) • "Cold Freon" effect • High oropharyngeal deposition
pMDI + spacer	• Easier to coordinate • Large drug doses delivered more conveniently than a pMDI alone • Less oropharyngeal deposition • Higher lung deposition than a pMDI	• Bulkier and less portable than a pMDI alone • Plastic spacers may acquire static charge • Additional cost to pMDIs
BA pMDI	• Portable and compact • Multidose device • Quick to use • Breath actuated (no coordination needed) • Cannot contaminate contents	• Contains propellants • "Cold Freon" effect • Requires moderate inspiratory flow to be triggered • More bulky and noisier than a pMDI
DPI	• Portable and compact; quick to use • Breath actuated (no coordination needed) • Usually higher lung deposition than a pMDI • Do not contain propellants	• Require an adequate inspiratory flow • May not be appropriate for emergency situations • Many patients cannot use them correctly • Most types are moisture sensitive
SMI (Respimat)	• Portable and compact • Multidose device • Probably easier to use than a pMDI • High lung deposition • Does not contain propellants	• Not breath actuated • Not currently available in most countries • Relatively expensive
Nebulizers	• May be used at any age • Do not require a specific inhalation technique • Vibrating mesh types are portable and do not require an outside energy source • May be used to dispense drugs that are not available for delivery with pMDIs or DPIs	• Jet and ultrasonic nebulizers require an outside energy source • Treatment times can be long • Performance varies between nebulizers • Jet nebulizers are wasteful since a certain volume of solution cannot be aerosolized • Risk of bacterial contamination • Newer nebulizers are expensive

Note: pMDI, pressurized metered-dose inhalers; BA pMDI, breath-actuated metered-dose inhaler; DPI, dry powder inhaler; SMI, soft mist inhaler.

Improvement Team (ADMIT) for inhaler selection, as well as an algorithm for asthma therapy adjustment.[5]

PRESSURIZED METERED-DOSE INHALERS

pMDIs were introduced in the 1950s as the first portable, multidose delivery system for bronchodilators. They are still the most widely prescribed inhalers for the treatment of asthma and chronic obstructive pulmonary disease.[8] The pMDI is a portable multidose device that utilizes a propellant under pressure to generate a metered dose of an aerosol through an atomization nozzle (Figure 15.1). Until recently, pMDIs used chlorofluorocarbons (CFC) as propellants to deliver drugs; however, in accordance with the Montreal Protocol of 1987, CFC propellants have, in most cases, been replaced by hydrofluoroalkane (HFA) propellants that do not have ozone-depleting properties.[9] The key components of the CFC-driven pMDIs (i.e., canister, metering valve, actuator, and propellant) have been retained in the HFA-driven pMDIs, but some of the elements required redesigning. Two approaches were used in the formulation of HFA-driven pMDIs. The first

approach was to show its equivalence with the CFC-driven pMDI, which was necessary for regulatory approval; this was used for salbutamol pMDIs and some of the corticosteroid pMDIs. Some HFA formulations were matched to their CFC counterparts on a microgram for microgram basis; therefore, no dosage modification was needed when switching from a CFC to a HFA formulation. The second approach involved extensive changes, particularly for corticosteroid inhalers containing beclomethasone dipropionate, and resulted in the development of solution aerosols with extra-fine particle size distributions and high lung deposition.[10,11] The exact dose equivalence of extra-fine HFA beclomethasone dipropionate and CFC beclomethasone dipropionate has not been established, but data from most trials have indicated a 2:1 dose ratio in favor of the HFA-driven pMDI.[10,11] Patients on regular long-term treatment with a CFC pMDI could be safely switched to a HFA pMDI without any deterioration in their pulmonary function, loss of disease control, increased frequency of hospital admissions, or other adverse effects.[9] However, when physicians prescribe HFA formulations in place of the CFC versions for the first time, they should

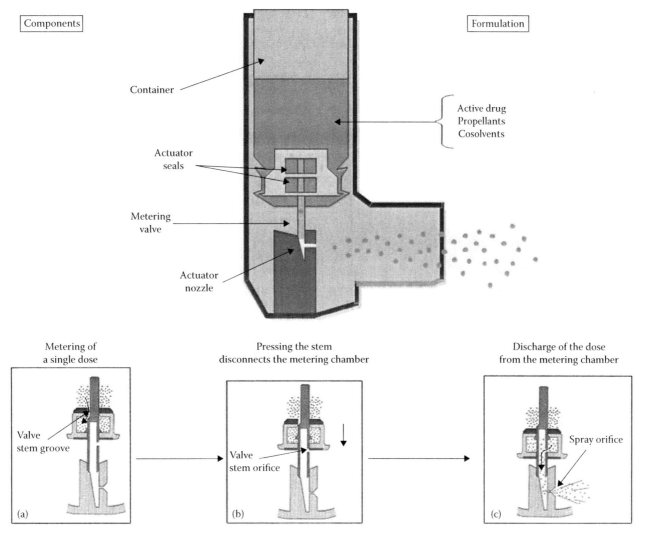

FIGURE 15.1 **(See color insert)** Schematic representation of the components of a pressurized metered-dose inhaler. The lower panels illustrate the process of aerosol generation.

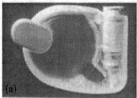 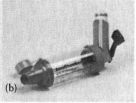 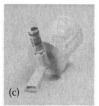

FIGURE 15.2 **(See color insert)** Examples of an open tube spacer (a: the Jet), a holding chamber (b: the AeroChamber Plus), and a reverse-flow spacer (c: the InspirEase).

inform their patients about the differences between these products. Two of the major differences between the CFC and HFA pMDIs are that the plume released from many HFA-driven pMDIs has a slower velocity and it is warmer.[6] These changes partially overcome the cold Freon effect[5] that has caused some patients to suddenly stop while in the process of inhaling their CFC pMDIs. Another difference is that many HFA-driven pMDIs contain a small amount of ethanol. This affects the taste, as well as further increasing the temperature and decreasing the velocity of the aerosol.

Despite the numerous advantages of pMDIs, most patients cannot use these inhalers correctly, even after repeated instruction (see Table 15.1).[5] This is because pMDIs require good coordination between the patient's inspiration and the timing of the device actuation to ensure the correct inhalation and deposition of the drug into the lungs. When using pMDIs, the correct inhalation technique involves firing the pMDI while breathing in deeply and slowly, continuing to inhale after firing, and then following inhalation with a breath-holding pause to allow particles to sediment on the airways.[12] The patient should also be instructed that, when used for the first time, and after several days of not using, the pMDI should be primed by actuating it before inhalation. Interestingly, patients frequently fail to continuously inhale slowly after activation of the inhaler and exhale fully before inhalation.[5,13] In addition, patients often get the timing wrong by activating the inhaler before inhalation, at the end of inhalation, or by initiating inhaler actuation while breath-holding.[5,13] Crompton et al.[7,13,14] showed that the proportion of patients capable of using their pMDI correctly after reading the package insert fell from 46% in 1982 to 21% in 2000, while only just over one-half of patients (52%) used a pMDI correctly even after receiving instruction. In a large (n = 4078) study, 71% of the patients were found to have difficulty using pMDIs, and almost one-half of them had poor coordination.[15] More importantly, an incorrect inhalation technique has been associated with poor asthma control.[13] The incorrect use of pMDIs is not confined to patients; both nurses and physicians also use pMDIs incorrectly.[5]

Even with the correct inhalation technique, pMDIs are inefficient since no more than 20% for CFC pMDIs[5] or 40% for HFA pMDIs producing extra-fine particles[10,11] of the emitted dose reaches the lungs, with a high proportion of the drug being deposited in the mouth and oropharynx, which can cause local as well as systemic side effects due to rapid absorption.[5,6]

pMDI ACCESSORY DEVICES: SPACERS AND VALVED HOLDING CHAMBERS

Spacer devices are attachments to the pMDI mouthpiece with volumes ranging from 50 to 800 mL (Figure 15.2). Many have a one-way valve that prevents the patient blowing the dose away after firing.[16] Spacers assist the patient to inhale without necessarily having to coordinate this with actuation of the device.[16] By acting as an aerosol reservoir, these devices slow the aerosol velocity and increase the transit time and distance between the pMDI actuator and the patient's mouth, allowing the particle size to decrease, with a consequent increased deposition of the aerosol particles in the lungs.[16] Moreover, because spacers trap large particles comprising up to 80% of the aerosol dose, only a small fraction of the dose is deposited in the oropharynx, thereby reducing the side effects, such as throat irritation, dysphonia, and oral candidiasis, associated with medications delivered by the pMDI alone.[16] There are three basic spacers designs: the open tube, the holding chamber, and the reverse flow design, in which the pMDI, placed close to the mouth, is fired in the direction away from the patient. A valved holding chamber fitted with an appropriate face mask is used to give pMDI drugs to neonates, young children, and elderly patients. The two key factors for optimum aerosol delivery are a tight but comfortable face mask fit and a reduced face mask dead space.[16] Because children have low tidal volumes and inspiratory flow rates, comfortable breathing through a face mask requires low-resistance inspiratory or expiratory valves. Of note, some spacers incorporate a whistle that makes a sound if inspiration is too fast; this feedback enables patients to improve drug delivery through optimizing their inhalation technique. There is evidence that spacers may improve the clinical effect of inhaled medications especially in patients who are unable to use a pMDI properly.[16] Indeed, spacers may increase the response to short-acting beta-adrenergic bronchodilators, even in patients with a correct inhalation technique.[17–20] While spacers are good drug-delivery devices, they suffer from the obvious disadvantage of making the entire delivery system less portable and compact than a pMDI alone. The size and the appearance of some spacers may detract from the appeal of the pMDI to patients, especially among the pediatric population, and negatively affect patients' compliance.[16] Furthermore, spacers may contribute to the inconsistent delivery of medication due to electrostatic charge, resulting in a buildup of drug deposits on the spacer wall.[16] Aerosols remain suspended for longer periods within holding chambers that are manufactured from nonelectrostatic materials compared with other materials. Thus, an inhalation might be delayed for 2–5 sec without substantial loss of the drug to the walls of metal or nonstatic spacers.[16] The electrostatic charge in plastic spacers can be substantially reduced by washing the spacer with a low concentration of dishwashing liquid and allowing it to drip dry rather than towel drying it. There is no consensus on how often a spacer should be cleaned, but recommendations range in general from once a week to once a month, and patients should be directed to the manufacturers' instructions.[6] The proportion of the drug dose that the patient inhales may vary greatly with different spacers, and the data about a spacer derived from studies with one drug and pMDI may not apply to other drugs.[16]

BREATH-ACTUATED pMDIs

BA pMDIs, such as the Autohaler and Easibreathe, are alternatives to standard pMDIs that have been developed to overcome the problem of poor coordination of pMDI actuation and inhalation.[21] BA pMDIs have a flow-triggered system driven by a spring that releases the dose during inhalation, so that firing and inhaling are automatically coordinated.[21] These inhalation devices can achieve good lung deposition and clinical efficacy in patients unable to use a pMDI correctly because of coordination difficulties.[22] Errors when using a BA pMDI are less frequent than when using a standard pMDI.[7] An increased use of BA pMDIs might improve asthma control and reduce the overall cost of asthma therapy compared with conventional pMDIs.[23] On the negative side, BA pMDIs do not solve the cold Freon effect and would be unsuitable for a patient who has this kind of difficulty using a pMDI. In addition, in order to trigger an actuation, these devices require a relatively higher inspiratory flow than pMDIs. Furthermore, oropharyngeal deposition with BA pMDIs is as high as that observed with CFC pMDIs.

DRY POWDER INHALERS

DPIs were first introduced in 1970, the earliest being single-dose devices containing the powder formulation in a gelatine capsule, which the patient loaded into the device prior to use. Since the late 1980s, multidose DPIs have been available, providing the same degree of convenience as a pMDI.[24] These devices have been further modified for the treatment of asthma and other conditions by delivering a range of drugs that are usually given by injection, such as peptides, proteins, and vaccines. The use of DPIs is expected to increase following the phasing out of CFC production along with the increased availability of dry powder inhalers and the development of novel powder devices.[25] DPI doses can be premetered in the form of single capsules or foil blisters or as multi-single unit dose disks (Figure 15.3); alternatively, device metering of bulk powder can be achieved through the use of reservoir devices.[24,25]

Generally, DPIs have many advantages over pMDIs. DPIs are actuated and driven by the patient's inspiratory flow; consequently, DPIs do not require propellants to generate the aerosol, removing the need to coordinate inhaler actuation with inhalation.[26] However, a forceful and deep inhalation through the DPI is needed to deaggregate the powder formulation into respirable-sized particles as efficiently as possible and, consequently, to ensure that the drug is delivered to the lungs.[26,27] Although most patients are capable of generating enough flow

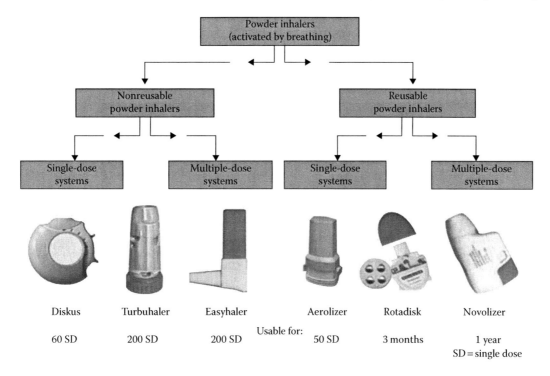

FIGURE 15.3 (See color insert) A variety of dry powder inhalers. (From Aerosol Drug Management Improvement Team (ADMIT). www.admit-online.info.)

to operate a DPI efficiently,[26] the need to inhale forcefully to generate sufficient inspiratory flow could be a problem for very young children or patients with severe airflow limitation.[28] For this reason, DPIs are not generally recommended for children under the age of 5.[26] The newer active or power-assisted DPIs incorporate battery-driven impellers and vibrating piezoelectric crystals that reduce the need for the patient to generate a high inspiratory flow rate, which is an advantage for many patients.[25] Drug delivery to the lungs ranges between 10% and 40% of the emitted dose for several DPIs.[25] The physical design of a DPI establishes its specific resistance to airflow (measured as the square root of the pressure drop across the device divided by the flow rate through the device), with current designs having specific resistance values ranging from about 0.02 to 0.2 cmH$_2$O/(L min).[27] To produce a fine powder aerosol with increased delivery to the lungs, a DPI that is characterized as having a low resistance requires an inspiratory flow of >90 L/min, a medium-resistance DPI requires 50–60 L/min, and a high-resistance DPI requires <50 L/min.[27] Of note, DPIs with a high resistance tend to produce greater lung deposition than those with a lower resistance,[27] but the clinical significance of this is not known.

Although DPIs offer advantages over pMDIs, they do have some limitations in their design, cost effectiveness, and user friendliness.[6] For instance, capsule-based DPIs, such as the Handihaler and the Aerolizer, require that single doses are individually loaded into the inhaler immediately before use. This is inconvenient for some patients, and difficult for those with problems related to manual dexterity; furthermore, these do not record the doses taken by the patient. In addition, the inhalation maneuver has to be repeated until the capsule is empty, which may give rise to underdosing and high-dose variability. Other DPIs are multiple unit dose devices, such as the Diskhaler, or multidose devices, such as the Diskus and the Turbuhaler. These devices do not have any triggering mechanism, which makes optimal drug delivery entirely dependent on an individual patient's inspiratory maneuver. Because of variations in the design and performance of DPIs, patients might not use all DPIs equally well; therefore, different types of DPIs might not be readily interchangeable, despite dispensing the same drug.[27] Studies have also shown that the dose emission is reduced when some DPIs are exposed to extremely low and high temperatures and humidity[25,26]; therefore, DPIs should be stored in a cool dry place.

A recent systematic literature review revealed that up to 90% of patients did not use their DPI correctly.[29] Common errors made by patients included lack of exhalation before inhalation, incorrect positioning and loading of the inhaler, failure to inhale forcefully and deeply through the device, and patients' failure to breath-hold after inhalation.[29] All these errors may lead to insufficient drug delivery, which adversely influences drug efficacy and may contribute to inadequate disease control.[29] It is not surprising that such a high proportion of patients were unable to use DPIs correctly as the devices have many inherent design limitations. The Diskhaler, for example, is a multiple unit dose device as it contains a series of foil blisters on a disk. It is complicated to use, requiring eight steps to

effect one correct inhalation; approximately 70% of patients are unable to use it correctly.[29] The disks have to be changed frequently and the device has to be cleaned before refilling. In addition, it provides no feedback to the patient of a successful inhalation, except a sweet taste in the mouth, which may simply be indicative of oral drug deposition. The Turbuhaler, a multidose reservoir device, is the most frequently prescribed DPI as it produces a good deposition of the drug in the lungs provided that a sufficient (about 60 L/min) inspiratory flow has been achieved by the patient. However, approximately 80% of patients are unable to use it correctly[29]; common mistakes made by patients using this inhaler are failure to rotate the base fully in both directions, and failure to keep the device upright until loaded. In addition, due to its high intrinsic resistance, patients who have a reduced inspiratory flow may encounter problems using this device. The Diskus (or Accuhaler) is another example of a multidose device that uses a foil blister strip. Up to 50% of patients use this DPI incorrectly. Common errors include failure or difficulty in loading the device before inhalation, and exhaling into the device.[29] The Diskus has a low intrinsic resistance but, like the Turbuhaler, it does not have any triggering mechanism, which makes optimal drug delivery entirely dependent on an individual patient's forceful inspiratory maneuver.[29] Additionally, as with other DPI devices employing drug blisters, incomplete emptying of the metered dose may occur, which could reduce the amount of drug delivered to the lungs and hence reduce its clinical efficacy.[29]

SOFT MIST INHALERS

The development of SMIs has opened up new opportunities for inhaled drug delivery. These inhalation devices use liquid formulations similar to those in nebulizers, but they are generally multidose devices that have the potential to compete with pMDIs and DPIs in the portable inhaler market. Currently, the only SMI marketed in some European countries is the Respimat inhaler. This device does not require propellants since it is powered by the energy of a compressed spring inside the inhaler. Individual doses are delivered via a precisely engineered nozzle system as a slow-moving aerosol cloud (hence the term *soft mist*).[30] Scintigraphic studies have shown that lung deposition is higher (up to 50%) than that from a CFC-based pMDI.[30] Although the Respimat has been used relatively little in clinical practice to date, clinical trials seem to confirm that drugs delivered by the Respimat are effective in correspondingly smaller doses in patients with obstructive airway disease.[31] The Respimat is a "press and breathe" device, and the correct inhalation technique closely resembles that used with a pMDI. However, although coordination between firing and inhaling is required, the low spray velocity and the long duration of the aerosol cloud (typically 1–1.5 sec) could enable patients to coordinate firing and inhaling more easily than with a pMDI.[30]

NEBULIZERS

Various types of nebulizers are available, and several studies have indicated that their performance varies between manufacturers and also between nebulizers from the same manufacturer.[32–34] There are two basic types of nebulizers: the pneumatic or jet nebulizer, and the ultrasonic nebulizer (Figure 15.4).[32–34]

The jet nebulizer generates aerosol particles as a result of the impact between a liquid and a jet of high-velocity gas (usually air or oxygen) in the nebulizer chamber. In a jet nebulizer, the driving gas passes through a very narrow opening from a high-pressure system. This driving gas passes at high velocity over the end of a narrow liquid feed tube or concentric feeding system creating a negative pressure. As a result of this fall in pressure, the liquid is sucked up by the Bernoulli effect and is broken into small droplets. The majority of the liquid mass produced during this process is in the form of large (15–500 μm) nonrespirable droplets; coarse droplets impact on the baffles of the nebulizer while smaller droplets may be inhaled or may land on the internal walls of the nebulizer, returning to the reservoir for renebulization.[32–34] The impaction of the large particles generates small, respirable particles, and therefore the baffle design has a critical effect on the droplet size. Concentric liquid feeds minimize blockage by residual drug buildup with repeated nebulization. A flat pick-up plate may allow some nebulizers to be tilted during treatment while maintaining the liquid flow from the reservoir. There are four different designs of jet nebulizers: a jet nebulizer with a reservoir tube, a jet nebulizer with a collection bag, a breath-enhanced jet nebulizer, and a BA jet nebulizer.[32–34] Both the breath-enhanced and the BA jet nebulizers are modifications of the "conventional" jet nebulizers specifically designed to improve their efficiency by increasing the amount of aerosol delivered to the patient with less wastage of the aerosol during exhalation. Different types of jet nebulizers have different output characteristics that are determined by the design of the air jet and the capillary tube orifices, their geometric relationship with each other, and the internal baffles; for a given design, the major determinant of the output is the driving pressure of gas (air or oxygen). The jet nebulizer with a reservoir tube provides continuous aerosolization during the entire breathing cycle, causing the release and wastage of the aerosol into the air during exhalation and anytime when the

patient is not breathing. Consequently, no more than 20% of the emitted aerosol is inhaled.[32–34] The jet nebulizer with a collection bag generates the aerosol by continuously filling a collection bag that acts as a reservoir. The patient inhales the aerosol from the reservoir through a one-way inspiratory valve and exhales to the environment through an exhalation port between the one-way inspiratory valve and the mouthpiece. The breath-enhanced jet nebulizer (e.g., the PARI LC Plus) uses two one-way valves to prevent the loss of the aerosol to the environment; when the patient inhales, the inspiratory valve opens and the aerosol vents through the nebulizer; the exhaled aerosol passes through an expiratory valve in the mouthpiece. BA jet nebulizers are designed to increase the aerosol delivery to the patient by means of a BA valve that triggers aerosol generation only during inspiration. Both the breath-enhanced and BA nebulizers increase the amount of inspired aerosol with a shorter nebulization time than "conventional" jet nebulizers.[32]

Ultrasonic nebulizers use a rapidly vibrating (>1 MHz) piezoelectric crystal to produce aerosol particles.[32–34] High-frequency ultrasonic waves induce vibrations from the crystal, which are transmitted to the surface of the drug solution where droplets break free from the crest of these waves and are released as an aerosol. The size of the droplets produced by an ultrasonic nebulizer is related to the frequency of the oscillation.[32–34] Although ultrasonic nebulizers can nebulize solutions more quickly than jet nebulizers, they are not suitable for suspensions and the piezoelectric crystal may heat the drug to be aerosolized. Vibrating mesh nebulizers are a relatively new form of ultrasonic nebulizer.[6] These nebulizers use electricity to create an aerosol by actively vibrating an aperture plate to pump liquid through funnel-shaped apertures or using an ultrasonic horn to push liquid through an aperture plate.[6] Vibrating mesh nebulizers have a number of advantages over the classic ultrasonic nebulizer systems: they are efficient, quiet, and generally portable. However, they are also significantly more expensive than other types of nebulizers, and require a significant amount of maintenance and cleaning after each use to prevent a buildup of deposits and a blockage of the apertures.[6]

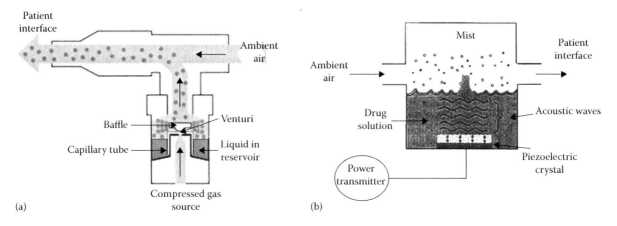

FIGURE 15.4 Schematic illustrations of the components of a jet nebulizer (a) and an ultrasonic nebulizer (b). (From O'Callaghan, C., Barry, P.W. *Thorax*, 52[Suppl. 2], s31–s44, 1997.)

Unlike pMDIs and DPIs, no special inhalation techniques are needed for optimum delivery with nebulizers; tidal breathing with only occasional deep breaths is sufficient. Thus, for patients who are unable to master the proper pMDI technique despite repeated instruction, the proper use of a nebulizer probably improves drug delivery. However, nebulizers have some distinct disadvantages. Patients must load the device with the medication solution for each treatment, and bacterial contamination of the reservoir can cause respiratory infections,[6,32–34] making regular cleaning important. Also, nebulizer treatments take longer than pMDIs and DPIs to administer (10–15 min for a jet nebulizer, 5 min for an ultrasonic or mesh nebulizer). Although they are relatively portable, a typical jet nebulizer must be plugged into a wall outlet or a power adaptor, and thus cannot be used easily in transit. Newer nebulizer designs have enhanced patients' convenience. Ultrasonic and vibrating mesh nebulizers are quieter and more efficient at generating an aerosol[6] and shortening treatment times. In addition, they do not require a compressor, making them lighter in weight, battery powered, and easier to use on the go.

CHOICE OF AN INHALER DEVICE FOR ASTHMA THERAPY

More than 100 inhaled device–drug combinations are currently available for the treatment of asthma patients.[35] The number is likely to increase with the development of generic inhaled drugs delivered by relatively low-cost pMDIs and DPIs. Consequently, the level of confusion experienced by clinicians, nurses, and pharmacists when trying to choose the most appropriate device for each patient is increased. Thus, physicians' experience is among the most important factors that influence decision making in the choice of inhaler in asthma therapy. In fact, inhalers are often prescribed on an empirical basis rather than an evidence-based approach. Following their own experience, doctors are much more likely to prescribe the same old inhaler that they have always prescribed rather than new, improved inhaler devices.

Asthma management guidelines provide guidance for prescribing inhalers to children; however, this is not the case for adult patients. The Global Initiative for Asthma (GINA) guidelines[1] recommend pMDIs with a spacer and a face mask for children younger than 4 years (or pMDIs with a spacer and a mouthpiece for those aged 4–6 years) and, in addition to pMDIs alone, DPIs or BA pMDIs for children older than 6 years. However, for adults, the same guidelines state that inhalers should be portable and simple to use, should not require an external power source, require minimal cooperation and coordination, and have minimal maintenance requirements.[1] The British Thoracic Society guidelines[36] also include the patient's preference and ability to use the device correctly. However, the advice relating to patient preference is not supported by scientific evidence that patients will correctly use their preferred inhaler.

The criteria to be considered when choosing an inhaler device differ depending on the audience being addressed.[37]

From the viewpoint of the respiratory therapist, consistent and safe dosing, sufficient drug deposition, and clinical effect guide the inhaler choice. The patient's ability to inhale through the device, the intrinsic airflow resistance of the device, and the degree of dependence of the drug release on inspiratory airflow variability are all important determinants when considering the constancy of dosing.[37] From the point of view of the clinician, clinical efficacy and safety should take precedence when choosing an inhaler.[37] However, in the real world, clinical efficacy must be balanced against cost effectiveness, and inhalers with an insufficient performance may be prescribed simply because they are cheap. Patients' preferences and acceptance of the inhaler should also be considered when deciding on a specific inhaler, since these will have major implications for compliance.

Several general principles of inhaler selection and use have been reviewed in detail by a joint committee of the American College of Chest Physicians and the American College of Asthma, Allergy and Immunology.[38] These guidelines conclude that pMDIs are convenient for delivering a wide variety of drugs to a broad spectrum of patients. For patients who have trouble coordinating inhalation with inhaler actuation, the use of spacers may obviate this difficulty, though most of these devices are cumbersome to store and transport.[38] The use of a spacer, however, is mandatory for infants and young children. DPIs are usually easier for patients to handle than pMDIs and a growing number of drug types are available in several DPI formats.[38] The key issue for dry powder inhalation is the minimum inspiratory flow rate below which deagglomeration is inefficient, resulting in a reduced drug delivered dose. The most ill patients and the very young may not be candidates for a DPI. A nebulizer could be used as an adequate alternative to a pMDI with a spacer by almost any patient in a variety of clinical settings from the home to the intensive care unit. However, nebulizers are more expensive, cumbersome, and relatively time consuming to use compared with handheld inhalers. These attributes should limit the use of nebulizers whose effect can be matched by handheld devices in almost all clinical settings.

Recently, Chapman and coworkers[39] proposed an algorithm approach to inhaler selection that considers the patient's ability to generate an inspiratory flow rate >30 L/min, to coordinate inhaler actuation and inspiration, and to prepare and actuate the device (Table 15.2).

When choosing an inhaler for children, it is essential that the individual child receives the appropriate instructions and training necessary for the management of the disease.[40] Furthermore, the child should be prescribed the correct medication tailored to the severity of their disease and, most importantly, the prescribed inhaler should suit the individual needs and preference of the child.[40] Contrary to general opinion, using an inhaler may be difficult for children[40]; many children with asthma use their inhaler incorrectly, which may result in unreliable drug delivery, even after instruction and training for correct inhalation. In addition, previous inhalation instruction may be forgotten; therefore, training

TABLE 15.2

Suitability of Inhaler Devices According to the Patient's Inspiratory Flow Rate and Ability to Coordinate Inhaler Actuation and Inhalation

Good Hand–Lung Coordination		Poor Hand–Lung Coordination	
Inspiratory Flow >30 L/min	Inspiratory Flow <30 L/min	Inspiratory Flow >30 L/min	Inspiratory Flow <30 L/min
pMDI	pMDI	pMDI + spacer	pMDI + spacer
BA pMDI	Nebulizer	BA pMDI	Nebulizer
DPI	SMI	DPI	SMI
Nebulizer		Nebulizer	
SMI		SMI	

Source: Modified from Chapman, K.R., Voshaar, T.H., Virchow, J.C., *Eur. Respir. Rev.,* 14, 117–122, 2005.

Note: pMDI, pressurized metered-dose inhalers; BA pMDI, breath-actuated metered-dose inhaler; DPI, dry powder inhaler; SMI, soft mist inhaler.

should be repeated regularly to maintain the correct inhalation technique in children with asthma.[40]

ADMIT RECOMMENDATIONS

Many physicians in Europe are fully aware of the difficulties that patients have using prescribed inhaler devices correctly and the negative impact that this may have on asthma control. ADMIT,[35] a consortium of European respiratory physicians with a common interest in promoting the excellent delivery of inhaled drugs, was formed with the goal to examine ways of improving the treatment of asthma and chronic obstructive pulmonary disease in Europe, with specific reference to inhalers. ADMIT has made a number of recommendations related to the delivery instructions for a correct inhalation technique for each inhaler device. These evidence-based recommendations are summarized in Table 15.3.

ADMIT[35] has also proposed a practical algorithm in order to improve the instruction given to patients regarding the optimal use of their inhalers (Figure 15.5). At each consultation, the physician should establish the patient's current level of symptoms and control, ideally using a composite measure such as the GINA control assessment or the Asthma Control Test,[1] and if the patient's asthma is well controlled for at least 3 months, therapy should be stepped down gradually according to the treatment guidelines. Conversely, if the patient answers "no" to any of these checklist questions, then compliance and aggravating (trigger) factors should be assessed. Most importantly, the patient's inhalation technique should be assessed. If the patient is unable to use a particular inhaler correctly despite repeated attempts, a change in inhaler device should be considered. In the cases where ongoing, uncontrolled asthma persists in the face of a correct inhaler technique, then asthma therapy should be stepped up according to the treatment guidelines and another appointment scheduled in order to recheck the symptoms.

TABLE 15.3

Recommendations from ADMIT for Inhaler Choice and Correct Inhalation Technique

- Inhalers should be matched to the patient as much as possible.
- In young children, if pMDIs are prescribed, they should be used with a spacer device.
- An alternative to a pMDI should be considered in elderly patients with a mini-mental test score <23/30 or an ideomotor dyspraxia score <14/20, as they are unlikely to have a correct inhalation technique through a pMDI.
- The patient's PIF values should be considered before prescribing a DPI. Those patients with severe airflow obstruction, children, and the elderly would benefit from an inhaler device with a low airflow resistance.
- Before prescribing a DPI, check that the patient can inhale deeply and forcibly at the start of the inhalation maneuver because the airflow profile affects the particle size produced and hence drug deposition and efficacy.
- Where possible, one patient should have one type of inhaler.
- Establish an official board to compile instructions for the correct inhalation technique for each inhaler device currently on the market.
- Instructions for correct inhaler use should be made readily accessible on a dedicated website.
- Training in the correct inhalation technique is essential for patients and health-care professionals.
- Inhalation techniques should be checked and reinforced at regular intervals.
- Teaching correct inhalation techniques should be tailored to the patient's needs and preferences: group instruction in correct inhalation techniques appears to be more effective than personal one-to-one instruction and equally as effective as video instruction; younger patients may benefit more from multimedia teaching methods; elderly patients respond well to one-to-one tuition.

Source: Modified from Crompton, G.K., Barnes, P.J., Broeders, M., et al., *Respir. Med.,* 100, 1479–1494, 2006.

Note: DPI, dry powder inhaler; PIF, peak inspiratory flow; pMDI, pressurized metered-dose inhaler.

CONCLUSIONS

The prevalence of asthma continues to rise throughout the world, particularly among children. Despite the publication of both national and international guidelines and the widespread availability of effective pharmacological therapy, asthma is frequently uncontrolled, and still causes death. There are a number of reasons for this anomalous situation. First, the guidelines are complex and too long for most physicians to absorb and implement. Second, patients frequently do not adhere to their treatment regimen for a variety of reasons including incorrect use of their inhaler and underestimation of the severity of their disease. In addition, asthma severity is often misclassified, leading to inappropriate or insufficient prescribed therapy. Finally, although the guidelines agree on the most appropriate therapy to control asthma, the method by which this therapy is delivered to the lungs often lacks sufficient detail.

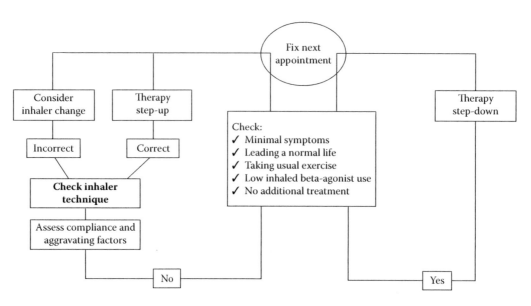

FIGURE 15.5 Asthma therapy adjustment flow chart. (Reprinted from Crompton, G.K., Barnes, P.J., Broeders, M., et al. *Respir. Med.*, 100, 1479–1494, 2006.)

To date, the advancement in asthma management has been pharmacologically driven rather than device driven. Since it is likely that inhaled bronchodilators and corticosteroids will remain the cornerstone of asthma therapy, the development of inhaler devices may become more important than the development of new drugs. In the past 10–15 years, several innovative developments have advanced the field of inhaler design. There are many choices in all device categories that incorporate features providing efficient aerosol delivery to treat obstructive airway diseases. The problems with drug delivery have been identified due to the inappropriate use of inhaler devices, particularly pMDIs where patients need to coordinate inhaler activation with inspiration. There is clearly a need to develop inhaler devices that are easy to use and capable of delivering consistent doses of drugs to the lungs, which may in turn improve patient compliance with treatment, leading to better asthma control.

The continued and repeated education of both health-care professionals and patients regarding the correct inhalation technique is essential, with reassessment at regular intervals. Substantial changes in educational efforts are clearly required and should be particularly addressed toward the general practitioner and the asthma nurse who are usually charged with teaching patients how to use their inhaler correctly. Finally, it is important to remember that continually changing inhaler devices that deliver the same drug is not the answer, as patients lose confidence in both the device and the drug, and compliance with therapy drops. An inhaler should only be prescribed with the absolute certainty that the patient can use it correctly.

REFERENCES

1. Global Initiative for Asthma. Global strategy for asthma management and prevention. http://www.ginaasthma.com. Updated Dec 2007.

2. Rabe K, Vermeire P, Soriano J, Maier W. Clinical management of asthma in 1999: The Asthma Insights and Reality in Europe (AIRE) study. *Eur Respir J* 2000;16:802–807.

3. Gruffydd-Jones K. Measuring pulmonary function in practice. *Practitioner* 2002;246:445–449.

4. Barnes PJ, Jonsson B, Klim JB. The costs of asthma. *Eur Respir J* 1996;9:636–642.

5. Crompton GK, Barnes PJ, Broeders M, et al. The need to improve inhalation technique in Europe: A report from the Aerosol Drug Management Improvement Team. *Respir Med* 2006;100:1479–1494.

6. Laube BL, Janssens HM, de Jongh FHC, et al. What the pulmonary specialist should know about the new inhalation therapies. *Eur Respir J* 2011;37:1308–1331.

7. Lenny J, Innes J, Crompton G. Inappropriate inhaler use: Assessment of use and patient preference of seven inhalation devices. *Respir Med* 2000;94:496–500.

8. Lavorini F, Corrigan CJ, Barnes PJ, et al. Retail sales of inhalation devices in European countries: So much for a global policy. *Respir Med* 2011;98:1099–1013.

9. Hendeles L, Colice GL, Meyer RJ. Withdrawal of albuterol inhalers containing chlorofluorocarbon propellants. *N Engl J Med* 2007;356:1344–1351.

10. Ganderton D, Lewis D, Davies R, et al. Modulite: A means of designing the aerosols generated by pressurized metered dose inhalers. *Respir Med* 2002;96(Suppl. D):S3–S8.

11. Leach CL. The CFC to HFA transition and its impact on pulmonary drug development. *Respir Care* 2005;50:1201–1208.

12. Newman SP, Pavia D, Clarke SW. How should a pressurized beta-adrenergic bronchodilator be inhaled? *Eur J Respir Dis* 1981;62:3–21.

13. Crompton GK. How to achieve good compliance with inhaled asthma therapy. *Respir Med* 2004;98(Suppl. B):S35–S40.

14. Crompton GK, The adult patient's difficulties with inhalers. *Lung* 1990;168(Suppl.):658–662.

15. Giraud V, Roche N. Misuse of corticosteroid metered-dose inhaler is associated with decreased asthma stability. *Eur Respir J* 2002;19:246–251.

16. Lavorini F, Fontana GA. Targeting drugs to the airways: The role of spacer devices. *Expert Opin Drug Deliv* 2009;6:91–102.

17. Fontana GA, Lavorini F, Chiostri M, et al. Large and small airway responses to procaterol hydrochloride administered through different extension devices in asthmatic patients. *J Aerosol Med* 1999;12:177–185.

18. Lavorini F, Geri P, Luperini M, et al. Clinical and functional responses to salbutamol inhaled via different devices in asthmatic patients with induced bronchoconstriction. *Brit J Clin Pharmacol* 2004;58:512–520.

19. Lavorini F, Geri P, Mariani L, et al. Speed of onset of bronchodilator response to salbutamol inhaled via different devices in asthmatics. A bioassay based on functional antagonism *Brit J Clin Pharmacol* 2006;62:403–411.

20. Lavorini F, Geri P, Camiciottoli G, Pistolesi M, Fontana GA. Agreement between two methods for assessing bioequivalence *Pulm Pharmacol Ther* 2008;21:380–384.

21. Crompton G, Duncan J. Clinical assessment of a new breath-actuated inhaler. *Pratictioner* 1989; 233:268–269.

22. Gross G, Cohen RM, Guy H. Efficacy response of inhaled HFA–albuterol delivered via the breath-actuated autohaler inhalation device is comparable to dose in patients with asthma. *J Asthma* 2003;40:487–495.

23. Price D, Thomas M, Mitchell G, et al. Improvement of asthma control with a breath-actuated pressurised metered dose inhaler (BAI): A prescribing claims study of 5556 patients using a traditional pressurised metered dose inhaler (MDI) or a breath-actuated device. *Respir Med* 2003;97:12–19.

24. Newman SP, Busse WW. Evolution of dry powder inhaler design, formulation, and performance. *Respir Med* 2002;96:293–304.

25. Islam N, Gladki E. Dry powder inhalers (DPIs): A review of device reliability and innovation. *Int J Pharm* 2008;360:1–11.

26. Atkins PJ. Dry powder inhalers: An overview. *Respir Care* 2005;50:1304–1312.

27. Azouza W, Chrystyn H. Clarifying the dilemmas about inhalation techniques for dry powder inhalers: Integrating science with clinical practice. *Prim Care Respir J* 2012;21:208–213.

28. Janssens W, VandenBrande P, Hardeman E, et al. Inspiratory flow rates at different levels of resistance in elderly COPD patients. *Eur Respir J* 2008;31:78–83.

29. Lavorini F, Magnan A, Dubus JC, et al. Effect of incorrect use of dry powder inhalers on management of patients with asthma and COPD. *Respir Med* 2008;102:593–604.

30. Dalby R, Spallek M, Voshaar T. A review of the development of Respimat Soft Mist Inhaler. *Int J Pharm* 2004;283:1–9.

31. Kassner F, Hodder R, Bateman ED. A review of ipratropium bromide/fenoterol hydrobromide (Berodual) delivered via Respimat Soft Mist Inhaler in patients with asthma and chronic obstructive pulmonary disease. *Drugs* 2004;64:1671–1682.

32. O'Callaghan C, Barry PW. The science of nebulised drug delivery. *Thorax* 1997;52(Suppl. 2):S31–S44.

33. Hess DR. Nebulizers: Principles and performance. *Respir Care* 2000;45:609–622.

34. Boe J, Dennis JH, O'Driscoll BR, et al. European Respiratory Society Guidelines on the use of nebulizers. *Eur Respir J* 2001;18:228–242.

35. Aerosol Drug Management Improvement Team (ADMIT). www.admit-online.info.

36. British Thoracic Society Scottish Intercollegiate Guidelines Network. British Guideline on the Management of Asthma. *Thorax.* 2008;63:1–121.

37. Virchow JC. What plays a role in the choice of inhaler device for asthma therapy? *Curr Med Res Opin* 2005;21(Suppl.):s19–s25.

38. Dolovich MB, Ahrens RC, Hess DR, et al. Device selection and outcomes of aerosol therapy: Evidence-based guidelines: American College of Chest Physicians/American College of Asthma, Allergy and Immunology. *Chest* 2005;127:335–371.

39. Chapman KR, Voshaar TH, Virchow JC. Inhaler choice in primary care. *Eur Respir Rev* 2005;14:117–122.

40. Brand PLP. Key issues in inhalation therapy in children. *Curr Med Res Opin* 2005;21(Suppl.):s27–s32.

16 Assessment of Asthma Control in Adults

Claude S. Farah and Helen K. Reddel

CONTENTS

CASE PRESENTATION

A 28-year-old female requests a repeat prescription for her asthma inhaler during a consultation for a simple upper respiratory tract infection. She describes having asthma since childhood and had several hospitalizations while growing up. Her last presentation to the emergency department was 6 months ago. She states that her symptoms became less intense as an adult and she considers her asthma well controlled. She experiences chest tightness most mornings, but her symptoms resolve following inhalation of a short-acting bronchodilator.

She does not experience frequent daytime chest tightness or breathlessness. Although she has been prescribed a combination inhaler of inhaled corticosteroids (ICS) and a long-acting beta-agonist (LABA), she rarely uses it unless her symptoms worsen despite frequent short-acting bronchodilators. She also finds that her voice quality changes if she uses the combination inhaler regularly for a week. The triggers for her asthma include a change of weather, respiratory infections, and exercise. She works at a busy stock brokerage firm as a clerical assistant and finds it difficult to allocate time for any exercise. Her weight has gradually increased over the last 5 years and her body mass index (BMI) is currently 31 kg/m². She smokes cigarettes socially mostly on weekends and usually less than five a day. Her chest examination does not reveal any focal signs. Her peak flow is 358 L/min (87% predicted). Her spirometry parameters are a forced expiratory volume in 1 sec (FEV₁) of 1.63 L (54% predicted), a forced vital capacity (FVC) of 2.85 L (82% predicted), and a FEV₁/FVC ratio of 57%. Her FEV₁ improved to 1.89 L following inhalation of a short-acting bronchodilator representing a 16% and 260 mL improvement.

INTRODUCTION

This case is not an uncommon presentation of someone with asthma in primary care. It highlights a number of pertinent issues regarding the assessment of asthma control. Importantly, the patient perceives her condition as well controlled despite frequent symptoms and the need for daily reliever medication, which from a medical perspective are features of poorly controlled asthma. Furthermore, the patient is not taking a regular preventer medication, she has suffered from a recent exacerbation, has low lung function, and is a smoker, all of which lead to an increased likelihood of future exacerbations. This future risk is another important component of the assessment of the patient's asthma control. Finally, there are other issues that will also need to be addressed as part of the assessment of her asthma control, including her increasing weight and her sedentary lifestyle. Obese patients with asthma may experience suboptimal control of their symptoms despite improvements in their spirometry and airway inflammation.

WHAT IS ASTHMA AND ASTHMA CONTROL? REVIEWING THE DEFINITION

DEFINITION OF ASTHMA

Asthma is defined as a chronic inflammatory disorder associated with physiological abnormalities in the airways, namely, variable airflow limitation and airway hyperresponsiveness (AHR).[1] The physiological perturbations in the airways are associated with the variable symptoms of breathlessness, chest tightness, wheeze, or cough. At times, these symptoms may be mild or even absent. On the other hand, symptoms may worsen acutely or subacutely leading to an asthmatic flare-up or exacerbation.

WHAT IS ASTHMA CONTROL?

Asthma control is defined as the extent to which the effects of the disease are reduced or removed by treatment.[2] Asthma that is well controlled is characterized by infrequent daytime symptoms, no activity limitation, no nocturnal symptoms, and normal lung function (Table 16.1). It is important

TABLE 16.1
Levels of Asthma Control in Adults and Children over 5 Years

A. Assessment of Current Clinical Control (Preferably over 4 weeks)

Characteristic	Controlled (All of the Following)	Partly Controlled (Any Measure Present)	Uncontrolled
Daytime symptoms	None (twice or less/week)	More than twice/week	Three or more features of partly controlled asthma[a,b]
Limitation of activities	None	Any	
Nocturnal symptoms/ awakening	None	Any	
Need for reliever/rescue treatment	None (twice or less/week)	More than twice/week	
Lung function (PEF or FEV₁)[c]	Normal	<80% predicted or personal best (if known)	

B. Assessment of Future Risk (Risk of Exacerbations, Instability, Rapid Decline in Lung Function, Side Effects)

Features that are associated with an increased risk of adverse events in the future include: poor clinical control, frequent exacerbations in the past year,[a] ever admitted to critical care for asthma, low FEV₁, exposure to cigarette smoke, and high-dose medications

Source: Global Strategy for Asthma Management and Prevention, Global Initiative for Asthma (GINA) Report: Global strategy for asthma management and prevention, 2011, http://www.ginasthma.org.

Note: The GINA Report is currently undergoing review and is due for publication in 2014. Refer to the website for the latest guidelines, http://www.ginasthma.org.

[a] Any exacerbation should prompt a review of the maintenance treatment to ensure that it is adequate.

[b] By definition, an exacerbation in any week makes that an uncontrolled asthma week.

[c] Without the administration of a bronchodilator.

to recognize that some patients can achieve this state with relatively low doses of ICS, while others may require more intense therapy. Since the disease is inherently variable over time, an assessment of asthma control should address both the current state of a person's asthma as well as accounting for the risk of problems in the future. Hence, the terms *current control* and *future risk* have been advocated.[2,3]

The concept of future risk is intended to highlight the potential limitations of focusing solely on current symptoms, which would fail to address the known factors that affect the clinical course of this disease over time. Future risk refers to the risk of adverse outcomes in the future, including exacerbations, the risk of accelerated lung function decline, or even the risk of side effects from medications. Poorly controlled asthma is a known risk factor for future exacerbations. In particular, nighttime symptoms and more frequent short-acting beta-agonist (SABA) use are strongly associated with an increased risk for a future exacerbation.[4] However, other risk factors for adverse outcomes, independent of the patient's level of current control, have also been identified. Asthma exacerbations can be triggered by a number of factors, including allergens, pollution, and infections. Viral infections account for most asthma exacerbations in adults,[5] which is reflected by a peak in the hospitalization rate every winter.[6] Furthermore, a recent exacerbation is a risk factor for future exacerbations, highlighting the complex interaction of future events and their relationship to airway function in the past. The relationship between current control and future exacerbations is another reason why an assessment of asthma control should be conducted at every clinical encounter.

The current emphasis on asthma control in clinical management differs from the earlier emphasis on asthma severity. Asthma severity was previously defined in terms of its clinical features *before* any treatment; this was thought to reflect the intrinsic qualities of the disease.[2] However, this definition was impractical once patients started regular treatment.

WHY IS AN ASSESSMENT OF ASTHMA CONTROL IMPORTANT?

TO UNDERSTAND THE IMPACT OF ASTHMA ON THE PATIENT

The assessment of asthma control should identify the frequency and/or intensity of asthma-related symptoms. Through this process, the clinician is able to appreciate the effect of asthma on the individual patient and how it may be impacting on his or her quality of life.

TO PREDICT THE RISK OF FUTURE ADVERSE OUTCOMES

As mentioned previously, poor asthma control is a risk factor for future exacerbations. Furthermore, other risk factors for future exacerbations as well as the risk for accelerated lung function decline or medication side effects should be identified at the time of the assessment. These future events are

clinically important since they can cause significant morbidity to the patient and impart a significant health burden to the community.

TO GUIDE TREATMENT AND MONITOR TREATMENT RESPONSE

Guidelines recommend an assessment of asthma control to guide therapy.[1] Specifically, patients with poorly controlled asthma should have their treatment increased but only after addressing other contributing factors such as adherence and device technique. On the other hand, patients with well-controlled asthma should have their ICS treatment down-titrated. Hence, the assessment of asthma control is integral to the management decisions made during follow-up.

TO FACILITATE PATIENT–DOCTOR COMMUNICATION ABOUT ASTHMA MANAGEMENT

During the process of assessing asthma control, the clinician is able to identify issues that may be contributing to suboptimal control. Categorizing the patient's level of asthma control may be used as a means of educating the patient about the disease and establishing treatment aims. A comprehensive assessment of asthma control addressing symptom frequency, lung function, and risk factors allows the clinician to tailor treatment type and dose to the individual patient.

HOW CAN WE MEASURE ASTHMA CONTROL?

Since the publication of the first asthma guidelines, the goals of treatment have been described in terms of controlling symptoms; reliever use; and avoiding activity limitation, exacerbations, and side effects. The concepts of asthma control have thus been accepted by consensus for many years, although there is no gold standard for measuring asthma control.

The measurement of current control should include an assessment of symptoms as well as some measure of lung function. Inevitably, there is a subjective component to asthma control and it can be regarded as a patient-centered outcome in asthma. Although asthma symptoms relate to lung function abnormalities, these correlations are weak. This is partly due to the lack of specificity of asthma symptoms. However, it is unlikely that a single physiological parameter will adequately reflect asthma control in its entirety. Ultimately, a multimodal assessment is advocated, one that measures some aspect of airway function as well as the measurement of more subjective parameters such as patient-reported symptoms.

When a discrepancy is found between symptoms and objective lung function, this should prompt the consideration of alternative or additional diagnoses; for example, in patients with frequent symptoms but normal lung function, the symptoms may be found to be due to a comorbidity such as vocal cord dysfunction (VCD) or obesity; and in patients with few symptoms but abnormal lung function, chronic obstructive pulmonary disease (COPD) may coexist, or they may have a poor perception of airway obstruction. In instances where such a discrepancy does exist, the choice of medication and dose should be guided by the abnormality or abnormalities that are identified, rather than simply increasing the treatment when the symptoms remain uncontrolled. Such patients should be referred for further investigation.

CLASSIFYING ASTHMA CONTROL: POORLY CONTROLLED, PARTLY CONTROLLED, WELL CONTROLLED

Categorizing a patient's level of asthma control can be useful to facilitate communication between clinicians, for educating the patient as well as for use in research. In general, three categories of asthma control have been used in the guidelines (Table 16.1). However, the degree of asthma control should be viewed as a continuum along a spectrum. Different guidelines have used different terminology to categorize the degree of control. Commonly used terms are *controlled*, *partly controlled*, and *poorly controlled*, as recommended by the Global Initiative for Asthma (GINA). Some have used the terms *totally controlled*, *well controlled*, and *uncontrolled*, whereas others prefer terms such as *optimal* and *suboptimal control*. The GINA controlled/partly controlled categories together correspond to a score of <1.0 on the five-item Asthma Control Questionnaire (ACQ-5).[7] A numeric score, however, may be more responsive to a change in the level of control over time.[7]

SYMPTOMS

It is recognized that the assessment of asthma control in primary care is predominantly based on asthma symptoms. To help facilitate this, a checklist of the relevant symptoms may be useful (Table 16.2). The frequency of asthma symptoms can be assessed over the preceding week or month, but the same time period should be used in follow-up for comparison. The triggers for patient symptoms, such as allergens, pollution, exercise, and respiratory tract infections, should also be ascertained.

Asthma symptoms can be difficult to distinguish from other respiratory causes. The British Guideline on the

---

TABLE 16.2

The Royal College of Physicians "Three Question" Screening Tool

In the Last Week or Month ...	Yes	No
1. Have you had difficulty sleeping because of your asthma symptoms (including cough)?		
2. Have you had your usual asthma symptoms during the day (cough, wheeze, chest tightness, or breathlessness)?		
3. Has your asthma interfered with your usual activities (e.g., housework, work, or school)?		

Management of Asthma[8] provides a useful summary of the features that make the diagnosis of asthma more or less likely. It should also be emphasized that not all respiratory symptoms reported by a patient with asthma are due to asthma itself (see the section "Who Benefits from Regular Assessment?"). Hence, an overreliance on symptoms for the assessment of asthma control could potentially lead to overtreatment. On the other hand, symptoms may be underreported by those with a sedentary lifestyle since exercise-induced bronchoconstriction leading to symptoms occurs less frequently in these individuals. Finally, symptom perception is heterogeneous and is affected by airway inflammation and ICS treatment.[9]

Symptoms can be recorded either prospectively in patient diaries or retrospectively by patient recall. The latter is most commonly employed in clinical practice. Symptoms are often recorded along a severity scale. On the other hand, documenting specific numeric variables such as the "number of days per week with symptoms" or "number of stairs that may be climbed without stopping" is often useful for comparison at follow-up visits.

The variability of the disease is important when assessing symptoms at any time point. Such an assessment must account for the change in symptoms from week to week. Hence, an assessment of control over shorter time periods may overestimate the degree of asthma control. For example, patients with daily symptoms and poorly controlled asthma at recruitment into a 3-month study who received as-needed SABA alone had a well-controlled asthma week on average every 4 weeks during the study.[10]

NIGHT WAKING DUE TO ASTHMA

Asthma symptoms tend to follow a diurnal pattern. In particular, symptoms at night or in the early morning are an indication that asthma may be suboptimally controlled. The The development of nighttime asthma symptoms may herald the onset of an exacerbation and should prompt a review of asthma management with appropriate follow-up.

Other conditions may also cause respiratory symptoms at night. Patients with cardiac disease may be woken up with breathlessness that slowly abates over several minutes by sitting upright and, in some cases, using sublingual nitrates. Patients with obstructive sleep apnea (OSA) may wake up with a choking sensation but this tends to resolve within seconds unless there is a superimposed anxiety component. Nocturnal cough should also prompt an investigation for gastroesophageal reflux disease (GERD).

SABA USE

The frequent use of SABA is another marker of poor asthma control. Traditionally, it is assumed that frequent symptoms lead to frequent reliever medication use behavior. However, the frequent inhalation of SABA can be associated with tachyphylaxis as well as airway reactivity and airway inflammation, and may, in fact, lead to frequent symptoms; that is, the frequent use of SABA may not only be a marker of poor asthma control but may also be a cause of poor asthma control.[11] Hence, the habitual overuse of SABA should be discouraged. On the other hand, SABA use is still advocated for the short-term relief of bronchospasm, and it may be lifesaving in acute severe asthma. Making such a distinction can be difficult for both the patient and the clinician.

The clues that suggest the inappropriate overuse of SABA include normal lung function during symptoms or despite frequent symptoms, the lack of an acute bronchodilator improvement on spirometry, and a decrease in the duration of the perceived effectiveness of SABA. The use of peak flow monitoring may help some subjects distinguish symptoms that are not related to asthma. The corollary, however, does not hold since peak flow readings can be reduced due to several factors including poor effort, inadequate inspiration, or upper airway pathology. The frequency of the symptoms and the need for reliever medication are also influenced by the concurrent use of LABA.

ACTIVITY LIMITATION

An appreciation of the impact of asthma on daily activity is also important when assessing asthma control. Patients with asthma should be encouraged to engage in all aspects of physical activity. However, some patients avoid activity due to uncontrolled asthma, while others may report minimal limitation due to a sedentary lifestyle. Comorbidities such as lack of fitness and obesity may also impact on the extent of physical activity and the intensity of the symptoms experienced.

Exercise-induced breathlessness is commonly reported, and the contribution of asthma in this context may be difficult to determine. However, exercise-induced bronchoconstriction typically starts after 5–8 min of exercise and may worsen after the cessation of exercise; it is particularly responsive to pretreatment with SABAs, and is substantially reduced by maintenance ICS treatment.

In some instances, exercise-based complex lung function testing may help clarify the underlying mechanism for the patient symptoms.[12] In older patients or those with cardiac risk factors, a stress exercise test may also be needed to exclude a cardiac cause for exercise-induced breathlessness and provide reassurance to the clinician and patient that the patient can exercise safely in the community.

COMPOSITE ASTHMA CONTROL SCORES

The composite "scores" of asthma control using validated patient questionnaires with or without lung function measurement have been widely used in research and may be used in a clinical setting.[13,14] These questionnaires refer to patient symptom frequency and/or intensity over the preceding 1–4 weeks. These tools have several advantages including ease of use; they can be completed by the patient; and they provide a standardized means of assessing asthma control from visit to visit (Table 16.3).

TABLE 16.3
Composite Tools to Assess Asthma Control

	Description	Duration of Scoring Period (Week)	Scoring
Asthma Control Questionnaire (ACQ)	Seven, six, or five items comprising: 1. Symptom frequency or severity (five items) 2. Reliever use 3. Percentage of FEV_1 predicted	1	Score range 0–6 Optimal cut point for well-controlled <0.75 and for poorly controlled > 1.5
Asthma Control Test (ACT)	Five items comprising: 1. Symptom frequency (four items) 2. Patient global assessment of asthma control	4	Score range 5–25 Optimal cut point for well-controlled ≥20 and for poorly controlled <15
Asthma Treatment Assessment Questionnaire (ATAQ)	Four domains comprising: 1. Self-perception 2. Impact 3. Symptoms 4. Reliever use	4	Score range 0 (complete control) to 4 (poor control)
Asthma Control Scoring System (ACSS)	Three components comprising: 1. Symptoms/reliever use 2. Percentage of FEV predicted 3. Inflammation	1	Score range 0% (poor control)–100% (optimal control). Final score is based on an average of the three individual components.

The ACQ is one of the most frequently used tools to measure asthma control in research and it has also been used in clinical practice.[13] This seven-item questionnaire includes five questions about symptoms in the previous week, one about rescue bronchodilator use, and one about prebronchodilator FEV_1. The ACQ is sensitive to within-patient changes and correlates well with other patient-related health measures, such as the Asthma Quality of Life Questionnaire. The symptom-only five-item ACQ (ACQ-5) correlates very closely to the full-length ACQ and has been commonly used in patients taking regular ICS/LABA, since prebronchodilator FEV_1 is not usually available.[15,16] While this could be viewed as evidence that both versions are measuring the same construct, it is more likely a consequence of mathematical averaging since FEV_1 contributes proportionally less to the overall ACQ score than the five symptom items.[17] A change in the ACQ score of 0.5 is considered clinically important.[16]

The Asthma Control Test (ACT) is another commonly used questionnaire for the assessment of asthma control. The ACT is administered by the patient and is composed of five items; four relate to the clinical features of asthma and the fifth is a global self-assessment of asthma control.[14] In contrast to the ACQ, the ACT measures symptoms over the preceding 4 weeks and does not include a physiological measurement, with the authors retaining this as an independent component of the asthma control assessment. The ACT has also been validated in research and in clinical practice. A change in the ACT score of 3 is considered clinically important.[18]

The Royal College of Physicians (RCP) has published a brief three-question screening tool to assess asthma control (RCP "3 questions") in people over the age of 16 (Table 16.2).[8] The questions can be applied to either the last week or the last month (but, again, the same time period should be consistently used so that comparisons can be made over time and between patients). This tool is feasible for use in primary care and can identify patients who need more thorough assessment of their symptoms.[19]

One pragmatic approach in the assessment of asthma control is to measure the ACQ-5 or ACT, as a measure of symptom control, and separately consider FEV_1 as a measure that provides independent information relevant to asthma control.

PATIENT-PERCEIVED ASTHMA CONTROL

Clinical surveys often report that patients underestimate their level of poor control.[20] However, a patient's understanding of the term *asthma control* may be at odds with the medical meaning of the term. Patients might consider their disease well controlled if their symptoms are rapidly relieved (or controlled) by a SABA. This discrepancy between the patients' perception and the clinicians' approach suggests that education efforts need to continue to improve patient outcome. An important limitation in the care of someone with asthma is the low attendance rate for

follow-up. It is possible that patients might return for clinical review more consistently if there was an expectation on the part of the patients that their lung function would be routinely measured in addition to receiving a clinical examination and an assessment of their symptom control. In doing so, the numeric feedback from measuring one's lung function, something akin to measuring the blood pressure, serves as an incentive for the patient to return for review again.

SIMPLE LUNG FUNCTION TESTING

Measuring lung function is essential for the diagnosis as well as the ongoing monitoring of asthma.

LIMITATIONS OF PEAK FLOW METERS

Peak flow devices are commonly used in primary care but they have significant limitations. The devices are not calibrated and readings may differ on different devices. A single peak expiratory flow (PEF) measurement is neither sensitive nor specific for a diagnosis of asthma.

The serial measurement of PEF readings over time may indicate a significant diurnal variability and this may be sufficient to confirm a diagnosis of asthma in patients with typical asthma symptoms.[1] Similarly, in a patient with a confirmed diagnosis of asthma, serial peak flow recordings performed on the same device by the same patient may provide very useful information about the trend over time. For example, a peak flow trend may provide a clue about occupational or recreational exposures. On the other hand, the presence of increased diurnal variability would be consistent with suboptimal control.[21] Furthermore, a downward trend in the peak flow readings may herald the onset of an exacerbation.

The most common method of calculating *within-day* variability (diurnal variability) is amplitude percent mean (day's highest minus lowest/mean), averaged over 7 days; the upper limit of normal with twice-daily PEF readings is 8%. A common method of calculating *between-day* PEF variability is the lowest PEF (or lowest morning PEF) over 1 or 2 weeks, divided by the highest PEF.[2] There is a moderate relationship between diurnal variability and AHR.

SPIROMETRY SHOULD BE MEASURED WHEN ASSESSING ASTHMA CONTROL

Spirometry is a reliable and standardized test of airway function. It measures flow and volume and predominantly reflects the physiology of the larger, more central airways. The main parameters measured are FEV_1, FVC, the spirometric ratio FEV_1/FVC, and, if performed before and after the inhalation of a short-acting bronchodilator, the amount of acute bronchodilator reversibility measured as the change in FEV_1 or FVC. There are several well-calibrated, handheld spirometry devices.

Guidelines exist for the performance of the test and acceptability criteria in primary care,[22] and for safety considerations.[23] However, the maneuver is effort dependent and some patients are unable to perform the test adequately. Hence, caution is needed when interpreting the results from a test that does not meet the acceptability criteria.

Although basic interpretative strategies can easily be learned, confidence in the interpretation of spirometry remains poor among primary care providers. In general terms, a reduced FEV_1/FVC ratio indicates airway obstruction and the FEV_1 declines with the worsening severity of the disease. The presence of significant reversibility (>200 mL improvement *and* >12% improvement in either FEV_1 or FVC) on spirometry in a patient established on ICS might be an indication of suboptimal treatment. FEV_1 improves within 2 months of treatment with ICS, whereas AHR continues to improve beyond 1 year of continuous anti-inflammatory treatment.[24]

A single spirometry measurement correlates only weakly with patient symptoms,[25] but low lung function has been consistently found to be an independent predictor of the risk of exacerbations,[26] and discordance between spirometry and symptoms may prompt the consideration of alternative or additional diagnoses that are contributing to the symptoms. Hence, the combination of a spirometry measurement and the patient's symptom profile provides a more comprehensive assessment of the disease status. Respiratory symptoms may also persist despite normal spirometry and in these cases referral for further lung function tests and specialist input would be indicated.

In a patient with asthma, spirometry should be performed to confirm the diagnosis, and then, if possible, it should be repeated 3–6 months after the commencement of regular treatment to document the patient's best lung function. Subsequently, spirometry should ideally be repeated once a year so that an accelerated lung function decline can be identified, or if worsening asthma symptoms fail to respond to a step-up in treatment.

WHO BENEFITS FROM REGULAR ASSESSMENT?

Everyone with asthma should be reviewed regularly. At the first clinical encounter, the diagnosis should be confirmed. If there is doubt about the diagnosis, the patient should be referred for a second opinion and further testing to ascertain the nature of the lung abnormality. Such an approach should reduce the risk of misdiagnosis, incorrect treatment, and an incorrect label of "severe" or "refractory" disease if the symptoms are not due to asthma itself. At each subsequent visit, an assessment of asthma control allows the clinician to review the treatment prescribed and adjust the dose of medication as appropriate. In this way, over- and undertreatment can be avoided.

It is suggested that asthma control be assessed at least annually and ideally twice per year, in all patients with asthma. Asthma control should also be reviewed 1–3 months after any change in treatment (step-up or step-down) or if worsening symptoms develop at any time. Patients with severe and difficult-to-treat asthma should be reviewed every 2–3 months. Spirometry should at least be measured at diagnosis and then annually in clinically stable patients.

ASTHMA CONTROL IN SPECIAL POPULATIONS

Some patients are more likely to have suboptimally controlled asthma and may benefit from a more frequent or intense review.

RHINOSINUSITIS

Asthma and rhinitis often coexist. Patients with untreated rhinosinusitis report more frequent symptoms, and treatment of their upper airway disease may improve their asthma control.[27]

ELDERLY

Elderly patients with asthma are also more likely to live with poorly controlled disease.[28] The exact reasons may be multifactorial and include inadequate education, poor inhaler use, the effects of aging on the physiology of the lung and the airways, and the lack of fitness. It is also possible that perception may be altered in the elderly.

OBESITY

Obesity is an increasingly common problem, which has been associated with increased asthma prevalence[29] and worse asthma control.[30] Importantly, an effect on asthma control is seen even in the "overweight" range (BMI 25–30 kg/m^2). An appreciation of the physiological determinants of the symptoms in any particular patient should guide treatment while minimizing the risk of overtreatment with ICS.

There appears to be a corticosteroid-responsive and corticosteroid-unresponsive component to the symptoms in this group of patients. An obese patient with asthma is exposed to the additive effects of an altered respiratory system physiology associated with obesity as well as an altered airway physiology associated with asthma.[31] Specifically there is some evidence that an expiratory flow limitation is more likely to develop during tidal breathing in the presence of bronchoconstriction, and this may be associated with persistent asthma symptoms despite ICS treatment.[32] Treatment strategies such as exercise and weight reduction should be advocated since studies also suggest that these have a beneficial effect on asthma control.

OBSTRUCTIVE SLEEP APNEA

OSA has also been associated with poor asthma control independent of obesity,[33] and there is some evidence that asthma control improves with sleep apnea treatment.

The mechanism for this is unclear, but the mechanical effects of breathing at low lung volumes during sleep may be important. Patients with symptoms suggestive of OSA, such as excessive daytime somnolence, snoring, and witnessed apneic episodes during sleep, should be referred for a monitored overnight sleep study. Other patients with poorly controlled asthma, especially patients with nocturnal symptoms, may also benefit from an assessment of any coexisting sleep-disordered breathing although this should be made on a case-by-case basis since there is no clear guidance in this regard.

Gastroesophageal Reflux Disease

GERD may either contribute to poor asthma control or lead to symptoms that are incorrectly attributed as asthma related. The treatment of symptomatic GERD with proton-pump inhibitors results in an improvement in asthma quality of life measures especially in patients experiencing nocturnal asthma symptoms.[34] However, clinically significant improvements in lung function are minimal and no benefit for asthma has been seen with the treatment of asymptomatic GERD.

Vocal Cord Dysfunction

VCD, or upper airway dysfunction, is another condition that may coexist with asthma or lead to a false-positive diagnosis of asthma.[35] Patients may experience breathlessness mainly on inspiration or they may report a choking sensation, throat tightness, voice hoarseness, stridor, and wheeze. The symptoms typically respond poorly to beta-agonists and patients often utilize more medical resources with repeated attendances for clinical review. Although the diagnosis of VCD may be difficult between acute episodes, normal spirometry with a suggestive history should alert the clinician to this possibility. In such circumstances, ICS dose escalation should be avoided. Instead, an assessment of the upper airway in a dedicated voice clinic with an ear, nose, and throat (ENT) surgeon and a speech pathologist can be helpful.[36]

Smoking

Smoking is, unfortunately, common among asthmatics. It is an important comorbidity that should be assessed in every patient with asthma. Smoking is associated with worse asthma control, more severe symptoms, and increased SABA use.[37] The detrimental effects of smoking on lung function are well known.[38] However, patients with asthma who smoke are also particularly susceptible to accelerated lung function decline.[39] Furthermore, smoking is associated with a reduction in the effectiveness of inhaled and oral corticosteroids[40] and patients with asthma who smoke may require an increased ICS dose for a similar benefit compared with nonsmoking patients. Hence, smoking can adversely affect the current control and future risk of the disease.

REFERRAL FOR SPECIALIST INVESTIGATIONS

The majority of patients with asthma have mild to moderate disease and can be managed in primary care. However, some patients benefit from referral to a respiratory specialist for assessment and management. Specifically, patients should be referred if they experience recurrent exacerbations, significant limitation of activity due to asthma, frequent symptoms despite normal lung function, or frequent symptoms despite treatment with ICS/LABA after confirming that their inhaler technique and adherence are adequate. Patients with more severe or difficult-to-treat asthma may benefit from more detailed lung function testing to optimally assess their asthma control and guide treatment strategies.

Chest X-Ray

A chest roentgenogram (CXR) is not usually needed as part of the assessment of asthma except in the context of acute severe asthma when a pneumothorax or pneumonia may need to be excluded.

High-Resolution Computed Tomography Chest Scans

High-resolution computed tomography (CT) scans of the chest provide better resolution of the large and medium airways as well as the lung parenchyma compared with a CXR. However, the potential benefit in clinical practice must be weighed against the radiation risk that is associated with such a scan. Patients that may warrant imaging as part of their assessment include patients with chronic sputum production to exclude bronchiectasis associated with allergic bronchopulmonary aspergillosis (ABPA) or common variable immunodeficiency; patients with fever, malaise, or haemoptysis to exclude tumors; patients who also smoke to exclude emphysema; and patients with recurrent exacerbations to exclude an abnormal airway anatomy. In all cases, the CT scan should ideally be performed several weeks after the resolution of an acute infection.

Bronchial Provocation Testing

Documenting the presence of AHR may be important when confirming the diagnosis of asthma in a new patient. Once regular treatment is underway, the absence of AHR does not exclude asthma, but it may permit more confidence in stepping down treatment even if some nonspecific symptoms persist. AHR is a physiological abnormality characteristic of asthma that can be measured in a laboratory using direct or indirect bronchial provocation tests. It is often measured as the dose or concentration of an inhaled spasmogen that causes a predefined fall in FEV_1 (usually 15% or 20%). The degree of AHR is variable over time and the abnormality is usually responsive to ICS treatment.[24] The sensitivity and specificity of the provocation tests depend on the population being studied (general population screening vs. selecting those with respiratory symptoms). Thus, the test results must be interpreted in the clinical context. Nevertheless, AHR has prognostic significance in asthma and correlates with long-term morbidity.[41]

Breath Testing for Exhaled Nitric Oxide

Measuring exhaled nitric oxide (FeNO) may be useful as a nonspecific marker of corticosteroid-responsive airway inflammation. There are several commercially available handheld devices but their performance characteristics differ. Hence, repeat measures are most useful when they are performed on the same device.[42]

In some patients, the FeNO level is elevated at diagnosis, reduces with ICS treatment, and correlates with clinical asthma control over time.[43,44] During monitoring, a significant rise in the FeNO level might indicate an increased risk of loss of control. An FeNO measurement is useful in patients where the contribution of eosinophilic airway inflammation to poor asthma control is unclear due to other comorbidities and it is useful to identify the likelihood of a response to ICS treatment.[45]

Sputum Induction for Inflammatory Cell Count

Patients with difficult-to-treat or severe asthma may be referred for a sputum cell count analysis as part of a range of second-line investigations. The availability of sputum sampling remains limited to certain tertiary and research centers. The knowledge of a patient's inflammatory profile can help tailor his or her treatment since eosinophilic asthma is typically more responsive to ICS treatment compared with neutrophilic asthma.[46] An ICS treatment algorithm guided by the presence of sputum eosinophilia was associated with reduced exacerbations. Interestingly, in the same study, the symptoms and quality of life measures did not significantly differ from treatment with a usual care algorithm. Hence, reducing eosinophilic airway inflammation may be of greater importance for the reduction of future risk than the assessment of current control, especially in patients in whom the symptoms are discordant with the degree of airway inflammation.

Complex Lung Function Testing

The small airways are clinically relevant for assessing current symptoms and predicting future asthma control. The degree of ventilation inhomogeneity, a sensitive marker of small airway dysfunction, correlates with symptom control measured using the ACQ-5 and it is a stronger determinant of current symptoms than spirometry or FeNO.[47] Furthermore, abnormal ventilation in the distal intra-acinar airways predicts an increased likelihood for loss of control following ICS down-titration in otherwise well-controlled patients.[48] Other, less sensitive

measures of small airway dysfunction, such as the degree of air trapping[49] and the propensity for airway closure,[50] have also been associated with the severity of asthma, the risk of exacerbations, and poor asthma control. These detailed lung function tests allow us to better understand the behavior of the airway in asthma. They are easy to perform and are used in certain clinical situations, such as pediatrics cystic fibrosis, as a monitoring tool. However, most of these tests are currently confined to research and tertiary care centers.

OTHER FACTORS MAY CONTRIBUTE TO POOR ASTHMA CONTROL

An assessment of asthma control in clinical practice is not complete without also assessing the patient's inhaler device technique, adherence with controller medication, and ownership and understanding of a written asthma action plan.

SUMMARY

Asthma is a common condition that continues to cause significant morbidity in the community, but the burden of the disease is often hidden as patients perceive asthma symptoms as "normal" and do not mention them unless prompted. An assessment of asthma control should address both current control and future risk. Current asthma control should be assessed at every consultation using several modalities if possible. In primary care, an assessment of the symptoms as well as a spirometry is advocated. Poor asthma control and previous exacerbations are among the risk factors for a future exacerbation. Comorbidities should be addressed to optimize asthma control. A suggested checklist for the assessment of asthma control is shown in Table 16.4. Novel measures of lung function may prove to be more useful for the assessment of asthma control but they remain largely as research tools. Patients with a poor response to standard inhaled treatment should be referred for further lung function testing and specialist advice.

TABLE 16.4
Quick Checklist for Assessing Asthma Control

A	Adherence
B	Bronchodilator use (reliever use >2 per week)
C	Control of symptoms (subjective assessment by patient)
D	Disability (limitation of activity)
E	Exacerbations recently
F	FEV$_1$

REFERENCES

1. Global Strategy for Asthma Management and Prevention. Global Initiative for Asthma (GINA) report: Global strategy for asthma management and prevention. 2011 [cited 2012 July]. Available from: http://www.ginasthma.org.

2. Reddel HK, Taylor DR, Bateman ED, et al. An Official American Thoracic Society/European Respiratory Society Statement: Asthma control and exacerbations–standardizing endpoints for clinical asthma trials and clinical practice. *Am J Respir Crit Care Med.* 2009;180:59–99.

3. Taylor DR, Bateman ED, Boulet LP, et al. A new perspective on concepts of asthma severity and control. *Eur Respir J.* 2008;32:545–554.

4. Meltzer EO, Busse WW, Wenzel SE, et al. Use of the Asthma Control Questionnaire to predict future risk of asthma exacerbation. *J Allergy Clin Immunol.* 2011;127:167–172.

5. Busse WW, Lemanske Jr RF, Gern JE. Role of viral respiratory infections in asthma and asthma exacerbations. *Lancet.* 2010;376:826–834.

6. Australian Centre for Asthma Monitoring. *Asthma in Australia 2011.* Canberra: Australian Institute of Health and Welfare, 2011.

7. O'Byrne PM, Reddel HK, Eriksson G, et al. Measuring asthma control: A comparison of three classification systems. *Eur Respir J.* 2010;36:269–276.

8. British Thoracic Society and Scottish Intercollegiate Guidelines Network. *Managing Asthma in Adults.* 2011 [cited 2012 July]. Available from: http://www.brit-thoracic.org.uk/Guidelines/Asthma-Guidelines.aspx.

9. Salome CM, Reddel HK, Ware SI, et al. Effect of budesonide on the perception of induced airway narrowing in subjects with asthma. *Am J Respir Crit Care Med.* 2002;165:15–21.

10. Calhoun WJ, Sutton LB, Emmett A, et al. Asthma variability in patients previously treated with beta2-agonists alone. *J Allergy Clin Immunol.* 2003;112:1088–1094.

11. Taylor DR. The beta-agonist saga and its clinical relevance: On and on it goes. *Am J Respir Crit Care Med.* 2009;179:976–978.

12. McNicholl DM, Megarry J, McGarvey LP, et al. The utility of cardiopulmonary exercise testing in difficult asthma. *Chest.* 2011;139:1117–1123.

13. Juniper EF, O'Byrne PM, Guyatt GH, et al. Development and validation of a questionnaire to measure asthma control. *Eur Respir J.* 1999;14:902–907.

14. Nathan RA, Sorkness CA, Kosinski M, et al. Development of the asthma control test: A survey for assessing asthma control. *J Allergy Clin Immunol.* 2004;113:59–65.

15. Juniper EF, O'Byrne PM, Roberts JN. Measuring asthma control in group studies: Do we need airway calibre and rescue beta2-agonist use? *Respir Med.* 2001;95:319–323.

16. Juniper EF, Bousquet J, Abetz L, et al. Identifying "well-controlled" and "not well-controlled" asthma using the Asthma Control Questionnaire. *Respir Med.* 2006;100:616–621.

17. Jenkins CR, Thien FC, Wheatley JR, et al. Traditional and patient-centred outcomes with three classes of asthma medication. *Eur Respir J.* 2005;26:36–44.

18. Schatz M, Kosinski M, Yarlas AS, et al. The minimally important difference of the Asthma Control Test. *J Allergy Clin Immunol.* 2009;124:719–723. e1.

19. Pinnock H, Burton C, Campbell S et al. Clinical implications of the Royal College of Physicians three questions in routine asthma care: a real-life validation study. *Prim Care Respir J.* 2012;21:288–294.

20. Rabe KF, Adachi M, Lai CKW, et al. Worldwide severity and control of asthma in children and adults: The global asthma insights and reality surveys. *J Allergy Clin Immunol.* 2004;114:40–47.

21. Reddel H, Ware S, Marks G, et al. Differences between asthma exacerbations and poor asthma control. *Lancet.* 1999;353:364–369.

22. Levy ML, Quanjer PH, Booker R, et al. Diagnostic spirometry in primary care: Proposed standards for general practice compliant with American Thoracic Society and European Respiratory Society recommendations: A General Practice Airways Group (GPIAG)1 document, in association with the Association for Respiratory Technology & Physiology (ARTP)2 and Education for Health3. www.gpiag.org, www.artp.org, and www.educationforhealth.org.uk. *Prim Care Respir J.* 2009;18:130–147.

23. Cooper BG. An update on contraindications for lung function testing. *Thorax.* 2011;66:714–723.

24. Reddel HK, Jenkins CR, Marks GB, et al. Optimal asthma control, starting with high doses of inhaled budesonide. *Eur Respir J.* 2000;16:226–235.

25. Shingo S, Zhang J, Reiss TF. Correlation of airway obstruction and patient-reported endpoints in clinical studies. *Eur Respir J.* 2001;17:220–224.

26. Kitch BT, Paltiel AD, Kuntz KM, et al. A single measure of FEV1 is associated with risk of asthma attacks in long-term follow-up. *Chest.* 2004;126:1875–1882.

27. Magnan A, Meunier JP, Saugnac C, et al. Frequency and impact of allergic rhinitis in asthma patients in everyday general medical practice: A French observational cross-sectional study. *Allergy.* 2008;63:292–298.

28. Talreja N, Baptist AP. Effect of age on asthma control: Results from the National Asthma Survey. *Ann Allergy Asthma Immunol.* 2011;106:24–29.

29. Ford ES, Mannino DM. Time trends in obesity among adults with asthma in the United States: Findings from three national surveys. *J Asthma.* 2005;42:91–95.

30. Farah CS, Kermode JA, Downie SR, et al. Obesity is a determinant of asthma control, independent of inflammation and lung mechanics. *Chest.* 2011;140:659–666.

31. Nicolacakis K, Skowronski ME, Coreno AJ, et al. Observations on the physiological interactions between obesity and asthma. *J Appl Physiol.* 2008;105:1533–1541.

32. Mahadev S, Farah CS, King GG, et al. Obesity, expiratory flow limitation and asthma symptoms. *Pulm Pharmacol Ther.* 2013;26(4):438–443.

33. Teodorescu M, Polomis DA, Hall SV, et al. Association of obstructive sleep apnea risk with asthma Control in Adults. *Chest.* 2010;138:543–550.

34. Kiljander TO, Harding SM, Field SK, et al. Effects of esomeprazole 40 mg twice daily on asthma: A randomized placebo-controlled trial. *Am J Respir Crit Care Med.* 2006;173:1091–1097.

35. Parsons JP, Benninger C, Hawley MP, et al. Vocal cord dysfunction: Beyond severe asthma. *Respir Med.* 2010;104:504–509.

36. Morris MJ, Christopher KL. Diagnostic criteria for the classification of vocal cord dysfunction. *Chest.* 2010;138:1213–1223.

37. Althuis MD, Sexton M, Prybylski D. Cigarette smoking and asthma symptom severity among adult asthmatics. *J Asthma.* 1999;36:257–264.

38. Fletcher C, Peto R. The natural history of chronic airflow obstruction. *Br Med J.* 1977;1:1645–1648.
39. Lange P, Parner J, Vestbo J, et al. A 15-year follow-up study of ventilatory function in adults with asthma. *N Engl J Med.* 1998;339:1194–1200.
40. Chalmers GW, Macleod KJ, Little SA, et al. Influence of cigarette smoking on inhaled corticosteroid treatment in mild asthma. *Thorax.* 2002;57:226–230.
41. Xuan W, Peat JK, Toelle BG, et al. Lung function growth and its relation to airway hyperresponsiveness and recent wheeze. Results from a longitudinal population study. *Am J Respir Crit Care Med.* 2000;161:1820–1824.
42. Taylor DR, Palmay R, Cowan JO, et al. Long term performance characteristics of an electrochemical nitric oxide analyser. *Respir Med.* 2011;105:211–217.
43. Jones SL, Kittelson J, Cowan JO, et al. The predictive value of exhaled nitric oxide measurements in assessing changes in asthma control. *Am J Respir Crit Care Med.* 2001;164:738–743.
44. Michils A, Baldassarre S, Van Muylem A. Exhaled nitric oxide and asthma control: A longitudinal study in unselected patients. *Eur Respir J.* 2008;31:539–546.
45. Dweik RA, Boggs PB, Erzurum SC, et al. An official ATS clinical practice guideline: Interpretation of exhaled nitric oxide levels (FENO) for clinical applications. *Am J Respir Crit Care Med.* 2011;184:602–615.
46. Pavord ID, Pizzichini MM, Pizzichini E, et al. The use of induced sputum to investigate airway inflammation. *Thorax.* 1997;52:498–501.
47. Farah CS, King GG, Brown NJ, et al. The role of the small airways in the clinical expression of asthma in adults. *J Allergy Clin Immunol.* 2012;129:381–387.
48. Farah CS, King GG, Brown NJ, et al. Ventilation heterogeneity predicts asthma control in adults following inhaled corticosteroid dose titration. *J Allergy Clin Immunol.* 2012;130:61–68.
49. Sorkness RL, Bleecker ER, Busse WW, et al. Lung function in adults with stable but severe asthma: Air trapping and incomplete reversal of obstruction with bronchodilation. *J Appl Physiol.* 2008;104:394–403.
50. in't Veen JCCM, Beekman AJ, Bel EH, et al. Recurrent exacerbations in severe asthma are associated with enhanced airway closure during stable episodes. *Am J Respir Crit Care Med.* 2000;161:1902–1906.

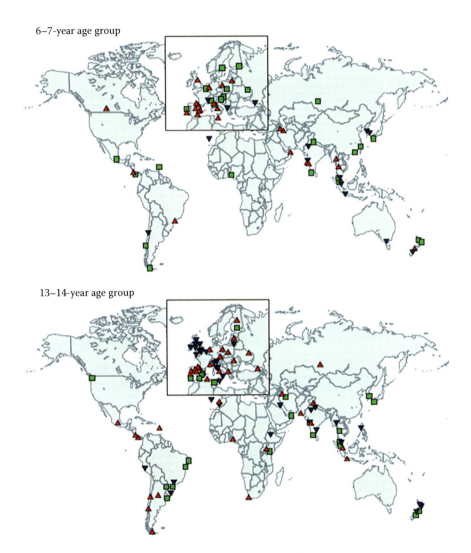

6–7-year age group

13–14-year age group

FIGURE 1.3 World map showing the direction of change in the prevalence of asthma symptoms for the 6–7-year age group and the 13–14-year age group. Each symbol represents a center. Blue triangle, prevalence reduced by ≥1 SE per year. Green square, little change (<1 SE). Red triangle, prevalence increased by ≥1 SE per year. (Reproduced from Asher, M.I., Montefort, S., Björkstén, B., et al., *Lancet*, 368, 733–743, 2006. With permission.)

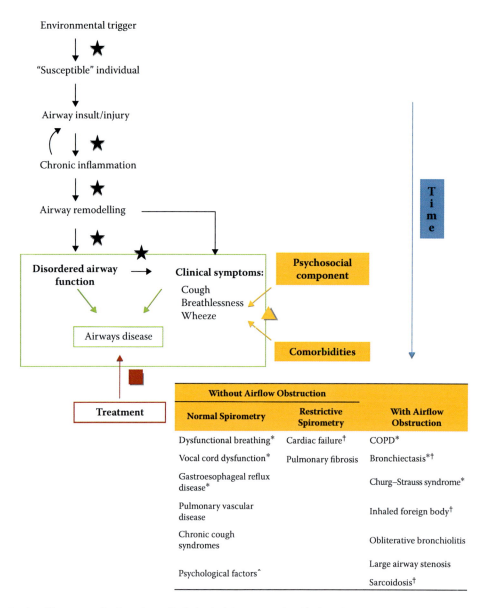

FIGURE 4.1 The basis of heterogeneity in asthma. Pathological heterogeneity (★) is a function of the spectrum of possible expressions at each proposed step of the disease pathogenesis. Clinical heterogeneity originates from pathological heterogeneity and is modified by a spectrum of responses to treatment (■) together with the confounding effect of comorbidities, psychosocial factors (▲), and time (long arrow). The table summarizes the commonly recognized disorders that may mimic or aggravate the clinical symptoms of asthma. *These conditions may coexist with asthma. †These conditions may be associated with normal spirometry. ^Psychological factors are also associated with behavioral traits that lead to increased disease activity in asthma. These include poor treatment adherence, failure to attend medical appointments, and smoking.

	Factor Analysis	**Cluster Analysis**
Plotting data for reduction	The population sum for each variable is calculated and plotted as a vector in space	The geometrical position of each data point is computed from the vectorial sum of the clustering variables
Measuring similarity	Angular relationship between constructed vectors	Geometrical distance in space between plotted data point(s)
Grouping	Defined according to the angular relationship between vectors and constructed factor axes	*Hierarchical methods:* Either group together or divide preformed groups according to threshold distances between pairs of data point(s)
		Nonhierarchical methods: Construct a prespecified number of cluster centers. Clusters are defined according to the geometrical distance between data point(s) and cluster centers
Outcome	Useful for characterising relationships between variables within a data set	Useful for grouping cases within a data set on the basis of shared similarity for chosen variables

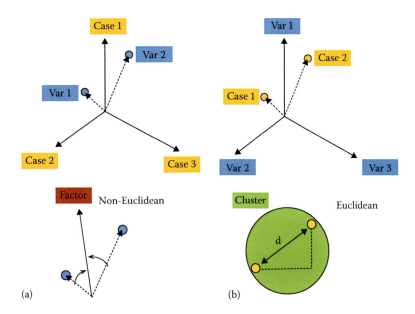

FIGURE 4.3 An overview and a comparison of (a) factor analysis and (b) cluster analysis.

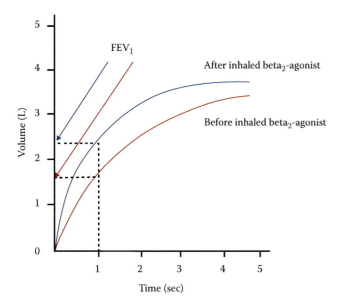

FIGURE 7.1 Measurements of FEV1 before and 10 minutes after an inhaled beta2-agonist in an asthmatic patient. The FEV1 value was 1.7 L before and 2.3 L after the inhaled beta2-agonist. This reversibility is consistent with a diagnosis of asthma.

FIGURE 7.2 Dose–response curves obtained during inhalation challenges with methacholine in a severe asthmatic, a mild asthmatic, and a normal subject. The response to increasing inhaled doses of methacholine is measured by a change in FEV1 from baseline. Asthmatics have (a) a lower threshold, (b) a steeper slope of the dose–response curve, and (c) a greater maximal response to inhaled methacholine. The response is expressed as the provocative concentration of methacholine causing a 20% fall in FEV1 (PC_{20}).

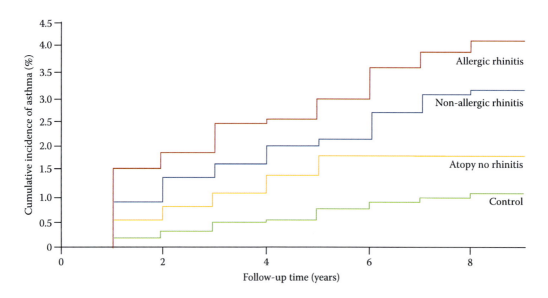

FIGURE 8.2 Association of rhinitis with the onset and incidence of asthma. (From Shaaban, R., Zureik, M., Soussan, D., et al., *Am. J. Respir. Crit. Care Med.*, 176, 659–666, 2007. With permission.)

Potential problems with technique	pMDI	pMDI + holding chamber	DPI
Decreased PIF	✔	✔	⊘
Impaired cognition	?	?	?
Decreased manual dexterity	⊘	?	
Decreased press and breathe coordination	⊘	✔	✔

Key: pMDI, pressurized-metered dose inhaler; DPI, dry powder inhaler; PIF, peak inspiratory flow.

 The patient should be able to master the technique in the presence of the impairment.

 The patient may possibly master the technique in the presence of the impairment.

 The device is not recommended when the impairment is present.

Regardless of the device selection, the practitioner must demonstrate the technique, and provide regular reassessment and instruction. Minimization of inhaler device polypharmacy is recommended.

FIGURE 13.2 A guide to inhaler device selection recognizing the potential problems associated with the optimal technique. (Reprinted from *The Lancet*, 374, Gibson, P.G., McDonald, V.M., and Marks, G.B., Asthma in the older adult, 803–813, ©2010, with permission from Elsevier.)

Case Study: Lucy's Written Asthma Action Plan

When Well
Seretide 250/25 mcg _____ Dose: Two puffs via your spacer morning and night
Ventolin* 100 mcg _____ Dose: Two puffs as needed
Take Ventolin two puffs 10 minutes before exercise

When Not Well

- If your peak flow reading does not reach 80% of your best value, which is **320 L/m** following your medication for a 24 hour period.

or

- If you are waking at night due to your asthma or have symptoms when you wake in the morning.

or

- If you require your Ventolin more frequently than usual and are not getting the same effect.

or

- You are getting a cold.

Then

- Increase your Ventolin: Take two extra puffs as needed.
- Start prednisone 37.5 mg a day for 14 days.
- See your doctor if you are no better in 2–3 days of increased treatment.

For a Severe Attack

- If your peak flow does not reach 50% of best value, which is **200 L/m.**

or

- If you have a severe shortness of breath and can only speak in short sentences.

or

- If you are having a severe attack of asthma and are frightened.

or

- If you need to take your Ventolin more than four puffs hourly and do not gain an effect.

Then

- Take Ventolin four puffs in your spacer: repeat if you do not improve.
- Take 50 mg of prednisone.
- Seek medical attention immediately by calling an ambulance on 000.
- Continue to use your Ventolin in your spacer four puffs every 4 minutes until help arrives.

Signature_____   Date_____

*Changed from terbutaline due to poor technique and inhaler poly device pharmacy.

FIGURE 13.3   An example of a written asthma action plan. (©Department of Respiratory and Sleep Medicine, John Hunter Hospital. Adapted from McDonald, V.M. and Gibson, P.G. Asthma patient education. In: Pawankar, R., Holgate, S., and Rosenwaser, L. (eds), *Allergy Frontiers: Diagnosis and Health Economics*, Japan: Springer, 2009 with permission.) *Note:* Trade names have been used to represent the language used in patient communication.

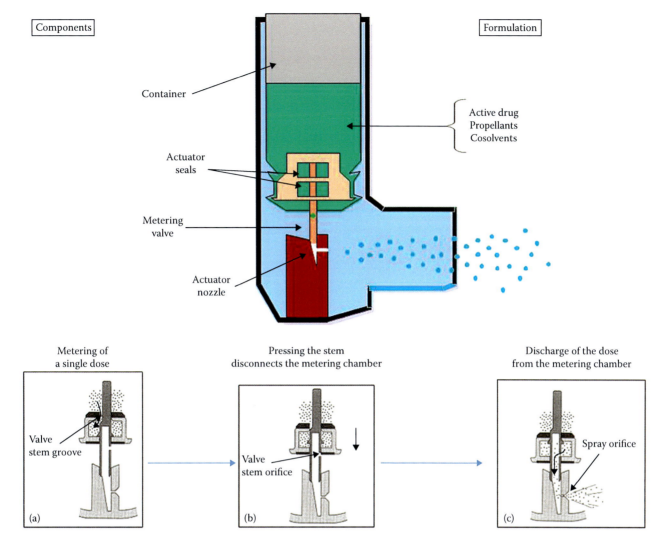

Components

Formulation

Container

Active drug
Propellants
Cosolvents

Actuator
seals

Metering
valve

Actuator
nozzle

Metering of
a single dose

Pressing the stem
disconnects the metering chamber

Discharge of the dose
from the metering chamber

Valve
stem groove

Valve
stem orifice

Spray orifice

(a)

(b)

(c)

FIGURE 15.1   Schematic representation of the components of a pressurized metered-dose inhaler. The lower panels illustrate the process of aerosol generation.

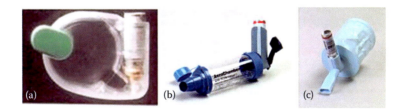

(a)

(b)

(c)

FIGURE 15.2   Examples of an open tube spacer (a: the Jet), a holding chamber (b: the AeroChamber Plus), and a reverse-flow spacer (c: the InspirEase).

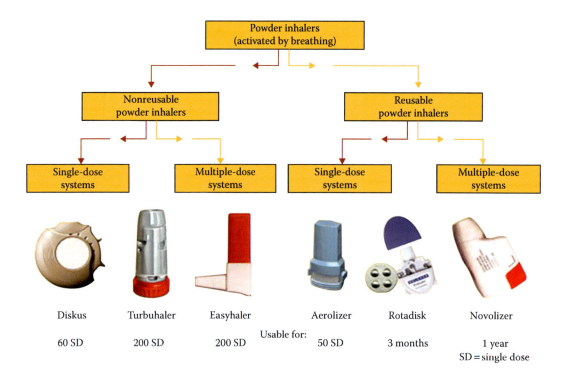

FIGURE 15.3   A variety of dry powder inhalers. (From www.admit-online.info.)

Section V

Asthma Management and Treatments

17 Management of Pediatric Asthma

Leonard B. Bacharier

CONTENTS

CASE PRESENTATION

A 4-year-old boy presents for an evaluation of recurrent episodes of cough and wheezing since 1 year of age. His initial episode, at age 3 months, was in the setting of a viral illness that was characterized by coryza, low-grade fever, and wheezing. For the past 2 years, he experienced cough and wheeze with nearly all upper respiratory tract infections. Over the past year, his mother has noticed him coughing and wheezing while playing soccer in addition to similar symptoms during upper respiratory tract infections. He awakens due to cough or wheeze approximately twice monthly. Albuterol consistently provides him with prompt, albeit transient, symptom relief. Oral corticosteroids have been prescribed twice yearly for the most significant episodes. No emergency department visits or hospitalizations have been required.

His past medical history is notable for an itchy rash over the antecubital and popliteal fossae since 1 year of age, which improved with topical corticosteroids. He has never

had pneumonia or croup. His only current medication is albuterol by nebulization as needed. His environment contains a cat and wall-to-wall carpeting throughout the home. The family history is notable for asthma in the father and allergic rhinitis in the mother.

On physical examination, he is alert, interactive, and not distressed. His weight is at the 45th percentile and his height is at the 40th percentile. His heart rate is 100/ min and his respiratory rate is 16/min. He has infraorbital shiners, edematous and pale nasal turbinates, no tonsillar enlargement, and his chest examination is clear without adventitious lung sounds or evidence of increased work of breathing. His skin examination discloses erythematous papules and excoriation in the antecubital fossae bilaterally. His chest radiograph is normal without infiltrates or hyperinflation. His parents wonder what can be done to prevent him from experiencing further episodes of cough and wheeze.

GOALS OF ASTHMA MANAGEMENT IN PRESCHOOL- AND SCHOOL-AGE CHILDREN

The principles of asthma management in preschool- and school-age children have evolved substantially over the past two decades to the current approach that is guided by the goals of the attainment and maintenance of asthma control (see Chapter 16). In contrast to asthma severity, which defines the intrinsic intensity of asthma as assessed without the use of a controller therapy, asthma control reflects the degree to which the signs and symptoms of asthma are minimized. Thus, successful asthma management achieves multiple goals, including (1) the minimization of day-to-day asthma-related symptomatology (i.e., a reduction in the current impairment domain of asthma); (2) the reduction or elimination of asthma exacerbations; (3) the minimization of treatment-related side effects; and (4) ideally, the prevention of impaired lung growth and progressive decline in lung function (i.e., a reduction in the future risk domain of asthma).

Preschool-age children often exhibit asthma that is more exacerbation prone than impairment dominant, while school-age children begin to demonstrate elements of both impairment and risk. The recognition of these different phenotypes and patterns of asthma expression has directed the research examining different treatment strategies in these two age groups, with exacerbation prevention and disease modification being the major focuses in preschool-age children while exacerbation prevention has been coupled with impairment reduction and interventions to prevent declines in lung function among school-age children.

HETEROGENEITY OF EARLY CHILDHOOD WHEEZING AND ASTHMA

Recurrent wheezing in the preschool-age group is a highly heterogeneous disorder, with multiple disease phenotypes based on the age of onset, age and likelihood of remission, concomitant risk factors (especially atopy), and triggering factors (such as viral infections). These multiple different phenotypic expressions of early childhood asthma are likely due to different underlying immunopathophysiological mechanisms, which may confer differential responses to therapeutic strategies. The heterogeneity of early childhood wheezing and asthma complicates the interpretation of much of the early research done in this population, as most of the early studies enrolled very heterogeneous populations of subjects rather than specific wheezing phenotypes. Fortunately, several recent studies have begun to focus on more well-defined and homogeneous populations, providing evidence to guide decision making in this challenging age group.

STEPWISE APPROACH TO ASTHMA CARE

Over the past decade, several asthma guidelines have been developed that provide carefully developed treatment recommendations for children with asthma, including the National Asthma Education and Prevention Program (NAEPP),[1] the Global Initiative for Asthma (GINA),[2] and the European Respiratory Society (ERS) task force.[3] All of these guidelines have proposed algorithms for the pharmacological management of asthma using stepwise approaches, with the steps of care being aligned with the levels of both the asthma severity and control. While the guidelines differ in terms of the number of steps of care and the order of preferences of treatments within each step,[4] there is a consensus that the achievement of asthma control is the major goal of therapy and that an individualized approach for each child is necessary based on the level of control achieved.

MANAGEMENT OF INTERMITTENT DISEASE (STEP 1 CARE)

According to the NAEPP guidelines, children with intermittent asthma under the age of 12 should receive Step 1 care (Figure 17.1), which includes as-needed use of a short-acting beta-agonist (SABA). The phenotype of intermittent asthma is most apparent in the preschool population, where it has been referred to using various terminology, including *severe intermittent asthma* and *episodic viral wheeze*. This phenotype exemplifies an exacerbation-dominant disease with minimal to no intercurrent symptomatology. However, given the substantial morbidity experienced during these episodes, therapeutic strategies aiming to prevent or attenuate episode severity, ranging from daily preventative therapy to episodic therapy, have been studied. In recognition of this symptom pattern, and since publication of the NAEPP guidelines in 2007, several studies have clarified and broadened the treatment possibilities for young children with intermittent/episodic disease, including the episodic use of controller medications at episode onset to attenuate symptom progression as well as the examination of daily controller therapy intended to prevent exacerbations.

EPISODIC CONTROLLER THERAPY

The intermittent and episodic nature of this condition has led parents, physicians, and investigators to consider the potential efficacy of the intermittent use of controller therapies just during periods of increased asthma symptomatology, such as viral respiratory tract infections. The use of high-dose inhaled corticosteroid (ICS) therapy (fluticasone propionate 750 mcg twice daily) in 1- to 6-year-old children started at the early signs of a developing respiratory tract illness reduced the risk of oral corticosteroid use by approximately 50%, but was associated with statistically significant reductions in both height and weight gain.[5] In contrast, two studies examining budesonide used intermittently (either 1 mg twice daily for 7 days at the earliest signs of a respiratory tract illness or 400 mcg daily beginning 3 days after the onset of respiratory tract symptoms) did not demonstrate a reduction in exacerbations requiring oral corticosteroids,[6,7] but it did result in modest reductions in symptomatology during illnesses.[6] The episodic use of montelukast at the early signs of respiratory tract illnesses also produced modest reductions

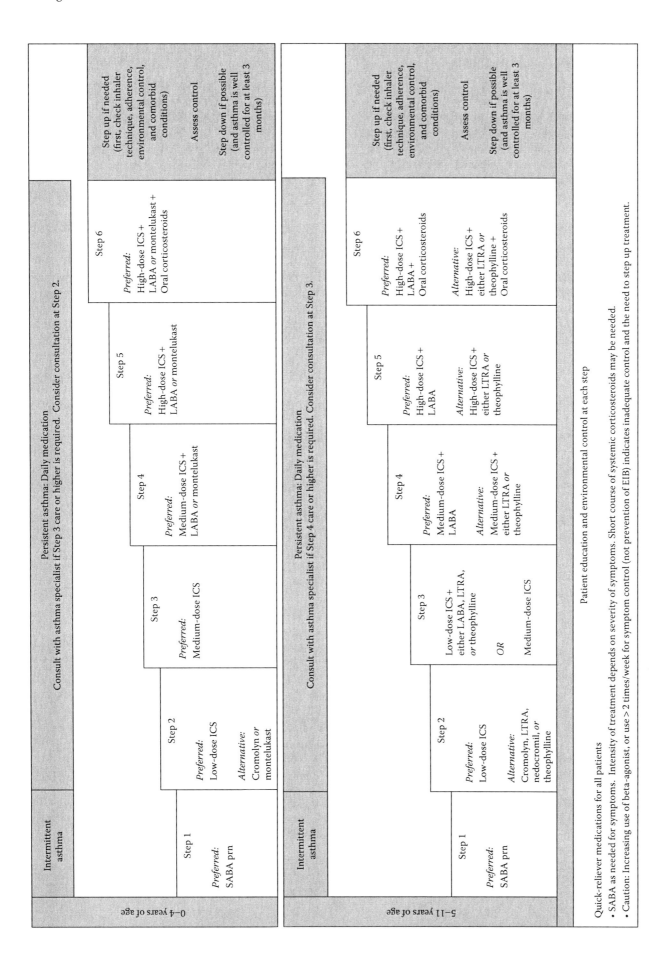

FIGURE 17.1 **(See color insert)** NAEPP stepwise approach for the long-term management of asthma in children aged 0–4 years (*upper panel*) and 5–11 years (*lower panel*). (Modified from National Asthma Education and Prevention Program. Expert Panel Report III: Guidelines for the diagnosis and management of asthma. Bethesda, MD: US Department of Health and Human Services; 2007.)

in symptomatology without reducing the need for systemic corticosteroids.[6]

DAILY CONTROLLER THERAPY

Given the severity of the episodes that are experienced by many children with intermittent disease, studies of daily controller therapy aimed at episode prevention have also been conducted. Daily treatment with low-dose ICS (fluticasone propionate 88 mcg twice daily) for 2 years in children aged 2–3 years with a recurrent wheeze, the absence of evidence of ongoing asthma impairment, and risk factors for the persistence of asthma (positive modified Asthma Predictive Index) resulted in significantly fewer oral corticosteroid courses and more episode-free days than did a placebo over the 2-year period.[8] A meta-analysis of 29 studies of infants and preschool-age children with recurrent wheeze or asthma demonstrated a reduction of approximately 40% in the risk of exacerbations associated with daily ICS therapy as well as an improved symptom burden and lung function.[9] Daily therapy with montelukast produced a significant reduction in asthma exacerbations relative to a placebo among 2- to 5-year-old children with intermittent asthma, but it did not impact the frequency of oral corticosteroid use.[10] A recent study compared the efficacy of daily low-dose ICS (budesonide 0.5 mg daily) with the episodic use of high-dose ICS (budesonide 1 mg twice daily started at the early signs of a respiratory illness) among 12- to 53-month-old children with recurrent wheeze, positive modified Asthma Predictive Indices, and an exacerbation in the previous year, and demonstrated no difference between the two treatment strategies in terms of oral corticosteroid use, episode severity, indicators of daily asthma impairment, or linear growth.[11] Currently, there are no studies directly comparing daily ICS and daily leukotriene receptor antagonist (LTRA) therapy in intermittent asthma in preschool-age children to determine the relative efficacies of these approaches.

MANAGEMENT OF PERSISTENT ASTHMA (STEP 2 CARE)

DAILY ICS THERAPY

There is consensus among guidelines that children with persistent asthma should receive daily controller therapy in an effort to reduce the elements of asthma impairment and risk. Nearly all guidelines endorse low-dose ICS therapy as the preferred controller for the management of mild persistent asthma (Step 2), based on a multitude of trials in preschool and school-age populations that demonstrate improvements in nearly all facets of asthma impairment and risk. Daily ICS therapy has consistently been shown to reduce days and nights with asthma symptoms, exacerbations requiring oral corticosteroids, health-care utilization, urgent care visits, hospitalizations, as well as physiological measures such as bronchial hyperresponsiveness and exhaled nitric oxide levels. While many studies have shown an improvement in

lung function (forced expiratory volume in 1 sec [FEV_1]) over relatively short time intervals (12 weeks), the Childhood Asthma Management Program (CAMP) demonstrated that among children aged 5–12 years with mild to moderate asthma, and despite significant improvements in multiple clinical measures of asthma control, there was no significant difference in lung function after 4.3 years of low-dose ICS therapy (budesonide 200 mcg twice daily) relative to a placebo,[12] nor was there a difference in lung function 4.8 years after stopping daily ICS therapy.[13]

ICS therapy is generally well tolerated by the majority of pediatric patients. However, the potential side effects of ICS therapy, which are generally dose dependent, include alterations in skeletal growth, bone density, hypothalamic-pituitary-adrenal (HPA) axis function, and local side effects including oral candidiasis and hoarseness. The clearly established clinical benefits provided by daily ICS therapy must be weighed against the potential risks associated with this approach in preschool-age children. The effect of ICS therapy on linear growth may be dependent on multiple factors, including age, weight, ICS dosing, the specific ICS product, and the delivery system. Multiple studies in school-age children have consistently demonstrated a clinically modest but statistically significant effect on linear growth (typically ~1.1 cm over the first year of therapy) with budesonide and beclomethasone, while studies in preschool-age children have been less consistent, demonstrating either similar growth effects[8,14] or no statistically significant effects of ICS therapy[15–17] on growth velocity. Long-term follow-up reveals that the growth-suppressive effects of ICS therapy on children are generally small on average, and appear to improve over time in most children, but there remain subgroups of children who experience greater than expected reductions in linear growth. The regular monitoring of growth in children receiving ICS therapy remains appropriate, with titration of the ICS dosing to the minimally effective dose.

DAILY LTRA THERAPY

Among preschool-age children with persistent asthma, montelukast given daily over 12 weeks significantly reduces asthma symptom frequency, rescue albuterol use, oral corticosteroid use, peripheral blood eosinophil levels, bronchial hyperreactivity, and fractional exhaled nitric oxide levels.[18–20] Similarly, among school-age children, montelukast therapy reduced asthma symptoms and rescue albuterol use while improving pulmonary function, quality of life, and peripheral blood eosinophil counts over an 8-week period in children aged 6–14 years with moderate asthma compared with a placebo,[21] as well as inhibiting exercise-induced bronchoconstriction in school-aged children with mild to moderate asthma.[22]

Montelukast therapy has demonstrated an excellent overall safety profile in pediatric patients, with upper respiratory tract infection, worsening asthma, pharyngitis, and fever as the most commonly reported side effects.[23] Neuropsychiatric events have been reported infrequently in patients of all ages taking montelukast, with preschool and school-age children not appearing to be more susceptible to such effects than older individuals.[24]

The NAEPP/Expert Panel Report 3 (EPR3) guidelines recommend ICS as the preferred controller at Step 2, with montelukast identified as an alternative based on several comparative trials and supported by a meta-analysis demonstrating greater efficacy for ICS therapy in general compared with LTRA therapy in terms of markers of asthma control, including symptom reduction, exacerbation prevention, and lung function improvement.[25–30] However, not all patients achieve superior asthma control with ICS relative to LTRA, with recent research confirming that patient characteristics may identify patients who may experience a differential response to ICS and LTRA. A crossover trial found that children with lower levels of lung function or high levels of markers of allergic inflammation (exhaled nitric oxide levels or greater airway hyperresponsiveness) were more likely to experience greater improvements in lung function (FEV_1) and other indicators of asthma control with ICS therapy than with LTRA therapy,[25,26] suggesting that ICS may be preferred over LTRA in children with these features. However, children less than 10 years of age and those with urinary leukotriene C4 levels >100 pg/mg were more likely to experience at least a 7.5% improvement in FEV_1 while receiving montelukast over an 8-week period, but did not experience comparable improvements while receiving ICS, further emphasizing the significant heterogeneity in response to asthma therapies. Based on their overall efficacy relative to ICS, LTRA may be considered as an alternative to ICS as a monotherapy at Step 2, if for some reason ICS therapy is not desirable.

APPROACHES FOR CHILDREN NOT WELL CONTROLLED WITH STEP 2 (AND ABOVE) THERAPY

Among children with persistent asthma, most will achieve asthma control with Step 2 therapy. When children fail to achieve asthma control with either daily low-dose ICS or LTRA therapy, considerations should include: (1) heterogeneity of the drug response (and thus a trial of an alternate agent in Step 2); (2) suboptimal adherence to the medical regimen; (3) improper drug administration techniques (e.g., an ineffective or incorrect inhalation technique); (4) comorbid conditions (e.g., rhinosinusitis, gastroesophageal reflux, and obesity); (5) ongoing trigger exposure (e.g., aeroallergens, environmental tobacco smoke, and viral infections); and (6) psychosocial factors (e.g., maternal and/or child stress and/or depression). If the consideration and modification of these factors do not produce asthma control, a step-up to Step 3 is indicated.

STEP 3 CARE AND ABOVE

For children aged 0–4 years, the NAEPP/EPR3 guidelines recommend escalating therapy to medium-dose ICS therapy in patients not controlled with low-dose ICS therapy (Step 3),

rather than instituting the combination therapy that is recommended in school-age children, in an effort to maximize the likelihood that an effective dose of ICS will be delivered to the lower airways before consideration of adjunctive (i.e., combination) therapy.[1] If the use of medium-dose ICS therapy does not achieve well-controlled asthma in children aged 0–4 years, the NAEPP/EPR3 guidelines suggest the following options for Step 4 care: the initiation of a combination controller therapy with a medium-dose ICS along with either a long-acting beta-agonist (LABA) or montelukast. There are limited data in this age group to firmly support these recommendations, and thus these recommendations are largely based on extrapolation from studies in older children and adults. One recent randomized trial demonstrated an improvement in lung function but not a reduction in asthma symptoms or rescue medication use among 4- to 7-year-old children with multiple-trigger wheeze treated with ICS plus a LABA relative to ICS treatment alone, although participants who received ICS within the previous 6 months were excluded from this trial and thus it is not clear if these participants would have demonstrated inadequate control while receiving ICS alone to warrant consideration of the addition of the LABA salmeterol.[31] Clearly, additional, adequately designed and powered, prospective, controlled trials of ICS + LABA therapy must be conducted in this age group in order to determine the appropriate role for LABA therapy in this age group.

In school-age children (5–11 years) not adequately controlled with low-dose ICS therapy, the NAEPP/EPR3 guidelines recommend the following as treatment options at Step 3: (1) low-dose ICS + LABA, (2) low-dose ICS + LTRA, (3) low-dose ICS + theophylline, or (4) medium-dose ICS, although relatively limited data for these approaches are available in this age group.

The role of the addition of LABA to ICS therapy in school-age children has been clarified over the past decade. An early trial demonstrated no difference in clinical or physiological outcomes among children who received medium-dose ICS compared with those treated with low-dose ICS + LABA,[32] and a more recent noninferiority study demonstrated no differences in lung function, exacerbations, or adverse events between children treated with low-dose ICS + LABA and those treated with medium-dose ICS.[33] Two recent Cochrane reviews concluded that the effect of the addition of LABA therapy to ICS, when compared with either the same dose of ICS alone or a higher dose of ICS alone, is not certain and may be associated with an increased risk of oral corticosteroid-treated exacerbations and hospitalizations.[34,35] Similarly, a recent meta-analysis concluded that there is insufficient evidence to determine if the addition of LTRA to ICS improves asthma outcomes.[30] However, since the publication of these Cochrane reviews and the meta-analysis, a prospective trial examined three step-up options among children aged 6–18 years with asthma inadequately controlled with low-dose ICS.[36] The addition of LABA to low-dose ICS was the approach most likely to produce the best response in terms of a composite outcome, which included asthma exacerbations, episode-free days, and lung function. However, either of the other two therapies studied, the addition of an LTRA to low-dose ICS or an increase to medium-dose ICS, was the therapy most likely to produce the best response among substantial proportions of participants. These findings suggest that these three treatment strategies are indeed effective as step-up strategies among children with asthma inadequately controlled with low-dose ICS, since nearly all children respond best to one of these strategies. African American children were least likely to show the best response to the addition of LTRA, and children without eczema were most likely to have the best response to LABA. Unfortunately, other predictors for which therapy is best for a given individual could not be clearly delineated. Thus, if a patient is inadequately controlled with a given Step 3 regimen, these data suggest changing to a different Step 3 approach before moving to Step 4.

The benefits associated with LABA therapy must be balanced against the potential risks of this class of therapeutics. Largely based on trials in adolescents and adults, there appears to be an increased risk of asthma-related death among patients who are treated with a LABA relative to those not treated with a LABA, although the largest studies demonstrating this effect did not mandate concomitant ICS use and provided LABA in a separate inhaler device, making it unclear whether concurrent ICS use mitigates the increased risk associated with LABA. As noted earlier, while the evidence for the efficacy of LABA therapy in school-age children appears generally supportive of this approach, several studies failed to demonstrate a significant improvement with ICS + LABA therapy. A recent study from the U.S. Food and Drug Administration concluded that the use of a LABA-containing therapy was associated with an increased likelihood of asthma-related death, hospitalization, and intubation among children, and that additional data are required to determine the risks of LABA in conjunction with ICS therapy.[37] Based on these findings, step-down therapy should be routinely considered, although no prospective clinical trial data are available to guide how to accomplish step-down in children in the safest and most effective manner.

TEMPORARY STEP-UP IN ANTICIPATION OF EXPOSURE TO PREDICTABLE TRIGGERS

Asthma exacerbations consistently increase in prevalence in September, presumably due to a combination of the return to school and the emergence of fall allergens and viral infections. Given the predictability of this increase, the augmentation of therapy with montelukast in anticipation of this increase in risk has been evaluated. While one trial studying the addition of montelukast or a placebo to the usual asthma therapy from September 1 to October 15 among 2- to 14-year-olds demonstrated significant reductions in days with worse asthma symptoms (53% fewer) and unscheduled physician visits (78% fewer),[38] a second trial was unable to identify a clinically relevant effect of the addition of montelukast to

standard therapy just prior to return to school in school-age children.[39] Thus, it is unclear if such a temporary step-up provides consistent protection from the falltime increase in asthma exacerbations.

IMMUNOTHERAPY

The NAEPP/ERP3 guidelines suggest that allergen immunotherapy be considered for patients with persistent asthma for whom there is a clear relationship between symptoms and exposure to the allergens to which the patients are sensitive.[1] A recent meta-analysis and an evidence-based review both concluded that specific immunotherapy is effective in the management of selected patients with allergic asthma,[40,41] particularly those with a sensitization to a single allergen. In contrast, a large placebo-controlled trial evaluating the efficacy of multiallergen immunotherapy for 2 years in asthmatic children did not demonstrate a benefit among children receiving appropriate medical treatment for asthma.[42] A recent trial demonstrated that immunotherapy in monosensitized children with seasonal allergic rhinitis without asthma may prevent the subsequent development of asthma,[43] suggesting that immunotherapy may allow for asthma prevention in children with sensitization to inhalant allergens.

MANAGEMENT OF SEVERE ASTHMA IN CHILDREN

The evaluation and management of children who appear to have asthma that does not respond as expected to the stepwise approach to asthma care involve several considerations, as described in the section Approaches for Children Not Well Controlled with Step 2 (and Above) Therapy, prior to a further escalation of stepwise care. However, should these additional strategies fail to bring asthma under control, any further escalation of care becomes challenging due to the relative paucity of data to guide decision making.

For children aged 0–4 years with severe asthma (i.e., those requiring Step 5 or 6 care), the NAEPP/EPR3 guidelines recommend, based on extrapolation from limited data in older children, the use of high-dose ICS therapy in combination with either a LABA or LTRA, and the addition of oral corticosteroids in the most extreme cases.[1]

Similarly, for children aged 5–11 years with severe asthma, the NAEPP/EPR3 guidelines recommend, based largely on extrapolation from data in older children, the use of high-dose ICS therapy in combination with a LABA as the preferred therapy at Step 5, with ICS + LTRA or ICS + theophylline as alternatives, and the addition of oral corticosteroids to ICS + LABA in those patients requiring Step 6 care.[1]

OMALIZUMAB

The anti-immunoglobulin E (IgE) monoclonal antibody omalizumab is currently not included in the NAEPP/EPR3 guidelines Steps 5 and 6 for children under the age of 12 years,[1] largely due to the lack of U.S. Food and Drug Administration (FDA) approval in this age group. Omalizumab effectively, rapidly, and significantly reduces circulating levels of IgE. Repeated subcutaneous administration of omalizumab has been demonstrated to be safe[44] and effective in permitting a reduction of ICS dosing while preventing asthma exacerbations[45,46] and improving asthma-related quality of life[47] in a placebo-controlled trial involving children aged 6–12 years with moderate to severe persistent allergic asthma receiving ICS. A large trial conducted in inner-city children and adolescents with asthma demonstrated that omalizumab therapy for 60 weeks produced a significant reduction in days with asthma symptoms and risk of exacerbation despite reductions in ICS and LABA use.[48] A recent small trial also demonstrated the ability of omalizumab to permit a reduction in oral corticosteroid dosing in children aged 5–16 years receiving maintenance oral corticosteroids therapy.[49] Omalizumab is currently approved in the United States as an adjunctive therapy for children aged 12 years and older with moderate to severe persistent allergic asthma whose symptoms are inadequately controlled with ICS therapy.

MANAGEMENT OF ASTHMA EXACERBATIONS

Exacerbations are often the dominant manifestation of asthma in young children (i.e., preschool-age), and while exacerbations tend to become less frequent as children mature through adolescence, they remain a major source of morbidity. Viral infections, most notably human rhinoviruses, are the dominant trigger for acute exacerbations in childhood, with allergen-triggered exacerbations occurring less frequently.

An exacerbation may be defined as either moderate or severe,[50] with moderate exacerbations consisting of events that are troublesome to the patient, do not represent the patient's usual day-to-day symptom variation, are not severe, but require prompt modification of treatment. A severe exacerbation is one that requires urgent action in order to prevent a serious outcome, such as asthma-related hospitalization or death.

The development of an exacerbation generally evolves over a period of days, highlighting the importance of recognizing the early changes in asthma status as antecedents to exacerbations. In addition to increases in the typical asthma symptoms such as cough, wheeze, and shortness of breath, other signs and symptoms often precede asthma exacerbations, including the emergence of upper respiratory tract infectious symptoms, behavioral changes, and other nonspecific symptoms.[51,52] Thus, attention should be focused on the occurrence of such factors as warning signs of an impending worsening of asthma.

QUICK RELIEVER MEDICATIONS

Beta$_2$-Adrenergic Agonists

Rapid-acting inhaled beta$_2$-adrenergic receptor agonists produce bronchodilation and serve as the preferred treatment for acute symptoms and exacerbations of asthma. Several different beta$_2$-agonists are currently available, and have comparable efficacy and safety properties.

Anticholinergic Agents

The parasympathetic nervous system contributes to the control of the airway tone. In general, the degree of bronchodilation achieved with anticholinergic agents (such as atropine and ipratropium bromide) is less than that produced by inhaled beta$_2$-agonists. The addition of ipratropium bromide to inhaled beta$_2$-agonists during moderate to severe acute exacerbations of asthma in children presenting in the emergency department decreases the rates of hospitalization[53] and the duration of time in the emergency department,[54] but there is no evidence to support the use of ipratropium in hospitalized patients.

Systemic Corticosteroids

Systemic corticosteroids may be considered as quick-reliever medications due to their efficacy in moderate to severe acute exacerbations of asthma among school-age children. Systemic corticosteroids accelerate the resolution of acute exacerbations of asthma in school-age children, and an emergency department administration of corticosteroids decreases asthma admission rates[55] and shortens the duration of hospitalization. In contrast, recent studies in preschool-age children with recurrent wheezing do not consistently demonstrate a clinical improvement with systemic corticosteroids,[56] and thus their use in wheezing exacerbations in this age group is currently uncertain.[57] The dosing recommendations for acute asthma range from 1 to 2 mg/kg of body weight per day of prednisone, with no significant difference in the efficacy of oral or parenteral corticosteroids in acute asthma,[58] unless the child is unable to tolerate oral medications due to vomiting. The clinically relevant suppression of the HPA axis does not typically occur following short "bursts" of systemic corticosteroids for acute exacerbations of asthma, and tapering of the dose is not required with courses of less than 10–14 days' duration.

MONITORING AND REASSESSMENT

The effective management of children with asthma is an ongoing process, requiring frequent reassessments to determine the degree of asthma control achieved with a treatment regimen. In addition to a general inquiry into parents' and patients' perceptions of the patients' asthma status, several validated tools allow for the longitudinal quantification of asthma control, including the Test for Respiratory and Asthma Control in Kids (TRACK),[59] the Childhood Asthma Control Test (C-ACT),[60,61] and the Asthma Control Questionnaire (ACQ).[62]

The serial examination of the pulmonary function via spirometry is an integral component of asthma monitoring and can generally be performed well on children over 5 years of age, and occasionally on 4-year-old children. Spirometry measures the forced vital capacity (FVC), FEV$_1$, the ratio of

FEV_1/FVC, as well as other measures of airflow including the forced expiratory flow between 25% and 75% of FVC (FEF_{25-75}). The FEV_1 is the most commonly used and reproducible measure of pulmonary function, whereas the FEF_{25-75} demonstrates much more intrapatient variability. Standards are widely available for most spirometric measures and allow for correction based on the patient's age, gender, race, and height. The FEV_1/FVC ratio is an indicator of airflow obstruction and may be more sensitive in identifying airflow abnormalities in asthma than the FEV_1 is, as most children with asthma have an FEV_1 within the normal range, even in the presence of severe disease (see Chapter 6). An effective asthma therapy should lead to an improvement in, and ideally a normalization of, the FEV_1 and the FEV_1/FVC ratio.

An assessment of the level of asthma symptom control, asthma-related morbidity as reflected by activity limitation, and school absences should be an integral component of every asthma visit. The frequency of rescue albuterol use and how frequently a canister of albuterol needs to be refilled due to use of the contents of a canister (200 actuations = 100 doses) are effective surrogate indicators of asthma control. The effect on the clinical course caused when the patient misses a dose (or several doses) of medications often provides a valuable insight into the disease activity.

STEP-DOWN THERAPY

If asthma is well controlled for a period of at least 3 months, consideration should be given to a step-down in therapy.[1] Circumstances that may preclude a step-down even in the setting of well-controlled asthma include the impending exposure to a known trigger, such as the return to school or an upcoming allergen or viral season, which has historically been associated with declines in asthma control. The general approach for step-down is to reduce therapy one step at a time, although very little clinical trial evidence provides guidance as to the best strategy for this approach or how best to identify the patients who are most likely to tolerate a step-down without a deterioration in their asthma control.

STEP-DOWN TO AS-NEEDED ADMINISTRATION OF ICS IN CHILDREN WITH MILD ASTHMA

Attention has recently been directed to the use of ICS therapy on an as-needed basis, with ICS being administered whenever children have asthma symptoms that require SABA rescue therapy. In a trial involving 288 children aged 5–18 years with mild persistent asthma that was demonstrated to be well controlled on low-dose ICS therapy alone (beclomethasone 40 mcg twice daily), the continuation of daily low-dose ICS therapy was superior to the discontinuation of ICS in terms of exacerbations requiring oral corticosteroids, but it was associated with a 1.1 cm reduction in linear growth over the 44-week trial.[63] However, stepping down from daily ICS therapy to an ICS + SABA (beclomethasone 80 mcg whenever albuterol was used) resulted in fewer exacerbations than

did the discontinuation of ICS and was not associated with an adverse effect on linear growth. This study suggests that among school-age children with mild asthma that is well controlled on low-dose ICS, the use of ICS as a rescue medication with albuterol might be an effective step-down strategy as it is more effective than albuterol alone and avoids the ICS-related growth effects seen with daily ICS therapy. Similarly, in a trial involving 276 children aged 1–4 years with frequent wheeze, daily treatment with ICS (beclomethasone 400 mcg twice daily) was superior to as-needed SABA alone in terms of symptom-free days, SABA use, nocturnal awakenings, and time to first oral corticosteroid use.[64] However, there was no statistically significant difference in the outcomes between the as-needed ICS + SABA group (beclomethasone 800 mcg each time albuterol was used) and the daily ICS group.

CONCLUSIONS

The evidence supporting treatment decision making in children with asthma has expanded substantially over the past decade. The optimal management of asthma entails continual reassessment, focusing on the appropriate recognition and classification of the disease severity and the level of control, which will result in the minimization of asthma-related impairment and risk. Using an approach to stepwise care, attention should be paid to the need for a step-up in care in the setting of suboptimal control as well as the potential step-down in care when disease control is achieved and maintained.

REFERENCES

1. National Asthma Education and Prevention Program. Expert Panel Report III: Guidelines for the diagnosis and management of asthma. Bethesda, MD: US Department of Health and Human Services; 2007.
2. Global Initiative for Asthma. Global Strategy for Asthma Management and Prevention, 2011. Available from www.gin-asthma.org.
3. Brand PL, Baraldi E, Bisgaard H, Boner AL, Castro-Rodriguez JA, Custovic A, et al. Definition, assessment and treatment of wheezing disorders in preschool children: An evidence-based approach. *Eur Respir J* 2008; 32:1096–1110.
4. Cope SF, Ungar WJ, Glazier RH. International differences in asthma guidelines for children. *Int Arch Allergy Immunol* 2009; 148:265–278.
5. Ducharme FM, Lemire C, Noya FJ, Davis GM, Alos N, Leblond H, et al. Preemptive use of high-dose fluticasone for virus-induced wheezing in young children. *N Engl J Med* 2009; 360:339–353.
6. Bacharier LB, Phillips BR, Zeiger RS, Szefler SJ, Martinez FD, Lemanske RF Jr., et al. Episodic use of an inhaled corticosteroid or leukotriene receptor antagonist in preschool children with moderate-to-severe intermittent wheezing. *J Allergy Clin Immunol* 2008; 122:1127–1135. e8.
7. Bisgaard H, Hermansen MN, Loland L, Halkjaer LB, Buchvald F. Intermittent inhaled corticosteroids in infants with episodic wheezing. *N Engl J Med* 2006; 354:1998–2005.

8. Guilbert TW, Morgan WJ, Zeiger RS, Mauger DT, Boehmer SJ, Szefler SJ, et al. Long-term inhaled corticosteroids in preschool children at high risk for asthma. *N Engl J Med* 2006; 354:1985–1997.

9. Castro-Rodriguez JA, Rodrigo GJ. Efficacy of inhaled corticosteroids in infants and preschoolers with recurrent wheezing and asthma: A systematic review with meta-analysis. *Pediatrics* 2009; 123:e519–e525.

10. Bisgaard H, Zielen S, Garcia-Garcia ML, Johnston SL, Gilles L, Menten J, et al. Montelukast reduces asthma exacerbations in 2- to 5-year-old children with intermittent asthma. *Am J Respir Crit Care Med* 2005; 171:315–322.

11. Zeiger RS, Mauger D, Bacharier LB, Guilbert TW, Martinez FD, Lemanske RF Jr., et al. Daily or intermittent budesonide in preschool children with recurrent wheezing. *N Engl J Med* 2011; 365:1990–2001.

12. Childhood Asthma Management Program Research Group. Long-term effects of budesonide or nedocromil in children with asthma. *N Engl J Med* 2000; 343:1054–1063.

13. Strunk RC, Weiss ST, Yates KP, Tonascia J, Zeiger RS, Szefler SJ. Mild to moderate asthma affects lung growth in children and adolescents. *J Allergy Clin Immunol* 2006; 118:1040–1047.

14. Skoner DP, Szefler SJ, Welch M, Walton-Bowen K, Cruz-Rivera M, Smith JA. Longitudinal growth in infants and young children treated with budesonide inhalation suspension for persistent asthma. *J Allergy Clin Immunol* 2000; 105:259–268.

15. Bisgaard H, Allen D, Milanowski J, Kalev I, Willits L, Davies P. Twelve-month safety and efficacy of inhaled fluticasone propionate in children aged 1 to 3 years with recurrent wheezing. *Pediatrics* 2004; 113:e87–e94.

16. Baker J, Mellon M, Wald J, Welch M, Cruz-Rivera M, Walton-Bowen K. A multiple-dosing, placebo-controlled study of budesonide inhalation suspension given once or twice daily for treatment of persistent asthma in young children and infants. *Pediatrics* 1999; 103:414–421.

17. Shapiro G, Mendelson L, Kraemer M, Cruz-Rivera M, Walton-Brown K, Smith J. Efficacy and safety of budesonide inhalation suspension (Pulmicort Respules) in young children with inhaled steroid-dependent asthma. *J Allergy Clin Immunol* 1998; 102:789–796.

18. Knorr B, Franchi LM, Bisgaard H, Vermeulen JH, LeSouef P, Santanello N, et al. Montelukast, a leukotriene receptor antagonist, for the treatment of persistent asthma in children aged 2 to 5 years. *Pediatrics* 2001; 108:E48.

19. Hakim F, Vilozni D, Adler A, Livnat G, Tal A, Bentur L. The effect of montelukast on bronchial hyperreactivity in preschool children. *Chest* 2007; 131:180–186.

20. Moeller A, Lehmann A, Knauer N, Albisetti M, Rochat M, Johannes W. Effects of montelukast on subjective and objective outcome measures in preschool asthmatic children. *Pediatr Pulmonol* 2008; 43:179–186.

21. Knorr B, Matz J, Bernstein JA, Nguyen H, Seidenberg BC, Reiss TF, et al. Montelukast for chronic asthma in 6- to 14-year-old children: A randomized, double-blind trial. Pediatric Montelukast Study Group. *JAMA* 1998; 279:1181–1186.

22. Kemp JP, Dockhorn RJ, Shapiro GG, Nguyen HH, Reiss TF, Seidenberg BC, et al. Montelukast once daily inhibits exercise-induced bronchoconstriction in 6- to 14-year-old children with asthma. *J Pediatr* 1998; 133:424–428.

23. Bisgaard H, Skoner D, Boza ML, Tozzi CA, Newcomb K, Reiss TF, et al. Safety and tolerability of montelukast in placebo-controlled pediatric studies and their open-label extensions. *Pediatr Pulmonol* 2009; 44:568–579.

24. Philip G, Hustad CM, Malice MP, Noonan G, Ezekowitz A, Reiss TF, et al. Analysis of behavior-related adverse experiences in clinical trials of montelukast. *J Allergy Clin Immunol* 2009; 124:699–706. e8.

25. Szefler SJ, Phillips BR, Martinez FD, Chinchilli VM, Lemanske RF, Strunk RC, et al. Characterization of within-subject responses to fluticasone and montelukast in childhood asthma. *J Allergy Clin Immunol* 2005; 115:233–242.

26. Zeiger RS, Szefler SJ, Phillips BR, Schatz M, Martinez FD, Chinchilli VM, et al. Response profiles to fluticasone and montelukast in mild-to-moderate persistent childhood asthma. *J Allergy Clin Immunol* 2006; 117:45–52.

27. Garcia Garcia ML, Wahn U, Gilles L, Swern A, Tozzi CA, Polos P. Montelukast, compared with fluticasone, for control of asthma among 6- to 14-year-old patients with mild asthma: The MOSAIC study. *Pediatrics* 2005; 116:360–369.

28. Ostrom NK, Decotiis BA, Lincourt WR, Edwards LD, Hanson KM, Carranza Rosenzweig JR, et al. Comparative efficacy and safety of low-dose fluticasone propionate and montelukast in children with persistent asthma. *J Pediatr* 2005; 147:213–220.

29. Sorkness CA, Lemanske RF Jr., Mauger DT, Boehmer SJ, Chinchilli VM, Martinez FD, et al. Long-term comparison of 3 controller regimens for mild-moderate persistent childhood asthma: The pediatric asthma controller trial. *J Allergy Clin Immunol* 2007; 119:64–72.

30. Castro-Rodriguez JA, Rodrigo GJ. The role of inhaled corticosteroids and montelukast in children with mild-moderate asthma: Results of a systematic review with meta-analysis. *Arch Dis Child* 2010; 95:365–370.

31. Makela MJ, Malmberg LP, Csonka P, Klemola T, Kajosaari M, Pelkonen AS. Salmeterol and fluticasone in young children with multiple-trigger wheeze. *Ann Allergy Asthma Immunol* 2012; 109:65–70.

32. Verberne AA, Frost C, Duiverman EJ, Grol MH, Kerrebijn KF. Addition of salmeterol versus doubling the dose of beclomethasone in children with asthma. The Dutch Asthma Study Group. *Am J Respir Crit Care Med* 1998; 158:213–219.

33. Vaessen-Verberne AA, van den Berg NJ, van Nierop JC, Brackel HJ, Gerrits GP, Hop WC, et al. Combination therapy salmeterol/fluticasone versus doubling dose of fluticasone in children with asthma. *Am J Respir Crit Care Med* 2010; 182:1221–1227.

34. Ducharme FM, Ni Chroinin M, Greenstone I, Lasserson TJ. Addition of long-acting beta2-agonists to inhaled corticosteroids versus same dose inhaled corticosteroids for chronic asthma in adults and children. *Cochrane Database Syst Rev* 2010; 5:CD005535.

35. Ducharme FM, Ni Chroinin M, Greenstone I, Lasserson TJ. Addition of long-acting beta2-agonists to inhaled steroids versus higher dose inhaled steroids in adults and children with persistent asthma. *Cochrane Database Syst Rev* 2010; 14:CD005533.

36. Lemanske RF Jr., Mauger DT, Sorkness CA, Jackson DJ, Boehmer SJ, Martinez FD, et al. Step-up therapy for children with uncontrolled asthma receiving inhaled corticosteroids. *N Engl J Med* 2010; 362:975–985.

37. McMahon AW, Levenson MS, McEvoy BW, Mosholder AD, Murphy D. Age and risks of FDA-approved long-acting beta(2)-adrenergic receptor agonists. *Pediatrics* 2011; 128:e1147–e1154.

38. Johnston NW, Mandhane PJ, Dai J, Duncan JM, Greene JM, Lambert K, et al. Attenuation of the September epidemic of asthma exacerbations in children: A randomized, controlled trial of montelukast added to usual therapy. *Pediatrics* 2007; 120:e702–e712.

39. Weiss KB, Gern JE, Johnston NW, Sears MR, Jones CA, Jia G, et al. The back to school asthma study: The effect of montelukast on asthma burden when initiated prophylactically at the start of the school year. *Ann Allergy Asthma Immunol* 2010; 105:174–181.

40. Abramson MJ, Puy RM, Weiner JM. Injection allergen immunotherapy for asthma. *Cochrane Database Syst Rev* 2010; 4:CD001186.

41. Larenas-Linnemann DE, Pietropaolo-Cienfuegos DR, Calderon MA. Evidence of effect of subcutaneous immunotherapy in children: Complete and updated review from 2006 onward. *Ann Allergy Asthma Immunol* 2011; 107:407–416. e11.

42. Adkinson NF Jr., Eggleston PA, Eney D, Goldstein EO, Schuberth KC, Bacon JR, et al. A controlled trial of immunotherapy for asthma in allergic children. *N Engl J Med* 1997; 336:324–331.

43. Jacobsen L, Niggemann B, Dreborg S, Ferdousi HA, Halken S, Host A, et al. Specific immunotherapy has long-term preventive effect of seasonal and perennial asthma: 10-year follow-up on the PAT study. *Allergy* 2007; 62:943–948.

44. Berger W, Gupta N, McAlary M, Fowler-Taylor A. Evaluation of long-term safety of the anti-IgE antibody, omalizumab, in children with allergic asthma. *Ann Allergy Asthma Immunol* 2003; 91:182–188.

45. Milgrom H, Berger W, Nayak A, Gupta N, Pollard S, McAlary M, et al. Treatment of childhood asthma with anti-immunoglobulin E antibody (omalizumab). *Pediatrics* 2001; 108:E36.

46. Lanier B, Bridges T, Kulus M, Taylor AF, Berhane I, Vidaurre CF. Omalizumab for the treatment of exacerbations in children with inadequately controlled allergic (IgE-mediated) asthma. *J Allergy Clin Immunol* 2009; 124:1210–1216.

47. Lemanske RF Jr., Nayak A, McAlary M, Everhard F, Fowler-Taylor A, Gupta N. Omalizumab improves asthma-related quality of life in children with allergic asthma. *Pediatrics* 2002; 110:e55.

48. Busse WW, Morgan WJ, Gergen PJ, Mitchell HE, Gern JE, Liu AH, et al. Randomized trial of omalizumab (anti-IgE) for asthma in inner-city children. *N Engl J Med* 2011; 364:1005–1015.

49. Brodlie M, McKean MC, Moss S, Spencer DA. The oral corticosteroid-sparing effect of omalizumab in children with severe asthma. *Arch Dis Child* 2012; 97:604–609.

50. Reddel HK, Taylor DR, Bateman ED, Boulet LP, Boushey HA, Busse WW, et al. An official American Thoracic Society/European Respiratory Society statement: Asthma control and exacerbations: Standardizing endpoints for clinical asthma trials and clinical practice. *Am J Respir Crit Care Med* 2009; 180:59–99.

51. Rivera-Spoljaric K, Jaenicke M, Sridhar S, Krauss MJ, Garbutt JM, Bacharier LB, et al. Caregivers report a wide variety of early signs and symptoms of impending asthma exacerbations that are not different between preschool and school-aged children. *J Allergy Clin Immunol* 2011; 128:1109–1111. e1-5.

52. Garbutt J, Highstein G, Nelson KA, Rivera-Spoljaric K, Strunk R. Detection and home management of worsening asthma symptoms. *Ann Allergy Asthma Immunol* 2009; 103:469–473.

53. Qureshi F, Pestian J, Davis P, Zaritsky A. Effect of nebulized ipratropium on the hospitalization rates of children with asthma. *N Engl J Med* 1998; 339:1030–1035.

54. Zorc JJ, Pusic MV, Ogborn CJ, Lebet R, Duggan AK. Ipratropium bromide added to asthma treatment in the pediatric emergency department. *Pediatrics* 1999; 103:748–752.

55. Scarfone RJ, Fuchs SM, Nager AL, Shane SA. Controlled trial of oral prednisone in the emergency department treatment of children with acute asthma. *Pediatrics* 1993; 92:513–518.

56. Panickar J, Lakhanpaul M, Lambert PC, Kenia P, Stephenson T, Smyth A, et al. Oral prednisolone for preschool children with acute virus-induced wheezing. *N Engl J Med* 2009; 360:329–338.

57. Guilbert TW, Bacharier LB. Controversies in the treatment of the acutely wheezing infant. *Am J Respir Crit Care Med* 2011; 183:1284–1285.

58. Becker JM, Arora A, Scarfone RJ, Spector ND, Fontana-Penn ME, Gracely E, et al. Oral versus intravenous corticosteroids in children hospitalized with asthma. *J Allergy Clin Immunol* 1999; 103:586–590.

59. Murphy KR, Zeiger RS, Kosinski M, Chipps B, Mellon M, Schatz M, et al. Test for respiratory and asthma control in kids (TRACK): A caregiver-completed questionnaire for preschool-aged children. *J Allergy Clin Immunol* 2009; 123:833–839. e9.

60. Liu AH, Zeiger R, Sorkness C, Mahr T, Ostrom N, Burgess S, et al. Development and cross-sectional validation of the childhood asthma control test. *J Allergy Clin Immunol* 2007; 119:817–825.

61. Liu AH, Zeiger RS, Sorkness CA, Ostrom NK, Chipps BE, Rosa K, et al. The childhood asthma control test: Retrospective determination and clinical validation of a cut point to identify children with very poorly controlled asthma. *J Allergy Clin Immunol* 2010; 126:267–273. 73 e1.

62. Juniper EF, O'Byrne PM, Guyatt GH, Ferrie PJ, King DR. Development and validation of a questionnaire to measure asthma control. *Eur Respir J* 1999; 14:902–907.

63. Martinez FD, Chinchilli VM, Morgan WJ, Boehmer SJ, Lemanske RF Jr., Mauger DT, et al. Use of beclomethasone dipropionate as rescue treatment for children with mild persistent asthma (TREXA): A randomised, double-blind, placebo-controlled trial. *Lancet* 2011; 377:650–657.

64. Papi A, Nicolini G, Baraldi E, Boner AL, Cutrera R, Rossi GA, et al. Regular vs prn nebulized treatment in wheeze preschool children. *Allergy* 2009; 64:1463–1471.

18 Management of Adolescent Asthma

Gina T. Cosia, Beverley J. Sheares, and Jean-Marie Bruzzese

CONTENTS

CASE PRESENTATION

Jessica is a 15-year-old female who was diagnosed with asthma at 5 years of age. She has never had a severe asthma exacerbation or been hospitalized. Her mother, Anna, had consistently administered her daughter's daily inhaled corticosteroid. Anna was vigilant about monitoring Jessica's symptoms until a year ago when Jessica started high school.

Jessica has now started her sophomore year and has just made the basketball team. She leaves for school very early in the morning and often misses dinner due to basketball practice. On the weekends, she spends time with her friends. Because Jessica has been a straight-A student, her mother believes that she is responsibly balancing school with extracurricular activities. She assumes that Jessica is also taking her asthma medications and is symptom-free as she is able to participate in sports and has not complained of symptoms.

One day, Anna receives a call from Jessica's basketball coach telling her that Jessica is in an ambulance en route to the local emergency department. He reports that while at practice, Jessica started coughing, became short of breath, and could barely speak. He also notes that Jessica has been coughing during practice since she had a cold 2 weeks

previously and has had wheezing and shortness of breath on occasion, but she rests and the symptoms abate. At the emergency department, Jessica is evaluated and treated for status asthmaticus. She is admitted to the pediatric intensive care unit for further management.

When her condition improves, after repeated questioning by the medical team, she casually acknowledges that with her long days and rigorous schedule, she often forgets to take her controller medication. Since she was feeling well and was able to succeed at basketball, she did not think much about missing the doses. In retrospect, Jessica recalls that she had noticed some increased nighttime cough, as well as cough, chest tightness, and shortness of breath during basketball practice, but she did not link this to her asthma. She also reported that while she has never smoked cigarettes, her new group of friends smoke after practice. Although the smoke caused her to cough, she was too embarrassed to leave for fear of being teased and left out. During the time when she realized she needed albuterol, she was too embarrassed to take it in the presence of her peers.

Jessica's condition improves and she is ready for discharge. Her mother threatens to resume responsibility for administering Jessica's asthma medications; however, Jessica protests that she is too old to have her mother give her medicine like she is a child. Both Jessica and her mother are left with many questions on how to manage Jessica's asthma at this stage in her development.

INTRODUCTION

The successful, ongoing treatment of asthma in adolescents presents numerous challenges because adolescence is a time of profound change. It is marked by the development of new cognitive skills, independent decision making, and increased peer pressure. Delivering effective care to reduce asthma morbidity and mortality in adolescence, and improve the quality of life and health of adolescents with asthma requires clinicians to have knowledge of the state-of-the-art asthma care as well as an understanding of the role that cognitive and psychosocial development plays in asthma management in this age group. To that end, this chapter reviews the epidemiology and natural history of asthma related to adolescents, discusses appropriate clinical management and examines how the developmental features of adolescence affect self-management and the treatment of asthma.

EPIDEMIOLOGY

Adolescence is defined as individuals aged 11–21 years and is divided into three age groups: (1) early adolescents (11–14 years), (2) middle adolescents (15–17 years), and (3) late adolescents (18–21 years).[1] In this chapter, we will focus on the early and middle adolescent age groups because their development is distinctly different from younger children and from older adolescents, whose behavior more closely resembles adults.

Compared with children aged 0–10 years, early and middle adolescents have a higher asthma prevalence,[2] ranging from 12% to 17%.[3,4] They also experience more frequent[5] and more severe[6] exacerbations, and have higher asthma-related mortality rates.[2] In fact, among youth, asthma-related deaths occur most frequently during the teenage years, and a history of prior, severe exacerbations is a significant risk factor for fatal asthma.[7] During early to mid-adolescence, the childhood trend that boys have higher rates of asthma than girls is reversed with female adolescents having higher asthma rates.[8]

Despite this increased morbidity and mortality, adolescents have fewer emergency department visits and hospitalizations for asthma compared with their younger counterparts[2]; they also have fewer ambulatory care visits each year and, as a result, they receive less ongoing care where their symptoms and lung function can be monitored.[9] This suggests that even in the face of significant complications from asthma, including persistent symptoms and severe exacerbations, patients in this age group may not seek or receive the care they need, which may be because they underrecognize their symptoms and their relationship to worsening asthma,[10] or because they underestimate the severity of their disease.[11,12]

NATURAL HISTORY OF ASTHMA IN ADOLESCENCE

The commonly held notion that asthma "remits in adolescence" is based on anecdotal clinical experience rather than the evidence from longitudinal cohort studies of children with asthma. While there are few studies documenting the natural history of asthma from childhood through adolescence,[13–15] these studies show that children with asthma are at increased risk for the persistence of respiratory symptoms into adulthood. Because the hormonal, behavioral, and physical changes that occur during adolescence can affect the course of asthma, it is important to delineate the risk factors associated with asthma symptoms that persist as children get older.

In a longitudinal birth cohort of children enrolled in the Tucson Children's Respiratory Study, investigators demonstrated that 60% of children with asthma, defined as the presence of frequent or continuous wheezing, prior to puberty, continued to experience wheezing episodes during early adolescence, and this persistence of the symptoms was due to several prepubertal risk factors, including an elevated body mass index; the early onset of puberty (characterized by voice change in males and menarche in females); and a physician diagnosis of sinusitis prior to the onset of puberty, and allergic sensitization to *Alternaria*.[13] Other studies have reported similar factors.[14–16]

In a longitudinal, population-based cohort study of children, who were studied at age 6–8 years and again at age 14–16 years, Withers et al. showed that greater than 50% of children with wheeze and more than one-third with cough at age 6–8 years continued to have these symptoms into their teenage years.[15] They demonstrated that a history of atopy was independently associated with persistent asthma symptoms. Additionally, maternal asthma was associated with wheeze that persisted into adolescence for females, but not males. The authors proposed that females may inherit genes associated with wheeze, and these genes may be expressed in later adolescence. This theory could explain the increased rate of asthma among female adolescents.

Other significant risk factors that Withers et al. identified to explain the persistence of respiratory symptoms into adolescence were active and passive smoking, particularly among males.[15] Regular, active smoking was strongly associated with persistent wheeze. The investigators suggest that the adverse effect of passive smoking in early life on the small caliber airways of males and the continued exposure of the airways through active smoking result in persistent cough and late-onset wheeze.[15]

Low socioeconomic class has also been found to be associated with the persistence of asthma symptoms into adolescence.[17] Also, a negative association has been found between the number of children in a household and wheeze that persists into adolescence.[18] The mechanism responsible for this relationship is thought to be an immunologically mediated protective effect of increased exposure to viral infections in early childhood, which may prevent the proliferation of T-helper type 2 (Th2) cells.[18]

When determining if asthma is in remission in an adolescent patient, the absence of asthma symptoms or the lack of need for asthma medications may not be sufficient determinants of the patient's asthma status.[7] During periods of clinical remission characterized by no asthma symptoms and no use of inhaled corticosteroids, bronchial hyperresponsiveness was tested and subjects were found to have subclinical but significant airway obstruction and airway inflammation. This suggests that some individuals who seem to be free of asthma symptoms in fact have persistent asthma.[19] Therefore, complete remission includes an absence of asthma symptoms and bronchial hyperresponsiveness, not needing to use inhaled corticosteroids, and normal lung function.

GUIDELINES FOR THE TREATMENT OF ADOLESCENT ASTHMA

The most recent guidelines from the Expert Panel Report 3 (EPR-3) in the United States[20] and the International Global Initiative for Asthma[21] guidelines emphasize the need to achieve control of asthma symptoms, thereby reducing impairment and risk for future morbidity—all goals that are most pertinent to the adolescent patient. These guidelines provide tools to help clinicians assess the patient's level of asthma severity prior to the start of treatment, as well as the patient's level of asthma control once on medications. Figures 18.1 and 18.2 provide the EPR-3 criteria to assess the severity and control of asthma, respectively, in adolescents.

		Classification of Asthma Severity ≥ 12 Years of Age			
			Persistent		
Components of Severity		**Intermittent**	**Mild**	**Moderate**	**Severe**
Impairment	Symptoms	≤ 2 days/week	> 2 days/week but not daily	Daily	Throughout the day
Normal FEV₁/FVC:	Nighttime awakenings	≤ 2 ×/month	3–4 ×/month	> 1 ×/week but not nightly	Often 7 ×/week
8–19 years 85%					
20–39 years 80%	Short-acting beta₂-adrenergic agonist use for symptom control (not prevention of EIB)	≤ 2 days/week	> 2 days/week but not daily, and not more than 1 × on any day	Daily	Several times per day
40–59 years 75%					
60–80 years 70%					
	Interference with normal activity	None	Minor limitation	Some limitation	Extremely limited
	Lung function	• Normal FEV₁ between exacerbations • FEV₁ > 80% predicted • FEV₁/FVC normal	• FEV₁ > 80% predicted • FEV₁/FVC normal	• FEV₁ > 60% but < 80% predicted • FEV₁/FVC reduced 5%	• FEV₁ < 60% predicted • FEV₁/FVC reduced > 5%
Risk	Exacerbations requiring oral systemic corticosteroids	0–1/year (see note)	≥ 2/year (see note) ──────────────→		
		←──────── Consider severity and interval since last exacerbation. ────────→			
		Frequency and severity may fluctuate over time for patients in any severity category.			
		Relative annual risk of exacerbations may be related to FEV₁.			
Recommended step for initiating treatment		Step 1	Step 2	Step 3	Step 4 or 5
					and consider short course of oral systemic corticosteriods
(See figure 18.3 for treatment steps.)		In 2–6 weeks, evaluate level of asthma control that is achieved and adjust therapy accordingly.			

FIGURE 18.1 Classifying asthma severity and initiating treatment in youths ≥12 years of age and adults. (From National Heart, Lung, and Blood Institute; National Institutes of Health; U.S. Department of Health and Human Services.) Abbreviation: FEV₁, forced expiratory volume in 1 second; FVC, forced vital capacity; ICU, intensive care unit. *Notes:* The stepwise approach is meant to assist, not replace, the clinical decision making required to meet individual patient needs. Level of severity is determined by assessment of both impairment and risk. Assess impairment domain by patient's/caregiver's recall of previous 2–4 weeks and spirometry. Assign severity to the most severe category in which any feature occurs. At present, there are inadequate data to correspond frequencies of exacerbations with different levels of asthma severity. In general, more frequent and intense exacerbations (e.g., requiring urgent, unscheduled care, hospitalization, or ICU admission) indicate greater underlying disease severity. For treatment purposes, patients who had ≥2 exacerbations requiring oral systemic corticosteroids in the past year may be considered the same as patients who have persistent asthma, even in the absence of impairment levels consistent with persistent asthma.

As detailed in Figure 18.2, the two main domains of asthma control are impairment and risk. The prevention of chronic, recurrent symptoms, the reduction in beta-agonist use, the maintenance of normal or near normal lung function, the resumption or maintenance of activities of daily living (including exercise), and meeting the patient's and his or her family's expectations and satisfaction with care are the goals of reducing the patient's impairment from asthma. Reducing

the risk for future adverse effects includes the prevention of recurrent exacerbations and a reduction in the need for emergency department visits and hospitalizations, the prevention of the loss of lung function, and the provision of an optimal medication regimen with minimal adverse effects that the patient can follow.[20]

A stepwise approach to medications is recommended in order to get asthma symptoms under control (see Figure 18.3

	Components of Control	Classification of Asthma Control (≥ 2 Years of Age)		
		Well Controlled	Not Well Controlled	Very Poorly Controlled
Impairment	Symptoms	≤ 2 days/week	> 2 days/week	Throughout the day
	Nighttime awakenings	≤ 2×/month	1–3×/week	≥ 4×/week
	Interference with normal activity	None	Some limitation	Extremely limited
	Short-acting beta$_2$-adrenergic agonist use for symptom control (not prevention of EIB)	≤ 2 days/week	> 2 days/week	Several times per day
	FEV$_1$ or peak flow	> 80% predicted/ personal best	60%–80% predicted/ personal best	< 60% predicted/ personal best
	Validated questionnaires			
	ATAQ	0	1–2	3–4
	ACQ	≤ 0.75*	≥ 1.5	N/A
	ACT	≥ 20	16–19	≤ 15
Risk	Exacerbations requiring oral systemic corticosteroids	0–1/year	≥ 2/year (see note)	
		Consider severity and interval since last exacerbation		
	Progressive loss of lung function	Evaluation requires long-term follow up care		
	Treatment-related adverse effects	Medication side effects can vary in intensity from none to very troublesome and worrisome. The level of intensity does not correlate to specific levels of control but should be considered in the overall assessment of risk.		
Recommended action for treatment (See figure 18.3 for treatment steps.)		• Maintain current step • Regular follow ups every 1–6 months to maintain control • Consider step down if well controlled for at least 3 months	• Step up 1 step and • Reevaluate in 2–6 weeks • For side effects, consider alternative treatment options	• Consider short course of oral systemic corticosteroids • Step up 1–2 steps, and • Reevaluate in 2 weeks • For side effects, consider alternative treatment options

FIGURE 18.2 Assessing asthma control and adjusting therapy in youths ≥12 years of age and adults. (From National Heart, Lung, and Blood Institute; National Institutes of Health; U.S. Department of Health and Human Services.) *ACQ values of 0.76–1.4 are indeterminate regarding well-controlled asthma. Abbreviation: EIB, exercise-induced bronchospasm; ICU, intensive care unit. *Notes:* The stepwise approach is meant to assist, not replace, the clinical decision making required to meet individual patient needs. The level of control is based on the most severe impairment or risk category. Assess impairment domain by patient's recall of previous 2–4 weeks and by spirometry/ or peak flow measures. Symptom assessment for longer periods should reflect a global assessment, such as inquiring whether the patient's asthma is better or worse since the last visit. At present, there are inadequate data to correspond frequencies of exacerbations with different levels of asthma control. In general, more frequent and intense exacerbations (e.g., requiring urgent, unscheduled care, hospitalization, or ICU admission) indicate poorer disease control. For treatment purposes, patients who had ≥2 exacerbations requiring oral systemic corticosteroids in the past year may be considered the same as patients who have not-well-controlled asthma, even in the absence of impairment levels consistent with not-well-controlled asthma. Validated Questionnaires for the impairment domain (the questionnaires do not assess lung function or the risk domain). ATAQ = Asthma Therapy Assessment Questionnaire© (See sample in "Component 1: Measures of Asthma Assessment and Monitoring."); ACQ = Asthma Control Questionnaire© (user package may be obtained at www.qoltech.co.uk or juniper@qoltech.co.uk); ACT = Asthma Control Test™ (See sample in "Component 1: Measures of Asthma Assessment and Monitoring."). Minimal Important Difference: 1.0 for the ATAQ; 0.5 for the ACQ; not determined for the ACT. Before step up in therapy: Review adherence to medication, inhaler technique, environmental control, and comorbid conditions. If an alternative treatment option was used in a step, discontinue and use the preferred treatment for that step.

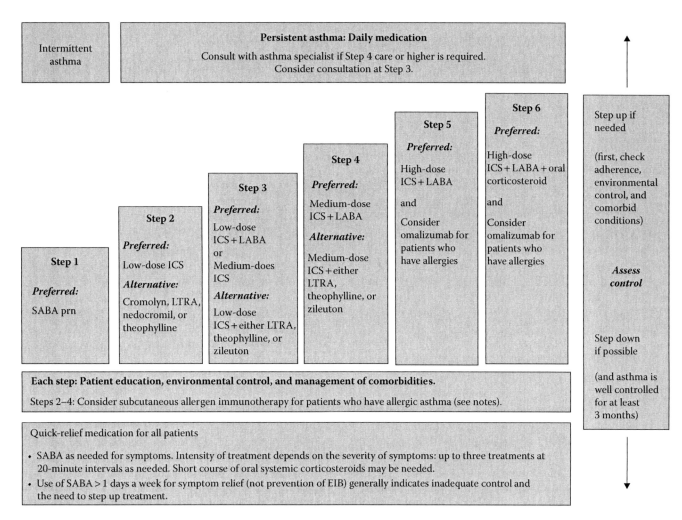

FIGURE 18.3 Stepwise approach for managing asthma in youths ≥12 years of age and adults. (From National Heart, Lung, and Blood Institute; National Institutes of Health; U.S. Department of Health and Human Services.) Abbreviation: EIB, exercise-induced bronchospasm; ICS, inhaled corticosteroid; LABA, long-acting inhaled beta$_2$-agonist; LTRA, leukotriene receptor antagonist; SABA, inhaled short-acting beta$_2$-adrenergic agonist. Alphabetical order is used when more than one treatment option is listed within either preferred or alternative therapy. *Notes:* The stepwise approach is meant to assist, not replace, the clinical decision making required to meet individual patient needs. If alternative treatment is used and response is inadequate, discontinue it and use the preferred treatment before stepping up. Zileuton is a less desirable alternative due to limited studies as adjunctive therapy and the need to monitor liver function. Theophylline requires monitoring of serum concentration levels. In Step 6, before oral systemic corticosteroids are introduced, a trial of high-dose ICS + LABA + either LTRA, theophylline, or zileuton may be considered, although this approach has not been studied in clinical trials. Steps 1, 2, and 3 preferred therapies are based on Evidence A; Step 3 alternative therapy is based on Evidence A for LTRA, Evidence B for theophylline, and Evidence D for zileuton. Step 4 preferred therapy is based on Evidence B, and alternative therapy is based on Evidence B for LTRA and theophylline and Evidence D for zileuton. Step 5 preferred therapy is based on Evidence B. Step 6 preferred therapy is based on (EPR-2 1997) and Evidence B for omalizumab. Immunotherapy for steps 2–4 is based on Evidence B for house-dust mites, animal danders, and pollens; evidence is weak or lacking for molds and cockroaches. Evidence is strongest for immunotherapy with single allergens. The role of allergy in asthma is greater in children than in adults. Clinicians who administer immunotherapy or omalizumab should be prepared and equipped to identify and treat anaphylaxis that may occur.

for a sample stepwise plan).[20] The type, amount, and frequency of medications are determined by the level of asthma severity. The level of severity provides a guide for the initiation of therapy in a patient who is not currently taking long-term controller medications. A key approach to reducing asthma symptoms is to select a medication regimen corresponding to the highest level of asthma severity for the patient, and once their asthma symptoms, lung function, and activity levels are optimized, step down the therapy to the least amount of

medicine required to maintain adequate asthma control and to reduce medication side effects. Once the patient is taking long-term controller medications, the response to the therapy and the control of the symptoms should guide the clinician's decision making regarding which step of care is appropriate. Close monitoring is essential to ensure that asthma control is achieved. Lung function monitoring is an invaluable tool in the adolescent population when symptoms may be unrecognized and underreported. It is also useful for monitoring disease progression over time, and for monitoring the response and adherence to medications.[20,21] As studies show that adolescents with asthma demonstrate a tendency toward underperception of their symptoms and inaccurate perception of asthma control,[12] objective measures of lung function are helpful.

It is recommended that patients receive a written asthma action plan that details the day-to-day management of their asthma, how to recognize and respond to specific symptoms, and when to seek medical care.[20,21] Specific instructions for the administration of medications, the management of exercise-induced symptoms, and the identification and avoidance of specific triggers should be included in the plan and discussed with the adolescent,[10] and a copy should be provided to the patient's school nurse.[20,21]

The adolescent patient should be directly involved in the formulation of the asthma treatment plan in establishing goals for therapy, and the plan should be realistic and achievable. To accomplish these goals, it is recommended that the adolescent meet with the clinician without the parents present at the beginning of the visit. This allows adolescent patients to assume more control and take more responsibility for their asthma management. The parents should be brought in at the end of the visit to review the plan together so that they can support the patient's efforts. The plan should encompass goals that personally benefit the adolescent, such as looking and feeling better (self-image), fully participating in physical activities and organized sports, and reducing symptoms when around friends (peer acceptance). These types of rewards are important to adolescent patients, and achieving asthma control provides positive feedback that reinforces their efforts.

ADOLESCENTS WHO DO NOT RESPOND TO THERAPY

Asthma is characterised by obstruction, hyperresponsiveness, and inflammation of the airways that is at least partially reversible. The symptoms may occur episodically. Additionally, alternative diagnoses should be excluded. Although patients with asthma present in different ways, most share common clinical and historical features that support the diagnosis. The use of lung function measurements, bronchial challenges, exercise challenges, and allergy skin tests to support the diagnosis is helpful, and in some cases it is necessary. Adolescent patients often describe symptoms of chest tightness with colds, chest congestion, and bronchitis. The symptoms occur more often at night and in the early morning hours, and improve throughout the day.[11] However, because many adolescents either deny their symptoms, or they underestimate or are unaware of the severity of their symptoms, the respiratory problem may not be diagnosed or, if it is diagnosed, it may be undertreated.[7]

For some adolescents, their history, clinical findings, response to therapy, and ancillary test results are inconsistent with a diagnosis of asthma. In these cases, alternative diagnoses should be considered, including cystic fibrosis, primary ciliary dyskinesia, immunodeficiency, and congenital heart disease.[11] Special attention should be given to vocal cord dysfunction (VCD) and habit-cough syndrome in this population.

VCD is a condition characterized by paradoxical closure of the vocal cords that can result in wheezing and shortness of breath during the respiratory cycle,[22] and can be mistaken for asthma or may coexist with it. It is more common in adolescent females and has been seen in elite athletes.[23,24] It is sometimes associated with social stressors, such as anxiety associated with participating in high-performance or competitive sports.[24] Patients with VCD exhibit loud wheezing over the trachea, they often have supraglottic retractions and complain of chest tightness. Despite the wheezing, patients with VCD have a poor response to bronchodilators and their oxygen saturations are usually normal.[11] Diagnostic studies during an acute episode include: (1) spirometry, which may demonstrate a flat inspiratory loop of the flow volume curve; and (2) flexible laryngoscopy, which may demonstrate adduction of the vocal cords during phonation. These findings are frequently absent when patients are asymptomatic.[11] The treatment of VCD focuses on the relaxation of the vocal cords, which can be taught by a speech pathologist or a psychologist with training in behavior modification. The accurate diagnosis and treatment of VCD can reduce morbidity, prevent the inappropriate use of inhaled corticosteroids, and improve patients' quality of life.[23]

Another disorder that is commonly mistaken for asthma in adolescents is habit-cough syndrome.[25] A habit cough usually begins during an upper respiratory illness, and persists after the acute illness has resolved. The cough in this syndrome is distinctive in that it is generally loud, barky, repetitive, abrasive, and attracts considerable attention. It is highly disruptive to both patients and families. The characteristic finding in habit-cough syndrome is the cessation of the cough during sleep as well as when patients believe that they are not under observation, which helps to differentiate habit-cough syndrome from other etiologies.[11,25] Appropriate behavioral intervention is the treatment of choice and includes suggestion therapy,[25] self-hypnosis,[26] and using a tightly wrapped bedsheet around the patient's chest combined with suggestion therapy.[27] These treatments distract the patient from the cough, and serve to reassure the patient that he or she can break the coughing cycle.

GENDER DIFFERENCES IN ASTHMA SELF-MANAGEMENT

Gender differences have been observed in two groups of urban, early adolescents, with males more likely to engage in asthma prevention.[28,29] Among Latino and African American urban youth aged 11–14 years, males took more steps than females to prevent having asthma symptoms, including using controller medications.[28] A similar finding was demonstrated in a sample of early adolescent African Americans from Detroit, of which males were more likely to take preventative medications, and were more comfortable doing so in the presence of their peers.[29] As clinicians teach adolescents about asthma management, it may be useful to consider these gender differences. While females are more likely to employ social skills that focus on communal goals, incorporating cooperation and relationship enhancement with their peers,[30] this does not necessarily translate into better self-management.

ADOLESCENT ASTHMA MANAGEMENT: DEVELOPMENTAL CONSIDERATIONS

The developmental changes that define adolescence present unique opportunities as well as challenges to asthma management. Clinicians should consider these developmental changes when guiding the adolescent through asthma self-management. In this section, we focus on cognitive development, expansion of domain knowledge, peer relations, autonomy, risk-taking behavior, identity development, as well as the process of transitioning responsibility from parents to patients.

COGNITIVE DEVELOPMENT

Abstract Thinking

Over time, adolescents develop formal operational thinking, which encompasses the skills of abstract thinking, logical reasoning, and problem solving.[31] Unlike children, who cannot think beyond the observable, adolescents can think abstractly, reflect upon their thoughts, and develop solutions accordingly. The hallmarks of asthma are chronic airway inflammation and bronchoconstriction. With more sophisticated thinking, adolescents are able to understand inflammation, something that they cannot necessarily see or feel. They can also begin to link the sensation of chest tightness to the concept of airway constriction. Moreover, they can differentiate between rescue medications and daily anti-inflammatory medications, and understand the role of each. Although early adolescents may not be ready to assume responsibility for taking daily medication,[30] clinicians should begin to teach them about the pathophysiology of asthma and how bronchodilators and anti-inflammatory medications work.

Integration of Past, Present, and Future

Adolescents develop the ability to integrate the past, the present, and the future,[32] which enables them to reflect on current and prior beliefs and memories. As a result, they can understand the concept of chronicity as it relates to asthma, recognizing that asthma is a disorder that they may continue to experience in the future. When placed in the context of asthma treatment, this insight may help them to work with clinicians to develop long-term goals for the prevention of asthma symptoms. As adolescents experience the physical limitations caused by uncontrolled asthma, they may recognize that the prevention of these limitations may lead to

physical well-being and better performance now as well as in the future. The perspective of asthma as a chronic disease that may persist into the future but can be currently controlled may promote the avoidance of specific triggers.

Decision-Making Skills

A greater working memory capacity and the ability to employ more problem-solving strategies[33] are keys to self-management in asthma. An improved working memory means, in part, that adolescents can consider multiple factors simultaneously and act accordingly. Together, these cognitive gains lead to more refined decision-making skills, enabling them to assess and respond to symptoms and situations that vary over time. Adolescents are able to understand and use treatment plans that require stepping up or stepping down medications in response to changes in symptoms, peak flow, or exposure to specific triggers.[34] Similarly, decision-making skills are necessary to help adolescents negotiate social situations that could impair their health. For example, when in the presence of peers who are smoking or when faced with the pressure to smoke actively, adolescents with asthma must weigh the social benefits of staying in the situation knowing that the smoke will exacerbate their asthma symptoms versus leaving their group of peers and risk separation from the group. Under these types of circumstances, it is important for clinicians to recognize that highly stressful or emotionally charged situations may hinder good decision making in adolescents.[1] This underscores the need for continuous monitoring by clinicians and the supportive guidance of parents, particularly in the early stages of the burgeoning independence of adolescents.

Metacognition

An individual's awareness of and control over the way that he or she processes information is referred to as metacognition.[1] One acquires a set of strategies and compares their relative efficacy across different situations. Metacognition facilitates self-regulation, which is the process by which one can observe, judge, and react to one's actions.[35] Asthma self-regulation is crucial in achieving and maintaining adequate asthma control.[36] One of the most important skills in asthma management is recognizing changes in symptoms or peak flow, and instituting early and appropriate therapy to reduce asthma morbidity. Patients can reflect on their actions, determine if their perceptions were accurate, and if their response produced the desired effect. Ultimately, it is through this cognitive process that patients decide if their actions were appropriate and successful, and if they should be repeated in the future.

DOMAIN-SPECIFIC KNOWLEDGE

Cognitive and reasoning abilities develop in conjunction with new experiences and increased knowledge acquisition. An adolescent who develops expertise in a topic performs like an adult who is new to the subject, despite having otherwise limited cognitive skills compared with the adult.

Domain-specific knowledge allows adolescents to apply a complex set of rules and enhance their performance.[34] The extent to which one is familiar with a topic increases the effectiveness of one's reasoning skills in that area. Through science and health courses taken in school, adolescents acquire domain-specific knowledge about the human body and how it functions. When the pathophysiology and management of asthma are introduced, the adolescent with knowledge of physiology and anatomy will be better able to incorporate these concepts and apply that knowledge to managing asthma.[34]

PEER RELATIONS

Teenagers spend increased time with their peers, and the nature of these relationships changes such that peer groups increase in size and diversity, and friendships become more intense.[37] The awareness of oneself as a social being is a prominent feature of adolescence, and has consequences and effects on social behavior.[38] Adolescents with asthma are often concerned that having asthma will decrease their peer acceptance. Socially stressful experiences, when not addressed appropriately, can lead to poor decision making. Many adolescents believe that people are constantly watching them and that they are the center of attention when this may not be so. This objectification of oneself may be an impediment to asthma self-management. Although adolescents may be cognizant of their symptoms, they may be reluctant to take medication or avoid asthma triggers for fear that their peers may witness or question their behavior. As a result, even though the adolescent has an asthma plan and knows how to respond to symptoms appropriately, the social milieu may still result in medication nonadherence.

Four strategies that early adolescents use to cope with peer-related stress in asthma management have been described: (1) cognitive justifying—rationalizing the asthma management behavior to oneself regardless of a nonsupportive peer-related environment; (2) explaining—describing asthma to peers so that they understand why the adolescent needs to carry out asthma management behaviors; (3) outsourcing—seeking social support to buffer or influence nonsupportive peer-related environments, which involves having a close friend act or speak out on the adolescent's behalf; and (4) undisclosing—keeping asthma management behaviors private or lying about the behaviors if they are not supported by peers.[39] These coping strategies are not mutually exclusive, and adolescents use a mix of strategies to cope with their peers.

Clinicians can assist the adolescent by discussing the issues of social stress and peer relations as they relate to asthma management directly with the adolescent and his or her parents, exploring how the treatment can be modified to fit the adolescent's life, and guiding them through coping strategies that will promote healthy asthma self-management. Peer support is crucial if chronic illnesses such as asthma are to be managed successfully.

INCREASED AUTONOMY AND SEPARATION FROM PARENTS

As adolescents develop autonomy and begin the process of separation from their parents, conflict may ensue. The pattern of adolescent–parent conflict varies over time, with early adolescence marked by the most conflict, and late adolescence by the least conflict.[37] For adolescents with asthma, one potential source of conflict is autonomy with medical management. As they strive for autonomy and independence, adolescents may begin to resent parental reminders about taking their asthma medications and consider it nagging, which leads to the avoidance of taking medication.[40] Clinicians are encouraged to work with both adolescents and their parents to assist in gradually transferring the responsibility of taking medication to the adolescent in a way that is consistent with the teenager's level of asthma knowledge, maturation, and development. Since adolescents spend increased time outside the home and parents may not be fully aware of their child's symptoms, clinicians should spend the first part of the visit with the adolescent, eliciting a history of symptoms, medication use, and trigger avoidance techniques before engaging in a joint discussion with the parents.

RISK-TAKING IN ADOLESCENTS

Risk-taking behaviors, such as tobacco, alcohol, and drug use, increase during adolescence.[10] Among adolescents with asthma, the prevalence of smoking is equivalent to[41] or even higher than those without asthma.[42] Teenagers with asthma who actively smoke or who have passive smoke exposure have more asthma symptoms,[43] are more likely to be admitted to hospital and require critical care interventions, such as intubation for asthma exacerbations,[44] and have suboptimal lung growth and reduced lung function.[45]

It is suggested that clinicians ask the adolescent about his or her smoking exposures and behaviors, and provide appropriate counseling regarding the specific asthma-related dangers associated with smoking. Moreover, they should recommend antismoking interventions, or refer the patient to an appropriate smoking cessation program. Additionally, it is important to inquire about exposure to smoke not only in the home, but also in vehicles and in other places where the adolescent may frequent. Reviewing the strategies to avoid exposure is also recommended, including possible smoking cessation programs for parents and other family members who may smoke.

IDENTITY DEVELOPMENT

Identity formation is a lifelong process that peaks during adolescence when teenagers are confronted with multiple social and biological challenges. In order to cope with these challenges, adolescents must maintain a stable sense of self across different roles and responsibilities.[46] Adolescents with chronic medical conditions, including asthma, bear an additional burden in that they must incorporate an additional challenge in their quest for identity formation—that of being a person with a chronic illness. Once adolescents accept the illness as part of who they are, they may understand that taking care of their disease is an integral component of taking care of themselves.[34] In contrast, the development of a sickly identity may contribute to low self-esteem and poor self-image, and result in increased nonadherence and morbidity. The challenge for clinicians is to help adolescent patients to create a self-concept of a strong individual who is empowered to confront and manage a chronic illness.

IMPROVING ADHERENCE

Adherence can be defined as taking medications, monitoring disease progress, and incorporating lifestyle changes that are consistent with medical and health advice to achieve optimum health outcomes.[47] In adolescents with asthma, medication adherence, particularly inhaled corticosteroids, has been estimated to be 50%.[48] Studies on adherence in adolescents have consistently noted four specific barriers: (1) negative perceptions about treatments and providers, (2) cognitive difficulty in following medical instructions due to limited intellectual abilities or forgetfulness, (3) social barriers due to peer pressure, and (4) underestimation of asthma symptoms and minimization of the consequences of nonadherence.[49] Despite this, clinicians can take steps to help adolescents improve their adherence.

GRADUAL TRANSITIONING OF ASTHMA CARE TO ADOLESCENTS

The developmental changes previously described suggest that early adolescents are ready to begin assuming responsibility for their asthma care. However, the transfer from parents to teenagers should be done gradually and monitored closely by both clinicians and parents, as asthma management by early adolescents is often suboptimal.[30] This highlights the important role that clinicians play as teachers, coaches, and supporters of adolescent patients with asthma and their families. They can facilitate this process of transition for families by providing appropriate asthma education for adolescents and by teaching parents how to monitor asthma care that will ensure the safety of the patient. A strong partnership among all three parties—the adolescent patient, his or her parents, and his or her clinician—will promote and support the teenager's independence while ensuring that the level of responsibility is tailored to the adolescent's level of development and asthma management skills.[30]

FORMING A THERAPEUTIC ALLIANCE WITH ADOLESCENT PATIENTS

Effective communication and a patient–clinician alliance are critical aspects of successful medical care. There is a positive relationship between a therapeutic alliance and treatment adherence. Research on the communication between physicians and adolescents with chronic illness has demonstrated that a relationship viewed as equal between the patient and the clinician is crucial to delivering effective care. Adolescents expressed that the use of age-appropriate language, an emphasis on the individual rather than on the disease, and a patient-focused rather than a parent-focused discussion contributed to their overall feeling of being a respected partner, rather than an ignored bystander in their care.[50] The establishment of a secure and trusting relationship is the foundation for open communication, which is essential when discussing sensitive matters, such as risk-taking behavior and peer relationships.

SUMMARY

The management of asthma in adolescents is a complex undertaking, which requires clinicians' awareness of medical therapies and sophisticated diagnostic tests, as well as a deep understanding of the psychosocial changes that adolescents experience. As knowledge of these intricate issues increases, clinicians can work with adolescent patients and their families to help the adolescent live a healthy, active, and symptom-free life.

REFERENCES

1. Adams GR, Berzonsky MD. *Blackwell Handbook of Adolescence*. Malden, MA: Blackwell; 2003.
2. Akinbami LJ, Moorman JE, Garbe PL, Sondik EJ. Status of childhood asthma in the United States, 1980–2007. *Pediatrics* 2009;123(Suppl 3):S131–S145.
3. Eaton DK, Kann L, Kinchen S, et al. Youth risk behavior surveillance: United States, 2005. *J Sch Health* 2006;76:353–372.
4. Fagan JK, Scheff PA, Hryhorczuk D, Ramakrishnan V, Ross M, Persky V. Prevalence of asthma and other allergic diseases in an adolescent population: Association with gender and race. *Ann Allergy Asthma Immunol* 2001;86:177–184.
5. Akinbami LJ, Schoendorf KC. Trends in childhood asthma: Prevalence, health care utilization, and mortality. *Pediatrics* 2002;110(2 Pt 1):315–322.
6. Calmes D, Leake BD, Carlisle DM. Adverse asthma outcomes among children hospitalized with asthma in California. *Pediatrics* 1998;101:845–850.
7. de Benedictis D, Bush A. The challenge of asthma in adolescence. *Pediatr Pulmonol* 2007;42:683–692.
8. Osman M, Hansell AL, Simpson CR, Hollowell J, Helms PJ. Gender-specific presentations for asthma, allergic rhinitis and eczema in primary care. *Prim Care Respir J* 2007;16:28–35.
9. Akinbami LJ, Schoendorf KC, Parker J. US childhood asthma prevalence estimates: The Impact of the 1997 National Health Interview Survey redesign. *Am J Epidemiol* 2003;158:99–104.
10. Sadof M, Kaslovsky R. Adolescent asthma: A developmental approach. *Curr Opin Pediatr* 2011;23:373–378.
11. Kendig EL, Wilmott RW. *Kendig and Chernick's Disorders of the Respiratory Tract in Children*, 8th edn. Philadelphia, PA: Saunders/Elsevier; 2012.
12. Rhee H, Belyea MJ, Elward KS. Patterns of asthma control perception in adolescents: Associations with psychosocial functioning. *J Asthma* 2008;45:600–606.

13. Guerra S, Wright AL, Morgan WJ, Sherrill DL, Holberg CJ, Martinez FD. Persistence of asthma symptoms during adolescence: Role of obesity and age at the onset of puberty. *Am J Respir Crit Care Med* 2004;170:78–85.

14. Nicolai T, Illi S, Tenborg J, Kiess W, v Mutius E. Puberty and prognosis of asthma and bronchial hyper-reactivity. *Pediatr Allergy Immunol* 2001;12:142–148.

15. Withers NJ, Low L, Holgate ST, Clough JB. The natural history of respiratory symptoms in a cohort of adolescents. *Am J Respir Crit Care Med* 1998;158:352–357.

16. Phelan PD, Robertson CF, Olinsky A. The Melbourne Asthma Study: 1964–1999. *J Allergy Clin Immunol* 2002;109:189–194.

17. von Mutius E. Progression of allergy and asthma through childhood to adolescence. *Thorax* 1996;51(Suppl 1):S3–S6.

18. von Mutius E, Martinez FD, Fritzsch C, Nicolai T, Reitmeir P, Thiemann HH. Skin test reactivity and number of siblings. *BMJ* 1994;308:692–695.

19. van Den Toorn LM, Prins JB, Overbeek SE, Hoogsteden HC, de Jongste JC. Adolescents in clinical remission of atopic asthma have elevated exhaled nitric oxide levels and bronchial hyperresponsiveness. *Am J Respir Crit Care Med* 2000;162(3 Pt 1):953–957.

20. Expert Panel Report 3 (EPR-3): Guidelines for the Diagnosis and Management of Asthma-Summary Report 2007. *J Allergy Clin Immunol* 2007;120(5 Suppl):S94–S138.

21. Bateman ED, Hurd SS, Barnes PJ, et al. Global strategy for asthma management and prevention: GINA executive summary. *Eur Respir J* 2008;31:143–178.

22. Newman KB, Mason UG 3rd, Schmaling KB. Clinical features of vocal cord dysfunction. *Am J Respir Crit Care Med* 1995;152(4 Pt 1):1382–1386.

23. Ibrahim WH, Gheriani HA, Almohamed AA, Raza T. Paradoxical vocal cord motion disorder: Past, present and future. *Postgrad Med J* 2007;83:164–172.

24. Powell DM, Karanfilov BI, Beechler KB, Treole K, Trudeau MD, Forrest LA. Paradoxical vocal cord dysfunction in juveniles. *Arch Otolaryngol Head Neck Surg* 2000;126(1):29–34.

25. Weinberger M, Abu-Hasan M. Pseudo-asthma: When cough, wheezing, and dyspnea are not asthma. *Pediatrics* 2007;120:855–864.

26. Anbar RD, Hall HR. Childhood habit cough treated with self-hypnosis. *J Pediatr* 2004;144:213–217.

27. Cohlan SQ, Stone SM. The cough and the bedsheet. *Pediatrics* 1984;74:11–15.

28. Bruzzese JM, Stepney C, Fiorino EK, et al. Asthma self-management is sub-optimal in urban Hispanic and African American/black early adolescents with uncontrolled persistent asthma. *J Asthma* 2012;49:90–97.

29. Clark NM, Dodge JA, Thomas LJ, Andridge RR, Awad D, Paton JY. Asthma in 10- to 13-year-olds: Challenges at a time of transition. *Clin Pediatr* 2010;49:931–937.

30. Bruzzese JM, Sheares BJ, Vincent EJ, et al. Effects of a school-based intervention for urban adolescents with asthma. A controlled trial. *Am J Respir Crit Care Med* 2011;183:998–1006.

31. Piaget J, Inhelder B. *The Psychology of the Child.* New York: Basic Books; 1969.

32. Gemelli RJ. *Normal Child and Adolescent Development.* Washington, DC: American Psychiatric Press; 1996.

33. Smith L, Vonèche JJ. *Norms in Human Development.* New York: Cambridge University Press; 2006.

34. Bruzzese JM, Bonner S, Vincent EJ, et al. Asthma education: The adolescent experience. *Patient Educ Couns* 2004;55(3):396–406.

35. Bandura A, Adams NE, Beyer J. Cognitive processes mediating behavioral change. *J Pers Soc Psychol* 1977;35(3):125–139.

36. Newman S, Steed L, Mulligan K. *Chronic Physical Illness: Self-Management and Behavioral Interventions.* Maidenhead, UK: McGraw-Hill Open University Press; 2009.

37. Lightfoot C, Cole M, Cole S. *The Development of Children,* 6th edn. New York: Worth Publishers; 2009.

38. Elkind D. Egocentrism in adolescence. *Child Dev* 1967;38(4):1025–1034.

39. Yang TO, Lunt I, Sylva K. Peer stress-related coping activities in young adolescents' asthma management. *J Asthma* 2009;46(6):613–617.

40. Penza-Clyve SM, Mansell C, McQuaid EL. Why don't children take their asthma medications? A qualitative analysis of children's perspectives on adherence. *J Asthma* 2004;41(2):189–197.

41. Backer V, Nepper-Christensen S, Ulrik CS, von Linstow ML, Porsbjerg C. Factors associated with asthma in young Danish adults. *Ann Allergy Asthma Immunol* 2002;89(2):148–154.

42. Tercyak KP. Psychosocial risk factors for tobacco use among adolescents with asthma. *J Pediatr Psychol* 2003;28(7):495–504.

43. Mak KK, Ho RC, Day JR. The associations of asthma symptoms with active and passive smoking in Hong Kong adolescents. *Respir Care* 2012;57(9):1398–1404.

44. LeSon S, Gershwin ME. Risk factors for asthmatic patients requiring intubation. II. Observations in teenagers. *J Asthma* 1995;32(5):379–389.

45. Joad JP. Smoking and pediatric respiratory health. *Clin Chest Med* 2000;21:37–46, vii–viii.

46. Erikson EH. *Identity, Youth, and Crisis,* 1st edn. New York: W.W. Norton; 1968.

47. Logan D, Zelikovsky N, Labay L, Spergel J. The illness management survey: Identifying adolescents' perceptions of barriers to adherence. *J Pediatr Psychol* 2003;28:383–392.

48. Desai M, Oppenheimer JJ. Medication adherence in the asthmatic child and adolescent. *Curr Allergy Asthma Rep* 2011;11:454–464.

49. Rhee H, Belyea MJ, Brasch J. Family support and asthma outcomes in adolescents: Barriers to adherence as a mediator. *J Adolesc Health* 2010;47(5):472–478.

50. Beresford BA, Sloper P. Chronically ill adolescents' experiences of communicating with doctors: A qualitative study. *J Adolesc Health* 2003;33(3):172–179.

19 Management of Adult Asthma

Pallavi Bellamkonda and Thomas B. Casale

CONTENTS

CASE PRESENTATION

A 47-year-old female presented to the clinic complaining of shortness of breath. Although she had not previously been diagnosed with asthma, she had been prescribed an albuterol inhaler 5 months earlier. In addition, she had seen a pulmonologist 1 year prior to this consultation for difficulty in breathing and she had been diagnosed with allergic rhinitis. A measurement of her lung function was not done at that time.

Her current symptoms consisted of coughing, wheezing, shortness of breath, chest tightness, and clear mucus production. Her screening Asthma Control Test (ACT) revealed a score of six (i.e., severely impaired asthma control). She complained of significant coughing and wheezing both at rest and with exercise. Her activity was limited due to shortness of breath. She also had significant nocturnal symptoms.

She stated that she had taken approximately 80 puffs of albuterol over the previous week.

In addition to her lower airway symptoms, she also complained of postnasal drip, nasal congestion, and itchy, watery eyes. Her family history was positive for allergic rhinitis, but there was no history of asthma.

Her past medical history was significant for hyperlipidemia treated with Lipitor 20 mg daily and allergic rhinitis treated with loratadine 10 mg daily. Her review of systems was unremarkable other than her upper and lower respiratory tract symptoms. She is a nonsmoker, but she is exposed to cigarette smoke passively.

Examination of the patient's vital signs revealed the following: pulse = 88 beats/min, respiratory rate = 18 breaths/min, blood pressure (BP) = 130/80 mmHg, height 65 in., and weight 155 lbs. She appeared anxious, but not in distress. Her head, eyes, ears, nose, and throat examination was remarkable for pale, boggy nasal turbinates and posterior pharyngeal cobblestoning consistent with postnasal drainage. Her cardiac examination was within the normal limits. Her lung examination revealed a prolonged expiratory phase and bilateral wheezing diffusely throughout all lung fields.

An exhaled nitric oxide reading was high at 69 ppb. A spirometry revealed a forced expiratory volume in 1 sec (FEV₁) of 1.23 L (45% predicted), a forced vital capacity (FVC) of 2.08 L (62% predicted), and an FEV₁/FVC ratio of 0.59. She received bronchodilator treatment with four puffs of albuterol and her FEV₁ improved to 1.52 (55% predicted), indicating significant reversibility. The patient was assessed as having severe asthma, allergic rhinitis, and conjunctivitis.

The patient was treated with prednisone 40 mg orally every morning for 7 days; Advair 250/50 (fluticasone/salmeterol) one puff twice daily; and fluticasone nasal spray two sprays in each nostril once per day, and continuation of loratadine.

One week later, she returned to the clinic and had a marked decrease in her asthma symptoms. She denied any coughing, shortness of breath, wheezing, or chest tightness. She was able to sleep through the night. Her physical examination was positive for a slight decrease in air movement bilaterally on auscultation of the lungs, but was otherwise unremarkable. A spirometry revealed an FEV₁ of 2.26 L (76% predicted), a FVC of 2.75 L (69% predicted), and an FEV₁/FVC ratio of 0.88. Her exhaled nitric oxide level was 29 ppb. The patient was treated with Advair 500/50 one puff twice daily, prednisone was discontinued, and the remainder of her medications remained the same.

The patient was seen 6 weeks later, and at that time she indicated that her breathing was better than it had been in the last 4 years. Her ACT was 25. She had only used her rescue inhaler once in the previous 6 weeks and she denied any daytime or nocturnal symptoms. Her physical examination was unremarkable with clear lung fields. Her spirometry revealed an FEV₁ of 2.48 L (84% of predicted).

This case illustrates several important points.

1. *The importance of spirometry in diagnosing and assessing the severity of asthma. This patient never had a spirometry prior to her initial visit to the clinic. If a spirometry had been obtained when she was first prescribed albuterol, the diagnosis and the assessment of her asthma severity could have been made sooner, thereby preventing the marked impairment and risk factors that she presented.*
2. *The utility of the Expert Panel Report 3 (EPR-3) asthma classification for judging asthma severity and guiding therapy decisions, including the assessment of impairment using standardized patient questionnaires such as the ACT.*
3. *The potential utility of exhaled nitric oxide in assessing lung inflammation and responsiveness to corticosteroids. This patient presented with a*

very high exhaled nitric oxide that was significantly lower after just 1 week of treatment with oral and inhaled corticosteroids (ICS). Typically, higher exhaled nitric oxide levels occur with an eosinophilic asthma phenotype, which tends to respond better to corticosteroids.
4. *The overuse of albuterol associated with uncontrolled asthma. Patients using as much albuterol as this patient reported are at a higher risk for catastrophic asthma events.*
5. *The utility of oral corticosteroid and ICS to quickly reduce the symptoms of asthma and improve spirometry and lower lung inflammation as assessed by exhaled nitric oxide.*
6. *The utility of spirometry and ACT to monitor control in patients.*
7. *Appropriate treatment can considerably improve the quality of life for patients and reverse many of the impairments and risk factors.*

OVERVIEW

Asthma is an inflammatory airway disease, with a complicated pathophysiology and is multifactorial in etiology. The onset of the disease can occur at any time during a person's lifetime, but it commonly occurs in childhood or early adolescence. According to data from the United States Centers for Disease Control, the disease burden has been on the rise for the past 20 years. In the United Sates, asthma prevalence increased from 7.3% in 2001 to 8.4% in 2010, an increase of 25.7 million persons.[1] Approximately 3800 deaths per year are from asthma and asthma has been a contributing factor in another 7000 deaths per year. In adults, asthma is the fourth leading cause of work absenteeism and results in almost $3 billion per year in lost productivity. Lower socioeconomic classes and African American populations have higher rates of mortality and morbidity.[1]

Close monitoring of disease progression, timely intervention in acute settings, and making sure that patients are on adequate therapy for their stage of disease to prevent exacerbations all contribute to the prevention of morbidity and mortality.

CLINICAL PRESENTATION AND EVALUATION

Asthma is manifested symptomatically as wheezing, chest tightness, dyspnea, and cough, typically at night or early in the morning. These symptoms tend to be episodic in nature with near complete remission between episodes in many cases. Atypical presentations can occur in adults, including dyspnea on exertion. It is important to keep in mind the following differential diagnoses, since these disorders can present with similar signs and symptoms: chronic obstructive pulmonary disease (COPD; emphysema and chronic bronchitis); pulmonary embolism; mechanical obstruction of the upper or lower airways (malignant and benign tumors); obstructive sleep apnea (OSA); vocal cord dysfunction; tracheomalacia;

congestive heart failure; herpetic tracheobronchitis; hyperventilation with panic attacks; cough due to angiotensin converting enzyme (ACE) inhibitors; and pulmonary infiltration with eosinophilia. In patients with difficult-to-control asthma, comorbid conditions such as gastroesophageal reflux disease (GERD), rhinosinusitis, OSA, obesity, and allergic bronchopulmonary aspergillosis (ABPA) should be recognized early and adequately treated. The triggers for worsening asthma should be documented, and include allergens, irritants (e.g., environmental and tobacco smoke), respiratory viruses, and medications (beta-blockers and ACE inhibitors). Each clinic visit should include an evaluation of asthma control, self-management skills, adherence, and the success of pharmacotherapy. A questionnaire encompassing various symptoms, duration, frequency, and severity can be used.

A physical examination during routine visits might not yield much, but it is useful in recognizing an exacerbation and in identifying comorbid conditions. On nasopharyngeal examination, there could be increased induration and erythema in the nasal turbinates and cobblestoning in the retropharynx from a postnasal drip in patients with chronic rhinosinusitis. On lung examination, patients can have wheezing, prolonged end-expiration, and decreased air movement. Patients could also present with a normal lung examination. A silent chest may actually indicate a severe exacerbation.

In the initial evaluation of new onset of asthma symptoms in adults, a chest x-ray should be done to rule out other etiologies of dyspnea. In asthma, the chest x-ray is usually within normal limits or occasionally shows hyperinflation and air trapping from mucus plugs. No further imaging studies are required for evaluating asthma.

Spirometry is an integral part of assessing asthma severity and control. Spirometry should be performed prior to initiating treatment in order to establish the presence and severity of baseline airway obstruction. The initial spirometry should also include measurements before and after inhalation of a short-acting bronchodilator to assess reversibility. Spirometry is generally recommended over measurements by a peak flow meter. Peak expiratory flow (PEF) meters are more appropriate for monitoring than they are as diagnostic tools; however, a home PEF diary may be helpful in diagnosing patients with a suggestive history of asthma when the lung function is normal in the clinic. The ratio of FEV_1/FVC is typically less than 70%. The FEV_1 is characteristically low in asthma. Reversibility is defined as a 12% improvement and an increase of 200 cc in FEV_1 in comparison to the baseline. Spirometry should be done to determine airflow obstruction and should be matched with the symptom profile. Many patients do not perceive airway obstruction; therefore, spirometry is especially useful in this population. There are guidelines for the technique and the equipment to be used while performing office spirometry.[2,3] Patient age, gender, height, and ethnic background should be taken into account when interpreting the results. In patients with a normal spirometry, airway hyperresponsiveness can be assessed using methacholine or mannitol bronchoprovocation challenge testing. A positive bronchoprovocation test does not confirm the diagnosis of asthma. Normal subjects without asthma, patients with rhinitis or COPD, and others may sometimes have a positive test. However, a negative test excludes the diagnosis of asthma, except in patients with a high pretest probability of asthma.

Laboratory testing is generally not helpful in the diagnosis or management of asthma. Total immunoglobulin E (IgE) can be elevated or normal, but population studies indicate a higher probability of airway hyperresponsiveness and asthma with elevated IgE levels.[4] Elevated blood eosinophil levels are not diagnostic for asthma but are predictive of better responses to ICS.[5]

All patients with persistent asthma are recommended for an evaluation of allergens as possible contributing factors, especially perennial allergens. This can be done through skin or *in vitro* testing. Allergies are significant triggers for asthma in ≥80% of children and 50%–60% of adults.

Exhaled nitric oxide can be helpful in certain instances. Recent guidelines[6] indicate that it can be used to assist in assessing the etiology of respiratory symptoms; to help in identifying the eosinophilic asthma phenotype; to assess the potential response or failure to respond to anti-inflammatory agents, notably corticosteroids; to establish a baseline during clinical stability for subsequent monitoring of persistent asthma; to guide changes in doses of anti-inflammatory medications: step-down dosing, step-up dosing, or discontinuation of anti-inflammatory medications; to assist in the evaluation of adherence to anti-inflammatory medications; and to assess whether airway inflammation is contributing to poor asthma control.

CLASSIFICATION OF ASTHMA

The initial step in the management of asthma is to accurately assess the patient and to classify the patient based on the severity of the symptoms.[7] Classification is based on an assessment of the impairment domain, which includes the duration, frequency, and severity of the symptoms and lung function, and the risk domain, which includes the presence and frequency of acute exacerbations (Figures 19.1 and 19.2).

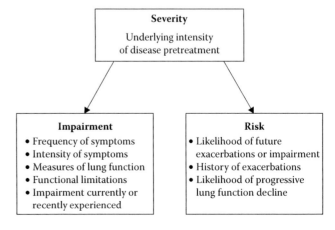

FIGURE 19.1 Asthma disease severity.

Components of Severity		Intermittent	Classification of Asthma Severity ≥ 12 Years of Age		
			Persistent		
			Mild	**Moderate**	**Severe**
Impairment	Symptoms	≤ 2 days/week	> 2 days/week but not daily	Daily	Throughout the day
Normal FEV₁/FVC:	Nighttime awakenings	≤ 2 ×/month	3–4 ×/month	>1 ×/week but not nightly	Often 7 ×/week
8–19 years 85%					
20–39 years 80%	Short-acting beta₂-adrenergic agonist use for symptom control (not prevention of EIB)	≤ 2 days/week	> 2 days/week but not > 1 × /day	Daily	Several times per day
40–59 years 75%					
60–80 years 70%					
	Interference with normal activity	None	Minor limitation	Some limitation	Extremely limited
	Lung function	• Normal FEV₁ between exacerbations • FEV₁ > 80% predicted • FEV₁/FVC normal	• FEV₁ ≥ 80% predicted • FEV₁/FVC normal	• FEV₁ > 60% but < 80% predicted • FEV₁/FVC reduced 5%	• FEV₁ < 60% predicted • FEV₁/FVC reduced > 5%
Risk	Exacerbations requiring oral systemic corticosteroids	0–1/year (see note)	≥ 2/year (see note) ───────────────────────────►		

Consider severity and interval since last exacerbation. ──────►
Frequency and severity may fluctuate over time for patients in any severity category.

Relative annual risk of exacerbations may be related to FEV₁.

FIGURE 19.2 Classification of asthma severity in patients ≥12 years of age. (From National Heart, Lung, and Blood Institute, National Institutes of Health, National Asthma Education and Prevention Program, Expert Panel Report 3: Guidelines for the diagnosis and management of asthma, 2007.)

DEFINITIONS

Severity is the intrinsic intensity of the disease process that is measured before receiving long-term control therapy. Control is the degree to which asthma's manifestations are minimized and the goals of therapy are met.

As rapid-acting bronchodilating medications are used by patients to control their symptoms, the domain of responsiveness can be assessed by evaluating the frequency of rescue inhaler use, the duration of relief of symptoms, and the extent of relief from symptoms. A deterioration of asthma control should be suspected if there is increased frequency of use, incomplete relief of symptoms, and shorter duration of symptom relief.[8] An awareness of the symptoms and self-management of the disease are essential to decrease the number of exacerbations, to increase exercise tolerance, and to improve quality of life. At every clinic visit, questions about inhalation use should be asked, and techniques should be checked.

The risk domain of asthma, which involves assessing the future risk of adverse reactions, the onset of critical exacerbations, and the loss of lung function, should be assessed on an individual basis.[7] A combination of the patient's history, comparative lung function assessment at each visit, and monitoring for deterioration and control should be studied.

GUIDELINE-DRIVEN CARE (SEE FIGURE 18.3)

INTERMITTENT ASTHMA

The treatment of mild intermittent asthma is essentially short-acting beta-agonists (SABAs), which are used for bronchodilation, as a rescue inhaler.

MILD AND MODERATE PERSISTENT ASTHMA

ICS are key controller agents for patients with chronic persistent asthma[9] and should be used in all patients with moderate to severe asthma. For mild asthma, ICS are the preferred treatment, but leukotriene modifiers (leukotriene receptor antagonists [LTRA] and zileuton) and theophylline can also be used. If symptoms are still uncontrolled, the dosage of ICS can be increased or long-acting beta-agonists (LABAs) can be added. The addition of a LABA to ICS compared with increasing the dose of ICS has shown better outcomes,

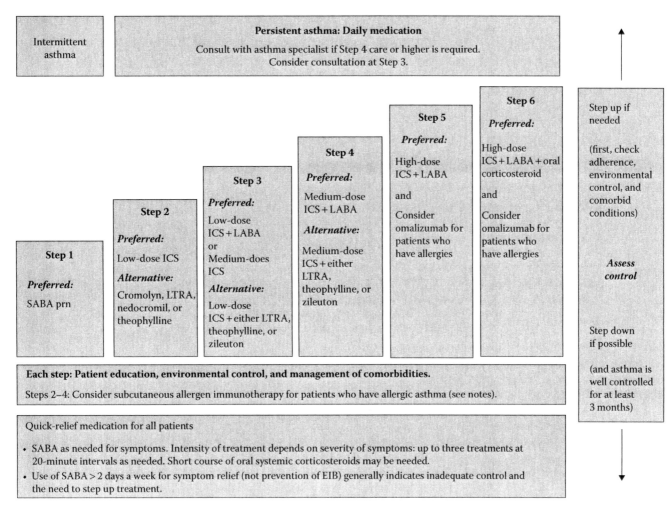

FIGURE 19.3 Asthma treatment recommendations in patients ≥12 years of age. (From National Heart, Lung, and Blood Institute, National Institutes of Health, National Asthma Education and Prevention Program, Expert Panel Report 3: Guidelines for the diagnosis and management of asthma, 2007.)

including an increase in symptom-free days, a decrease in the rate of exacerbations, and a decrease in the number of sick days and days away from work and school.[10,11]

SEVERE PERSISTENT ASTHMA

In patients who do not achieve adequate control with high doses of ICS plus LABAs, omalizumab can be considered in patients with perennial allergies.[12]

PHARMACOTHERAPY

The following is a summary of the individual asthma therapies.

SHORT-ACTING BETA₂-ADRENERGIC AGONISTS (SABAS)

Beta₂-agonists stimulate beta-adrenergic receptors and increase cyclic adenosine monophosphate (cAMP), causing a relaxation of the airway smooth muscles and thus reversing bronchoconstriction. Albuterol, salbutamol, levalbuterol, and pirbuterol are all drugs of choice for the immediate relief of symptoms. SABAs should only be used as rescue medications and not continuously for disease control. Higher frequency usage is a warning sign for loss of disease control and an increased risk for an exacerbation.

LONG-ACTING BETA₂-ADRENERGIC AGONISTS (LABAS)

LABAs have an increased lipophilic nature and thus have prolonged retention in the lung tissue with a duration of action of up to 12 h.[13] Salmeterol has a slower onset of action than formoterol, which some studies support using as a rescue inhaler when combined with ICS. Side effects include tachycardia, a prolonged QTC interval, and hypokalemia.[14,15] LABAs should not be used as monotherapy, and when used with ICS there is an improvement in both the impairment and risk domains. The U.S. Food and Drug Administration (FDA) has issued a black box warning about LABAs, noting that their use may increase the risk of severe asthma exacerbation or death.

CORTICOSTEROIDS

Corticosteroids have multiple mechanisms of action: suppressing cytokine release, decreasing the recruitment of airway eosinophils, and inhibiting the release of inflammatory mediators. They help diminish airway hyperresponsiveness and decrease lung inflammation.[9] Corticosteroids can be administered via different routes: inhaled, oral, intramuscular, or intravenous. There is an increased bioavailability of ICS, requiring lower doses and thus lowering the incidence of adverse reactions with their usage. Local adverse effects include oral candidiasis, dysphonia (seen in higher doses and in vocal stress), reflex cough, and bronchospasm (from the faster rate of inhalation). Oral candidiasis and dysphonia can be controlled by washing the mouth after each use and by using a spacer. Severe and difficult-to-control asthma warrants the possibility of using oral corticosteroids for long-term symptom control. However, there are many other options and the risk/benefit ratio of placing a patient on prolonged oral corticosteroids must be carefully weighed. Systemic side effects, seen more commonly with the prolonged use of oral corticosteroids, include cushingoid features associated with adrenal gland suppression, hypertension, uncontrolled blood sugars, cataracts, a fatty liver, and proximal muscle weakness.[7] Chronic usage can suppress immunity and may increase the risk of infection and cause the potential reactivation of tuberculosis.

Corticosteroid insensitivity or a variation in sensitivity is a result of various molecular mechanisms and the preponderance varies in different patient phenotypes. If asthma is poorly controlled despite high-dose ICS and oral steroids, corticosteroid insensitivity should be considered.[16] Decreased responsiveness has been shown with smoking (active and passive) or asthma with predominantly neutrophilic inflammation.

LEUKOTRIENE MODIFIERS

Montelukast and zafirlukast block the effects of the CysLT1 receptor (approved for use in childhood asthma) and zileuton inhibits the 5-lipoxygenase pathway. The use of zileuton requires close monitoring of liver function tests. Leukotriene modifiers can be used in mild persistent asthma as a monotherapy and in addition to ICS for more severe disease. Certain phenotypes show a better response, including patients with a smoking history, obesity, aspirin-exacerbated disease, and ICS insensitivity.

METHYLXANTHINES

Sustained-release theophylline is a mild to moderate bronchodilator that can be used for mild asthma or in addition to ICS in more severe disease. It is essential to monitor the serum levels of theophylline because of its narrow therapeutic range and side effects, including arrhythmias and seizures. Theophylline levels between 8 and 13 μg/mL are considered therapeutically effective and safe.

OMALIZUMAB

Omalizumab is a recombinant IgG humanized monoclonal antibody to the Fc3 portion of the IgE antibody. It decreases the binding of IgE to the surface of mast cells, leading to a decrease in the release of mediators, in response to exposure to any allergen. Omalizumab decreases the FcϵRI expression on basophils, mast cells, dendritic cells, monocytes, and airway submucosal cells. It is recommended as an adjunctive therapy for patients with perennial allergies and those who have moderate to severe persistent asthma. There is a small but significant improvement in lung function (approximately 6%), a decrease in the number of exacerbations, and in the capacity to decrease the dose of oral corticosteroids.[12] Injection-site pain and bruising are common and anaphylactic reactions are seen in about 0.1% of cases.

ANTICHOLINERGIC AGENTS

Ipratropium bromide inhibits muscarinic cholinergic receptors and reduces the intrinsic vagal tone of airways. This is a quick-relief medication used either as an additive to SABA or as an alternative to SABA in patients who cannot tolerate SABAs. Recently, long-acting muscarinic antagonists (tiotropium) have shown benefits equivalent to LABAs in patients on ICS.[17,18] The addition of tiotropium to a combination therapy with ICS plus LABA has shown improved FEV$_1$ values.[18]

CROMOLYN SODIUM AND NEDOCROMIL

Here, the mechanism of action is through blocking chloride channels and modulating the release of mast cell mediators and eosinophil recruitment. Both agents inhibit bronchospasm caused by exercise or cold air and prophylactically prevent allergen-induced asthma worsening. Their safety profile is very good and they can be used as a maintenance therapy especially in childhood asthma. However, they are no longer available in the United States because nonchlorofluorocarbon (CFC) formulations have not been approved.

ALLERGY IMMUNOTHERAPY

Both subcutaneous and sublingual immunotherapy have been shown to decrease asthma-related symptoms and improve lung function and bronchial hyperreactivity. However, anaphylactic reactions (primarily in subcutaneous immunotherapy) can occur and therefore immunotherapy should only be used in patients whose asthma is controlled and who have an FEV$_1$ of >70% predicted normal. Studies in children have shown a decrease in the incidence of asthma exacerbations with immunotherapy and the ability to prevent new sensitizations and the progression to newly diagnosed asthma in patients with allergic rhinitis.[19]

BRONCHIAL THERMOPLASTY

A novel approach to treating severe asthma is through bronchial thermoplasty, which involves a bronchoscopy and

administering thermal energy to the airways. It is believed to work by reducing the airway smooth muscle mass. While there has been no decrease in airway hyperresponsiveness or an improvement in FEV_1, there has been a significant improvement in patients' quality of life. Most studies are done on patients with no more than three exacerbations per year and the very strict inclusion criteria mean that this intervention might not be applicable to all patients.

EMERGENCY MANAGEMENT

The evaluation of an acute exacerbation of asthma starts with a history. Recent multiple emergency room visits and current oral corticosteroids may indicate an exacerbation that has become refractory to outpatient management, mandating a hospital admission. A previous exacerbation leading to respiratory failure requiring intubation and ventilator support or an attack that has previously caused seizures may indicate that the disease has progressed to severe uncontrolled asthma (see Chapters 21 and 22).

A rapid assessment should be completed for those who require immediate intervention. A severe attack may be suggested by the patient's difficulty in completing sentences and diaphoresis. Respiratory distress at rest can present with using the accessory muscles of respiration, an increased respiratory rate of >28, and tachycardia. Impending respiratory failure could present as a depressed respiratory effort, a paroxysmal diaphragmatic movement, and alternating abdominal and ribcage breathing.

The severity of an attack cannot be clearly assessed by the intensity of wheezing and sometimes a fatal attack can present without any wheezing and with only silent lung sounds on auscultation. Pulsus paradoxus is another indicator of the severity of the disease. An altered mental status in a patient with an acute exacerbation may require intubation.

If possible, spirometry should be done to assess the severity of the airway obstruction and to determine if admission is needed. A FEV_1 of <30% of predicted values (<1 L) or a FEV_1 showing a <40% improvement after 1 h of vigorous bronchodilator therapy is an indication for admission into hospital. A laboratory evaluation should be focused on finding the cause of the exacerbation and also on an assessment of severity. A complete blood count should be done to exclude any infectious processes. A chest x-ray should be obtained to rule out other causes of dyspnea and respiratory distress if suspected. The arterial blood gases should be considered if there is a severe attack. Hospitalization is required if PaO_2 is <60 mmHg. $PaCO_2$ may initially be low due to an increased respiratory rate, and later increase as the patient begins to fatigue and go into respiratory distress, which might necessitate the need for intubation. Management consists of intensive bronchodilator therapy, oxygen, and systemic corticosteroids. Approximately one-third of patients in the emergency department (ED) might show no bronchodilator response to albuterol. This unresponsiveness could be secondary to an increased airway inflammation, a distortion of the airways, and the presence of mucus in the airways.

Spirometry is warranted in the ED and a decision regarding admission could be made sooner based on response or no-response to albuterol inhalation after 30 and 60 min. In accordance with the National Institutes of Health (NIH) guidelines, responders could potentially be discharged from the ED.[20] Patients who have an intermediate response to albuterol, defined as persistent symptoms of dyspnea and a FEV_1 between 50% and 70% of predicted, should be considered for hospital admission.[20]

Even though there are several complications associated with mechanical ventilation, such as barotrauma, hypotension, and infections, it can be lifesaving in patients with severe exacerbations. Identifying the precipitating cause of the exacerbation is the next step after stabilizing the patient, in order to dictate the most appropriate immediate and prophylactic therapies.

THERAPY DECISION PARADIGMS

The asthma guidelines provide the basis for medical decision-making in treating patients. However, the therapy for each patient must be individualized. Moreover, there are alternative therapies listed under each category of asthma severity and asthma control in Figure 19.4. How does one make an appropriate choice? The following are some data to help with the decision-making process.

In patients with mild persistent asthma, the guidelines list low-dose ICS as the preferred choice. Several alternatives are listed, but only LTRA are commonly used. What do the data say?
The National Heart, Lung, and Blood Institute (NHLBI) and the Global Initiatives for Asthma (GINA) guidelines as well as Cochrane analyses all support the use of low-dose ICS over LTRAs. However, some patients are placed on a combination inhaler with ICS plus LABA. Although this will improve their asthma, it is frequently not necessary or recommended. In the OPTIMA trial, patients were randomized to budesonide versus budesonide at the same dose and formoterol or a placebo for 1 year. The patients had mild disease and were corticosteroid-free at baseline. After 1 year, the rate of severe exacerbations was equivalent for the combination therapy versus ICS monotherapy.[21]

Another decision that physicians often face is when and which controller medications can be stopped in mild persistent asthma patients who are well controlled. This was addressed in the salmeterol or corticosteroids (SOCS) trial published in 2001.[22] In this study, patients with mild persistent asthma who were well controlled on ICS were randomized to continued treatment with ICS, salmeterol alone, or a placebo. Patients on ICS did much better than either of the other two groups. These data suggested that some patients might need continued long-term controller therapy and that salmeterol monotherapy should not be used in patients with chronic persistent asthma.

Indeed, because of the controversy surrounding the potential deleterious effect of LABAs, both the asthma guidelines

	Components of Control	Classification of Asthma Control (≥ 12 Years of Age)		
		Well Controlled	**Not Well Controlled**	**Very Poorly Controlled**
Impairment	Symptoms	≤ 2 days/week	> 2 days/week	Throughout the day
	Nighttime awakenings	≤ 2×/month	1–3×/week	≥ 4×/week
	Interference with normal activity	None	Some limitation	Extremely limited
	Short-acting beta$_2$-adrenergic agonist use for symptom control (not prevention of EIB)	≤ 2 days/week	> 2 days/week	Several times per day
	FEV_1 or peak flow	> 80% predicted/ personal best	60%–80% predicted/ personal best	< 60% predicted/ personal best
	Validated questionnaires			
	ATAQ	0	1–2	3–4
	ACQ	≤ 0.75*	≥ 1.5	N/A
	ACT	≥ 20	16–19	≤ 15
Risk	Exacerbations requiring oral systemic corticosteroids	0–1/year	≥ 2/year (see note)	
		Consider severity and interval since last exacerbation		
	Progressive loss of lung function	Evaluation requires long-term follow up care		
	Treatment-related adverse effects	Medication side effects can vary in intensity from none to very troublesome and worrisome. The level of intensity does not correlate to specific levels of control but should be considered in the overall assessment of risk.		
Recommended action for treatment		• Maintain current step • Regular follow ups every 1–6 months to maintain control • Consider step down if well controlled for at least 3 months	• Step up 1 step and • Reevaluate in 2–6 weeks • For side effects, consider alternative treatment options	• Consider short course of oral systemic corticosteroids • Step up 1–2 steps, and • Reevaluate in 2 weeks • For side effects, consider alternative treatment options

FIGURE 19.4 Classification of asthma control in patients >12 years of age. (From National Heart, Lung, and Blood Institute, National Institutes of Health, National Asthma Education and Prevention Program, Expert Panel Report 3: Guidelines for the diagnosis and management of asthma, 2007.)

and the FDA stress that LABAs should not be used as monotherapy for the long-term control of persistent asthma. LABAs should continue to be considered as an adjunctive therapy to ICS and their use in combination with ICS should be done with a single inhaler to ensure compliance with the aforementioned recommendation. Despite the FDA's concerns, there are extensive data supporting the use of LABAs in patients with moderate to severe asthma in combination with an ICS.[10,11,23,24]

Studies in the mid-1990s showed that adding salmeterol versus a higher dose of ICS in asthma patients with symptoms on ICS resulted in less impairment.[23,24] The formoterol and corticosteroids establishing therapy (FACET) international study group showed that the addition of formoterol to budesonide in patients either on low- or moderate-dose ICS reduced severe exacerbations. Overall, these data support the use of LABA in patients uncontrolled on ICS alone over the use of ICS in higher doses. This was further supported by the gaining optimal asthma control (GOAL) study published in 2004.[11] In patients who were not well controlled

on moderate to high doses of ICS, the achievement of well-controlled or completely controlled asthma was enhanced by the addition of a LABA.

What about patients who have uncontrolled asthma despite optimal therapy according to the guidelines? There are many potential reasons for this, including comorbid conditions that could aggravate their symptoms. Also, it is important to recognize and control environmental triggers. However, one of the most important factors in gaining better control of asthma is to improve adherence.

A recent study of a U.S. Medicaid pediatric population indicated that the average adherence was 20% for ICS-treated children and 28% for LTRA-treated children.[25] Furthermore, children in the highest adherence category had significantly lower odds of an ED visit than those in the lowest adherence category.

Perennial allergic asthma patients, who have well-managed, comorbid disorders, and verified good adherence to controller therapy and control of environmental triggers in the home and, when possible, the workplace, and who continue to have significant asthma symptoms, can be considered for treatment with omalizumab.

Recent data from European studies indicate that combination therapy with ICS plus formoterol can be used as needed in addition to maintenance therapy. This is because formoterol has a rapid onset of action and produces bronchodilation in less than 15 min. Several studies have demonstrated that patients have greater reductions in asthma exacerbations and lower overall corticosteroid loads compared with a fixed-dose ICS/LABA combination.[26] The so-called SMART therapy (salmeterol maintenance and reliever therapy) is approved by the European Union and Health Canada, but not in the United States. With the advent of Dulera on the market, there are currently two options for consideration as SMART therapy.

Finally, one can also consider the addition of tiotropium bromide. Recent studies indicate that the addition of tiotropium bromide improved FEV_1 and PEFs to a greater degree than LABA or doubling the dose of ICS.[17] Similar to LABAs, tiotropium improved asthma-control days over doubling the dose of ICS. More recently, adding tiotropium to maintenance therapy with high-dose ICS with LABA has been shown to improve the pulmonary function of patients with severe uncontrolled asthma.[18]

Therefore, in patients who are not controlled despite optimal therapy, there are many options to consider. These options need to be carefully weighed based on an individual's needs.

There is also controversy as to when to step down from asthma therapy. The guidelines recommend that the current step in asthma therapy be maintained until control is achieved for a minimum of 3 months. In patients who are on medium to high doses of ICS with a LABA, the question arises whether one should step off the LABA or step down the ICS. In 2010, the U.S. FDA recommended that the LABA should be stepped off. However, there are no data to support this approach. A systematic review published in the *Archives of Internal Medicine* in 2012[27] showed that a meta-analysis of studies to date favored the continued use of LABA. Thus, although there is controversy over the safety of LABAs, there is a considerable amount of evidence supporting their use for patients with asthma.

MISCELLANEOUS CONSIDERATIONS

ASPIRIN-EXACERBATED RESPIRATORY DISEASE

Aspirin (acetylsalicylic acid [ASA])-induced asthma is associated with rhinosinusitis, nasal polyps, and asthma (ASA triad or Sampter's triad), which is precipitated by aspirin and other nonsteroidal anti-inflammatory drugs. This is more commonly seen in females and often presents in patients around 30–40 years of age. Aspirin-sensitive patients are noted to have increased eosinophilic inflammation, and these patients have been found to have increased levels of urinary LTE4. Atopy is not a risk factor for ASA

triad. Aspirin and cross-reacting COX1 nonsteroidal anti-inflammatory agents should be avoided in such patients and, if this cannot be done, desensitization, preferably post-polypectomy, is an option.[28]

ASTHMA IN PREGNANCY (SEE CHAPTER 25)

Asthma has been shown to affect up to 8% of pregnant women and is probably one of the most common medical causes of morbidity in pregnancy. Better control of asthma lowers the risk of pregnancy complications and mortality associated with asthma. Limited information is available on pharmacotherapy in pregnancy. Most studies have shown that it is safer to use medications to keep asthma under control, rather than have an acute exacerbation during pregnancy. It is essential to identify and avoid any exacerbating factors, including exposure to tobacco smoke and GERD.[29]

OCCUPATIONAL ASTHMA (SEE CHAPTER 24)

Exposure to high molecular weight proteins and low molecular weight chemicals followed by a latency period before symptom onset has been demonstrated to cause occupational asthma in a previously healthy, susceptible worker or to exacerbate preexisting asthma. Furthermore, acute or chronic exposure to irritants in the workplace can cause airway hyperresponsiveness and bronchial constriction, referred to as irritant-induced asthma or reactive airways dysfunction syndrome (RADS). The early identification of occupational asthma is required to prevent further exposure and to obtain good long-term outcomes.[30]

EXERCISE-INDUCED BRONCHOCONSTRICTION (EIB) (SEE CHAPTER 12)

EIB is defined as a lower airway obstruction with symptoms of cough, wheezing, or dyspnea induced by exercise in patients without underlying asthma. Exercise-induced asthma is the same as EIB except that it occurs in patients with chronic asthma. Exercising causes hyperventilation of air that is dryer and cooler,[31] and this loss of heat and moisture causes bronchoconstriction. The onset of EIB is usually minutes after beginning exercise, peaks around 10 min after stopping exercise, and lasts around 30–40 min. The diagnosis is based on a history of chest tightness, cough, and wheezing after exercising; also, exercise-challenge testing can be done. A 15% decrease in FEV_1 postexercise is consistent with EIB.[32] Treatment usually involves the use of a SABA 15–30 min prior to exercise.

REFERENCES

1. Akinbami LJ, Moorman MS, Bailey C, et al. Trends in asthma prevalence, health care use and mortality in the United States, 2001–2010. *NCHS Data Brief* 2012; 94.
2. Miller MR, Hankinson V, Brusasco F, et al. Standardisation of spirometry. *Eur Respir J* 2005; 26:319–338.

3. Levy ML, Quanjer PH, Booker R, et al. Diagnostic spirometry in primary care: Proposed standards for general practice compliant with American Thoracic Society and European Respiratory Society recommendations. *Prim Care Respir J* 2009; 18(3):130–147.

4. Burrows B, Martinez FD, Halonen M, et al. Association of asthma with serum IgE levels and skin-test reactivity to allergens. *N Engl J Med* 1989; 320(5):271–277.

5. Meijer RJ, Postma DS, Kauffman HF, et al. Accuracy of eosinophils and eosinophil cationic protein to predict steroid improvement in asthma. *Clin Exp Allergy* 2002;32:1096–1103.

6. Dweik RA, Boggs PB, Erzurum SC, et al. An official ATS clinical practice guideline: Interpretation of exhaled nitric oxide levels (FENO) for clinical applications. *Am J Respir Crit Care Med* 2011;184(5):602–615.

7. National Heart, Lung, and Blood Institute, National Institutes of Health. National Asthma Education and Prevention Program. Expert Panel Report 3: Guidelines for the diagnosis and management of asthma. NIH Publication No. 07–4051, 2007.

8. Zeiger RS, Yegin A, Simons FE, et al. Evaluation of the National Heart, Lung, and Blood Institute guidelines impairment domain for classifying asthma control and predicting asthma exacerbations. *Ann Allergy Asthma Immunol* 2012; 108(2):81–87.

9. Masoli M, Beasley R. Asthma exacerbations and inhaled corticosteroids. *Lancet* 2004; 363(9416):1236.

10. Masoli M, Weatherall M, Holt S, et al. Moderate dose inhaled corticosteroids plus salmeterol versus higher doses of inhaled corticosteroids in symptomatic asthma. *Thorax* 2005; 60(9):730–734.

11. Bateman ED, Boushey HA, Bousquet J, et al. Can guideline-defined asthma control be achieved? The gaining optimal asthma control study. *Am J Respir Crit Care Med* 2004; 170(8):836–844.

12. Humbert M, Beasley R, Ayres J, et al. Benefits of omalizumab as add-on therapy in patients with severe persistent asthma who are inadequately controlled despite best available therapy (GINA 2002 step 4 treatment): INNOVATE. *Allergy* 2005; 60(3):309–316.

13. Grembiale RD, Pelaia G, Naty S, et al. Comparison of the bronchodilating effects of inhaled formoterol, salmeterol and salbutamol in asthmatic patients. *Pulm Pharmacol Ther* 2002; 15(5):463–466.

14. Nelson HS, Carr W, Nathan R, et al. Update on the safety of long-acting beta-agonists in combination with inhaled corticosteroids for the treatment of asthma. *Ann Allergy Asthma Immunol* 2009; 102(1):11–15.

15. Ostrom NK. Tolerability of short-term, high-dose formoterol in healthy volunteers and patients with asthma. *Clin Ther* 2003; 25(11):2635–2646.

16. Tantisira KG, Lasky-Su J, Harada M, et al. Genome-wide association between GLCCI1 and response to glucocorticoid therapy in asthma. *N Engl J Med* 2011; 365(13):1173–1183.

17. Peters SP, Kunselman SJ, Icitovic N, et al. Tiotropium bromide step-up therapy for adults with uncontrolled asthma. *N Engl J Med* 2010; 363(18):1715–1726.

18. Kerstjens HA, Disse B, Schroder-Babo W, et al. Tiotropium improves lung function in patients with severe uncontrolled asthma: A randomized controlled trial. *J Allergy Clin Immunol* 2011; 128(2):308–314.

19. Cox L, Li JT, Nelson H, et al. Allergen immunotherapy: A practice parameter second update. *J Allergy Clin Immunol* 2007; 120:S25–S85.

20. Camargo CA Jr, Rachelefsky G, Schatz M. Managing asthma exacerbations in the emergency department: Summary of the National Asthma Education and Prevention Program Expert Panel Report 3 guidelines for the management of asthma exacerbations. *J Allergy Clin Immunol* 2009; 124(2 Suppl):S5–S14.

21. O'Byrne PM, Barnes PJ, Rodriguez-Roisin R, et al. Low dose inhaled budesonide and formoterol in mild persistent asthma: The OPTIMA randomized trial. *Am J Respir Crit Care Med* 2001; 164(8 Pt 1):1392–1397.

22. Lazarus SC, Boushey HA, Fahy JV, et al. Long-acting beta2-agonist monotherapy vs continued therapy with inhaled corticosteroids in patients with persistent asthma: A randomized controlled trial. *JAMA* 2001; 285(20):2583–2593.

23. Greening AP, Ind PW, Northfield M, et al. Added salmeterol versus higher-dose corticosteroid in asthma patients with symptoms on existing inhaled corticosteroid. *Lancet* 1994; 344(8917):219–224.

24. Woolcock A, Lundback B, Ringdal N, et al. Comparison of addition of salmeterol to inhaled steroids with doubling of the dose of inhaled steroids. *Am J Respir Crit Care Med* 1996; 153(5):1481–1488.

25. Herndon JB, Mattke S, Evans Cuellar A, et al. Anti-inflammatory medication adherence, healthcare utilization and expenditures among Medicaid and children's health insurance program enrollees with asthma. *Pharmacoeconomics* 2012; 30(5):397–412.

26. Chapman KR, Barnes NC, Greening AP, et al. Single maintenance and reliever therapy (SMART) of asthma: A critical appraisal. *Thorax* 2010; 65(8):747–752.

27. Brozek J, Kraft M, Krishnan J, et al. Long-acting beta2-agonist step-off in patients with controlled asthma. *Arch Int Med* 2012; 172(18):1365–1375.

28. Chang JE, White A, Simon RA, et al. Aspirin-exacerbated respiratory disease: Burden of disease. *Allergy Asthma Proc* 2012; 33(2):117–121.

29. Louik C, Schatz M, Hernandez-Diaz S, et al. Asthma in pregnancy and its pharmacologic treatment. *Ann Allergy Asthma Immunol* 2010; 105(2):110–117.

30. Nicholson PJ, Cullinan P, Taylor AJ, et al. Evidence based guidelines for the prevention, identification, and management of occupational asthma. *Occup Environ Med* 2005; 62(5):290–299.

31. Anderson SD. Exercise-induced bronchoconstriction in the 21st century. *J Am Osteopath Assoc* 2011; 111(11 Suppl 7):S3–S10.

32. Anderson SD, Fitch K, Perry CP, et al. Responses to bronchial challenge submitted for approval to use inhaled beta2-agonists before an event at the 2002 Winter Olympics. *J Allergy Clin Immunol* 2003; 11(1):45–50.

20 Management of Asthma in Older Adults

Tolly G. Epstein

CONTENTS

CASE PRESENTATION

A 68-year-old white male is referred to an allergy clinic for chronic rhinitis. He initially focuses on his upper respiratory complaints, but mentions shortness of breath in the review of systems. Upon further questioning, the patient reports a history of childhood asthma and increased shortness of breath for several years, which he attributes to "old age." He smoked one pack of cigarettes per day for 20 years in the distant past. He has a history of diabetes and hypertension. On examination, he has faint expiratory wheezes. Pulmonary function testing (PFT) reveals a forced expiratory volume in 1 sec (FEV_1)/forced vital capacity (FVC) ratio of 62% and an FEV_1 of 65%, with a 20% improvement in FEV_1 with albuterol. His postbronchodilator FEV_1/FVC ratio is 71%. His initial Asthma Control Test (ACT) score is 13 (indicating uncontrolled asthma).

The patient receives extensive counseling regarding the diagnosis of probable asthma with a possible component of chronic obstructive pulmonary disease (COPD). He is started on mometasone two puffs at night, a dry powder steroid inhaler with a dose counter, and he receives counseling on the appropriate inhaler technique. His allergy skin testing is positive for several indoor and outdoor aeroallergens, for which he receives counseling on avoidance measures.

After 1 month, the patient's ACT has improved to 16 and his peak expiratory flow (PEF) is 70% of normal. However, he has developed thrush, which is treated with antifungal lozenges. The mometasone is changed to a beclometasone

hydrofluoroalkane (HFA) metered-dose inhaler (MDI), two puffs twice daily with a spacer device to optimize his inhaler technique. After extensive counseling, he demonstrates the appropriate technique. After 2 months, his thrush has not recurred, but his asthma symptoms are still uncontrolled, with a FEV_1 of 74%. His beclometasone is increased to four puffs twice daily (high dose) and he again develops recurrent thrush. He is subsequently changed to budesonide/formoterol, a combination inhaled corticosteroid (ICS) and long-acting beta-agonist (LABA), two puffs twice daily. After a few days, he is hospitalized for severe shortness of breath and is noted to be in atrial fibrillation with a rapid ventricular rate. He is taken off budesonide/formoterol, placed on a beta-blocker for control of the atrial fibrillation, and instructed to restart beclomethasone two puffs twice daily. He does not restart beclomethasone because of a concern for side effects. One month later, his PEF rate is 40% of normal and he is visibly short of breath. He receives a 5-day course of prednisone and is restarted on beclomethasone. His symptoms improve quickly but his asthma remains uncontrolled. He is started on tiotropium (in combination with beclomethasone). Six weeks later, his ACT has improved to 20 (controlled) and his FEV_1 is stable at 82%.

INTRODUCTION

The number of asthmatics aged 65 and older in the United States is expected to *double* to greater than 6 million in the next 25 years.[1] The prevalence of asthma in adults aged 65 and older is already as high as 10% and up to two-thirds of asthma-related deaths occur in this population.[2,3] While mortality from asthma overall is <2.2/100,000, asthma-related mortality among older adults is almost five times greater, with 10.5/100,000 seniors dying from asthma.[2] A recent study of emergency room and hospital visits in the United States found that 903 out of 1144 individuals who died from acute asthma exacerbations were adults over 55 years of age.[4] Older asthmatics are three times more likely to be classified as having a severe disease and to experience an asthma exacerbation requiring systemic corticosteroids.[5] Asthma-related quality of life is also lower among older asthmatics, medication use is higher, and health-care costs are double those for younger asthmatics.[5–7] Given the heavy burden of asthma in older adults, the development of strategies to optimize asthma management in this population is of great importance.

The management of asthma in older adults presents unique challenges. Aging is associated with physiological, anatomical, and psychosocial changes, all of which may impact treatment responses. Older asthmatics may also require greater assistance and possibly alternative strategies to achieve good inhaler technique and compliance with care regimens. Moreover, the existence of significant medical comorbidities in this population can lead to diagnostic delays and may limit management options. This chapter presents an evidence-based approach to tackling these issues in order to provide optimal care for older asthmatics.

DIAGNOSIS OF ASTHMA IN OLDER ADULTS

Despite the high morbidity and mortality from asthma in older adults, underrecognition of asthma in this age group remains a significant problem. Some studies have suggested that the diagnosis is missed in approximately 50% of asthmatics aged 65 and older.[8] This is in part because of the large differential diagnosis of diseases that can present with respiratory difficulties in this age group.[9] There is also a common misperception that asthma only begins in childhood or young to middle adulthood. In reality, the incidence of asthma remains approximately 1 in 1000 throughout adult life, with 40%–50% of asthmatics developing symptoms after age 40, and more than 10% reporting symptom-onset after age 65.[10,11] Another major reason for a delay in diagnosis is that older asthmatics, particularly those with a long-standing disease, are frequently "poor perceivers" of acute and chronic lung impairment.[12] Having a less active lifestyle may also contribute to underrecognition of symptoms. Moreover, cognitive impairment and depression, which occur more frequently with age, may prohibit the recognition of the disease by both the patient and his or her physician.[7] Despite the critical need for objective testing in such situations, PFTs are less frequently performed in older asthmatics.[13]

Some conditions that may confound the diagnosis of or occur concurrently with asthma in older adults include COPD, congestive heart failure, arrhythmias, pulmonary emboli, chronic aspiration, gastroesophageal reflux disease (GERD), bronchiectasis, tracheobronchial tumors, and postnasal drainage from chronic rhinitis. It can be particularly challenging to differentiate asthma from COPD in older adults. Both conditions can present with shortness of breath, chest tightness, wheezing, or cough. It is, nevertheless, important to establish the correct diagnosis, given that the prognosis and the ideal therapeutic regimens for these conditions may differ. For example, first-line therapy for patients with moderate COPD consists of a long-acting bronchodilator alone, which would be inappropriate and potentially dangerous for an individual with asthma.[14] Table 20.1 provides some helpful tips to distinguish COPD from asthma in older adults.

The Global Initiative for Chronic Obstructive Lung Disease (GOLD) defines COPD as a common preventable and treatable disease, characterized by persistent airflow limitation that is usually progressive and associated with an enhanced chronic inflammatory response in the airways and the lungs to noxious particles or gases.[14,15] The hallmark features of COPD include that it generally begins later in life, it is largely related to tobacco smoke exposure, and it is characterized by irreversible airflow obstruction (though there is often an element of reversibility present in COPD).[9,15] Based on the GOLD criteria, a cutoff of 70% for the FEV_1/FVC ratio defines the presence of an airflow obstruction. While it is less challenging to differentiate COPD from asthma in younger populations, older adults with tobacco exposure frequently have elements of both diseases.[16] It is not uncommon to encounter older asthmatics with substantial tobacco exposure, as the prevalence of previous tobacco use in older adults may be as high as 50%.[11] In addition, a previous smoking history does not necessarily indicate that an individual has COPD, as only a small minority of individuals who smoke go on to develop the disease.[17] Therefore, an older age of symptom onset does not exclude asthma. Furthermore, as lung function may become irreversible in chronic asthma, this condition needs to be differentiated from COPD.

PFTs to differentiate COPD from asthma can sometimes be misleading in older adults. Healthy aging is associated with a decline in FEV_1, and using a fixed cutoff value of 70% for the FEV_1/FVC ratio, rather than the lower limit of normal (LLN) to identify COPD, may result in misclassification. Thus, the American Thoracic Society (ATS)/European Respiratory Society (ERS) currently recommends that the LLN for the FEV_1/FVC ratio be adjusted for age.[18] Classically, a diagnosis of asthma is established by the combination of: (1) symptoms consistent with asthma; (2) spirometry showing obstruction with at least 12% and 200 mL reversibility in the FEV_1 or FVC with a bronchodilator (albuterol); or (3) a positive methacholine challenge test for airway hyperresponsiveness. These diagnostic criteria do not always serve to rule out COPD, however, as more than 50% of individuals with COPD may have significant reversibility.[15] Some individuals with COPD also have a positive methacholine challenge test.[19] Moreover, a low postbronchodilator FEV_1/FVC ratio does not reliably rule out asthma in older adults, as at least 16% of asthmatics may develop a fixed obstructive defect over time due to airway remodeling.[20] While a low

TABLE 20.1

Helpful Tools to Differentiate Asthma from COPD in Older Adults

	COPD	Asthma
Symptoms	Shortness of breath with exertion may be prominent and develops slowly over time	Intermittent flare-ups more common
Family history	Generally absent	May be present, especially if childhood onset
Exposure history	Tobacco exposure prominent	Tobacco does not rule out
Age of onset	Generally after age 40–50 years unless strong susceptibility	Any age; breathing problems in childhood increase suspicion
Common comorbid conditions	Osteoporosis, cardiovascular disease, depression, weight loss	Atopy (although many nonatopic); aspirin-exacerbated respiratory disease (AERD) with nasal polyposis
Classic pulmonary function test findings	Postbronchodilator FEV_1/FVC ratio <0.7 (GOLD criteria) or Postbronchodilator FEV_1/FVC ratio less than the lower limit of normal for age, gender, height, and race (ATS/ERS criteria) and/or Low diffusing capacity for carbon monoxide (DLCO)	FEV_1/FVC ratio consistent with obstruction and Increase in FEV_1 of 12% and 200 mL with bronchodilator or Positive methacholine challenge test

diffusing capacity for carbon monoxide (DLCO) can help point toward a diagnosis of COPD, patients with asthma and tobacco exposure may have a low DLCO but maintain many of the clinical characteristics of asthma.

The reluctance of some physicians to order PFTs in older asthmatics may be partly due to the increased difficulty of performing adequate spirometry in older adults.[13] Obtaining a good-quality PFT from an older adult may require an additional 20–30 min and a greater number of FVC maneuvers in order to achieve consistent results.[9] Nevertheless, at least 50%–90% of older adults are able to meet quality end points, and there are very few circumstances in which spirometry should not be attempted in order to establish the correct diagnosis.[9] Because they include increased numbers of older adults, the National Health and Nutrition Examination (NHANES) III reference equations should be used for spirometry in this age group.[21]

As mentioned previously, the interpretation of PFTs should take into account that it may be more difficult to demonstrate airway reversibility in older asthmatics. This may be due to airway remodeling or a blunted response to inhaled beta-agonists that can occur with age (see 'Inhaled Beta₂-Agonists'). Older age is not a contraindication to performing methacholine challenge testing for patients in whom the diagnosis of asthma cannot be established with spirometry alone. Methacholine testing has safely been performed in patients up to 92 years old with a baseline FEV_1 of >70%.[11] PEF monitoring can also be attempted in order to demonstrate 20% diurnal variability to establish a diagnosis of asthma in older patients; however, peak flow measurements are less reliable in patients with cognitive or physical impairments. Little is known regarding the utility of exhaled nitric oxide (ENO)

measurements to assist with the diagnosis of asthma in older adults. One study of 77 adults over 60 years of age found that ENO was not helpful to distinguish asthmatics from control subjects, although the findings may have been influenced by the use of ICS.[7]

TREATMENT OF ASTHMA IN OLDER ADULTS

Evidence-based guidelines should be used in the same way for the treatment of asthma in older adults as they are in younger individuals.[22] Older adults who are diagnosed with persistent asthma should be placed on a controller therapy according to their level of severity, and their medications should be adjusted at follow-up based on both domains of asthma control (i.e., impairment and risk). While the basic principles of "step-therapy" are the same regardless of age, optimal therapeutic strategies in older asthmatics may vary due to psychosocial factors and because of age-related differences in medication efficacy and side effects. Clinical trials for asthma frequently exclude older asthmatics, thus making it more difficult to develop evidence-based assessments of various pharmaceutical agents for this age group. Despite these challenges, some studies have found that older asthmatics who are appropriately managed can achieve comparable if not better asthma control than younger individuals.[23]

OVERCOMING BARRIERS TO ADHERENCE TO MEDICAL ADVICE IN OLDER ASTHMATICS

The Global Initiative for Asthma (GINA) framework emphasizes that the creation of a partnership between the clinician and the patient with asthma is critical to achieve and maintain good asthma control.[24] This partnership requires active participation by the patient in his or her care, which includes ongoing communication with the physician as well as daily compliance with medications. Patients must also learn to develop appropriate inhaler techniques and to monitor for signs of asthma exacerbations. As a starting point, patients and physicians must identify and agree on the goals of treatment. While improving asthma symptoms is generally recognized as an important treatment goal by both patients and physicians, many older patients do not appreciate the importance of developing self-management skills, improving airflow obstruction based on objective testing, and maintaining normal body weight.[25] Patients with significant cognitive, emotional, physical, or financial difficulties frequently find it difficult to maintain an active partnership with their physicians. Moreover, complicated treatment regimens that do not take these issues into account may become burdensome and overwhelming, leading to frustration and poor adherence. For most older patients, maintaining an acceptable quality of life requires that prescribed treatments must incur minimal side effects and financial burden. Physicians must recognize and accommodate these factors.

Older asthmatics may find it difficult to identify worsening asthma control because of a poor perception of dyspnea and confusion with symptoms related to comorbid diseases. Many older adults assume that shortness of breath is a routine part of aging, and do not report symptoms unless they are severe. Routinely performing objective measurements, including peak flow monitoring and spirometry are therefore particularly important in this age group.[12] Routine monitoring of asthma symptoms and rescue medication using standardized questionnaires such as the ACT are also recommended; however, these tests may be less reliable in patients with multiple comorbid conditions who sometimes cannot differentiate asthma symptoms from those related to other conditions.[21]

Another major issue impacting adherence is that many older asthmatics do not properly use commonly prescribed inhaler devices due to physical or cognitive limitations.[26] Using the correct inhaler technique, including shaking the device before use, administering a dose, and holding one's breath after the dose is administered, is critically important to ensure the proper delivery of medication to the lungs. MDIs in particular require some dexterity to coordinate the actuation of the device by pressing down on the canister, with inhalation followed by breath holding. One out of two patients is unable to demonstrate the proper MDI technique.[26] As few as 10% of adults aged 65 and older may be able to optimally use a MDI due to physical impairments such as hand arthritis, muscle weakness, visual problems, or cognitive difficulties that can limit one's ability to learn and retain information.[26] Cognitive impairment is a strong predictor of poor inhaler technique, with a score of 23/30 or lower on the Mini Mental Test identifying patients who are at risk of poor technique.[26]

There are several administration strategies that can reduce dosing administration errors in older asthmatics. First and foremost, adequate time and attention must be devoted to education and routine reevaluation of inhaler technique. Spacer devices for MDIs improve drug delivery in older patients who have difficulties with MDIs.[27] These devices, which can hold the administered dose in the chamber for more than one inspiration, eliminate the necessity of simultaneously coordinating dose actuation and deep inhalation.[26] While most studies have not shown improved medication delivery with nebulizer devices versus MDIs with spacers, using a nebulizer is a reasonable approach for patients who cannot achieve a good inhaler technique due to fatigue, frailty, or various other reasons. The use of breath-actuated inhalers, which are automatically triggered by inhalation, offers another alternative. Some studies have shown that breath-actuated inhalers are easier and more successfully used by older patients; however, others found more errors in the use of these devices compared to MDIs.[28] Dry powder inhalers, such as Turbuhalers and Diskus inhalers (Accuhalers), which also do not require simultaneous dose actuation and deep inhalation, have been associated with fewer administration errors in older adults.[29] The downside to these devices is that they require adequate peak inspiratory flow rates (60–90 L/min for Turbuhaler and 30–90 L/min for Diskus) to ensure deaggregation (in the case of the Turbuhaler) and drug delivery to the lungs.[29] Some older asthmatics are therefore not able to achieve adequate drug delivery using a dry powder inhaler due to the decline in the peak inspiratory flow that occurs with age.[29] Another consideration when selecting an inhaler device is whether or not the device has a dose counter. Having a dose counter is particularly useful for patients on multiple medications or those with cognitive difficulties who may have problems keeping track of when an MDI needs to be refilled. In addition, as for any age group, the ease of use of various delivery devices must be balanced against the likelihood of achieving asthma control based on other properties of the prescribed medication.

INHALED BETA$_2$-AGONISTS

Regardless of age, short-acting beta$_2$-adrenergic agonists (SABAs) such as albuterol are considered an essential, life-saving component of asthma management by allowing for rapid bronchodilation during acute asthma exacerbations. Long-acting beta$_2$-adrenergic agonists (LABAs), including salmeterol and formoterol, also play an important role together with ICS controller therapy for individuals who require Step three or higher care.[22] It is important to be aware of the potential for age-related differences in responses to beta$_2$-agonists.[26] The activity of the sympathetic nervous system increases by about 10%–15% per decade of life. In addition, age-related changes in beta$_2$-receptor density, affinity, and signaling have been suggested. Data regarding the relationship between the density of beta$_2$-receptors and age are complex; however, the administration of corticosteroids to older individuals is known to induce an increased response to beta$_2$-agonists due to an increase in the density of beta$_2$-receptors. In addition, the percentage of high-affinity beta-receptors on target tissues declines with age.[30–32] Age-related abnormalities in cyclic adenosine mono-phosphate (cAMP) levels and activity, which is important for beta-receptor signaling, have also been identified.[33]

While studies involving SABAs and LABAs have shown efficacy and good tolerability among older asthmatics, some have suggested that they may be less effective than they are in younger individuals. One study found that older asthmatics had a decreased FEV_1 response to SABAs with age.[34] Another study showed a decreased ability of SABAs to return the FEV_1 to normal after methacholine testing in healthy individuals aged 60–76 years.[35] In contrast, age did not affect the impact of SABAs on FEV_1 improvement after methacholine challenge testing in a third study.[36] In addition, another study found that age was not a predictor of response to SABAs for acute severe asthma attacks.[37] A recent study comparing the efficacy of budesonide/formoterol (a com-bination inhaled steroid and a LABA) therapy in asthmat-ics over 65 years of age versus younger patients found that both groups showed similar improvements in asthma control based on asthma control questionnaire (ACQ) scores and exacerbations.[38] In addition, the age of asthma onset did not impact treatment responses among older asthmatics.

The side effects related to beta₂-agonists tend to be more pro-nounced in older patients. Oral beta₂-agonists should be avoided in favor of inhaled medications. Inhaled beta₂-agonists can cause an increase in the heart rate, blood pressure, myocardial oxygen demand, hypokalemia, nausea, and tremor in patients of any age. Older patients are more susceptible to adverse events related to these effects due to preexisting comorbid conditions such as ischemic heart disease and arrhythmias, as well as the increased potential for medication interactions due to poly-pharmacy. In a study of 7599 patients with symptomatic heart failure, the use of inhaled bronchodilators was associated with increased all-cause mortality, cardiovascular death, heart fail-ure hospitalization, and major adverse cardiovascular events.[39] Another study of 1244 heart failure patients found no increased risk of long-term mortality associated with beta₂-agonist use.[40] Future prospective studies may clarify the risks of beta₂-agonist use in patients with cardiac disease. For now, a careful consider-ation of the potential risks and benefits of beta₂-agonists in older patients with cardiac conditions should be undertaken.

Separate from the cardiac risks, some studies have also described an increased risk for asthma-related death with LABAs. This led the U.S. Food and Drug Administration to require labeling in 2010 indicating that LABAs should only be used (1) in combination with an ICS for asthmatics, (2) in individuals who cannot achieve adequate control with other controller medications, and (3) for the shortest duration of time required to achieve asthma control and then discontin-ued if possible. The risks for adverse effects with LABAs may be greatest in children, although the aforementioned recommendations apply to individuals of all age groups.

ANTICHOLINERGIC AGENTS

Both short-acting and long-acting inhaled anticholinergic antimuscarinic agents can be used in addition to ICS for the

treatment of asthma. These agents lead to airway smooth muscle relaxation (bronchodilation) and decreased mucus secretion. Existing asthma guidelines provide little informa-tion regarding the appropriate use of these drugs. In addition, age-related changes in the efficacy and safety of anticholin-ergics are less well studied than those for beta₂-agonists. It is known that parasympathetic activity decreases with age, and animal studies have shown changes in anticholinergic responses due to reduced receptor numbers or postreceptor coupling.[41,42] The safety profile of anticholinergics in older adults is generally favorable, with a dry mouth and occa-sional prostate-related symptoms being the most commonly reported side effects. While, in general, SABAs are thought to be better bronchodilators than anticholinergics, one study found that asthmatics over 60 years of age had a bet-ter response to the short-acting anticholinergic, ipratropium bromide, than a SABA.[43] Another study found that the short-acting anticholinergic, oxitropium, led to improved asthma control in older asthmatics who were already taking high-dose ICS.[44]

In recent years, tiotropium, a long-acting antimuscarinic agent (LAMA), has become increasingly utilized as a ther-apy for asthma. In 2010, a high-profile study of 210 asthmat-ics found that tiotropium led to an equivalent improvement in symptoms and lung function as a LABA when used as an add-on therapy with ICS.[45] Another study involving 107 severe asthmatics found that tiotropium improved lung function among patients who were already taking high-dose inhaled steroids and a LABA.[46] Studies regarding the use of LAMAs in older asthmatics are lacking; however, they may turn out to be an especially useful therapy in this population, given their generally favorable side-effect profile and theoretical potential for age-related superiority over LABAs. It should be noted, however, that several studies have raised concerns regarding the safety of tiotropium in cardiac patients with COPD.[47] Further study to clarify the efficacy and safety of short-acting and long-acting anticholinergics in older asth-matics is warranted.

LEUKOTRIENE RECEPTOR ANTAGONISTS (LTRAs)

LTRAs, such as montelukast, are considered an appropriate add-on therapy in combination with ICS for asthmatics of all ages, and may be considered as a monotherapy in mild asthmatics.[22,24] The efficacy of antileukotrienes for older asthmatics has not been extensively studied. A recent study of 513 asthmatics over 60 years of age found that montelu-kast decreased exacerbations and the need for rescue inhaler use among severe asthmatics who were taking ICS and a LABA.[48] In addition, a study of 41 asthmatics over 65 years of age found that pranlukast was equivalent to an ICS as a monotherapy for mild asthma.[49] LTRAs thus appear to be useful for some older asthmatics. In particular, a trial of these medications for older asthmatics with nasal polyposis and/or aspirin-exacerbated respiratory disease (AERD) is reason-able, given that AERD patients have been shown to incur greater improvements in asthma control with LTRAs than can be achieved with ICS alone. In addition, because they are in pill form, LTRAs are easier to use for older patients who have difficulties with inhalers. While they are generally well tolerated, a potential increased risk of Churg–Strauss vasculitis has been reported among patients taking leukotriene antagonists. In addition, concerns have been raised regarding psychological side effects, including a potentially increased risk of suicide.[50] Physicians prescribing these medications in older asthmatics, who are at increased risk of depression and cognitive impairment, must be aware of these risks.

METHYLXANTHINES

Theophylline is a phosphodiesterase inhibitor that has been used as a bronchodilator and anti-inflammatory agent for asthma for over 75 years. It has become less popular in recent years because of its narrow therapeutic window (10–20 mg/L) and its potential for life-threatening arrhythmias. Several important changes occur with aging that impact theophylline responses, including (1) decreased activity of phosphodiesterases, and (2) reduced clearance of the drug by the liver and kidneys with a resultant increased half-life.[51] The decline in theophylline clearance becomes especially prominent beginning in the seventh decade of life. In addition, theophylline has the potential for multiple drug interactions, which is problematic in older asthmatics on multiple medications. While theophylline can be effective for older asthmatics, it should be used cautiously in this population given the aforementioned concerns.

INHALED CORTICOSTEROIDS

While ICS are the cornerstone of asthma management for asthmatics of any age, the side effects related to these medications can be more prominent in older adults.[52] Oral candidiasis associated with ICS may occur more frequently in older asthmatics, particularly among those with dentures. The measures to minimize candida infection, including the use of spacers and mouth-rinsing after ICS dosing, should be emphasized. The risk of osteoporosis related to oral and inhaled steroids increases with age, and routine monitoring for its development should be conducted. Screening for cataracts among older asthmatics with previous oral or high-dose ICS should be considered. In addition, consideration should also be given to measuring vitamin D levels in this population, both for bone health and because of the association between low vitamin D levels, which are common in older adults, and poorer asthma control.

OTHER TREATMENT CONSIDERATIONS IN OLDER ASTHMATICS

Other therapies that are effective for younger asthmatics can also be considered in older asthmatics. Subcutaneous allergen immunotherapy may be appropriate for atopic asthmatics of any age, although the presence of comorbid conditions and medications that impact the safety of immunotherapy (e.g., beta-blockers) must be considered. The humanized

monoclonal anti-immunoglobulin E (IgE) antibody, omalizumab, has been shown to improve asthma symptoms and lung function and to decrease exacerbations in atopic, severe asthmatics with a median age of 60 years; seven patients studied were over 64 years of age.[53] Another study also showed clinical improvements among severe, atopic asthmatics aged 50 and older.[54] Omalizumab can thus also be considered in older, severe asthmatics with atopy who are refractory to other therapies and meet the dosing criteria involving body weight and total IgE level.

Obesity in Older Adults

Obesity may be a risk factor for more severe asthma in older adults. A study of 104 asthmatics aged 65 and older found that obesity was significantly associated with poorer asthma control based on ACQ scores; this finding remained after adjusting for multiple other potential risk factors.[11] It is unclear if the association between obesity and asthma is related to changes that occur in the lung mechanics with increased weight, versus the potential effects of obesity on the immune system. Studies in younger age groups have shown that weight loss improves asthma control and decreases airway hyperresponsiveness.[55]

Exercise and Pulmonary Rehabilitation

Exercise programs tailored for asthmatics have been shown to improve both physical and psychosocial functioning in younger patients. Programs that encourage increased physical activity and especially those that increase respiratory muscle strength may lead to improved quality of life in older asthmatics.[56] Pulmonary rehabilitation is a standard of care for patients with COPD, and may be considered in appropriate older asthmatics.[21] Some of the key aspects of the treatment of asthma in older adults are summarized in Table 20.2.

CONTROLLING TRIGGERS FOR ASTHMA IN OLDER ASTHMATICS

Environmental control measures are recognized as an important component of care in asthma treatment guidelines.[24] Because of the increased time that they spend at home relative to younger adults, older adults may have greater exposure to residential air pollutants and indoor aeroallergens. Controlling home environmental exposures, if possible, is therefore especially important in this population.

Relevant air pollution exposures may include those from outdoor sources that penetrate most dwellings, as well as indoor pollutants from tobacco smoke, cooking, and heating.[9,11] Asthmatics aged 65 and older may be disproportionately impacted by traffic-related air pollution relative to younger asthmatics. A recent study showed that chronic residential exposure to traffic pollution was among the strongest predictors of poorer asthma control in older adults.[11] Multiple other studies support the strong relationship between traffic pollution exposure and poor asthma control in older adults, including: a systematic review of admissions for respiratory diseases and particulate air pollution indicating that children

TABLE 20.2

Key Aspects of Asthma Treatment in Older Adults

Overcoming barriers to adherence	Form a partnership between patient and physician
	Identify barriers and goals of treatment
	Establish a plan for routine monitoring of symptoms and objective testing
	Provide effective teaching and routine reeducation regarding inhaler techniques
	Tailor therapies to physical, cognitive, and psychosocial abilities
Consider risk/benefit of treatments	Inhaled beta$_2$-agonists are still a cornerstone of care, but some studies suggest that they may be less effective and have increased cardiac side effects
	Short-acting and long-acting anticholinergics may be effective and their side-effect profile appears to be good overall, but more study is needed
	Antileukotrienes have not been extensively studied in older asthmatics, but a few studies have shown good efficacy; psychological side effects may be problematic
	Methylxanthines are still effective but have an increased risk for side effects in older adults
	Oral steroids and high-dose inhaled steroids may cause increased side effects in older adults, including exacerbation of heart failure, oral candidiasis, cataracts, and osteoporosis
	Allergen immunotherapy and omalizumab can be considered in appropriate patients
	Weight loss and pulmonary rehabilitation are therapeutic considerations in appropriate patients
	Consideration may also be given to clinical phenotypes and biomarkers when selecting medications
Environmental controls	Minimize indoor and outdoor air pollution exposure
	Methods that are used to reduce indoor aeroallergen exposure in younger patients should be considered in sensitized older asthmatics
	Minimize risk for viral infections, including vaccination when available, and isolating infected individuals in institutional and hospital settings

and older adults were at greatest risk[57]; an ecological study showing that asthmatics aged 65 and older have a shorter "lag time" to hospitalization when exposed to outdoor air pollutants[58]; and a study indicating that higher traffic density and ozone levels have a greater impact on older asthmatics relative to younger asthmatics.[59] Currently, there is unfortunately little that can be recommended to limit exposure to outdoor air pollutants that penetrate the home environment. It is recommended that older asthmatics minimize the time that they spend outdoors and keep windows closed on days that the air quality index (AQI) is greater than 100.[60]

Little is known about the impact of pollutants from indoor sources on asthma in older adults. Wood-burning stoves and biomass contribute to COPD, and probably to asthma in rural areas and developing countries. In addition, higher levels of respirable particles, such as those from tobacco smoke, are associated with increased acute respiratory symptoms and lower PEFs among adults aged 65 years and older.[61] Decreasing their exposure to pollutants from indoor sources should be attempted in older asthmatics.

Aeroallergen exposures can impact asthma control in sensitized older asthmatics, although possibly to a lesser extent than in younger individuals. While the prevalence of allergy-related symptoms may be lower in older versus younger asthmatics, two recent studies found that at least 70% of older asthmatics were atopic based on having at least one positive allergy skin prick test.[7,11] No studies have specifically addressed the impact of environmental control measures designed to decrease aeroallergen exposures, such as those from pets, dust mites, or mold, in older asthmatics. Despite a lack of evidence in this age group, it may be reasonable to attempt environmental

control measures for older, allergen-sensitive asthmatics based on their demonstrated efficacy in younger asthmatics.[62]

Respiratory virus infections are an important, potentially modifiable environmental risk factor for asthma exacerbations in older asthmatics. The rate of infection with viral pathogens may be as high as 11% among older adults living in institutional settings.[21] In contrast, seniors living at home appear to have lower infection rates than the general adult population. While most data related to viral infections and asthma exacerbations are extrapolated from younger populations, it is reasonable to assume that older asthmatics who are exposed to these pathogens are at increased risk for exacerbations.[21] As with asthmatics of any age, older asthmatics should be encouraged to undergo vaccination for influenza. Measures should also be taken in institutional and hospital settings to minimize the spread of viral infections, including the isolation of infected patients, hand washing, and wearing masks when appropriate.

ASTHMA PHENOTYPES IN OLDER ADULTS

Questions involving asthma phenotypes in older adults frequently focus on the clinical significance of the age of asthma onset as it relates to prognosis and treatment. In a recent cross-sectional study of 104 asthmatics aged 65 years and older, 28% of subjects developed asthma before age 18, 27% between ages 19 and 40, 33% between ages 41 and 64, and 12% after age 64.[11] In general, patients with onset of asthma before 40 years of age (early onset) are more likely to have genetic risk factors for the disease, and are more likely to be atopic and to exhibit T-helper type 2 (Th2)-driven, eosinophilic inflammation.[21] In contrast, in patients who develop asthma after age 40, epigenetic mechanisms may predominate, inflammation may be neutrophilic or eosinophilic, and other pathways of inflammation, including T-helper type 1 (Th1) and Th17 pathways may predominate.[63]

Studies are lacking in older asthmatics regarding biomarkers that might predict corticosteroid responsiveness, such as peripheral and sputum eosinophils, ENO, and sensitivity to methacholine. A few studies have suggested that neutrophilic inflammation becomes more prominent in the respiratory track of older asthmatics; however, the relevance of this finding to treatment responsiveness is not clear.[64] In addition, studies are lacking regarding the responsiveness of older asthmatics with AERD to tailored treatment regimens involving antileukotrienes and potentially aspirin desensitization. Research studies to address the impact of clinical and biological phenotypes in older asthmatics on treatment responses are needed.

CONCLUSION

In summary, the diagnosis and management of asthma in older adults is complicated by age-related changes in physiology and psychosocial functioning, as well as by the presence of comorbid medical conditions. A rigorous approach to diagnosis using objective testing is needed in order to differentiate asthma from other prevalent conditions in this population. Establishing good communication and shared goals with the older asthmatic patient is critical to maintaining good asthma control. Medication choices for older asthmatics should be informed by accepted asthma guidelines; however, consideration must be given to the potential for the decreased efficacy of some treatments, an increased rate of side effects, and factors such as the delivery method of a medication that may impact compliance. Controlling exposure to triggers such as viral infections, aeroallergens, and air pollution should be attempted. Future studies are needed to determine which treatments provide the greatest efficacy and safety in older asthmatics in general, as well as to identify clinical and biological predictors of treatment responses to particular therapies in this population.

REFERENCES

1. US Census Bureau. United States, Age and Sex; 2007 American Community Survey 1-Year Estimates, 2007. http://factfinder.census.gov. Accessed 10/1/2010.
2. Moorman JE, Rudd RA, Johnson CA, et al. National surveillance for asthma: United States, 1980–2004. *MMWR Surveill Summ* 2007; 56:1–54.
3. Australian Centre for Asthma Monitoring. Asthma in Australia 2008. Canberra: Australian Centre for Asthma Monitoring, 2008.
4. Tsai CL, Lee WY, Hanania NA, et al. Age-related differences in clinical outcomes for acute asthma in the United States, 2006–2008. *J Allergy Clin Immunol* 2012; 129:1252–1258 e1.
5. Plaza V, Serra-Batlles J, Ferrer M, et al. Quality of life and economic features in elderly asthmatics. *Respiration* 2000; 67:65–70.
6. Stupka E, deShazo R. Asthma in seniors: Part 1. Evidence for underdiagnosis, undertreatment, and increasing morbidity and mortality. *Am J Med* 2009; 122:6–11.
7. Smith AM, Villareal M, Bernstein DI, et al. Asthma in the elderly: Risk factors and impact on physical function. *Ann Allergy Asthma Immunol* 2012; 108:305–310.
8. Enright PL, McClelland RL, Newman AB, et al. Underdiagnosis and undertreatment of asthma in the elderly. Cardiovascular Health Study Research Group. *Chest* 1999; 116:603–613.
9. Diaz-Guzman E, Mannino DM. Airway obstructive diseases in older adults: From detection to treatment. *J Allergy Clin Immunol* 2010; 126:702–709.
10. Reed CE. Asthma in the elderly: What we do not know yet but should find out. *J Allergy Clin Immunol* 2011; 128:S1–S3.
11. Epstein TG, Ryan PH, LeMasters GK, et al. Poor asthma control and exposure to traffic pollutants and obesity in older adults. *Ann Allergy Asthma Immunol* 2012; 108:423–428 e2.
12. Battaglia S, Sandrini MC, Catalano F, et al. Effects of aging on sensation of dyspnea and health-related quality of life in elderly asthmatics. *Aging Clin Exp Res* 2005; 17:287–292.
13. Gershon AS, Victor JC, Guan J, et al. Pulmonary function testing in the diagnosis of asthma: A population study. *Chest* 2011; 141:1190–1196.
14. Global Strategy for the Diagnosis, Management and Prevention of COPD. Global Initiative for Chronic Obstructive Lung Disease (GOLD), 2013. http://www.goldcopd.org/.
15. Perng DW, Huang HY, Chen HM, et al. Characteristics of airway inflammation and bronchodilator reversibility in COPD: A potential guide to treatment. *Chest* 2004; 126:375–381.
16. Shaya FT, Dongyi D, Akazawa MO, et al. Burden of concomitant asthma and COPD in a Medicaid population. *Chest* 2008; 134:14–19.
17. Jordan RE, Miller MR, Lam KB, et al. Sex, susceptibility to smoking and chronic obstructive pulmonary disease: The effect of different diagnostic criteria. Analysis of the Health Survey for England. *Thorax* 2012; 67:600–605.
18. Pellegrino R, Viegi G, Brusasco V, et al. Interpretative strategies for lung function tests. *Eur Respir J* 2005; 26:948–968.
19. Yang SC, Lin BY. Comparison of airway hyperreactivity in chronic obstructive pulmonary disease and asthma. *Chang Gung Med J* 2010; 33:515–523.
20. Vonk JM, Jongepier H, Panhuysen CI, et al. Risk factors associated with the presence of irreversible airflow limitation and reduced transfer coefficient in patients with asthma after 26 years of follow up. *Thorax* 2003; 58:322–327.
21. Hanania NA, King MJ, Braman SS, et al. Asthma in the elderly: Current understanding and future research needs—A report of a National Institute on Aging (NIA) workshop. *J Allergy Clin Immunol* 2011; 128:S4–S24.
22. National Heart, Lung, and Blood Institute, National Asthma Education and Prevention Program, Expert Panel Report 3: Guidelines for the Diagnosis and Management of Asthma. U.S. Department of Health and Human Services, National Institutes of Health, 2007.
23. Slavin RG, Haselkorn T, Lee JH, et al. Asthma in older adults: Observations from the epidemiology and natural history of asthma—Outcomes and treatment regimens (TENOR) study. *Ann Allergy Asthma Immunol* 2006; 96:406–414.
24. Global Initiative for Asthma (GINA). Global Strategy for Asthma Management and Prevention, 2010.
25. McDonald VM, Higgins I, Simpson JL, et al. The importance of clinical management problems in older people with COPD and asthma: Do patients and physicians agree? *Prim Care Respir J* 2011; 20:389–395.

26. Bellia V, Battaglia S, Matera MG, et al. The use of bronchodilators in the treatment of airway obstruction in elderly patients. *Pulm Pharmacol Ther* 2006; 19:311–319.

27. Connolly MJ. Inhaler technique of elderly patients: Comparison of metered-dose inhalers and large volume spacer devices. *Age Ageing* 1995; 24:190–192.

28. Chapman KR, Love L, Brubaker H. A comparison of breath-actuated and conventional metered-dose inhaler inhalation techniques in elderly subjects. *Chest* 1993; 104:1332–1337.

29. Baba K, Tanaka H, Nishimura M, et al. Age-dependent deterioration of peak inspiratory flow with two kinds of dry powder corticosteroid inhalers (Diskus and Turbuhaler) and relationships with asthma control. *J Aerosol Med Pulm Drug Deliv* 2011; 24:293–301.

30. Takayanagi I, Kawano K, Koike K. Effect of aging on the response of guinea pig trachea to isoprenaline. *Jap J Pharmacol* 1990;53:359–366.

31. Feldman RD, Limbird LE, Nadeau J, et al. Leukocyte beta-receptor alterations in hypertensive subjects. *J Clin Invest* 1984;73:648–653.

32. Scarpace PJ, Baresi LA. Increased beta-adrenergic receptors in the light-density membrane fraction in lungs from senescent rats. *J Gerontology* 1988;43:B163–B167.

33. Ericsson E, Lundholm L. Adrenergic beta-receptor activity and cyclic AMP metabolism in vascular smooth muscle; variations with age. *Mech Ageing Dev* 1975;4:1–6.

34. Teramoto S. Evaluating the bronchodilator response in elderly who have asthma. *Chest* 1996;109:589–590.

35. Connolly MJ, Crowley JJ, Charan NB, et al. Impaired bronchodilator response to albuterol in healthy elderly men and women. *Chest* 1995;108:401–406.

36. Parker AL. Aging does not affect beta-agonist responsiveness after methacholine-induced bronchoconstriction. *J Am Geriatr Soc* 2004;52:388–392.

37. Rodrigo G, Rodrigo C. Effect of age on bronchodilator response in acute severe asthma treatment. *Chest* 1997;112:19–23.

38. Haughney J, Aubier M, Jorgensen L, et al. Comparing asthma treatment in elderly versus younger patients. *Respir Med* 2011;105:838–845.

39. Hawkins NM, Wang D, Petrie MC, et al. Baseline characteristics and outcomes of patients with heart failure receiving bronchodilators in the CHARM programme. *Eur J Heart Fail* 2010;12:557–565.

40. Bermingham M, O'Callaghan E, Dawkins I, et al. Are beta2-agonists responsible for increased mortality in heart failure? *Eur J Heart Fail* 2011;13:885–891.

41. Goldstein DS. Plasma catecholamines and essential hypertension. An analytical review. *Hypertension* 1983;5:86–99.

42. Preuss JM, Goldie RG. Age-related changes in airway responsiveness to phosphodiesterase inhibitors and activators of adenyl cyclase and guanylyl cyclase. *Pulm Pharmacol Ther* 1999;12:237–243.

43. van Schayck CP, Folgering H, Harbers H, et al. Effects of allergy and age on responses to salbutamol and ipratropium bromide in moderate asthma and chronic bronchitis. *Thorax* 1991;46:355–359.

44. Nishimura K, Koyama H, Ishihara K, et al. Additive effect of oxitropium bromide in combination with inhaled corticosteroids in the treatment of elderly patients with chronic asthma. *Allergol Intern* 1999;48:85–88.

45. Peters SP, Kunselman SJ, Icitovic N, et al. Tiotropium bromide step-up therapy for adults with uncontrolled asthma. *N Engl J Med* 2010;363:1715–1726.

46. Kerstjens HA, Disse B, Schroder-Babo W, et al. Tiotropium improves lung function in patients with severe uncontrolled asthma: A randomized controlled trial. *J Allergy Clin Immunol* 2011;128:308–314.

47. Singh S, Loke YK, Enright P, Furberg CD. Pro-arrhythmic and pro-ischaemic effects of inhaled anticholinergic medications. *Thorax* 2013;68(1):114–116.

48. Bozek A, Warkocka-Szoltysek B, Filipowska-Gronska A, et al. Montelukast as an add-on therapy to inhaled corticosteroids in the treatment of severe asthma in elderly patients. *J Asthma* 2012;49:530–534.

49. Horiguchi T, Tachikawa S, Kondo R, et al. Comparative evaluation of the leukotriene receptor antagonist pranlukast versus the steroid inhalant fluticasone in the therapy of aged patients with mild bronchial asthma. *Arzneimittelforschung* 2007;57:87–91.

50. Schumock GT, Lee TA, Joo MJ, et al. Association between leukotriene-modifying agents and suicide: What is the evidence? *Drug Safety* 2011;34:533–544.

51. Gupta P, O'Mahony MS. Potential adverse effects of bronchodilators in the treatment of airways obstruction in older people: Recommendations for prescribing. *Drugs Aging* 2008;25:415–443.

52. Ohbayashi H, Adachi M. Influence of dentures on residual inhaled corticosteroids in the mouths of elderly asthma patients. *Resp Investig* 2012;50:54–61.

53. Verma P, Randhawa I, Klaustermeyer WB. Clinical efficacy of omalizumab in an elderly veteran population with severe asthma. *Allergy Asthma Proc* 2011;32:346–350.

54. Korn S, Schumann C, Kropf C, et al. Effectiveness of omalizumab in patients 50 years and older with severe persistent allergic asthma. *Ann Allergy Asthma Immunol* 2010;105:313–319.

55. Boulet LP, Turcotte H, Martin J, et al. Effect of bariatric surgery on airway response and lung function in obese subjects with asthma. *Respir Med* 2012;106:651–660.

56. Gomieiro LT, Nascimento A, Tanno LK, et al. Respiratory exercise program for elderly individuals with asthma. *Clinics* 2011;66:1163–1169.

57. Anderson HR, Atkinson RW, Bremner SA, et al. Particulate air pollution and hospital admissions for cardiorespiratory diseases: Are the elderly at greater risk? *Eur Respir J Suppl* 2003;40:39s–46s.

58. Ko FW, Tam W, Wong TW, et al. Effects of air pollution on asthma hospitalization rates in different age groups in Hong Kong. *Clin Exp Allergy* 2007;37:1312–1319.

59. Meng YY, Wilhelm M, Rull RP, et al. Traffic and outdoor air pollution levels near residences and poorly controlled asthma in adults. *Ann Allergy Asthma Immunol* 2007;98:455–463.

60. Air Quality Index (AQI): A Guide to Air Quality and Your Health. AirNow. United States Environmental Protection Agency, 2012. http://www.airnow.gov. Accessed 8/1/2012.

61. Simoni M, Jaakkola MS, Carrozzi L, et al. Indoor air pollution and respiratory health in the elderly. *Eur Respir J Suppl* 2003;40:15s–20s.

62. Busse PJ, Lurslurchachai L, Sampson HA, et al. Perennial allergen-specific immunoglobulin E levels among inner-city elderly asthmatics. *J Asthma* 2010;47:781–785.

63. Busse PJ, Mathur SK. Age-related changes in immune function: Effect on airway inflammation. *J Allergy Clin Immunol* 2010;126:690–699; quiz 700–701.

64. Nyenhuis SM, Schwantes EA, Evans MD, Mathur SK. Airway neutrophil inflammatory phenotype in older subjects with asthma. *J Allergy Clin Immunol* 2010;125:1163–1165.

21 Severe Acute and Life-Threatening Asthma in Children

Annabelle Quizon and Erick Forno

CONTENTS

CASE PRESENTATION

A 12-year-old girl is brought to the emergency room (ER) by her parents. She has a long-standing history of asthma; her usual medications include a combination inhaler with fluticasone and salmeterol as well as montelukast, both of which her parents admit she takes irregularly. She has had three hospital admissions for asthma in the past year (one of them in the pediatric intensive care unit [PICU]); the most recent being 4 months ago. Her last visit to the doctor was approximately 1 month ago; her mother says her lung functions at that time were "low," and the doctor insisted she needed to take her medicines daily and follow up in a month. Her parents report she had been doing quite well with only nighttime cough until the night before, when she visited a friend who has several cats, to which she is allergic. On returning home, she started coughing, and they gave her albuterol nebulizations every 2–3 h all day with no apparent response. In the past hour, they noticed that she was looking tired and lethargic, and decided to bring her to the ER.

On initial evaluation, she exhibited increased work of breathing with tachycardia, tachypnea, and O2 saturation of 88% despite being on oxygen at 10 Lpm via a nonrebreather mask. She was conscious but lethargic. Breath sounds were decreased bilaterally with no wheezing. Back-to-back nebulizations with albuterol and ipratropium bromide were administered. Auscultation revealed sporadic inspiratory and expiratory wheezes but still markedly decreased breath sounds and prolonged expiration; she remained tachypneic and was becoming less responsive. Continuous albuterol nebulizations were administered and intravenous (IV) access was obtained after which she received a dose of methylprednisolone and a normal saline bolus. Chest x-ray showed marked hyperinflation with some areas of atelectasis; arterial blood gas (ABG) showed a pH of 7.34 and partial pressure of carbon dioxide (pCO_2) of 44 torr. The patient then became progressively obtunded, and a repeat ABG showed pH of 7.30 and pCO_2 of 49 torr. She was intubated and *received IV terbutaline and magnesium sulfate. Heliox was started and the patient was transferred to the PICU.*

In the PICU, she was placed on mechanical ventilation and received continuous albuterol nebulization as well as IV terbutaline and methylprednisolone. Within 24 h, auscultatory findings improved with increased air entry; ABG normalized. She was extubated to positive pressure ventilation by the second day and eventually weaned to room air. She was switched to oral corticosteroids by the third day and tolerated weaning of nebulized albuterol to every 4 h. She was discharged home after 5 days with instructions to continue usual home medications and to follow up with her primary pediatrician and with the pulmonologist who saw her during the admission.

DEFINITION AND EPIDEMIOLOGY

Asthma affects over 7 million children in the United States, and status asthmaticus is the most common pediatric medical emergency in the country.[1] The exact prevalence of "near-fatal" asthma and of status asthmaticus is difficult to estimate, because definitions of both vary significantly, but mortality from the disease currently stands at approximately 28 deaths per year for every 1 million children with asthma, and can be as high as 34 per million depending on age and gender.[2] This translates into at least ~200–240 unnecessary deaths due to childhood asthma every year. In previous review articles, status asthmaticus was defined as the condition of a patient in progressive respiratory failure due to asthma in whom conventional forms of therapy have failed; for clinical purposes, a patient not responding to initial doses of nebulized bronchodilators is considered to have status asthmaticus.[3,4] A recent study of fatal and near-fatal asthma (defined as asthma requiring mechanical ventilation) reported that in 13% of such cases there was no previous diagnosis of asthma;[1] in those children the initial presentation of asthma was a life-threatening exacerbation, which underscores the importance of prompt recognition and aggressive treatment of such exacerbations.

PRESENTATION

Clinical characteristics (Table 21.1) of a severe asthma exacerbation include dyspnea at rest, severely increased work of breathing or respiratory distress, markedly decreased breath sounds, especially when wheezing is faint or inaudible (quiet lungs may mean there is simply no air movement and be a sign of impending respiratory failure), altered mental status, rising pCO_2 (pCO_2 levels are usually low initially due to tachypnea, but may tend to "normalize" as the patient becomes tired; this, too, may be a sign of impending respiratory failure), and, when feasible to perform, peak expiratory flows (PEF) under 40% of predicted or personal best. The Expert Panel Report 3 (EPR-3) from the National Institutes of Health (NIH) of the United States further describes life-threatening exacerbations as those in which patients are too dyspneic to speak and PEF falls under 25%

TABLE 21.1

Clinical Characteristics of a Severe or Life-Threatening Asthma Exacerbation

History
Sleepiness or lethargy
Dyspnea interferes with ability to talk

Physical Examination
Altered mental status
Significant respiratory distress
"Silent thorax" with markedly decreased air movement and scarce wheezing

Laboratory
Significant and/or refractory hypoxia
"Normalization" of pCO_2 in the setting of persistent respiratory distress
Respiratory acidosis
PEF less than 40% of predicted or personal best

of predicted or personal best.[5] However, the clinical presentation of severe or life-threatening status asthmaticus is variable, and it is paramount that the clinician be able to recognize severe cases rapidly and promptly escalate management to prevent potentially fatal complications. In the case described above, the patient presented with several of these characteristics, including significant dyspnea, hypoxia, progressively altered mental status, "silent" lungs on auscultation, and worsening respiratory acidosis. As is usually the case with these children, she failed to respond to appropriate initial therapy with bronchodilators, but prompt recognition of the severity of the exacerbation and aggressive treatment made it possible for her to recover without major complications.

RISK FACTORS

The EPR-3 lists several risk factors for death from asthma in children and adults (Table 21.2).[5] As evidenced by the table, perhaps the most important single risk factor for a severe (and potentially life-threatening) asthma exacerbation is a previous history of severe exacerbations, particularly when such exacerbations have occurred recently. Additionally, several studies have identified various risk factors such as gender (male predominance in childhood with a later switch to female predominance), low lung function despite treatment, longer duration of disease,[6,7] exacerbation triggered by allergens or irritants rather than exertion or viral illness, and more abrupt onset of the exacerbation.[8] In a study of PICU admissions for asthma, Carroll et al. found that children with multiple PICU admissions for asthma are more likely to be overweight and have public insurance and less likely to be Caucasian compared with other asthmatic children with only one PICU admission.[9] In the report by Newth et al. looking at children who required intubation for a life-threatening asthma exacerbation, there was an overrepresentation of African Americans.[1] In that study, mortality rate was 4%,

TABLE 21.2
Risk Factors for Death from Asthma (Children and Adults)

Asthma History

Previous severe exacerbation (e.g., intubation or PICU admission for asthma)

Two or more hospitalizations for asthma in the past year

Three or more ER visits for asthma in the past year

Hospitalization or ER visit for asthma in the past month

Using more than two canisters of albuterol per month

Difficulty perceiving asthma symptoms or severity of exacerbations

Other risk factors: lack of a written asthma action plan, sensitivity to *Alternaria*, etc.

Social History

Low socioeconomic status or inner-city residence

Illicit drug use

Major psychosocial problems

Comorbidities

Cardiovascular disease

Other chronic lung disease

Chronic psychiatric disease

Other chronic illnesses

Source: National Asthma Education and Prevention Program (NAEPP), *J. Allergy Clin. Immunol.*, 120, S94–S138, 2007.

and 10 of the 11 children who died had experienced cardiac arrest before admission to the PICU.

Given the known heritability of asthma, it is to be expected that genetic and genomic polymorphisms and variants will likely be associated with higher risk of severe or near-fatal asthma. Polymorphisms of the beta-adrenergic receptor gene *ADRB2*, for example, have been associated with the length of PICU stay for status asthmaticus in children.[10] Similarly, a higher level of African ancestry—determined using genetic methods—was recently associated with lower lung function in Puerto Rican children,[11] one of the ethnic groups with the highest prevalence, morbidity, and mortality related to asthma. As the field progresses, new genetic or epigenetic variants may be identified that could be used to personalize management, both acute and chronic, according to the patient's asthma severity or risk for complications.

Asthma is a complex, multifactorial disease, and the risk factors for severe and life-threatening asthma exacerbations are similarly complex. In summary, a past (and especially recent) history of a severe asthma exacerbation and poor asthma control are probably the two most portentous risk factors for future severe exacerbations. Still, a significant proportion of children who present with potentially fatal asthma have no recent history of similar attacks, and in many of them it may present their index presentation. Physicians and providers need to be aware of risk factors for severe asthma, but also should be able to recognize presenting signs and symptoms quickly even in children without prior history. Most importantly, once recognized, they need to be able to act swiftly and aggressively manage the patient to prevent complications or death.

MANAGEMENT

GENERAL MEASURES

Acute severe asthma in children is a common cause of admission to the PICU. Children with acute severe asthma require cardiorespiratory monitoring and stabilization that ensure that the treatment goals of adequate oxygenation and reversal of bronchial narrowing are achieved. Patients present with hypoxemia from ventilation–perfusion mismatch and benefit from high-flow supplemental oxygen delivered via a partial or nonrebreather mask. Signs of impending respiratory failure should be monitored and prompt management with ventilatory support should be provided once present. Fluid replacement should be provided to restore euvolemia for dehydrated patients as a result of vomiting, poor intake, and increased insensible fluid loss from the respiratory tract. Fluid balance should be monitored closely inasmuch as overhydration can result in pulmonary edema; patients can also develop the syndrome of inappropriate antidiuretic hormone secretion (SIADH).[3,4]

INITIAL LABORATORY STUDIES

The objective of laboratory studies is to detect actual or impending respiratory failure. However, the decision to intubate a patient and provide ventilatory support should not depend on laboratory measurements. ABG is useful for assessment of pulmonary gas exchange. With increasing airflow obstruction, hypercarbia develops and heralds impending respiratory failure. Venous levels of pCO_2 have been tested as a substitute for arterial measurements such that a venous $pCO_2 > 45$ mmHg may serve as a screening test but cannot substitute for ABG in the evaluation of respiratory function.[12] An indwelling arterial line facilitates frequent blood gas assessment in the intubated and mechanically ventilated patient.

Complete blood count (CBC) is not routinely required but may be considered in patients suspected to have concomitant infection, especially if they exhibit a fever or purulent sputum. However, leukocytosis can be present in patients with asthma exacerbations and can be further confounded by the use of systemic corticosteroids within a few hours of administration. Measurement of serum electrolytes is reasonable, especially for patients with cardiovascular disease and/or receiving diuretics inasmuch as frequent beta-agonist administration is associated with hypokalemia, hypomagnesemia, and hypophosphatemia.

CHEST RADIOGRAPHY

Chest radiographs are not routinely required but may be indicated when there is suspicion of another pulmonary process such as air leak or barotrauma (pneumothorax or pneumomediastinum), pneumonia, or lobar atelectasis, or when the underlying cause of wheezing is in doubt.

PHARMACOTHERAPY

Prompt administration of medications to reverse airflow obstruction is crucial in the management of acute severe asthma. In this section, medications used in the PICU setting are discussed; references to initial emergency department (ED) management are mentioned whenever applicable. The dosages of medications as described in the National Heart, Lung, and Blood Institute (NHLBI) guidelines and cited references are found in Table 21.3.

Beta-Receptor Agonists

Beta-receptor agonists are the mainstays of treatment of acute severe asthma. By binding to beta-receptors in the airway smooth muscles, short-acting beta-agonists (SABAs) produce smooth muscle relaxation. To avoid the risk of cardiotoxicity, selective SABAs are recommended such as albuterol; levalbuterol, the pure R enantiomer of albuterol, has also been used. These agents have rapid onsets of action and have been administered via several routes that include IV, nebulized, subcutaneous, and oral. In the PICU setting, the nebulized and IV routes are applicable. Of note is that the use of metered-dose inhalers with a valved holding chamber for delivery of albuterol has been found to be effective in

children with moderate to severe asthma exacerbations.[13–15] However, the nebulized route may be the preferred route in the PICU for patients unable to cooperate due to factors such as age and severity of presentation; the patient also derives benefit from the oxygen that is used to propel the nebulization device. For patients who require frequent doses of albuterol, continuous nebulization is preferred over intermittent doses. Continuous nebulization results in rapid improvement without the increased risk of toxicity.[16–19]

Levalbuterol is more potent in beta-receptor binding than S-albuterol and is responsible for the bronchodilating effects of the racemic compound—albuterol being an equal mixture of R-albuterol and S-albuterol. However, Gawchik et al. found no significant differences in efficacy or safety between levalbuterol and albuterol.[20] In a prospective study by Andrews et al., substituting high-dose continuous levalbuterol for racemic albuterol did not reduce the time on continuous therapy and had similar adverse effects in children presenting in status asthmaticus who have failed initial treatment with racemic albuterol.[21] No recommendation can presently be made regarding the use of the more expensive levalbuterol in children with acute severe asthma.

IV beta-agonists should be considered in patients unresponsive to treatment with continuous nebulization. Near-complete airway obstruction as well as decreased tidal volumes may affect delivery of aerosolized bronchodilator to the lung. Terbutaline is the IV beta-agonist that is currently used in the United States. In a prospective study conducted by Bogie et al. the addition of IV terbutaline to continuous high-dose nebulized albuterol in children with acute severe asthma resulted in a trend toward improvement regarding outcome measures consisting of asthma severity score, duration of continuous nebulized albuterol, and PICU stay.[22]

Adverse events related to beta-agonist use, via both inhalational and IV routes, are cardiac in nature. However, other than tachycardia or diastolic hypotension, neither albuterol nor terbutaline is associated with clinically significant cardiac toxicity in pediatric patients.[19,23] In a prospective study, Chiang et al. found no significant cardiac toxicity among pediatric patients with acute severe asthma who received IV terbutaline.[24] Other adverse events include tremors, worsening of ventilation/perfusion mismatch, and transient decreases in serum levels of potassium, magnesium, and phosphorus. On a cautionary note, severe hypokalemia may precipitate cardiac arrhythmias.

Anticholinergics

Increased acetylcholine release from parasympathetic nerves has been associated with increased smooth muscle tone and bronchoconstriction. Ipratropium bromide, a quaternary ammonium derivative of atropine, is a short-acting anticholinergic and has been used in the management of acute asthma exacerbations. It does not induce systemic or respiratory side effects due to minimal systemic absorption, the latter as a result of inefficient absorption from the lungs and gastrointestinal tract.[25] It has been demonstrated in several systematic reviews to significantly improve pulmonary

TABLE 21.3
Medications and Doses in Pediatric Acute Severe Asthma

Medication	Route	Dose
Beta-Receptor Agonists		
Albuterol (salbutamol)	Intermittent nebulization	0.15–0.3 mg/kg (up to 10 mg) every 1–4 h as needed[5]
	Continuous nebulization	0.5 mg/(kg h) (up to 10 mg/h)[5]
Levalbuterol	Intermittent nebulization	0.075–0.15 mg/kg (up to 5 mg) every 1–4 h as needed[5]
Terbutaline	Intravenous	0.4–10 (μg/kg min)[23]
Anticholinergics		
Ipratropium bromide	Intermittent nebulization	0.25–0.5 mg every 6 h[76,77]
Corticosteroids		
Methylprednisolone	Intravenous	1 mg/kg every 6 h (maximum 125 mg single dose)[34,78]
Hydrocortisone	Intravenous	2–4 mg/kg every 4–6 h[4]
Other		
Magnesium sulfate	Intravenous	25–40 mg/kg over 20 min (maximum 2 g/dose)[51,52]
Aminophylline	Intravenous	6–8 mg/kg initial followed by 0.7–1.2 mg/(kg h) to maintain serum concentrations of 10–15 mg/L[79,80]

function and clinical outcomes compared with the use of a beta-agonist alone.[26–28] In a pooled analysis combining adult and pediatric studies, Rodrigo and Castro-Rodriguez showed a dose–response relationship with a greater benefit being achieved in patients treated with more than two doses of anticholinergic agents in combination with a beta-agonist, as reflected in hospital admission rates and pulmonary function.[26] A few of the studies in children reported a significant improvement in clinical scores after combined treatment, with no apparent increase in side effects such as tremors or heart rate. Asthma clinical pathways carried out in EDs in the management of children presenting with acute severe asthma include administration of three doses of nebulized albuterol with ipratropium bromide within the first 60 min of treatment.[5] Anticholinergics are used in combination with beta-agonists to arrest progression to hypercapnic respiratory failure that requires PICU admission; once a patient is mechanically ventilated, anticholinergics offer little benefit.[29]

Corticosteroids

Asthma is an inflammatory disease and corticosteroids constitute first-line treatment for acute severe asthma. Mechanisms of action of corticosteroids that render them beneficial in asthma are discussed in previous chapters. The use of inhaled corticosteroids at higher than maintenance doses has been explored in mitigating an exacerbation when given at its onset; it has also been studied regarding its benefit in acute management of patients seen in the ED.[30,31] However, the data on the efficacy of inhaled corticosteroids in children in these settings are inconsistent,[32] perhaps due to inconsistency of dosing. Smith et al., in a meta-analysis on the use of corticosteroids in children with acute severe asthma, stated that inhaled or nebulized corticosteroids cannot be recommended as equivalent to systemic corticosteroids.[33]

For acute severe asthma, systemic corticosteroids should be given promptly; beneficial effect becomes evident at 1–3 h and maximal effects at 4–8 h after administration of the first dose in conjunction with administration of beta-agonists.[34] Moreover, frequent dosing, typically four times daily, has also been found to be efficacious. Oral or parenteral corticosteroids are equally efficacious; in the PICU setting however, parenteral corticosteroids are preferred for critically ill children, more so if they are intubated or unable to tolerate oral doses. Once the patient is extubated or stabilized and able to tolerate oral intake and provided gastrointestinal transit time and absorption are not impaired, switching from IV to oral corticosteroids may be considered.

The more commonly used systemic corticosteroids include IV hydrocortisone and methylprednisolone. Intramuscular dexamethasone has been studied but mostly in the ER setting and in comparison with oral prednisolone for treatment of moderate asthma exacerbations.[35–38] Given its pharmacologic properties (i.e., biologic half-life of 36–72 h and systemic bioavailability), it is usually given as a single intramuscular dose and on some occasions by oral or nebulized routes.[39] There is no extra advantage to administering higher than conventional doses of corticosteroids such as methylprednisolone.[40] In an adult study, hydrocortisone was found to be more effective than methylprednisolone regarding median duration of hospitalization and lung function.[41] The total course of systemic corticosteroids for acute severe asthma may last from 3 to 10 days. For courses of less than 1 week, there is no need to taper the dose; for slightly longer courses up to 10 days, there is probably no need to taper, especially if patients are concurrently using inhaled corticocosteroids.[5] If treatment is required for longer than 10 days, slow dosage taper is recommended.[42]

Short-term use of high-dose corticosteroids is usually not associated with significant adverse effects. Hyperglycemia, hypertension, and acute psychosis have been reported.[43] Concerns regarding the immunosuppressive effects of corticosteroids have been raised but are associated with long-term use. However, risk for fatal varicella has been reported with a single course of corticosteroids.[44]

Magnesium

Magnesium can inhibit calcium uptake and result in smooth muscle relaxation and has therefore been used in the management of acute asthma, particularly in the ER setting. It can be given intravenously or via nebulization. A Cochrane review by Blitz et al. that included two studies conducted exclusively in pediatric patients showed nebulized magnesium sulfate in addition to beta-agonist improved pulmonary function in patients with severe asthma and decreased hospitalization rates.[45] The use of IV magnesium for acute asthma was the subject of meta-analyses[46–49] as well as other studies conducted in pediatric patients.[50–52] These studies showed that IV magnesium may reduce hospitalization rates among pediatric patients in status asthmaticus seen in the ED and should be considered in refractory patients with impending respiratory failure. The EPR-3 NIH guidelines recommend that IV magnesium sulfate may be considered to avoid intubation, specifically in patients who continue to present with severe symptoms after an hour of intensive conventional therapy.[5]

Helium–Oxygen

Inhaled mixtures of helium–oxygen (heliox) containing up to 60%–80% helium fraction lower the density of a gas and reduce resistance during turbulent flow and, in the process, allow better oxygen delivery to the distal airways. Similar to the recommendation for the use of magnesium sulfate, the EPR-3 NIH guidelines state that for impending respiratory failure, heliox-driven albuterol nebulization should be considered for patients who have life-threatening exacerbation, specifically those who continue to present with severe symptoms after an hour of intensive conventional therapy.[5] Ho et al., in a systematic review that included two exclusively pediatric studies, found that heliox may offer mild to moderate benefits in patients with acute asthma within the first hour of use; its effect may be more pronounced in more severe cases.[53] Similarly, from a Cochrane review, heliox treatment was shown not to play a role in the initial treatment of patients with acute asthma; however, benefits were greater in patients with more severe obstruction.[54]

Methylxanthines

Methylxanthines act as phosphodiesterase inhibitors resulting in bronchodilation. In addition, other mechanisms of action have been invoked to be beneficial in improving respiratory status, such as their ability to stimulate endogenous catecholamine release and function as diuretics, beta-adrenergic agonists, and prostaglandin antagonists; they also augment diaphragmatic contractility. Their use, however, has been limited, not just by availability of therapeutic options, but by their narrow therapeutic range and well-known toxicities. Toxicities include nausea, vomiting, tachycardia, and agitation. Life-threatening toxicities have been documented and include cardiac arrhythmias, hypotension, seizures, and death.

Mitra et al. reviewed the use of IV aminophylline for acute severe asthma in children over 2 years receiving inhaled bronchodilators.[55] They found that the addition of IV aminophylline to beta-agonists and glucocorticoids (with or without anticholinergics) improved lung function within 6 h of treatment but with no reduction in symptoms, numbers of nebulized treatment, and length of hospital stay; there was insufficient evidence to assess its impact on oxygenation, PICU admission, and mechanical ventilation. Similar results were found by Yung and South insofar as improvements in lung function and oxygen saturation within 6 and 30 h, respectively, in children given aminophylline after large doses of beta-agonists and corticosteroids were observed.[56] However, the EPR-3 NIH guidelines did not recommend the use of methylxanthines for severe exacerbations in ER or hospital settings.[5]

Leukotriene Receptor Antagonists

These drugs, available as tablets, have been typically used as controller medications. Capsomidis and Tighe, in reviewing available studies in children, concluded that the use of oral montelukast is not currently recommended in moderate to severe asthma exacerbations in children.[57] The EPR-3 NIH guidelines affirm this conclusion, stating there are insufficient data to recommend the use of IV leukotriene receptor antagonists for moderate to severe exacerbations. A study conducted by Camargo et al. in adult asthmatics with moderate and severe exacerbations demonstrated improvement in lung function with the addition of IV montelukast to bronchodilators and corticosteroids.[58]

Inhalational Anesthetics

Volatile anesthetics have beneficial effects on airway tone and reactivity that include a direct effect on bronchial smooth muscle resulting in bronchodilatation.[59–61] Other physiological functions include decreased mean arterial pressure and myocardial contractility. The use of inhalational anesthetic agents, notably isoflurane and halothane, in children presenting with acute severe asthma refractory to conventional measures has been anecdotal.[61–65] In a case series consisting of six pediatric patients,[64] isoflurane was administered using a volume-limited Servo 900D ventilator with an attached vaporizer that delivered the anesthetic; the authors

recommended monitoring of end tidal CO_2 and placement of central venous and arterial catheters as well as consideration of inline monitoring of isoflurane concentration. More recently, in a retrospective review over 15 years that included patients with a mean age of 9.5 years, Turner et al. concluded that isoflurane appeared to be an effective therapy in patients with life-threatening bronchospasm refractory to conventional therapy, although the overall impact remained uncertain; the majority of patients developed hypotension but there was a low incidence of side effects.[66]

VENTILATORY SUPPORT

Absolute indications for intubation include cardiopulmonary arrest, severe hypoxia, and rapid deterioration in the patient's mental status.[3] Progressive respiratory fatigue despite maximal pharmacotherapy including noninvasive techniques constitutes a relative indication for intubation and mechanical ventilation. A cuffed or sufficiently large endotracheal tube is recommended to minimize air leak with the anticipated high inspiratory pressures. Newth et al. found no increased risk for postextubation complications in children who were intubated using cuffed endotracheal tubes.[67] The intubated patient receiving mechanical ventilation requires sedation (usually with opioids, benzodiazepines or propofol) to avoid ventilator dyssynchrony. The use of neuromuscular blockade should be considered for patients in whom adequate ventilation cannot be achieved despite acceptable ventilatory pressures or settings. Clinicians should pay close attention to maintaining or replacing intravascular volume given that hypotension commonly accompanies the initiation of positive pressure ventilation.

Noninvasive Ventilation (NIV)

In the study by Newth,[67] 23% of pediatric patients with severe asthma received noninvasive ventilation before intubation and after extubation; neither noninvasive nor invasive ventilation seemed to cause additional air leaks. In prospective and retrospective studies, the use of noninvasive positive pressure ventilation was found to be safe, well tolerated, and effective in the management of children presenting with acute severe asthma.[68,69]

Mechanical Ventilation

The EPR guidelines recommend the use of permissive hypercapnea or controlled hypoventilation as ventilator strategies.[5] This mode allows the provision of adequate oxygenation and ventilation while minimizing high airway pressures and barotrauma[4,70] with adjustments made to the tidal volume, ventilator rate, and inspiration-to-expiration ratio to minimize airway pressures.

Extracorporeal Life Support

In children with severe refractory acute asthma who use anesthetic therapies, the use of extracorporeal life support has been anecdotally reported. Data from the Life Support Organization registry show that only 64 children received extracorporeal membrane oxygenation (ECMO) for asthma over a 21-year period covering 1986–2007 with a 94% survival rate;[71] of the survivors, significant neurological complications were found in 4%.

COMPLICATIONS

Children presenting with acute severe asthma are often admitted to the PICU for impending or actual respiratory failure and are at risk for complications not just from the underlying condition but also as a result of interventions such as pharmacotherapy and ventilatory support. Adverse reactions caused by medications are discussed in the previous section on Management. In a retrospective study, Carroll and Zucker identified common complications such as aspiration pneumonia, ventilator-associated pneumonia, barotrauma (e.g., pneumomediastinum and pneumothorax), and rhabdomyolysis; intubated children were significantly more likely than nonintubated children to experience a complication with duration of mechanical ventilation being an important factor.[72] They found that the use of positive pressure is associated with an increased risk of barotrauma in children regardless of whether this was provided by noninvasive means or via mechanical ventilation through an endotracheal tube. In the Collaborative Pediatric Critical Care Research Network (CPCCRN) study, 12% of patients admitted to the PICU had complications; the majority of the complications consisted of central nervous system deficits and a quarter of the patients developed barotrauma.[1] Neuropathy was also reported in a few patients.

Mechanical ventilation has been found to be a risk factor for rhabdomyolysis, especially in older children, through a mechanism similar to the pathogenesis of exercise-related rhabdomyolysis,[73] and can present acutely. The use of systemic corticosteroids and neuromuscular blockers may add to the risk of rhabdomyolysis, such that creatine phosphikinase should be monitored in children with acute respiratory failure. A case of subarachnoid hemorrhage was reported in association with the use of permissive hypercapnia for acute respiratory failure.[74]

Regarding mortality, the CPCCRN study cited a mortality rate of 4% with cause of death listed as anoxic brain injury (in the majority), cardiac arrest, pneumonia, and multiple organ failure.[1]

PROGNOSIS AND FOLLOW-UP

Admission to the PICU for asthma is a predictor of hospital readmission. Moreover, risk factors for mortality from asthma have been discussed in 'Risk Factors' and listed in Table 21.2.

Using data from the Centers for Disease Control and Prevention, Akinbami et al. described trends among asthmatic children 0–17 years of age; they cited that asthma-related deaths increased through the mid-1990s but decreased after 1999.[2] In a study that followed up pediatric patients admitted to the PICU over a 15-year period, 5% of patients who received mechanical ventilation for asthma during their index admission died within 10 years of discharge;[75] risk factors for subsequent mortality included multiple ICU admissions, persistent asthma, and ventilation at admission. In the same study, risk factors for ICU admission were admission for asthma in the preceding year and ventilation at admission.

Thus, patients admitted to the PICU for acute severe asthma require close follow-up upon discharge, especially if they required mechanical ventilation, which increases the risk for subsequent mortality. It is imperative that all asthmatic patients who are discharged from the hospital are provided with adequate education and written plans that encompass a list of medications, follow-up appointments with primary care providers and specialists, and recognition and initial management of an exacerbation. The importance of patient and parent or caregiver education cannot be overemphasized. An acknowledgment of the life-threatening complications of asthma can be the starting point of the education process that will help underscore the importance of adherence to medications and follow-up, understanding of the concept of controller and rescue medications, and even renewed efforts toward environmental controls and attention to avoidable triggers. A review of medications should include a demonstration of inhaler technique and appropriate feedback, especially with regard to inhaled medications that require nebulization or the use of spacer devices. A peak flow meter may be considered in children who are at least 5 years of age (and their parents or caregivers), those who have a history of severe exacerbations, those who have moderate or severe persistent asthma, and those who poorly perceive airflow obstruction or worsening asthma.[5]

REFERENCES

1. Newth CJ, Meert KL, Clark AE, Moler FW, Zuppa AF, Berg RA, et al. Fatal and near-fatal asthma in children: The critical care perspective. J Pediatr. 2012;161:214–221.
2. Akinbami LJ, Moorman JE, Garbe PL, Sondik EJ. Status of childhood asthma in the United States, 1980–2007. Pediatrics. 2009;123(Suppl 3):S131–S145.
3. Mannix R, Bachur R. Status asthmaticus in children. Curr Opin Pediatr. 2007;19(3):281–287.
4. Werner HA. Status asthmaticus in children: A review. Chest. 2001;119(6):1913–1929.
5. National Asthma Education and Prevention Program (NAEPP). Expert Panel Report 3 (EPR-3): Guidelines for the Diagnosis and Management of Asthma-Summary Report 2007. J Allergy Clin Immunol. 2007;120(Suppl 5):S94–S138.
6. Lyell PJ, Villanueva E, Burton D, Freezer NJ, Bardin PG. Risk factors for intensive care in children with acute asthma. Respirology. 2005;10(4):436–441.
7. Moore WC, Peters SP. Severe asthma: An overview. J Allergy Clin Immunol. 2006;117(3):487–494; quiz 95.
8. Sala KA, Carroll CL, Tang YS, Aglio T, Dressler AM, Schramm CM. Factors associated with the development of severe asthma exacerbations in children. J Asthma. 2011;48(6):558–564.
9. Carroll CL, Uygungil B, Zucker AR, Schramm CM. Identifying an at-risk population of children with recurrent near-fatal asthma exacerbations. J Asthma. 2010;47(4):460–464.

10. Carroll CL, Sala KA, Zucker AR, Schramm CM. Beta-adrenergic receptor polymorphisms associated with length of ICU stay in pediatric status asthmaticus. *Pediatr Pulmonol.* 2012;47(3):233–239.

11. Brehm JM, Acosta-Perez E, Klei L, Roeder K, Barmada MM, Boutaoui N, et al. African ancestry and lung function in Puerto Rican children. *J Allergy Clin Immunol.* 2012;129(6):1484–1490.

12. Kelly AM, Kyle E, McAlpine R. Venous pCO(2) and pH can be used to screen for significant hypercarbia in emergency patients with acute respiratory disease. *J Emerg Med.* 2002;22(1):15–19.

13. Castro-Rodriguez JA, Rodrigo GJ. Beta-agonists through metered-dose inhaler with valved holding chamber versus nebulizer for acute exacerbation of wheezing or asthma in children under 5 years of age: A systematic review with meta-analysis. *J Pediatr.* 2004;145(2):172–177.

14. Cates CJ, Crilly JA, Rowe BH. Holding chambers (spacers) versus nebulisers for beta-agonist treatment of acute asthma. *Cochrane Database Syst Rev* (Online). 2006;(2)(2):CD000052.

15. Dolovich MB, Ahrens RC, Hess DR, Anderson P, Dhand R, Rau JL, et al. Device selection and outcomes of aerosol therapy: Evidence-based guidelines—American College of Chest Physicians/American College of Asthma, Allergy, and Immunology. *Chest.* 2005;127(1):335–371.

16. Craig VL, Bigos D, Brilli RJ. Efficacy and safety of continuous albuterol nebulization in children with severe status asthmaticus. *Pediatr Emerg Care.* 1996;12(1):1–5.

17. Papo MC, Frank J, Thompson AE. A prospective, randomized study of continuous versus intermittent nebulized albuterol for severe status asthmaticus in children. *Crit Care Med.* 1993;21(10):1479–1486.

18. Montgomery VL, Eid NS. Low-dose beta-agonist continuous nebulization therapy for status asthmaticus in children. *J Asthma.* 1994;31(3):201–207.

19. Katz RW, Kelly HW, Crowley MR, Grad R, McWilliams BC, Murphy SJ. Safety of continuous nebulized albuterol for bronchospasm in infants and children. *Pediatrics.* 1993;92(5):666–669.

20. Gawchik SM, Saccar CL, Noonan M, Reasner DS, DeGraw SS. The safety and efficacy of nebulized levalbuterol compared with racemic albuterol and placebo in the treatment of asthma in pediatric patients. *J Allergy Clin Immunol.* 1999;103(4):615–621.

21. Andrews T, McGintee E, Mittal MK, Tyler L, Chew A, Zhang X, et al. High-dose continuous neublized levalbuterol for pediatric status asthmaticus: A randomized trial. *J Pediatr.* 2009;155(2):205–210.

22. Bogie AL, Towne D, Luckett PM, Abramo TJ, Wiebe RA. Comparison of intravenous terbutaline versus normal saline in pediatric patients on continuous high-dose nebulized albuterol for status asthmaticus. *Pediatr Emerg Care.* 2007;23(6):355–361.

23. Stephanopoulos DE, Monge R, Schell KH, Wyckoff P, Peterson BM. Continuous intravenous terbutaline for pediatric status asthmaticus. *Crit Care Med.* 1998;26(10):1744–1748.

24. Chiang VW, Burns JP, Rifai N, Lipshultz SE, Adams MJ, Weiner DL. Cardiac toxicity of intravenous terbutaline for the treatment of severe asthma in children: A prospective assessment. *J Pediatr.* 2000;137(1):73–77.

25. Cugell DW. Clinical pharmacology and toxicology of ipratropium bromide. *Am J Med.* 1986;81(5A):18–22.

26. Rodrigo GJ, Castro-Rodriguez JA. Anticholinergics in the treatment of children and adults with acute asthma: A systematic review with meta-analysis. *Thorax.* 2005;60(9):740–746.

27. Stoodley RG, Aaron SD, Dales RE. The role of ipratropium bromide in the emergency management of acute asthma exacerbation: A metaanalysis of randomized clinical trials. *Ann Emerg Med.* 1999;34(1):8–18.

28. Plotnick LH, Ducharme FM. Should inhaled anticholinergics be added to beta2 agonists for treating acute childhood and adolescent asthma? A systematic review. *BMJ.* 1998;317(7164):971–977.

29. Papiris SA, Manali ED, Kolilekas L, Triantafillidou C, Tsangaris I. Acute severe asthma: New approaches to assessment and treatment. *Drugs.* 2009;69(17):2363–2391.

30. Volovitz B, Bentur L, Finkelstein Y, Mansour Y, Shalitin S, Nussinovitch M, et al. Effectiveness and safety of inhaled corticocorticosteroids in controlling acute asthma attacks in children who were treated in the emergency department: A controlled comparative study with oral prednisolone. *J Allergy Clin Immunol.* 1998;102(4 Pt 1):605–609.

31. Edmonds ML, Camargo CA Jr., Pollack CV Jr., Rowe BH. Early use of inhaled corticocorticosteroids in the emergency department treatment of acute asthma. *Cochrane Database Syst Rev* (Online). 2003;(3)(3):CD002308.

32. Rowe BH, Edmonds ML, Spooner CH, Diner B, Camargo CA Jr. Corticosteroid therapy for acute asthma. *Resp Med.* 2004;98(4):275–284.

33. Smith M, Iqbal S, Elliott TM, Everard M, Rowe BH. Corticosteroids for hospitalised children with acute asthma. *Cochrane Db Syst Rev* (Online). 2003;(2)(2):CD002886.

34. Chipps BE, Murphy KR. Assessment and treatment of acute asthma in children. *J Pediatr.* 2005;147:288–294.

35. Gordon S, Tompkins T, Dayan PS. Randomized trial of single-dose intramuscular dexamethasone compared with prednisolone for children with acute asthma. *Pediatr Emerg Care.* 2007;23(8):521–527.

36. Qureshi F, Zaritsky A, Poirier MP. Comparative efficacy of oral dexamethasone versus oral prednisone in acute pediatric asthma. *J Pediatr.* 2001;139(1):20–26.

37. Greenberg RA, Kerby G, Roosevelt GE. A comparison of oral dexamethasone with oral prednisone in pediatric asthma exacerbations treated in the emergency department. *Clin Pediatr.* 2008;47(8):817–823.

38. Gries DM, Moffitt DR, Pulos E, Carter ER. A single dose of intramuscularly administered dexamethasone acetate is as effective as oral prednisone to treat asthma exacerbations in young children. *J Pediatr.* 2000;136(3):298–303.

39. Scarfone RJ, Loiselle JM, Wiley JF 2nd, Decker JM, Henretig FM, Joffe MD. Nebulized dexamethasone versus oral prednisone in the emergency treatment of asthmatic children. *Ann Emerg Med.* 1995;26(4):480–486.

40. Harfi H, Hanissian AS, Crawford LV. Treatment of status asthmaticus in children with high doses and conventional doses of methylprednisolone. *Pediatrics.* 1978;61(6):829–831.

41. Hall CM, Louw SJ, Joubert G. Relative efficacy of hydrocortisone and methylprednisolone in acute severe asthma. *S Afr Med J.* 1995;85(11):1153–1156.

42. Warner JO, Naspitz CK. Third international pediatric consensus statement on the management of childhood asthma. International pediatric asthma consensus group. *Pediatr Pulmonol.* 1998;25(1):1–17.

43. Klein-Gitelman MS, Pachman LM. Intravenous corticosteroids: Adverse reactions are more variable than expected in children. *J Rheumatol.* 1998;25(10):1995–2002.

44. Kasper WJ, Howe PJ. Fatal varicella after a single course of corticosteroids. *Pediatr Infect Dis J.* 1990;9(10):729–732.

45. Blitz M, Blitz S, Beasely R, Diner BM, Hughes R, Knopp JA, et al. Inhaled magnesium sulfate in the treatment of acute asthma. *Cochrane Database Syst Rev* (Online). 2005;(4) (4):CD003898.

46. Rowe BH, Bretzlaff JA, Bourdon C, Bota GW, Camargo CA Jr. Intravenous magnesium sulfate treatment for acute asthma in the emergency department: A systematic review of the literature. *Ann Emerg Med.* 2000;36(3):181–190.

47. Alter HJ, Koepsell TD, Hilty WM. Intravenous magnesium as an adjuvant in acute bronchospasm: A meta-analysis. *Ann Emerg Med.* 2000;36(3):191–197.

48. Cheuk DK, Chau TC, Lee SL. A meta-analysis on intravenous magnesium sulphate for treating acute asthma. *Arch Dis Child.* 2005;90(1):74–77.

49. Mohammed S, Goodacre S. Intravenous and nebulised magnesium sulphate for acute asthma: Systematic review and meta-analysis. *Emerg Med J: EMJ.* 2007;24(12):823–830.

50. Scarfone RJ, Loiselle JM, Joffe MD, Mull CC, Stiller S, Thompson K, et al. A randomized trial of magnesium in the emergency department treatment of children with asthma. *Ann Emerg Med.* 2000;36(6):572–578.

51. Ciarallo L, Sauer AH, Shannon MW. Intravenous magnesium therapy for moderate to severe pediatric asthma: Results of a randomized, placebo-controlled trial. *J Pediatr.* 1996;129(6):809–814.

52. Ciarallo L, Brousseau D, Reinert S. Higher-dose intravenous magnesium therapy for children with moderate to severe acute asthma. *Arch Pediatr Adol Med.* 2000;154(10):979–983.

53. Ho AM, Lee A, Karmakar MK, Dion PW, Chung DC, Contardi LH. Heliox vs air-oxygen mixtures for the treatment of patients with acute asthma: A systematic overview. *Chest.* 2003;123(3):882–890.

54. Rodrigo G, Pollack C, Rodrigo C, Rowe BH. Heliox for non-intubated acute asthma patients. *Cochrane Database Syst Rev* (Online). 2006;(4)(4):CD002884.

55. Mitra A, Bassler D, Goodman K, Lasserson TJ, Ducharme FM. Intravenous aminophylline for acute severe asthma in children over two years receiving inhaled bronchodilators. *Cochrane Database Syst Rev* (Online). 2005;(2)(2):CD001276.

56. Yung M, South M. Randomised controlled trial of aminophylline for severe acute asthma. *Arch Dis Child.* 1998;79(5):405–410.

57. Capsomidis A, Tighe M. Archimedes. Question 2. Is oral montelukast beneficial in treating acute asthma exacerbations in children? *Arch Dis Child.* 2010;95(11):948–950.

58. Camargo CA Jr., Smithline HA, Malice MP, Green SA, Reiss TF. A randomized controlled trial of intravenous montelukast in acute asthma. *Am J Resp Crit Care Med.* 2003;167(4):528–533.

59. Vaschetto R, Bellotti E, Turucz E, Gregoretti C, Corte FD, Navalesi P. Inhalational anesthetics in acute severe asthma. *Curr Drug Tar.* 2009;10(9):826–832.

60. Tobias JD. Inhalational anesthesia: Basic pharmacology, end organ effects, and applications in the treatment of status asthmaticus. *J Intensive Care Med.* 2009;24(6):361–371.

61. Tobias JD, Garrett JS. Therapeutic options for severe, refractory status asthmaticus: Inhalational anaesthetic agents, extracorporeal membrane oxygenation and helium/oxygen ventilation. *Paediatr Anaesth.* 1997;7(1):47–57.

62. Johnston RG, Noseworthy TW, Friesen EG, Yule HA, Shustack A. Isoflurane therapy for status asthmaticus in children and adults. *Chest.* 1990;97(3):698–701.

63. Arnold JH, Truog RD, Rice SA. Prolonged administration of isoflurane to pediatric patients during mechanical ventilation. *Anesth Analg.* 1993;76(3):520–526.

64. Wheeler DS, Clapp CR, Ponaman ML, Bsn HM, Poss WB. Isoflurane therapy for status asthmaticus in children: A case series and protocol. *Pediatr Crit Care Med.* 2000;1(1):55–59.

65. Restrepo RD, Pettignano R, DeMeuse P. Halothane, an effective infrequently used drug, in treatment of pediatric status asthmaticus: A case report. *J Asthma.* 2005;42(8):649–651.

66. Turner DA, Heitz D, Cooper MK, Smith PB, Arnold JH, Bateman ST. Isoflurane for life-threatening bronchospasm: A 15 year single-center experience. *Respir Care.* 2012;57(11):1857–1864.

67. Newth CJ, Rachman B, Patel N, Hammer J. The use of cuffed versus uncuffed endotracheal tubes in pediatric intensive care. *J Pediatr.* 2004;144(3):333–337.

68. Carroll CL, Schramm CM. Noninvasive positive pressure ventilation for the treatment of status asthmaticus in children. *Ann Allergy Asthma Immunol.* 2006;96(3):454–459.

69. Basnet S, Mander G, Andoh J, Klaska H, Verhulst S, Koirala J. Safety, efficacy, and tolerability of early initiation of non-invasive positive pressure ventilation in pediatric patients admitted with status asthmaticus: A pilot study. *Pediatr Crit Care Med.* 2012;13(4):393–398.

70. Darioli R, Perret C. Mechanical controlled hypoventilation in status asthmaticus. *Am Rev Resp Dis.* 1984;129(3):385–387.

71. Hebbar KB, Petrillo-Albarano T, Coto-Puckett W, Heard M, Rycus PT, Fortenberry JD. Experience with use of extracorporeal life support for severe refractory status asthmaticus in children. *Crit Care.* 2009;13(2):R29.

72. Carroll CL, Zucker AR. The increased cost of complications in children with status asthmaticus. *Pediatr Pulmonol.* 2007;42(10):914–919.

73. Mehta R, Fisher LE Jr., Segeleon JE, Pearson-Shaver AL, Wheeler DS. Acute rhabdomyolysis complicating status asthmaticus in children: Case series and review. *Pediatr Emerg Care.* 2006;22(8):587–591.

74. Edmunds SM, Harrison R. Subarachnoid hemorrhage in a child with status asthmaticus: Significance of permissive hypercapnia. *Pediatr Crit Care Med.* 2003;4(1):100–103.

75. Triasih R, Duke T, Robertson CF. Outcomes following admission to intensive care for asthma. *Arch Dis Child.* 2011;96(8):729–734.

76. Davis A, Vickerson F, Worsley G, Mindorff C, Kazim F, Levison H. Determination of dose-response relationship for nebulized ipratropium in asthmatic children. *J Pediatr.* 1984;105(6):1002–1005.

77. Beakes DE. The use of anticholinergics in asthma. *J Asthma.* 1997;34(5):357–368.

78. Barnett PL, Caputo GL, Baskin M, Kuppermann N. Intravenous versus oral corticosteroids in the management of acute asthma in children. *Ann Emerg Med.* 1997;29(2):212–217.

79. Nuhoglu Y, Dai A, Barlan IB, Basaran MM. Efficacy of aminophylline in the treatment of acute asthma exacerbation in children. *Ann Allergy Asthma Immunol.* 1998;80(5):395–398.

80. Ream RS, Loftis LL, Albers GM, Becker BA, Lynch RE, Mink RB. Efficacy of IV theophylline in children with severe status asthmaticus. *Chest.* 2001;119(5):1480–1488.

22 Severe Acute and Life-Threatening Asthma in Adults

Brian H. Rowe

CONTENTS

CASE PRESENTATION

A 27-year-old female graduate student presented to the emergency department (ED) with dyspnoea, cough, and chest tightness following an upper respiratory infection for the past 3 days. Overnight, she became acutely dyspneic and presented via emergency medical services at 7 a.m. Her prehospital treatment included salbutamol (5.0 mg) and ipratropium bromide (250 μg) via nebulization with oxygen three times over 60 min. She admitted to recent nonadherence with her preventer agents (fluticasone 250 μg; two activations per day) and had used 20 puffs of salbutamol via a metered-dose inhaler (MDI) in the 24 h prior to presentation. She admitted to occasionally smoking marijuana and cigarettes and had recently purchased a kitten.

At presentation, she was speaking in short sentences, was alert although anxious, and she had the following vital signs: pulse = 124 beats/min; respiratory rate = 28 breaths/min; temperature = 37.5°C; SaO$_2$ = 89% on room air; and peak expiratory flow (PEF; expected = 455 L/min) = 150 L/min (33% predicted). In the ED, she was triaged as urgent and received oral prednisone (50 mg), intravenous (IV) magnesium sulfate (MgSO$_4$; 2 g), supplemental oxygen, and continued salbutamol and ipratropium bromide via a MDI and a spacer device every 20 min. After 4 h of treatment, her vitals had stabilized, her PEF had improved to 70% predicted, and she was able to maintain her oxygen saturation (SaO$_2$) at 93% without supplemental oxygen.

INTRODUCTION

Asthma is one of the most common chronic health conditions and is characterized by variable airflow obstruction. Not surprisingly, patients with asthma suffer intermittent exacerbations followed by variable degrees of "stability." Asthma is an inflammatory disease of the airways, with many symptoms resulting from secondary bronchoconstriction and is a classic example of a gene–environment interaction. It is a multifactorial disease influenced by geography (regional variation is well documented), heredity, early environmental influences and exposures, demographic factors (e.g., age, sex, and ethnicity), lifestyle choices (e.g., smoking status and body mass index), the environment (e.g., living conditions and air quality), and socioeconomic status. Not surprisingly, the prevalence of asthma varies widely within and among countries; however, acute severe asthma occurs everywhere and its management has evolved dramatically over the past two decades.

Despite rapid advances in the understanding of the pathophysiology and management of asthma, the control of asthma has proven to be difficult to achieve. A deterioration in asthma control is common when patients are exposed to airway irritants and viruses, and when adherence to chronic anti-inflammatory medications is suboptimal. The hallmark of an exacerbation includes a history of asthma, increasing symptoms of dyspnea, wheeze, and cough, and an increasing need for short-acting beta$_2$-adrenergic agonist (SABA) agents. Asthma exacerbations are common presentations to the ED in many parts of the world[1] and the costs associated with the care of asthma are significant.[2-4] For example, in the United States, approximately $14 billion per year is spent on asthma[5]; nearly one-quarter of all asthma expenses is related to acute exacerbations (ED visits and hospitalizations).[4] *Severe acute asthma* is a potentially life-threatening medical emergency that usually involves symptoms such as shortness of breath, cough, and wheeze, and signs such as accessory muscles use, tachypnea and tachycardia, airway outflow measures (PEF or forced expiratory volume in 1 sec [FEV$_1$]) <50% of predicted, and arterial saturation <90%.

Given this major economic and health burden, it is not surprising that a number of guidelines have been developed to guide the management of asthma and its severe exacerbations.[6-10] However, despite the widespread availability of asthma guidelines, there is a "care gap" between what is practiced and the published evidence. Frequently, evidence summaries are unavailable for guiding the management of patients in the ED or other acute care settings. This is due, in part, to the volume of literature and perhaps a lack of access to synthesized evidence by clinicians. Moreover, disparities in terms of health-care access (patients often cannot afford the appropriate medicines) and education (some patients do not know that it is possible to live well with asthma) continue to complicate the management of asthma.

This chapter focuses on summarizing the evidence for the management of severe acute asthma in the ED and following discharge. The approach outlined here may enable clinicians to help their asthma patients avoid ED visits and hospitalizations, limit airway interventions, reduce relapses, and improve long-term asthma control.

ACUTE ASTHMA ED FREQUENCY AND SEVERITY

Several large-scale studies have examined the presentations of patients with asthma to EDs. Using the National Hospital Ambulatory Medical Care Survey, investigators in the United States have demonstrated stable numbers of ED presentations,[11] while Canadian studies have shown a decreasing rate of asthma presentations to the ED.[12] In addition, two investigator groups have demonstrated various factors associated with hospitalization (see Table 22.1). Multivariate modeling techniques have provided a list of factors associated with admission. These results suggest that the patient's ethnicity, age, sex, asthma severity (respiratory rate, SaO$_2$, and triage scores), past history of asthma control (e.g., intubations and asthma admissions), and previous outpatient unscheduled office and ED visits requiring the use of oral corticosteroids are all factors associated with an increased risk for hospitalization. Overall, clinicians should consider these risk factors when making admission and discharge decisions for patients with asthma managed in the acute care setting.

ACUTE ASTHMA ASSESSMENT

Estimates of the disease severity, the need for hospitalization, and the risk of relapse following discharge by physicians are often inaccurate in acute asthma. Although the assessment of asthma severity is recommended by all major acute asthma guidelines,[6,7] there is disagreement on the most suitable approach. Some guidelines recommend that the severity be determined objectively using spirometry, PEF, or both.[7] While there is conflicting evidence regarding the psychometric properties of each of these measures,[13] many EDs measure the PEF rate rather than FEV$_1$, and follow this clinical measure of severity over the course of treatment. The cut points for severity vary among the different guidelines; however, all the guidelines suggest that <30%–50% predicted of either the PEF or FEV$_1$ indicates severe disease. A more important consideration for ED clinicians relates to the change in pulmonary function over the acute treatment period. Finally, most guidelines suggest that the ED target for discharge be at least 70% of the predicted lung function, which may not always be feasible especially in patients with moderate to severe fixed airway obstruction.[6,7]

Vital signs (temperature, pulse rate, respiratory rate, and blood pressure) may be helpful in assessing severe acute asthma. A "fifth vital sign," SaO$_2$ measured by pulse oximetry, should also be recorded. While vital signs are considered helpful, they may provide misleading information in adults. For example, normal or near normal vital signs do not exclude severe asthma or the possibility of a post-ED relapse. While the measurement of SaO$_2$ may help to guide treatment in adult patients, no studies have clearly demonstrated that SaO$_2$ predicts admission or relapse in adult asthmatic patients.

TABLE 22.1

Factors Associated with Hospital Admission for Acute Asthma Following ED Management in Large Multicentered Studies

Factors	U.S. Data	Canadian Data
Demographics		
Age	—	↑/10 years***
Sex	↑ if female**	—
Race/ethnicity	↑ if black*	—
Severity		
Pulmonary functions	↑ per increase of 10% predicted initial PEF***	—
Triage score	—	↑ if CTAS 1 or 2 at presentation***
Home SABA treatments	↑ if home nebulizer during past 4 weeks***	↑ if >8 activations in past 24 h*
Oxygen saturation		↑ if <95%***
Respiratory rate	↑ with every 5 breaths/min increment**	↑ if >22/min**
Past History		
Previous admissions	—	↑ if any admissions*
Ever intubated	↑ if intubated*	—
Corticosteroid use	↑ if on chronic CS*	—
	↑ if on pulse CS*	
Asthma medication	↑ if used more than ICS and SABA in past 4 weeks**	—
ED Treatment		
SABA treatment in the ED	↑ if any***	—
Pulmonary functions	↑ per decrease of 10% predicted final PEF***	—

Note: CS, corticosteroids; CTAS, Canadian Triage and Acuity Score; ICS, inhaled corticosteroids; ED, emergency department; PEF, peak expiratory flow; ABA, short-acting beta-agonists.

*$P < .5$; **$P < .01$; ***$P < .001$.

Sophisticated investigations are rarely required for the management of patients with acute asthma, and clinical assessment over time is far more important than wasting time and resources by ordering tests. Since patients presenting with acute asthma are generally young and have few comorbidities, laboratory tests, radiography, and other more sophisticated tests are less important than initiating the appropriate treatment.

In summary, the assessment of acute asthma severity requires a careful and multifactorial approach. The use of pulse oximetry, pulmonary function tests, vital signs, history, physical examination, previous and current responses to therapy, and current medications are all required to determine the need for hospitalization and the risk of relapse after discharge.

THERAPEUTIC MANAGEMENT OF SEVERE ACUTE ASTHMA IN THE ED

BETA₂-AGONIST BRONCHODILATORS

The early treatment of acute asthma has generally focused on the use of inhaled SABA agents because of their undisputed and generally rapid bronchodilation effect. The therapeutic advantages of the most common delivery methods, which are nebulizers or MDIs with a holding chamber or a spacer device, have been extensively investigated. A Cochrane library systematic review, updated in 2008, involving 614 adults from 27 trials from EDs and community settings suggested that the use of either delivery method for acute (but not acute severe) asthma yields similar clinical outcomes.[14] In adults, the relative risk (RR) of admission or poor outcome for a holding chamber versus a nebulizer was 0.97 (95% confidence interval [CI]: 0.63, 1.49). The ED length of stay for adults and FEV_1 or PEF measurements posttreatment were also similar for the two delivery methods (Figure 22.1). Furthermore, the use of a MDI with a holding chamber was associated with fewer side effects, such as tachycardia and tremor, compared with nebulizers, especially in children. An economic evaluation of these two delivery approaches has demonstrated that SABA delivery by a MDI with a holding chamber is more cost-effective compared with a nebulizer.[15] An important caveat is that the clinical trials included in the systematic review did not include patients with *status asthmaticus* or near-fatal asthma.

Review: Holding chambers (spacers) versus nebulizers for beta-agonist treatment of acute asthma
Comparison: One spacer (chamber) versus nebulizer (multiple treatment studies)
Outcome: One hospital admission

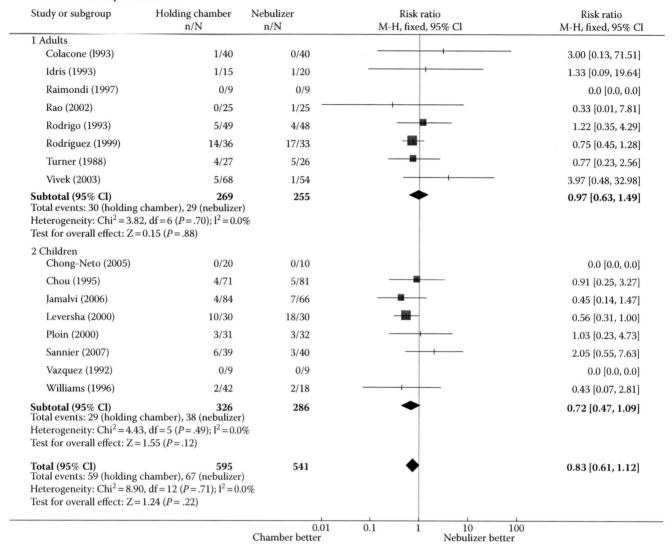

Study or subgroup	Holding chamber n/N	Nebulizer n/N	Risk ratio M-H, fixed, 95% CI	Risk ratio M-H, fixed, 95% CI
1 Adults				
Colacone (1993)	1/40	0/40		3.00 [0.13, 71.51]
Idris (1993)	1/15	1/20		1.33 [0.09, 19.64]
Raimondi (1997)	0/9	0/9		0.0 [0.0, 0.0]
Rao (2002)	0/25	1/25		0.33 [0.01, 7.81]
Rodrigo (1993)	5/49	4/48		1.22 [0.35, 4.29]
Rodriguez (1999)	14/36	17/33		0.75 [0.45, 1.28]
Turner (1988)	4/27	5/26		0.77 [0.23, 2.56]
Vivek (2003)	5/68	1/54		3.97 [0.48, 32.98]
Subtotal (95% CI)	**269**	**255**		**0.97 [0.63, 1.49]**

Total events: 30 (holding chamber), 29 (nebulizer)
Heterogeneity: Chi^2 = 3.82, df = 6 (P = .70); I^2 = 0.0%
Test for overall effect: Z = 0.15 (P = .88)

2 Children				
Chong-Neto (2005)	0/20	0/10		0.0 [0.0, 0.0]
Chou (1995)	4/71	5/81		0.91 [0.25, 3.27]
Jamalvi (2006)	4/84	7/66		0.45 [0.14, 1.47]
Leversha (2000)	10/30	18/30		0.56 [0.31, 1.00]
Ploin (2000)	3/31	3/32		1.03 [0.23, 4.73]
Sannier (2007)	6/39	3/40		2.05 [0.55, 7.63]
Vazquez (1992)	0/9	0/9		0.0 [0.0, 0.0]
Williams (1996)	2/42	2/18		0.43 [0.07, 2.81]
Subtotal (95% CI)	**326**	**286**		**0.72 [0.47, 1.09]**

Total events: 29 (holding chamber), 38 (nebulizer)
Heterogeneity: Chi^2 = 4.43, df = 5 (P = .49); I^2 = 0.0%
Test for overall effect: Z = 1.55 (P = .12)

| **Total (95% CI)** | **595** | **541** | | **0.83 [0.61, 1.12]** |

Total events: 59 (holding chamber), 67 (nebulizer)
Heterogeneity: Chi^2 = 8.90, df = 12 (P = .71); I^2 = 0.0%
Test for overall effect: Z = 1.24 (P = .22)

```
              0.01        0.1        1        10        100
              Chamber better                Nebulizer better
```

FIGURE 22.1   The effectiveness of short-acting beta-agonist delivery by an inhaler and a spacer device compared with a nebulizer (admission outcome). (From Cates, C.J., Crilly, J.A., and Rowe, B.H., *Cochrane Database Syst. Rev.*, CD000052, 2006. With permission.)

The attempts to identify optimal doses or treatment intervals to achieve maximal bronchodilation or symptom relief have not been successful.[16] In addition, lower SABA doses appear to be equivalent to higher doses of up to 5–10 mg via a nebulizer in achieving maximum clinical outcomes.[17] Clinicians often observe a "plateau" in bronchodilation, suggesting that continued SABA treatment may produce more adverse effects rather than additional bronchodilation. Some guidelines now recommend titrating SABA use to a plateau using an objective assessment of the airway obstruction with pulmonary function measures.[10]

DELIVERY METHODS FOR BETA-AGONISTS

The recommended delivery of SABA bronchodilators is through the inhaled route as previously described. The need to focus on other management issues may make nebulization the most attractive delivery method in patients with severe acute asthma. When patients present with severe acute asthma, clinicians attempt to maximize bronchodilation, and the penetration of an inhaled drug to the affected small airways may be limited. The evidence suggests that several alternative considerations are available, such as continuous nebulization and IV delivery. The theory behind the continuous delivery of SABA is that the bolus of intermittent administration may produce the bronchodilation required for the effective delivery of other inhaled agents. A systematic review involving the continuous delivery of beta-agonists supports this approach as one option for patients with severe acute asthma.[18] The theory behind the use of IV agents is that their effectiveness in acute severe asthma may be the result of beta$_2$-receptor activation through the systemic circulation. In these circumstances, if bronchodilation occurs predominantly in response to the systemic distribution of the drug, the addition of IV bronchodilators to the inhaled administration of bronchodilators may provide an earlier clinical response.[19]

A recent systematic review of the published literature in adult and pediatric cases suggests that the IV route should be used cautiously.[20] The evidence is based on the results of a few randomized controlled trials (RCTs), and the benefit appears to be limited to pediatric cases. Overall, the authors concluded that there is no apparent benefit to using IV SABA for adults with severe acute asthma. Until more robust evidence is available, the potential frequency and the severity of the adverse effects associated with IV SABA drug delivery preclude its use in most cases. Its role may be restricted to intubated patients where drug delivery is known to be significantly impaired.

In summary, there are a variety of delivery approaches for SABA agents for patients with acute severe asthma, each of which has advantages and disadvantages. The majority of patients should be managed with inhaled SABA delivery through a MDI and a holding chamber. Supporting this recommendation for limiting SABA treatment via a nebulizer is the recent worldwide severe acute respiratory syndrome (SARS) and H1N1 influenza pandemics and their apparent spread following nebulization,[21] which in some settings has facilitated the conversion to a MDI with a holding chamber.

Anticholinergic Bronchodilators

Short-acting anticholinergic agents (SAAC) are bronchodilators that also reduce pulmonary secretions. There is support for *adding* SAAC agents to SABA therapy in moderate to severe acute asthma in children[22] and adults.[23] A systematic review involving 2047 patients from 16 trials of acute asthma identified a beneficial effect of adding SAAC (most often ipratropium bromide) to inhaled SABA agents in the early treatment of adults with acute asthma. The risk of admission was decreased by 32% (RR: 0.68; 95% CI: 0.53, 0.99) and the number needed to treat (NNT) to prevent a single admission was 14 (95% CI: 9, 30). Multiple doses (more than two) of SAAC reduced the risk of hospital admission by 47% (RR: 0.53; 95% CI: 0.36, 0.7683) and the NNT to prevent a single admission was 6 (95% CI: 4, 13). The effect was not related to the use of systemic corticosteroids (SCs); however, the evidence regarding their role in severe asthma was inconclusive.

The review provided pooled results to suggest that pulmonary function also improved in patients treated with a SAAC/SABA combination compared with the control SABA group. Overall, short-term treatment with SAAC is exceedingly safe, inexpensive, and readily available in most centers. Although several questions regarding SAAC in acute asthma remain unresolved (such as the dose–response relationship), evidence supports adding SAAC to SABA for patients with severe acute asthma.

Corticosteroids

Most patients with severe acute asthma have impressive airway edema and increased secretions resulting from the inflammation cascade. Therefore, almost all of these patients warrant early, aggressive anti-inflammatory treatments. For example, SCs delivered early (i.e., within 2 h of arrival) is a first-line treatment in most current published asthma guidelines.[8,9,10,24–25] A Cochrane systematic review consisting of 12 RCTs and involving a total of 863 patients with acute asthma concluded that SCs significantly reduced admissions (odds ratio [OR] = 0.50; 95% CI: 0.31, 0.81) compared with a placebo or standard care; the NNT was 8 (95% CI: 5, 20).[26] This benefit was more pronounced for corticosteroid-naive patients (OR = 0.37; 95% CI: 0.19, 0.70) and those experiencing a severe attack (OR = 0.35; 95% CI: 0.21, 0.59). Overall, short-term treatment with SCs is exceedingly safe, inexpensive, and readily available in most centers. Moreover, the delivery of this treatment can be safely initiated by both triage nurses[27] and other health professionals prior to physician assessment,[28] in order to ensure drug delivery at the earliest possible time.

Current treatment options for physicians include using IV, intramuscular (IM), and oral SCs in severe disease. While most evidence-based clinicians use oral agents (e.g., prednisone or dexamethasone), in certain situations an IV route of administration may be preferable. For example, IV corticosteroids should be considered for patients who have severe or near-fatal asthma, are too dyspneic to swallow, have a decreased level of consciousness, are intubated or in the process of being intubated, and are unable to tolerate oral medications (e.g., severe nausea, gastrointestinal [GI] bleeding, and vomiting). Unfortunately, systematic reviews in hospitalized patients are underpowered to conclude superiority or equivalence regarding high versus moderate doses.

Overall, it seems appropriate to provide oral SCs to almost all other patients with acute asthma. The agent and dose of SC administered should be based on familiarity, availability, and patient factors. Most importantly, clinicians need to start SCs early and consistently for patients with severe acute asthma.

MgSO₄

IV $MgSO_4$ is a treatment option for a variety of severe acute diseases such as eclampsia, cardiac arrhythmias, and asthma. In asthma, it has both a direct effect on the smooth muscles through its influence on cellular calcium homeostasis, and a proposed airway anti-inflammatory effect. The use of IV $MgSO_4$ in unresponsive patients with acute asthma has gained support over the past decade. A number of systematic reviews have all concluded that IV magnesium is not only safe but it is also effective in those patients with severe disease.[29,30] Overall, 13 studies (8 adults; 5 children) involving 965 patients have examined the *addition* of IV $MgSO_4$ to SABA and SCs. Considering all the studies, the addition of $MgSO_4$ reduced hospitalization; however, significant heterogeneity was identified ($I^2 = 47.6\%$; Figure 22.2). When

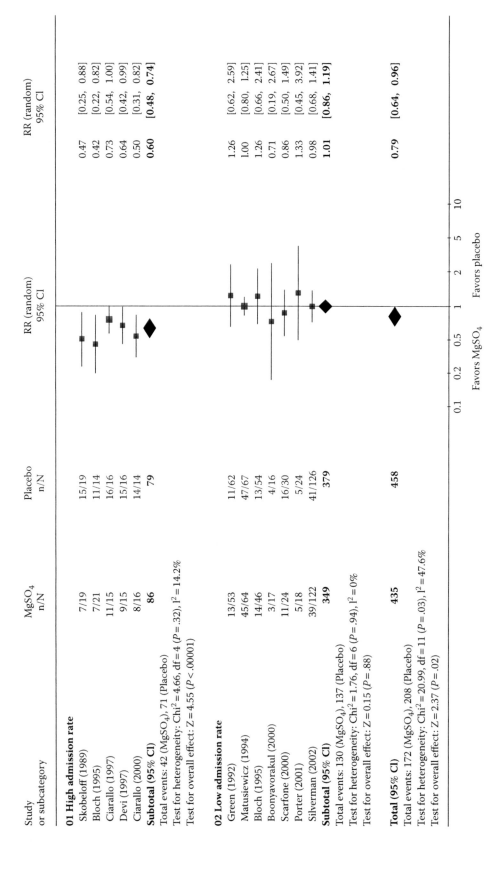

Study or subcategory	MgSO$_4$ n/N	Placebo n/N	RR (random) 95% CI	RR (random) 95% CI
01 High admission rate				
Skobeloff (1989)	7/19	15/19		0.47 [0.25, 0.88]
Bloch (1995)	7/21	11/14		0.42 [0.22, 0.82]
Ciarallo (1997)	11/15	16/16		0.73 [0.54, 1.00]
Devi (1997)	9/15	15/16		0.64 [0.42, 0.99]
Ciarallo (2000)	8/16	14/14		0.50 [0.31, 0.82]
Subtotal (95% CI)	**86**	**79**		**0.60 [0.48, 0.74]**
Total events: 42 (MgSO$_4$), 71 (Placebo)				
Test for heterogeneity: Chi^2 = 4.66, df = 4 (P = .32), I^2 = 14.2%				
Test for overall effect: Z = 4.55 (P < .00001)				
02 Low admission rate				
Green (1992)	13/53	11/62		1.26 [0.62, 2.59]
Matusiewicz (1994)	45/64	47/67		1.00 [0.80, 1.25]
Bloch (1995)	14/46	13/54		1.26 [0.66, 2.41]
Boonyavorakul (2000)	3/17	4/16		0.71 [0.19, 2.67]
Scarfone (2000)	11/24	16/30		0.86 [0.50, 1.49]
Porter (2001)	5/18	5/24		1.33 [0.45, 3.92]
Silverman (2002)	39/122	41/126		0.98 [0.68, 1.41]
Subtotal (95% CI)	**349**	**379**		**1.01 [0.86, 1.19]**
Total events: 130 (MgSO$_4$), 137 (Placebo)				
Test for heterogeneity: Chi^2 = 1.76, df = 6 (P = .94), I^2 = 0%				
Test for overall effect: Z = 0.15 (P = .88)				
Total (95% CI)	**435**	**458**		**0.79 [0.64, 0.96]**
Total events: 172 (MgSO$_4$), 208 (Placebo)				
Test for heterogeneity: Chi^2 = 20.99, df = 11 (P = .03), I^2 = 47.6%				
Test for overall effect: Z = 2.37 (P = .02)				

0.1   0.2   0.5   1   2   5   10

Favors MgSO$_4$ Favors placebo

FIGURE 22.2   The effectiveness of intravenous magnesium sulfate compared with a placebo in severe acute asthma (admission outcome).

the analysis was restricted to only adults, the treatment did not appear to reduce admissions (RR = 0.91; 95% CI: 0.77, 1.09). In the severe asthma subgroup, $MgSO_4$ did reduce hospitalization when all studies were considered (RR = 0.60; 95% CI: 0.48, 0.74), and it also improved pulmonary function (PEF = 26.8 L/min; 95% CI: 7.3, 45). Overall, adverse effects and side effects with this treatment were rare or minor, although these outcomes are poorly reported in most clinical trials.

Adult patients with clinically severe asthma (e.g., pulmonary function testing less than 30% predicted and those patients with severe symptoms who exhibit a poor response to initial bronchodilator therapy) appear to benefit most from IV $MgSO_4$ treatment. Since this agent has been shown to be easy to use, extremely safe, and inexpensive, its early use in severe acute asthma should be considered. Currently, the recommended dose is 2 g IV over 20 min in adults; this approach has been widely accepted by emergency physicians surveyed in North America.[31]

INHALED CORTICOSTEROIDS (ICS)

While ICS are considered standard treatment for chronic asthma, evidence has accumulated to indicate that ICS also influence outcomes in the acute phase of the illness.[32] Their efficacy is most likely linked to their acute vasoconstrictive properties, rather than their more chronic anti-inflammatory properties.

Cochrane systematic review evidence has identified trials examining the use of ICS alone or in combination with SCs in the treatment of acute asthma.[32] From 12 trials involving 960 patients, patients treated with ICS were less likely to be hospitalized (OR = 0.44; 95% CI: 0.31, 0.62). While this is compelling evidence, a clinically more important question involves the benefit of adding ICS to SCs. From 5 trials involving 433 patients, patients treated with a variety of ICS agents in combination with SCs were less likely to be hospitalized (OR = 0.54; 95% CI: 0.36, 0.81). Overall, the ICS treatments were well tolerated.

Since the combination subgroup exhibited moderate heterogeneity ($I^2 = 52\%$), caution when interpreting these results is advised. ICS agents should not be the first-line treatment in acute asthma; however, they may assist in more severe asthma, especially if patients have not previously been on SCs prior to ED presentation. The dose, frequency, and agents used in this review varied widely; however, there appears to be evidence of effect despite this heterogeneity. For example, various ICS agents were used (budesonide in 14 studies), the median single dose was 900 μg, the median frequency of treatment was two activations, and the median cumulative dose was 2 mg over up to 6 h of observation.[32]

ADJUVANT AGENTS

IM epinephrine injections have been recommended in acute allergic reactions and may benefit patients whose acute asthma is suspected or known to be due to possible anaphylaxis.[33]

While long-acting beta$_2$-adrenergic agonists (LABA) and leukotriene receptor antagonists (LTRA) are recommended as add-on therapy in chronic, poorly controlled asthma,[34] research in acute asthma is limited. An RCT of 201 patients treated with either a placebo or 7 or 14 mg of IV montelukast suggested a clinically significant improvement in FEV_1 within 10 min of administration;[35] however, other evidence-based treatments were not administered to all patients. Another study examined treatments in the ED and after discharge.[36] Overall, the evidence for this treatment is limited and whether its use should be encouraged *in addition* to SCs remains uncertain. As the evidence regarding the use of both LTRA and LABA agents accumulates, clinicians are encouraged to search for updates of existing systematic reviews.

AIRWAY INTERVENTIONS

Despite the use of aggressive management as outlined earlier, in rare cases some patients will continue to deteriorate and decisions regarding the need for assisted ventilation will be required.

NONINVASIVE VENTILATION (NIV)

Experienced clinicians in the ED setting have become accustomed to using NIV (also referred to as noninvasive positive pressure ventilation [NIPPV]) for patients with respiratory failure, especially in the setting of heart failure and chronic obstructive pulmonary disease (COPD).[37,38] NIV is usually delivered by a partial or full-face mask, in the form of biphasic respiratory support. While the evidence to support this intervention in COPD and heart failure, based on data pooled from multiple small RCTs, demonstrates homogeneous efficacious outcomes, the evidence in acute asthma is sparse. In fact, a Cochrane systematic review updated in 2012 identified 5 studies involving 206 participants; however, not all studies contributed to every outcome assessed. From two studies involving 90 patients, endotracheal intubation was not reduced using NIV (OR = 4.81; 95% CI: 0.22, 105.2). Hospital admissions were reduced using NIV in one study (OR = 0.13; 95% CI: 0.03, 0.64); however, a meta-analysis could not be performed on the length-of-stay data from two studies. There were no deaths reported in any studies. While the body of evidence is positive,[39] recent reviews have generated neutral recommendations.[40] The benefits of NIV in this setting and its success in similar respiratory failure cases due to other common acute conditions suggest a definitive trial of NIV in severe acute asthma may be warranted. The ultimate goal is to avoid intubation and NIV represents a last resort for some patients.

INTUBATION

If all else fails to improve the symptoms and signs for patients with severe acute asthma, an airway intervention (e.g., intubation) may be required. The decision to intubate patients with asthma should not be taken lightly, given the potential barotrauma and complications associated with this intervention. Limited comparative research has been performed in this setting and, fortunately, the need for intubation is rare. A decreasing level of consciousness and respiratory fatigue are clear signs of the need for airway control. While rapid sequence intubation with ketamine is recommended, it must be stressed that preparation and airway expertise are essential for a successful, nontraumatic intubation. The airway settings, the techniques of mechanical ventilation, the use of heliox, the timing of extubation, and other airway considerations are covered more comprehensively elsewhere.[41]

OTHER OPTIONS FOR MANAGING ACUTE SEVERE ASTHMA

Over the years, many treatments have been used and advocated that now require only a passing mention due to their lack of effectiveness. For example, while methylxanthines were often used in the treatment of acute severe asthma, the overall scientific evidence suggests that aminophylline (the main IV agent in this class) is ineffective.[42] Moreover, the side effects associated with this agent outweigh any benefit that may be observed; therefore, this agent is no longer considered an appropriate treatment for severe acute asthma.

Antibiotics have been used excessively and often inappropriately in the past in both emergency and primary care settings to treat bronchitis[43] and asthma. A summary of the evidence to date would suggest that antibiotics are ineffective in the treatment of severe acute asthma.[44] The use of antibiotics for severe acute asthma should therefore be limited to patients with documented fever, purulent sputum, and an infiltrate on chest radiography, or evidence of another source of bacterial infection requiring antibiotics (e.g., acute sinusitis).

Other agents such as heliox[45] and inhaled $MgSO_4$[46] are currently not recommended because the evidence is insufficient to demonstrate a clear benefit to treatment.

MANAGEMENT OF SEVERE ACUTE ASTHMA IN PREPARATION FOR ED DISCHARGE

While it could be argued that evidence-based management of severe presentations is the most important treatment of ED patients with acute asthma, the frequency of improvement leading to the eventual discharge of the majority of these patients suggests that this should also be an important focus for all emergency physicians.[47] In this regard, arranging follow-up with the patients' usual physician and/or family practitioner is essential for ensuring continuity of care and preventing recidivism to the ED (see also Chapter 29).

SYSTEMIC CORTICOSTEROIDS

Corticosteroids are nonspecific, anti-inflammatory agents commonly used in asthma. In a Cochrane systematic review of RCTs, the risk of relapse and the need for a rescue therapy were significantly reduced with SCs compared with a placebo.[48] In addition, the evidence would suggest that the benefit of SCs extends beyond the traditional 5–7 days of treatment and also reduces the need for rescue beta-agonists over the first 3 weeks postdischarge. Since oral corticosteroids are relatively safe, inexpensive, and effective, this should be the first-line agent for patients with moderate to severe asthma discharged from the ED after treatment.

At times, adherence with this treatment can be difficult and there is some evidence to suggest that in the case of patients where compliance or access to medications may be problematic, there is a role for IM injections of corticosteroids. Approximately five trials have been published in this area, which generally suggest a reduction in relapse following the use of IM agents such as triamcinolone, dexamethasone, and methylprednisolone.[49] As the majority of patients with acute severe asthma would prefer to ingest a tablet rather than receive an IM injection, this form of therapy is infrequently used. It is, however, an option in settings where access to medications or compliance may be problematic.

The duration of oral therapy is debated and while the current evidence is based on 7–10 days of treatment in the RCTs, including the Cochrane review, the current form of reduced therapy is more acceptable to patients and physicians. The evidence from large observational ED studies has demonstrated the use of a median of 5 days of therapy and rarely more than 7 days of therapy with oral agents.[47] In some cases, short courses of dexamethasone are used[50]; however, this is more common in the pediatric setting where the tolerance for SC agents is poor. While a recent questionnaire study investigating physician use of oral SCs demonstrated a heterogeneous approach, it also revealed that most physicians prescribed less than the upper dose recommended in the guidelines and many prescribed a total SC burst dose below the lower end of the recommended dose range.[51] Further studies should focus on the optimal treatment regimen of oral SCs in the management of acute severe asthma to help establish a better overall consensus among physicians. While the side-effect profile of oral SCs is reasonably safe, patients should still be advised of the potential side effects such as abdominal discomfort, and in some cases a GI bleed, insomnia, hyperphagia, and exacerbation of chronic mental health disorders.

INHALED CORTICOSTEROIDS

While moderate-dose ICS is considered standard treatment for chronic asthma, there are a surprising number of patients presenting with chronic, poorly controlled asthma who are not receiving ICS agents or are not adhering to the recommendations for using these agents.[47] The addition of ICS to SCs at discharge is now relatively common in some settings. The evidence for a management strategy originated from an RCT in the ED setting,[52] and was further fortified in a systematic review in the Cochrane library.[50] The first major clinical trial on this topic was conducted in Canada[52] and included 188 asthmatic patients presenting to a community ED. All patients received a concomitant 7-day course of prednisone daily at discharge. In addition, they were randomized in a double-blind fashion to 1600 mg/day of inhaled budesonide compared with a placebo. The study examined moderate to severe asthmatic patients considered well enough for discharge after treatment. The addition of high-dose budesonide decreased the 21-day relapse proportions (12.8% vs. 24.5%; $P = .04$; NNT = 9). An improved quality of life and a reduced SABA puffer use (2.4 vs. 4.2 puffs/day) were also observed.

Despite these early and promising results, similar trials have failed to confirm these findings. In a Cochrane systematic review summarizing the evidence for ICS treatment after discharge from the ED, three RCTs were identified and pooled. The meta-analysis provided a nonsignificant trend in favor of adding ICS to corticosteroids after discharge (OR = 0.68; 95% CI: 0.46, 1.02).[50] Combined with administrative data evidence[53] that suggests ICS agents should be added to reduce relapse after discharge and current guidelines for the control of patients with chronic asthma, the majority of patients seen in the ED with an acute exacerbation of their asthma qualify for treatment with moderate-dose ICS agents.

The exact agent, dose, and duration of ICS after discharge remain unclear. The current recommendation from the chronic asthma literature suggests that doses above moderate ICS are not beneficial.[54] The ICS recommendations following discharge from the ED are based on a consensus and likely should be moderate to high doses.

ADDITION OF LABA

In the treatment of chronic asthma, disease control may be achieved with the addition of inhaled LABA to the regular use of ICS agents.[55] The exact role of LABA in the ED remains a topic of debate. In an RCT of 137 patients discharged from a Canadian ED with acute asthma, patients administered LABA in combination with ICS, compared with ICS alone, fared no better after discharge.[56] In an *a priori* subgroup analysis, those patients who were not receiving ICS at presentation to the ED did not appear to benefit from the addition of ICS plus LABA after discharge. For example, approximately 5% of patients suffered relapse if administered ICS agents in combination with prednisone after discharge. Conversely, patients who were already receiving ICS agents at the time of presentation to the ED appeared to benefit more from a switch to an ICS/LABA combination agent. In this study, patients who were already receiving ICS agents at presentation to the ED had a nonsignificant 50% reduction in relapse in the subsequent 3 weeks and also an improvement in their quality of life.

Given the current guideline recommendations to add a LABA agent to ICS in patients with unstable asthma, including exacerbations, this may be an appropriate ED treatment option. Further research is clearly required and whether these patients need to remain on the ICS/LABA combination long term is still undetermined. Clearly, the majority of patients do not need ICS/LABA long term and it is important to ensure that asthma education, close follow-up, and compliance

with medications are included in a comprehensive effort to achieve asthma control.

POST-ED DISCHARGE MANAGEMENT

PREVENTING RELAPSE

Since relapse after discharge is an important outcome for patients with asthma, several studies have attempted to identify the factors associated with this outcome. A large, multicenter ED study of patients with acute asthma identified the factors associated with relapse after discharge[57]; however, standard evidence-based treatments were not provided in all cases. A prospective, observational study of patients discharged from Canadian EDs with high follow-up and frequent discharge treatment with SCs and ICS agents documented relapses in 9.2% of patients in 1 week (95% CI: 7.1%–12.0%) and nearly 14% (95% CI: 11%–17%) in 2 weeks.[47] Multivariate modeling of factors associated with relapse produced a list of factors associated with relapse after discharge. These results suggest that patient characteristics (i.e., ethnicity and sex), exacerbation frequency (i.e., prior ED visits and asthma admissions), and treatment (i.e., use of oral corticosteroids) factors were associated with asthma relapse. Overall, acute care providers should consider these risk factors in their discharge decisions.

PREVENTING FUTURE PRESENTATIONS TO THE ED

Despite applying the evidence as outlined in this chapter, asthma control can be elusive for many patients. Nonpharmacological management issues need to be considered in all patients seen in the ED. For example, many patients with asthma continue to actively smoke or inhale passive cigarette smoke, and referral to smoking cessation programs may be warranted. In addition, many patients have not received influenza immunization, do not have an asthma action plan,[58] have not received asthma education,[59] and have not been using a holding chamber or a spacer device for their inhalers.[40,47,56] Moreover, follow-up care is often delayed. In one Canadian study, despite national guidelines suggesting rapid follow-up after an ED presentation, the median follow-up after ED discharge was nearly 3 weeks.[12] Finally, compliance is a critical issue in the treatment of chronic diseases such as asthma.[60] Clinicians in acute care settings should recognize their role in the continuum of asthma care and identify opportunities to enhance these much-needed management strategies.

CONCLUSION

Asthma is a common, chronic, and often debilitating disease and exacerbations present frequently to acute care settings in most developed countries. In severe acute cases, the treatment approaches to control bronchial inflammation reflect the need for early, aggressive, multimodal intervention in order to avoid hospitalization, intubation, and other complications of the acute episode. Combining SABA bronchodilators and

TABLE 22.2

Summary of Drug Class, Agents, and Dosing Used in Severe Acute Asthma in Adults

Class	Most Frequent Agent	Most Frequent Dose
SABA	Salbutamol through a spacer device	4–8 puffs every 20 min for 3 doses
	Salbutamol via nebulization	2.5–5.0 mg every 20 min for 3 doses
SAAC	Ipratropium bromide (Atrovent) through a spacer device	4–8 puffs every 20 min for 3 doses
	Ipratropium bromide (Atrovent) via nebulization	250–500 µg every 20 min × 3 doses
Systemic Corticosteroids	Prednisone	40–60 mg oral
	Methylprednisolone (Solumedrol)	80–125 mg IV
	Hydrocortisone (Solucortef)	250–500 mg IV
	Dexamethasone (Decadron)	0.6 mg/kg oral or 0.3 mg IM
Inhaled Corticosteroids	Fluticasone (Flovent) through a spacer device	250–500 µg administered in variable frequencies
	Budesonide (Pulmicort) through a spacer device	400–800 µg administered in variable frequencies
	Budesonide (Pulmicort) via nebulization	1–2 mg administered in variable frequencies
Other Treatments for Acute Severe Asthma	Magnesium sulfate (MgSO$_4$)	2 g IV over 20 min
	Noninvasive ventilation	Variable
	Epinephrine	0.3 cc IM (1:1000 concentration); may be repeated, if necessary
	Oxygen	To maintain SaO$_2$ > 92%

Note: IM, intramuscular; IV, intravenous; MgSO$_4$, magnesium sulfate; SAAC, short-acting anticholinergics; SABA, short-acting beta-agonists.

corticosteroids is sufficient for most patients (Table 22.2); however, adjuncts such as inhaled SAAC, IV MgSO$_4$, ICS, and NIV provide patients with the best opportunity to avoid serious adverse events from the exacerbation episode.

Combining SCs and ICS (either alone or in combination with LABA agents) provides patients with the best opportunity to avoid relapses after ED discharge. Nonpharmacological issues, which are often ignored in the ED, remain important considerations for most patients. For example, smoking cessation, a discharge action plan, close follow-up with a primary care physician/general practitioner, immunization for influenza, and the delivery of asthma education (including an asthma action plan) are all important components of the efforts to regain asthma control in the future.

Despite the advancements in evidence-based asthma, additional research is required to improve the care of these patients. Future research should examine methods to measure severity, personalize treatment, disseminate and implement evidence-based treatments in the ED setting, evaluate the role of innovative health service delivery options (such as observation units and short-stay units), and identify additional management strategies.

KEY POINTS

- The use of inhaled SABA with a spacer device is safe and effective for most patients.
- The early treatment of acute asthma with SC and SABA agents combined with SAAC agents may be required.

- In more severe presentations, adjunctive treatments such as IV MgSO$_4$ and ICS may reduce the need for intubation.
- When patients remain distressed, NIV may be an option prior to intubation.
- If all treatments fail, securing the airway through intubation using rapid sequence intubation by experienced personnel with intubation skills and experience in mechanical ventilation is critical.
- Treatment following stabilization should include at least SC and ICS agents with urgent follow-up by an outpatient clinician charged with exploring interventions to reduce the risk of future exacerbations.

ACKNOWLEDGMENTS

The author would like to thank Diane Milette (Department of Emergency Medicine) for her assistance with the production of this chapter. Dr. Rowe is supported by a Tier I Canada Research Chair in Evidence-based Emergency Medicine through the Canadian Institutes of Health Research (CIHR) from the Government of Canada (Ottawa, ON). Dr. Rowe has received funding for investigator-initiated asthma and COPD research in the past 2 years from GlaxoSmithKline (Mississauga, ON, Canada) and for an industry-initiated asthma studies from MedImmune Inc. (Bethesda, MD); however, he is not a paid employee or consultant to either respiratory company.

ABBREVIATIONS

CI	Confidence interval
COPD	Chronic obstructive pulmonary disease
ED	Emergency department
FEV_1	Forced expiratory volume in 1 sec
ICS	Inhaled corticosteroids
IM	Intramuscular
IV	Intravenous
LABA	Long-acting $beta_2$-adrenergic agonists
LTRA	Leukotriene receptor antagonists
MDI	Metered-dose inhaler
$MgSO_4$	Magnesium sulfate
NIV	Noninvasive ventilation
NIPPV	Noninvasive positive pressure ventilation
NNT	Number needed to treat
OR	Odds ratio
PEF	Peak expiratory flow
RCT	Randomized controlled trials
RR	Relative risk
SAAC	Short-acting anticholinergics
SABA	Short-acting beta-agonist
SaO_2	Oxygen saturation
SARS	Severe acute respiratory syndrome
SCs	Systemic corticosteroids

REFERENCES

1. Mannino DM, Homa DM, Pertowski CA, et al. Surveillance for asthma—United States, 1960–1995. *MMWR CDC Surveill Summ* 1998; 47:1–27.
2. Weiss KB, Sullivan SD, Lyttle CS. Trends in the cost of illness for asthma in the United States, 1985–1994. *J Allergy Clin Immunol* 2000; 106:493–499.
3. Weiss KB, Sullivan SD. The health economics of asthma and rhinitis. I. Assessing the economic impact. *J Allergy Clin Immunol* 2001; 107:3–8.
4. Krahn MD, Berka C, Langlois P, Detsky AS. Direct and indirect costs of asthma in Canada, 1990. *CMAJ* 1996; 154:821–831.
5. American Lung Association. Trends in Asthma Morbidity and Mortality. November 2007.
6. Expert Panel Report 3 (EPR-3): Guidelines for the Diagnosis and Management of Asthma-Summary Report 2007. *J Allergy Clin Immunol* 2007; 120:S94–S138.
7. Hodder R, Lougheed MD, Rowe BH, FitzGerald JM, Kaplan AG, McIvor RA. Management of acute asthma in adults in the emergency department: Nonventilatory management. *CMAJ* 2010; 182:E55–E67.
8. Global Initiative for Asthma (GINA). Component 4: Manage asthma exacerbations. In: *Global Strategy for Asthma Management and Prevention*; 2010. Available at www.ginasthma.org (accessed September 9, 2013).
9. British Guideline on the Management of Asthma. *Thorax* 2008; 63(Suppl 4):iv1– iv121.
10. Boulet L-P, Becker A, Berube D, Beveridge RC, Ernst P, on behalf of the Canadian Asthma Consensus Group. Canadian asthma consensus report, 1999. *Can Med Assoc J* 1999; 161:S1–S61.
11. Niska R, Bhuiya F, Xu J. National Hospital Ambulatory Medical Care Survey: 2007 emergency department summary. *Natl Health Stat Rep* 2010; 26:1–31.
12. Rowe BH, Voaklander DC, Wang D, et al. Asthma presentations by adults to emergency departments in Alberta, Canada: A large population-based study. *Chest* 2009; 135:57–65.
13. Worthington JR, Ahuja J. The value of pulmonary function tests in the management of acute asthma. *CMAJ* 1989; 140:153–156.
14. Cates CJ, Crilly JA, Rowe BH. Holding chambers (spacers) versus nebulisers for beta-agonist treatment of acute asthma. *Cochrane Database Syst Rev* 2006:CD000052.
15. Turner MO, Gafni A, Swan D, FitzGerald JM. A review and economic evaluation of bronchodilator delivery methods in hospitalized patients. *Arch Intern Med* 1996; 156:2113–2118.
16. Emerman CL, Cydulka RK, McFadden ER. Comparison of 2.5 vs 7.5 mg of inhaled albuterol in the treatment of acute asthma. *Chest* 1999; 115:92–96.
17. Strauss L, Hejal R, Galan G, Dixon L, McFadden ER Jr. Observations on the effects of aerosolized albuterol in acute asthma. *Am J Respir Crit Care Med* 1997; 155:454–458.
18. Camargo CA Jr., Spooner CH, Rowe BH. Continuous versus intermittent beta-agonists in the treatment of acute asthma. *Cochrane Database Syst Rev* 2003:CD001115.
19. Browne GJ, Penna AS, Phung X, Soo M. Randomised trial of intravenous salbutamol in early management of acute asthma in children. *Lancet* 1997; 349:301–305.
20. Travers AH, Milan SJ, Jones AP, Camargo CA Jr., Rowe BH. Addition of intravenous beta2-agonists to inhaled beta2-agonists for acute asthma. *Cochrane Database Syst Rev* 2012; 12. DOI: 101002/14651858CD010179.
21. Varia M, Wilson S, Sarwal S, et al. Investigation of a nosocomial outbreak of severe acute respiratory syndrome (SARS) in Toronto, Canada. *CMAJ* 2003; 169:285–292.
22. Stoodley RG, Aaron SD, Dales RE. The role of ipratropium bromide in the emergency management of acute asthma exacerbation: A metaanalysis of randomized clinical trials. *Ann Emerg Med* 1999; 34:8–18.
23. Rodrigo GJ, Castro-Rodriguez JA. Anticholinergics in the treatment of children and adults with acute asthma: A systematic review with meta-analysis. *Thorax* 2005; 60:740–746.
24. National Asthma Education Prevention Program (NAEPP). Expert Panel Report 2: Guidelines for the Diagnosis and Management of Asthma (EPR-2 1997). NIH Publication No. 97–4051. Bethesda, MD: Department of Health and Human Services; National Institutes of Health; National Heart, Lung, and Blood Institute; National Asthma Education and Prevention Program; 1997 (Accessed October 17, 2012).
25. Network BTSSIG. British guideline on the management of asthma. *Thorax* 2003; 58:1–94.
26. Rowe BH, Spooner C, Ducharme FM, Bretzlaff JA, Bota GW. Early emergency department treatment of acute asthma with systemic corticosteroids. *Cochrane Database Syst Rev* 2001:CD002178.
27. Zemek R, Plint A, Osmond MH, et al. Triage nurse initiation of corticosteroids in pediatric asthma is associated with improved emergency department efficiency. *Pediatrics* 2012; 129:671–680.
28. Rowe BH, Chahal AM, Spooner CH, et al. Increasing the use of anti-inflammatory agents in acute asthma in the emergency department: Experience with an asthma care map. *Can Respir J* 2008; 15:20–26.
29. Rowe BH, Bretzlaff JA, Bourdon C, Bota GW, Camargo CA Jr. Magnesium sulfate for treating exacerbations of acute asthma in the emergency department. *Cochrane Database Syst Rev* 2000:CD001490.

30. Alter HJ, Koepsell TD, Hilty WM. Intravenous magnesium as an adjuvant in acute bronchospasm: A meta-analysis. *Ann Emerg Med* 2000; 36:191–197.

31. Rowe BH, Camargo CA Jr. The use of magnesium sulfate in acute asthma: Rapid uptake of evidence in North American emergency departments. *J Allergy Clin Immunol* 2006; 117:53–58.

32. Edmonds ML, Camargo CA, Pollack CV, Rowe BH. Early use of inhaled corticosteroids in the emergency department treatment of acute asthma. *Cochrane Database Syst Rev* 2000:CD002308; 2003.

33. Simons FE. Emergency treatment of anaphylaxis. *BMJ* 2008; 336:1141–1142.

34. Ducharme FM, Lasserson TJ, Cates CJ. Long-acting beta2-agonists versus anti-leukotrienes as add-on therapy to inhaled corticosteroids for chronic asthma. *Cochrane Database Syst Rev* 2006:CD003137.

35. Camargo CA Jr., Smithline HA, Malice MP, Green SA, Reiss TF. A randomized controlled trial of intravenous montelukast in acute asthma. *Am J Respir Crit Care Med* 2003; 167:528–533.

36. Silverman RA, Nowak RM, Korenblat PE, et al. Zafirlukast treatment for acute asthma: Evaluation in a randomized, double-blind, multicenter trial. *Chest* 2004; 126:1480–1489.

37. Browning J, Atwood B, Gray A. Use of non-invasive ventilation in UK emergency departments. *Emerg Med J* 2006; 23:920–921.

38. Hess DR, Pang JM, Camargo CA Jr. A survey of the use of noninvasive ventilation in academic emergency departments in the United States. *Respir Care* 2009; 54:1306–1312.

39. Ram FS, Wellington S, Rowe B, Wedzicha JA. Non-invasive positive pressure ventilation for treatment of respiratory failure due to severe acute exacerbations of asthma. *Cochrane Database Syst Rev* 2005:CD004360.

40. Penuelas O, Frutos-Vivar F, Esteban A. Noninvasive positive-pressure ventilation in acute respiratory failure. *CMAJ* 2007; 177:1211–1218.

41. Hodder R, Lougheed MD, FitzGerald JM, Rowe BH, Kaplan AG, McIvor RA. Management of acute asthma in adults in the emergency department: Assisted ventilation. *CMAJ* 2010; 182:265–272.

42. Parameswaran K, Belda J, Rowe BH. Addition of intravenous aminophylline to beta2-agonists in adults with acute asthma. *Cochrane Database Syst Rev* 2000:CD002742.

43. Smucny J, Fahey T, Becker L, Glazier R, McIsaac W. Antibiotics for acute bronchitis. *Cochrane Database Syst Rev* 2000:CD000245.

44. Graham VAL, Lasserson T, Rowe BH. Antibiotics for acute asthma. *Cochrane Database Syst Rev* 2001:CD002741.

45. Rodrigo G, Pollack C, Rodrigo C, Rowe BH. Heliox for non-intubated acute asthma patients. *Cochrane Database Syst Rev* 2006:CD002884.

46. Blitz M, Blitz S, Beasely R, et al. Inhaled magnesium sulfate in the treatment of acute asthma. *Cochrane Database Syst Rev* 2005; 19(4):CD003898.

47. Rowe BH, Villa-Roel C, Sivilottii M, et al. Relapse following emergency department discharge for acute asthma: A prospective multi-center study. *Acad Emerg Med* 2008; 15:709–717.

48. Rowe BH, Spooner C, Ducharme FM, Bretzlaff JA, Bota GW. Early emergency department treatment of acute asthma with systemic corticosteroids (Cochrane Review). *Cochrane Database Syst Rev.* 2001; Issue 1. DOI: 10.1002/14651858. CD002178.

49. Lahn M, Bijur P, Gallagher EJ. Randomized clinical trial of intramuscular vs oral methylprednisolone in the treatment of asthma exacerbations following discharge from an emergency department. *Chest* 2004; 126:362–368.

50. Edmonds ML, Camargo CA, Saunders LD, Brenner BE, Rowe BH. Inhaled steroids in acute asthma following emergency department discharge. *Cochrane Database Syst Rev* 2000:CD002316.

51. Fuhlbrigge AL, Lemanske RF Jr, Rasouliyan L, Sorkness CA, Fish JE. Practice patterns for oral corticosteroid burst therapy in the outpatient management of acute asthma exacerbations. *Allergy Asthma Proc* 2012; 33:82–9.

52. Rowe BH, Bota GW, Fabris L, Therrien SA, Milner RA, Jacono J. Inhaled budesonide in addition to oral corticosteroids to prevent relapse following discharge from the emergency department: A randomized controlled trial. *JAMA* 1999; 281:2119–2126.

53. Sin DD, Man SFP. Low-dose inhaled corticosteroid therapy and risk of emergency department visits for asthma. *Arch Intern Med* 2002; 162:1591–1595.

54. Lougheed MD, Lemiere C, Ducharme FM, et al. Canadian Thoracic Society 2012 guideline update: Diagnosis and management of asthma in preschoolers, children and adults. *Can Respir J* 2012; 19:127–164.

55. The Global Strategy for Asthma Management and Prevention (2011). Global Initiative for Asthma (GINA). Available at http://wwwginasthmaorg (accessed Octber 20, 2012).

56. Rowe BH, Wong E, Blitz S, et al. Adding long-acting beta-agonists to inhaled corticosteroids after discharge from the emergency department for acute asthma: A randomized controlled trial. *Acad Emerg Med* 2007; 14:833–840.

57. Emerman CL, Woodruff PG, Cydulka RK, et al. Prospective multicenter study of relapse following treatment for acute asthma among adults presenting to the emergency department. *Chest* 1999; 115:919–927.

58. Gibson PG, Powell H. Written action plans for asthma: An evidence-based review of the key components. *Thorax* 2004; 59:94–99.

59. Gibson PG, Coughlan J, Wilson AJ, et al. Self-management education and regular practitioner review for adults with asthma. *Cochrane Database Syst Rev* 2000:CD001117.

60. Haynes RB, Xao X, Degani A, Kripalani S, Garg A, McDonald HP. Interventions for enhancing medication adherence. *Cochrane Database Syst Rev* 2005; Issue 4. DOI: 101002/14651858CD000011pub2.

Section VI

Asthma and Special Populations

23 Asthma and Obesity
Clinical Implications

Fernando Holguin

CONTENTS

CASE PRESENTATION

JB is a 35-year-old black female who has had asthma since she was 6 years old. Over the years, she has had many trips to the emergency room and multiple corticosteroid tapers. She has been treated with inhaled corticosteroids (ICSs) and long-acting bronchodilators, but occasionally stops using them. She is atopic and is allergic to cats, dogs, several pollens, grass, dust mites, and more, to name a few. She was recently discharged from the intensive care unit after suffering from a severe asthma exacerbation, which was believed to be triggered by influenza virus H1N1. Her body mass index (BMI) is 30; she has gained weight slowly over time. Spirometry shows moderate airway obstruction with a large bronchodilator response. Her exhaled nitric oxide (NO) is 90 ppb and her IgE level is 316 IU/mL. On previous blood counts, her eosinophils were often 10% or less. In contrast, LB is a 40-year-old white female with asthma that was diagnosed in her late twenties. She has achieved poor control despite being on high-dose ICSs and a long-acting beta-agonist. She uses the emergency room frequently and her inhaled medications do not give her great relief. Her peripheral eosinophils are not elevated, she is nonatopic, and her total IgE is 80 IU/mL. Her exhaled NO is 24 ppb, and lung function testing only revealed mild airway obstruction with a 12% increase in forced expiratory volume in 1 sec (FEV$_1$) after bronchodilators. These subjects are both obese asthmatics, yet as this chapter will discuss, the association between asthma and obesity may be different in these cases. It is possible, for example, that, in the first case, obesity is a consequence of the underlying asthma severity; in the second case, being obese could potentially be playing a more causative role in lack of asthma control and disease severity.

INTRODUCTION

Given the continued rise in the average BMI among the general population, it is not surprising that a considerable number of subjects with asthma are also overweight or obese. Many studies have shown being overweight or obese is a risk factor for increased asthma severity, poor asthma control, and lower asthma-related quality of life.[1–4] Yet the strength of the obesity/asthma association seems less apparent when considering more objective clinical measures (i.e., those not depending on symptoms), such as bronchial hyperresponsiveness (BHR) and biomarkers of airway inflammation.[5] To further complicate things, obesity can increase the risk of being wrongly diagnosed with asthma, particularly among patients presenting in the urgent care setting.[6] This bias is not inconsequential, considering that in one study 30% of subjects diagnosed with asthma actually did not have it.[7] Taken together, this suggests that the obesity/asthma association is more complex than initially thought. This relationship is probably comprised by a heterogeneous population of subjects with asthma. For some, obesity mostly acts as a respiratory symptoms burden without affecting BHR or airway inflammation, while in more susceptible subjects obesity increases asthma severity by adversely modifying airway function, specific inflammatory/injury pathways, or both. For others, obesity may even be the result, rather than the cause, of increased asthma severity.[8] Understanding the heterogeneity of this relationship is essential for developing specific, phenotype-driven, weight-loss and pharmacologic interventions for asthmatics most susceptible to being obese.

This chapter will review the clinical implications of obesity and asthma; it will briefly discuss potential causal pathways linking both conditions, summarize the evidence relating obesity to asthma severity, and discuss the differential response of obesity to asthma medications. Throughout this chapter, asthma and obesity will be discussed in general terms; however, the last section will focus on the current understanding of the "obese asthma phenotype."

Although several epidemiological studies and a recent meta-analysis have shown that increasing BMI is a risk factor for incident asthma (i.e., new asthma medical diagnosis),[9] this is not the focus of this chapter and will therefore not be included in this review.

OBESITY, A HEAVY LOAD FOR THE RESPIRATORY SYSTEM

As adiposity increases, several well-known physiological changes occur. Restrictive lung physiology is induced by excess adipose deposition around the upper abdomen and chest wall and by diaphragmatic displacement due to increased abdominal fat. The reductions in fractional residual capacity and expiratory reserve volume mean breathing occurs in the less compliant part of the pressure–volume curve; thus, obese individuals require greater respiratory work of breathing in order to maintain adequate ventilation levels.[10] Obese patients also have increased airway resistance and closing volume, suggesting small airway closure and dynamic air trapping.[10,11] Further, obesity may alter airway mechanics and increase the risk for developing BHR.[12,13] Although an obesity-mediated increase in BHR has not been shown in all studies,[5] this inconsistency may be explained by using arbitrarily determined BHR cutoff levels instead of the area under the curve, and by studies using heterogeneous asthma phenotypes, some of which may be more or less susceptible to obesity-mediated BHR. Although there is probably construable heterogeneity across obese subjects, the combination of these obesity-mediated changes in lung function largely explain why obesity increases dyspnea and poor exercise tolerance.

Beyond the increased mechanical load on the respiratory system, adiposity may affect airway function through changes in adipokine levels. With increasing BMI, there is a concomitant increase in serum leptin and reduction in serum adiponectin. BMI-related changes in these adipokines may potentially be causatively related to obesity and asthma.[14] As shown in murine models, leptin and adiponectin respectively increase or decrease airway inflammation and BHR.[15,16] Airway leptin levels are also increased in relation to BMI and are highest among obese asthmatics.[17,18] Moreover, airway macrophages from obese asthmatics produced the highest levels of interferon-gamma and tumor necrosis factor-alpha (TNF-α) when treated with leptin.[17] These data would suggest that leptin may play a role in mediating airway inflammatory responses in asthma. In contrast to leptin, greater levels of adiponectin have been found to be protective in females with asthma, and to be inversely related to exhaled NO in cross-sectional studies.[19,20] Further studies are needed to determine whether modifying adipokines leads to clinical outcome changes among obese asthmatics. The metabolic syndrome may potentially be another mechanism linking obesity to asthma. Among school-age children, higher triglycerides and acanthosis nigricans (associated with insulin resistance) were associated with higher asthma prevalence rates.[21] Interestingly, in adults, hyperglycemia and dyslipidemia associated with the metabolic syndrome are associated with steeper loss of lung function over time. There are potential mechanisms linking the metabolic syndrome to asthma; insulin resistance has been shown to have a mitogenic effect on airway smooth muscle cells and to induce a hypercontractile phenotype in these cells.[22,23] In addition, leptin has been shown to stimulate inflammatory signaling in human airway epithelial cells.[24]

CLINICAL IMPLICATIONS

OBESITY AS A RISK FACTOR FOR ASTHMA CONTROL AND SEVERITY

Being overweight or obese has been shown in several studies to be a risk factor for increased asthma severity. Compared with lean asthmatics, obese and overweight asthmatics have more frequent respiratory symptoms, use rescue therapies more often, and have poorer asthma-related quality of life and asthma control. Further, obesity is associated with increased emergency room visits and hospitalizations for asthma exacerbations.[3] Yet the severity of asthma exacerbations between obese and nonobese individuals is similar.[25] This would suggest that, potentially, other factors, such as symptom perception and symptom intensity, contribute to obesity's association with greater numbers of emergency room visits. Regardless, there is strong evidence that changes in body weight influence asthma control, as shown in a longitudinal study of difficult-to-control asthma patients. In this study, patients who gained 5 lb (2.27 kg) during the 12-month interval between baseline and follow-up reported worse asthma control (adjusted odds ratio [OR]: 1.22; 95% CI: 1.01–1.49; $P = 0.04$) and quality of life (0.18; 95% CI: 0.30–0.06; $P = 0.003$), as well as a greater number of steroid bursts (OR: 1.31; 95% CI: 1.04–1.66; $P = 0.02$) than patients who either maintained or lost weight.[26]

OBESITY AND RESPONSE TO MEDICATIONS

Peters-Golden et al. reported, in a retrospective analysis of a clinical trial comparing ICS and montelukast versus placebo, that obese asthmatics have reduced responses to ICS therapy.[27] Increasing BMI was inversely associated with achieving adequate asthma control days while adjusting for potential confounders. Interestingly, the inverse association between asthma control days and BMI was less steep among subjects randomized to montelukast, which suggests that leukotriene blockers could potentially be more effective among the obese. However, a subsequent study showed that inhaled fluticasone, regardless of BMI category, was superior to montelukast in improving lung function, symptom scores, and morning peak flow and reducing albuterol use.[28] Even when adhering to treatment guidelines, having a higher BMI affects the response to therapy. As shown by Saint-Pierre et al., overweight asthmatics have a significantly lower probability of achieving asthma control when compared with those with a lower normal BMI.[29] Further, in a study of corticosteroid-naïve asthmatics randomized to inhaled budesonide or budesonide + salmeterol, obese and overweight asthmatics had lower odds ratios for achieving asthma control at 12 weeks regardless of the assigned treatment.[2] In children participating in the Childhood Asthma Management Program (CAMP), those who were overweight or obese had improvements in FEV_1 and bronchodilation in response to budesonide; however, this was a transient improvement that occurred during the early but not late stages of the trial.[30] Although it is unclear why obesity may render inhaled steroids less effective, there is evidence that it may increase steroid resistance. It has been demonstrated that with increasing BMI, the ability of dexamethasone to induce mitogen-activated protein kinase phosphatase-1 (MKP-1, a key factor for steroid activity) in peripheral blood monocytes (PBMC) and bronchoalveolar lavage cells is reduced. Also, the expression of TNF-α in PBMC of asthmatics increased in relation to BMI.[31]

OBESITY AND BIOMARKERS OF AIRWAY INFLAMMATION AND OXIDATIVE STRESS

Increasing BMI in asthmatics has either not been associated or, somewhat paradoxically, has been inversely related to airway biomarkers of eosinophilic inflammation. Several studies, for example, have shown that the fractional excretion of exhaled nitric oxide (FeNO) is inversely associated with BMI or that obese asthmatics have lower FeNO when compared with the leaner weight categories. More recently, it has been suggested that among late-onset asthmatics, the inverse association between FeNO and BMI may be partly determined by the L-arginine and the asymmetric di-methylarginine (ADMA) balance. ADMA is an endogenous inhibitor of nitric oxide synthase (NOS) that can uncouple NOS, reducing NO production while generating anion superoxide.[32] Among consecutive outpatient asthmatics, sputum eosinophils have not been shown to be different across the quintile BMI distribution; in contrast, among difficult-to-control asthmatics, increasing BMI has been inversely related to sputum eosinophils.[20,33–36] In contrast, some obese asthmatics have been shown to have greater airway neutrophilia.[37] Interestingly, after ingestion of a high-fat meal, there is an increase in airway neutrophilia in lean and obese asthmatics, which is also associated with reduced bronchodilation.[38] Higher BMI has also been linked to increased levels of 8-isoprostanes (a nonenzymatic biomarker of lipid peroxidation), higher levels of 4-hydroxynonenal, and reduced

airway pH.[34,39,40] A greater degree of airway neutrophilia and oxidative stress could potentially explain why some obese asthmatics are less ICS responsive.[41]

OBESITY AND WEIGHT LOSS IN ASTHMA

Weight loss is by all accounts beneficial to patients with asthma. As shown in a meta-analysis, weight loss randomized control studies (using diet, medication, and exercise) can lead to reductions in respiratory symptoms, lower rates of rescue medication use, and modest improvements in FEV_1.[42] However, issues related to small sample size and potential bias limit the interpretation of these results. Two studies have shown that bariatric surgery-induced weight loss improves asthma control, lessens asthma severity, and reduces BHR.[43,44] However, in a *post hoc* analysis, Dixon et al. showed an effect modification on BHR based on whether subjects had lower or normal versus high IgE. In other words, only among subjects with low or normal IgE (these patients are usually more likely to be late-onset asthma with less atopic patients) was weight loss effective in improving BHR. Boulet et al. did not find that age of asthma onset modified the effect that bariatric surgery-induced weight loss had on BHR; however, this study was very small.[44] Although it requires further evaluation, the study by Dixon et al. suggests that obesity may differentially affect airway function, depending on the underlying asthma clinical phenotype.[43]

IS THERE AN OBESE ASTHMA PHENOTYPE DETERMINED BY THE AGE OF ASTHMA ONSET?

Asthma that begins later in life is now recognized as more commonly occurring in women and consisting of multiple different phenotypes, but is often less associated with allergic/T-helper type 2 (Th2) inflammation than early-onset disease.[45,46] While aspirin-sensitive asthma and occupational asthma are considered adult-onset forms, more recent studies have suggested that some late-onset asthma is associated with obesity. These studies suggest that the physiology and even the pathobiology of adult-onset, obese asthma are different from those of childhood-onset asthma.[47] In fact, data from cluster analyses of asthma phenotypes studies suggest that obesity is associated with a cluster, characterized by late-onset asthma in patients who are primarily obese women with a high degree of symptoms, despite having relatively preserved lung function or low levels of airway inflammation.[45,46] However, the obese-asthma phenotype is not necessarily uniform across all obese individuals. Based on the combined analysis of two studies from the Asthma Clinical Research Network, there were two clusters with BMI in the obese range: an uncontrolled asthma cluster, characterized by higher exhaled NO, lower BMI, and a younger age of asthma onset (mean of 10 years); and a second, asthma-controlled cluster, characterized by older age of asthma onset (mean of 16.1 years), lower exhaled NO, and lower IgE levels.[48] These two obese clusters could represent two distinct obese phenotypes: an early-onset atopic one with more eosinophilic

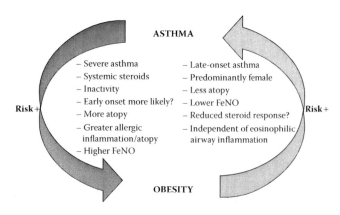

FIGURE 23.1 Obesity and asthma: a bidirectional association.

airway inflammation, and a second, less atopic and of later onset. The difficult question here is to determine in which of these phenotypes is obesity a factor for asthma severity or a consequence of increased asthma severity. Although cross-sectional studies cannot fully answer this question, a recent study from the Severe Asthma Research program (SARP) showed that among early-onset asthmatics (<12 years of age) BMI appears to linearly increase in relation to the duration of asthma; in contrast, there is no association between asthma duration and BMI among later-onset asthmatics.[8] This difference could potentially suggest that in early-onset asthma, increasing BMI may be the consequence of asthma (i.e., respiratory severity, inability to exercise, steroids, etc.), whereas in the late-onset disease obesity may be a primary determinant of the disease, rather than a response to the disease or its treatment (see Figure 23.1).

SUMMARY

The association between obesity and asthma is highly complex and potentially causative at many pathophysiological levels. Although it seems that obesity universally increases the respiratory symptoms' frequency or severity, it may be, in a subset of more susceptible patients (i.e., obese asthma phenotype), that obesity increases the exacerbation risk through mechanisms such as increased BHR and changes in noneosinophilic airway inflammation and oxidation. Identifying this asthma phenotype will be critical in developing specific therapies and public health interventions geared toward those that stand to benefit the most.

KEY PRACTICAL POINTS

- Obesity is a risk factor for increased respiratory symptom severity in subjects with asthma.
- The asthma phenotype (more susceptible asthmatics in whom obesity affects mechanisms or airway inflammation/function) may be characterized by those with late-onset asthma, probably after 12 years of age, that are less atopic and have low exhaled NO. This phenotype may be more frequent among females.

- Inhaled steroids (whether this is limited to only those with the "asthma phenotype" is unclear) may be less effective in obese asthmatics.
- Weight loss improves symptom scores and lung volumes, yet it appears that obesity-mediated BHR is potentially limited to those with less allergic inflammation.

REFERENCES

1. Vortmann M, Eisner MD. BMI and health status among adults with asthma. *Obesity.* 2008;16(1):146–152.
2. Sutherland ER, Lehman EB, Teodorescu M, Wechsler ME. Body mass index and phenotype in subjects with mild-to-moderate persistent asthma. *J Allergy Clin Immunol.* 2009;123(6):1328–1334.
3. Taylor B, Mannino D, Brown C, Crocker D, Twum-Baah N, Holguin F. Body mass index and asthma severity in the National Asthma Survey. *Thorax.* 2008;63(1):14–20.
4. Lessard A, Turcotte H, Cormier Y, Boulet LP. Obesity and asthma: A specific phenotype? *Chest.* 2008;134(2):317–323.
5. Dixon AE, Holguin F, Sood A, Salome CM, Pratley RE, Beuther DA, et al. An official American Thoracic Society Workshop report: Obesity and asthma. *Proc Am Thorac Soc.* 2010;7(5):325–335.
6. Pakhale S, Doucette S, Vandemheen K, Boulet LP, McIvor RA, Fitzgerald JM, et al. A comparison of obese and non-obese people with asthma: Exploring an asthma-obesity interaction. *Chest.* 2010;137(6):1316–1323.
7. Aaron SD, Vandemheen KL, Boulet LP, McIvor RA, Fitzgerald JM, Hernandez P, et al. Overdiagnosis of asthma in obese and nonobese adults. *CMAJ.* 2008;179(11):1121–1131.
8. Holguin F, Bleecker ER, Busse WW, Calhoun WJ, Castro M, Erzurum SC, et al. Obesity and asthma: An association modified by age of asthma onset. *J Allergy Clin Immunol.* 2011;127(6):1486–1493.
9. Beuther DA, Sutherland ER. Overweight, obesity, and incident asthma: A meta-analysis of prospective epidemiologic studies. *Am J Respir Crit Care Med.* 2007;175(7):661–666.
10. Lin CK, Lin CC. Work of breathing and respiratory drive in obesity. *Respirology.* 2012;17(3):402–411.
11. Sutherland TJ, Cowan JO, Taylor DR. Dynamic hyperinflation with bronchoconstriction: Differences between obese and non-obese women with asthma. *Am J Respir Crit Care Med.* 2008;177(9):970–975.
12. Holguin F, Cribbs S, Fitzpatrick AM, Ingram RH Jr., Jackson AC. A deep breath bronchoconstricts obese asthmatics. *J Asthma.* 2010;47(1):55–60.
13. Skloot G, Schechter C, Desai A, Togias A. Impaired response to deep inspiration in obesity. *J Appl Physiol.* 2011;111(3):726–734.
14. Dixon AE. Adipokines and asthma. *Chest.* 2009;135(2):255–256.
15. Shore SA, Schwartzman IN, Mellema MS, Flynt L, Imrich A, Johnston RA. Effect of leptin on allergic airway responses in mice. *J Allergy Clin Immunol.* 2005;115(1):103–109.
16. Shore SA, Terry RD, Flynt L, Xu A, Hug C. Adiponectin attenuates allergen-induced airway inflammation and hyperresponsiveness in mice. *J Allergy Clin Immunol.* 2006;118(2):389–395.
17. Lugogo NL, Hollingsworth JW, Howell DL, Que LG, Francisco D, Church TD, et al. Alveolar macrophages from overweight/obese subjects with asthma demonstrate a proinflammatory phenotype. *Am J Respir Crit Care Med.* 2012;186(5):404–411.

18. Holguin F, Fitzpatrick A, Anderson A, Brown LA. Airway adipokines and airway oxidative stress in lean and obese controls and asthmatics. *Am J Respir Crit Care Med.* 2009;179:A2510.

19. Sood A, Cui X, Qualls C, Beckett WS, Gross MD, Steffes MW, et al. Association between asthma and serum adiponectin concentration in women. *Thorax.* 2008;63(10):877–882.

20. Sutherland TJ, Sears MR, McLachlan CR, Poulton R, Hancox RJ. Leptin, adiponectin, and asthma: Findings from a population-based cohort study. *Ann Allergy Asthma Immunol.* 2009;103(2):101–107.

21. Cottrell L, Neal WA, Ice C, Perez MK, Piedimonte G. Metabolic abnormalities in children with asthma. *Am J Respir Crit Care Med.* 2011;183(4):441–448.

22. Schaafsma D, McNeill KD, Stelmack GL, Gosens R, Baarsma HA, Dekkers BG, et al. Insulin increases the expression of contractile phenotypic markers in airway smooth muscle. *Am J Physiol.* 2007;293(1):C429–C439.

23. Schaafsma D, Gosens R, Ris JM, Zaagsma J, Meurs H, Nelemans SA. Insulin induces airway smooth muscle contraction. *Br J Pharmacol.* 2007;150(2):136–142.

24. Papagianni M, Hatziefthimiou A, Chachami G, Gourgoulianis K, Molyvdas PA, Paraskeva E. Insulin causes a transient induction of proliferation via activation of the PI3-kinase pathway in airway smooth muscle cells. *Exp Clin Endocrinol Diabetes.* 2007;115(2):118–123.

25. Thomson CC, Clark S, Camargo CA Jr. Body mass index and asthma severity among adults presenting to the emergency department. *Chest.* 2003;124(3):795–802.

26. Haselkorn T, Fish JE, Chipps BE, Miller DP, Chen H, Weiss ST. Effect of weight change on asthma-related health outcomes in patients with severe or difficult-to-treat asthma. *Respir Med.* 2009;103(2):274–283.

27. Peters-Golden M, Swern A, Bird SS, Hustad CM, Grant E, Edelman JM. Influence of body mass index on the response to asthma controller agents. *Eur Respir J.* 2006;27(3):495–503.

28. Camargo CA Jr., Boulet LP, Sutherland ER, Busse WW, Yancey SW, Emmett AH, et al. Body mass index and response to asthma therapy: Fluticasone propionate/salmeterol versus montelukast. *J Asthma.* 2010;47(1):76–82.

29. Saint-Pierre P, Bourdin A, Chanez P, Daures JP, Godard P. Are overweight asthmatics more difficult to control? *Allergy.* 2006;61(1):79–84.

30. Forno E, Lescher R, Strunk R, Weiss S, Fuhlbrigge A, Celedon JC. Decreased response to inhaled steroids in overweight and obese asthmatic children. *J Allergy Clin Immunol.* 2011;127(3):741–749.

31. Sutherland ER, Goleva E, Strand M, Beuther DA, Leung DY. Body mass and glucocorticoid response in asthma. *Am J Respir Crit Care Med.* 2008;178(7):682–687.

32. Holguin F, Comhair SA, Hazen SL, Powers RW, Khatri SS, Bleecker ER, et al. An association between L-arginine/asymmetric dimethyl arginine balance, obesity, and the age of asthma onset phenotype. *Am J Respir Crit Care Med.* 2013;187(2):153–159.

33. Todd DC, Armstrong S, D'Silva L, Allen CJ, Hargreave FE, Parameswaran K. Effect of obesity on airway inflammation: A cross-sectional analysis of body mass index and sputum cell counts. *Clin Exp Allergy.* 2007;37(7):1049–1054.

34. Komakula S, Khatri S, Mermis J, Savill S, Haque S, Rojas M, et al. Body mass index is associated with reduced exhaled nitric oxide and higher exhaled 8-isoprostanes in asthmatics. *Respir Res.* 2007;8:32.

35. van Veen IH, Ten Brinke A, Sterk PJ, Rabe KF, Bel EH. Airway inflammation in obese and nonobese patients with difficult-to-treat asthma. *Allergy.* 2008;63(5):570–574.

36. Berg CM, Thelle DS, Rosengren A, Lissner L, Toren K, Olin AC. Decreased fraction of exhaled nitric oxide in obese subjects with asthma symptoms: Data from the population study INTERGENE/ADONIX. *Chest.* 2011;139(5):1109–1116.

37. Telenga ED, Tideman SW, Kerstjens HA, Hacken NH, Timens W, Postma DS, et al. Obesity in asthma: More neutrophilic inflammation as a possible explanation for a reduced treatment response. *Allergy.* 2012;67(8):1060–1068.

38. Wood LG, Garg ML, Gibson PG. A high-fat challenge increases airway inflammation and impairs bronchodilator recovery in asthma. *J Allergy Clin Immunol.* 2011;127(5):1133–1140.

39. Fernandez-Boyanapalli R, Goleva E, Kolakowski C, Min E, Day B, Leung DY, et al. Obesity impairs apoptotic cell clearance in asthma. *J Allergy Clin Immunol.* 2012;131(4):1041–1047.

40. Liu L, Teague WG, Erzurum S, Fitzpatrick A, Mantri S, Dweik RA, et al. Determinants of exhaled breath condensate pH in a large population with asthma. *Chest.* 2011;139(2):328–336.

41. Jatakanon A, Uasuf C, Maziak W, Lim S, Chung KF, Barnes PJ. Neutrophilic inflammation in severe persistent asthma. *Am J Respir Crit Care Med.* 1999;160(5 Pt 1):1532–1539.

42. Adeniyi FB, Young T. Weight loss interventions for chronic asthma. *Cochrane Database Syst Rev.* 2011;7:CD009339.

43. Dixon AE, Pratley RE, Forgione PM, Kaminsky DA, Whittaker-Leclair LA, Griffes LA, et al. Effects of obesity and bariatric surgery on airway hyperresponsiveness, asthma control, and inflammation. *J Allergy Clin Immunol.* 2011;128(3):508–515 e2.

44. Boulet LP, Turcotte H, Martin J, Poirier P. Effect of bariatric surgery on airway response and lung function in obese subjects with asthma. *Respir Med.* 2012;106(5):651–660.

45. Moore WC, Meyers DA, Wenzel SE, Teague WG, Li H, Li X, et al. Identification of asthma phenotypes using cluster analysis in the Severe Asthma Research Program. *Am J Respir Crit Care Med.* 2007;181(4):315–323.

46. Haldar P, Pavord ID, Shaw DE, Berry MA, Thomas M, Brightling CE, et al. Cluster analysis and clinical asthma phenotypes. *Am J Respir Crit Care Med.* 2008;178(3):218–224.

47. Miranda C, Busacker A, Balzar S, Trudeau J, Wenzel SE. Distinguishing severe asthma phenotypes: Role of age at onset and eosinophilic inflammation. *J Allergy Clin Immunol.* 2004;113(1):101–108.

48. Sutherland ER, Goleva E, King TS, Lehman E, Stevens AD, Jackson LP, et al. Cluster analysis of obesity and asthma phenotypes. *PLoS One.* 2012;7(5):e36631.

24 Occupational Asthma

Jonathan A. Bernstein

CONTENTS

CASE PRESENTATION

A 49-year-old male worker for a chemical manufacturing company presents with increased shortness of breath, chest tightness, and wheezing, which began approximately 7 months after starting his job. His symptoms begin within 1 h after arriving at work and persist throughout his shift. Initially the symptoms resolved after leaving the workplace, but over time persisted at home, causing him to wake up two to three times a night. His symptoms improve when the plant is closed for holidays and when he is on vacation, but resume immediately after returning to work. He has no history of asthma but has some spring and fall seasonal upper respiratory symptoms consisting of sneezing, nasal congestion, and rhinorrhea. Other than some mild hypertension and hypercholesterolemia controlled with diet, he is healthy. His work process involves operating a forklift in a warehouse where finished powdered chemicals in one-ton plastic bales are stored. He wears no personal protective equipment such as a respirator. His physical exam reveals some mild inspiratory wheezing but is otherwise normal. His peak expiratory flow (PEF) is 350, which is decreased for his age and height (normal for 72-inch male: 632 L/min). Spirometry reveals an FEV_1 of 2.4 L (60% predicted), which improves to 4 L (100% predicted) after bronchodilators. Exhaled nitric oxide level is 72 ppb (normal <20 ppb). The worker is provided with a PEF meter and diary and asked to record PEF every 2 h while in the workplace and every 3–4 h at home while awake. He is given an albuterol inhaler to use as needed for chest tightness and wheezing. He also is asked to obtain material safety data sheets (MSDSs) for review.

During his return visit 2 weeks later he is still very symptomatic. His PEF is 30% lower at work than at home. MSDSs reveal he is exposed to trimellitic anhydride (TMA), phthalic anhydride (PA), and maleic anhydride (MA) powders. Blood is obtained for specific IgE and IgG to TMA, PA, and MA from a commercial laboratory. He is started on an inhaled corticosteroid and instructed not to go into the warehouse. After discussion with the company safety supervisor, the worker is able to be placed in an area of the plant where there is no chemical exposure. A return visit 4 weeks later reveals that the worker is symptomatically much improved and his PEF has increased to 560 L/min; his FEV_1 has improved to 3.7 L and his exhaled nitric oxide has decreased to 20 ppb. Results of his blood testing reveal increased specific IgE and IgG to TMA only. The worker is instructed to continue to avoid exposure to TMA and continue his inhaled corticosteroid as prescribed. A return visit 8 weeks later reveals he is completely asymptomatic and his FEV_1 has increased to 4 L.

Diagnosis: *TMA-induced occupational asthma.*

INTRODUCTION

Occupational asthma (OA) is defined as "a disease characterized by variable airflow limitation and/or hyperresponsiveness and/or inflammation due to causes and conditions attributable to a particular occupational environment and not to stimuli encountered outside the workplace".[1] OA classically is characterized by a latency period during which time workers are exposed to either a high-molecular-weight (HMW) or low-molecular-weight (LMW) agent for a varying amount of time before becoming sensitized and subsequently developing asthma symptoms.[2,3] HMW agents include plant or animal proteins larger than 1000 kD, which include natural rubber latex, enzymes, or laboratory animal allergens.[3] LMW agents include chemicals smaller than 1000 kD that require conjugation with an endogenous protein (i.e., human serum albumin) to form a complete antigen capable of eliciting a specific immune response; they include isocyanates, acid anhydrides, and metallic salts.[3] However, it is now well recognized that OA can occur in the absence of a latency period after a large exposure to an irritating or toxic material, resulting in airway hyperresponsiveness (AHR) and asthma within 24 h, referred to as reactive airways dysfunction syndrome (RADS) or irritant-induced asthma.[4] The term *work-exacerbated asthma* has been recommended for patients with preexisting asthma that later develop worsening of asthma due to exposures in the workplace.[5]

EPIDEMIOLOGY

A description of breathing problems related to a worker's trade, which would be considered OA in modern times, was first provided by Hippocrates (460–370 BC) in reference to metalworkers, tailors, horsemen, farmhands, and fishermen.[1] Throughout history, physicians have increasingly recognized the relationship been asthma and a variety of occupations. The incidence of OA per year varies among countries, ranging from 10 to 114 cases per million per year. Differences in incidence are mainly due to methodological differences in calculating incidence and the types of occupations and employment opportunities in each country.[6] The Sentinel Event Notification System for Occupational Risks (SENSOR) was first developed in several U.S. states in the 1980s to encourage reporting of OA cases by physicians and to put them in contact with public health agencies responsible for investigating high-risk workplaces.[7] This program was successful at increasing awareness among physicians about OA, but underreporting of cases has been a continuous problem.[7] Other countries have developed voluntary reporting registries to identify the ongoing incidence and prevalence of OA with varying degrees of success.[8-12] The evaluation of asthma cases being considered for workers' compensation or disability benefits has been another source of estimated incidence rates of OA.

It is estimated that up to 15% of all new diagnoses of asthma begin in the workplace. More than 300 agents in the workplace have now been associated with causing OA.[13] Cross-sectional studies have provided prevalence data for a number of agents known to cause OA. Prevalence of OA varies widely between occupations. Studies have found the prevalence of OA for laboratory animal workers to be approximately 20%, for western red cedar-induced OA approximately 5%, for baker's asthma 7%–9%, for isocyanate-induced OA 5%–21%, platinum-exposed workers 20%–50%, and enzyme-exposed workers to be as high as 60%.[6,14-16] The prevalence of OA within a specific occupation depends on environmental conditions within the plant, exposure levels,

durations of exposure, and the effectiveness of procedures implemented in the workplace to reduce worker exposure.[6] Using cross-sectional studies to determine OA prevalence can result in an underestimation due to the "healthy worker effect," which refers to the occurrence of symptomatic workers leaving the workplace without documenting the work relatedness of their illness, leading to what appears to be a healthier workforce.[17] To obtain more accurate prevalence data information about the causes, risk factors, and natural course of OA, surveillance programs for some high-risk manufacturing industries have been established in developed countries, including the United Kingdom, United States, and Finland. The Surveillance of Work-Related and Occupational Respiratory Disease (SWORD) program established in the United Kingdom involves voluntary reporting of occupational illnesses from a variety of industries by pulmonologists and occupational medicine physicians.[18] This program has been very useful for generating prevalence data due to the excellent response rate from participating physicians. The SWORD database has found that OA is the most frequently reported occupational respiratory illness and that isocyanates are the most common specific cause of OA.[18] As mentioned, the SENSOR program established in the United States has not been as successful in obtaining useful epidemiologic data due to a poor response rate from participating physicians.[7] In contrast, the Finnish program has been successful over a relatively short period in estimating the country's yearly incidence of OA and hypersensitivity pneumonitis.[8]

IMMUNOPATHOGENESIS

The pathogenic features of OA are similar to those observed in non-OA patients. In general, lung biopsies of patients with OA demonstrate increased numbers of inflammatory cells with a predominance of eosinophils and lymphocytes, increased intercellular spaces between epithelial cells, and thickening of the reticular basement membrane due to deposition of types I, III, and V collagen.[19] It has been demonstrated that the degree of reticular basement membrane thickening differs between different forms of OA. For example, workers with RADS have been demonstrated to have basement membrane thickening as great as 30–40 μm compared with workers with diisocyanate-induced OA (6–15 μm) and normal subjects (3–8 μm).[20] Similar bioactive mediators and proinflammatory cytokines occur in OA and non-OA.[19] Interestingly, agents including natural rubber latex, mushroom spores, acrylates, and epoxy resins can cause work-related lower respiratory symptoms that manifest as eosinophilic bronchitis, characterized as a chronic cough with sputum eosinophilia, in the absence of bronchial AHR.[21] Although less common, OA can manifest as neutrophilic inflammation with some LMW agents.[22] For non-OA, the presence of neutrophils is believed to be a marker of severity, but their role in different causes of OA is still unclear.[23] Patients with OA and non-OA can exhibit similar inflammatory/physiologic phases of asthma.[24] However, different causes of OA characteristically exhibit different airway responses. For example, whereas an early airway response (EAR) is more characteristic of HMW agents, the late airway response (LAR) and dual airway response (DAR) are more commonly observed in workers with isocyanate-induced OA.[24] It is possible to miss a diagnosis of isocyanate-induced OA as workers who exhibit a LAR may not manifest clinical symptoms until leaving the workplace.[24]

MECHANISMS

HMW and LMW agents known to cause OA involve T-helper type 2 (Th2) proinflammatory cytokines characteristic of IgE-mediated allergic asthma.[19] Enzymes are a good example of HMW agents whereas acid anhydrides are a good example of LMW agents known to cause OA through an IgE-mediated mechanism. In contrast to HMW agents, most LMW chemicals (plicatic acid and diisocyanates) cause OA through as of yet unknown non-IgE-mediated mechanisms. Several mechanisms have been proposed for different clinical presentations associated with a number of causative agents.[19] For acid anhydrides, specific IgE, cytotoxic, immune complex, and cell-mediated immune responses have all been reported (Table 24.1).[25,26] The mechanism(s) for irritant-induced asthma or RADS caused by a single high exposure or chronic low exposure to a chemical (i.e., anhydrous ammonia) also remains elusive.[4] It is speculated that chronic inflammatory changes occur in these workers as a result of toxic injury to bronchial epithelial cells leading to loss of epithelial-derived relaxing factors combined with neurogenic inflammation and release of bioactive mediators and proinflammatory cytokines by nonspecific activation of mast cells.[4] A number of OA animal models have been developed in an attempt to better elucidate the role of innate and adaptive immune responses in causing a variety of IgE and non-IgE-mediated induced OA.[27-29]

GENETICS

Genetic associations in workers with OA have been reported. For example, workers who develop acid anhydride OA express the class II HLA molecule DQB1*501.[30] Interestingly, this genetic marker may be protective against developing OA secondary to isocyanates or plicatic acid.[31,32] In laboratory animal handlers, the HLADRB1*07 phenotype was more commonly expressed in workers sensitized to rat lipocalin allergens.[33] Glutathione-S transferase (GST) polymorphisms, associated with reduction in oxidative stress, have been reported to protect isocyanate-exposed workers from developing asthma in a way similar to what has been observed with non-OA induced by ozone and diesel exhaust particulate exposures.[34] Subsequently, GST, microsomal epoxide hydrolase, and manganese superoxide dismutase have been demonstrated to be associated with diisocyanate OA.[35] More recently, polymorphisms of α-catenin gene (CTNNA3), a key protein of the adherence junctional complex on epithelial cells important for cell adherence, have been found to be associated with diisocyanate OA.[36] In addition, previous studies have found that N-acetyltransferase genotypes, specifically the slow acetylator genotype, increased the risk of isocyanate-exposed workers for developing OA almost

---

TABLE 24.1
Trimellitic Acid Anhydride Clinical Syndromes

Characteristics	Rhinitis/Asthma	Late Asthma	Late Respiratory Systemic Syndrome (LRSS) aka TMA Flu	Pulmonary Disease-Anemia	Irritant-Induced Asthma
Latency period	Yes	Yes	Yes	Yes	No
Onset of symptoms after work exposure	Immediate (30–60 min)	4–12 h	4–12 h	Progressive with further work exposure	Variable depending on exposure
Clinical symptoms	Cough, wheeze, chest tightness, shortness of breath, rhinorrhea, nasal congestion, sneezing, postnasal drainage	Coughing, sneezing, tightness in chest, wheezing due to constriction of airways, sneezing, itching of nose	Resembles hypersensitivity pneumonitis. Coughing, wheezing and dyspnea often accompanied by malaise, chills, fever, muscle and joint pains	Hemoptysis, dyspnea, pulmonary infiltrates, restrictive lung disease, and anemia, as well as the same symptoms as LRSS	Cough, chest tightness, wheezing, shortness of breath and upper airway and eye irritation, lacrimation, sneezing, and nasal discharge
Specific IgE	+	±	−	−	−
Specific IgG	+	±	±	±	−
Gell-Coombs classification	IgE mediated	?Type I (late-phase asthmatic response)	Type III (Immune-complex-mediated hypersensitivity)	Type II (antibody-dependent cytotoxic hypersensitivity); type III (immune-complex-mediated hypersensitivity)	−

Source: Zeiss, C.R., Mitchell, J.H., Van Peenen, P.F., Kavich, D., Collins, M.J., Grammer, L. et al., *Allergy Proc.*, 13, 193–198, 1992; Zeiss, C.R., Patterson, R., Pruzansky, J.J., Miller, M.M., Rosenberg, M., Levitz, D., *J. Allergy Clin. Immunol.*, 60, 96–103, 1977.

eightfold.[37] Over the last several years, IL-4R gene polymorphisms have been found to be associated with isocyanate-induced OA, and more recently linkages with IL4RA, CD14, and IL-13 have been reported.[38,39]

DIAGNOSIS

HISTORY

The criteria for diagnosis of OA proposed by the American College of Chest Physicians are summarized in Table 24.2.[40] To successfully diagnose OA, the physician must be familiar with known causative HMW and LMW agents, which are continuously increasing each year. A comprehensive review of old and new causes of OA has recently been published.[13]

The classic presentation of a worker with OA consists of symptoms that begin while at work and resolve or improve either shortly after leaving the workplace at night, during weekends, or while on vacation.[41] However, a worker with OA may not improve away from the workplace because of chronic airway inflammation with or without fixed obstruction of the airways as a result of persistent workplace exposure to an agent for months or years after the initial onset of symptoms.[41] In addition, patients with RADS typically do not improve away from work.[4] Therefore, the diagnosis of OA should not be overlooked because of the apparent lack of correlation of symptoms with workplace exposure.

Omission or an inadequate history pertaining to the workplace can often delay the diagnosis of OA for months or years.

Figure 24.1 is an algorithmic approach for the evaluation and diagnosis of OA.[42] Structured occupational questionnaires have been developed as tools for determining the probability of OA.[40] The basic components of a structured occupational questionnaire include an employment history and medical history (Table 24.3).[40] The employment history should ascertain the following information: the worker's past and present employment history; their work process, including all jobs that could be related to specific exposures; work processes in adjacent areas; work-shift hours; previous jobs where the worker may have been exposed to similar or identical agents; relationship of symptoms experienced before, during, or after work to a specific exposure in the workplace; duration of symptoms after leaving the workplace; improvement of symptoms on weekends or vacations; associated upper respiratory and dermatologic symptoms; systemic symptoms such as fever, chills, and temperature; smoking history; preexisting allergy/asthma history; previous chemical spill exposure; and potential risk factors for OA.[40] Although occupational questionnaires are helpful in ascertaining invaluable information that determines the likelihood of workplace-related asthma, history alone is sensitive but not specific and therefore cannot be relied upon to make a definitive diagnosis of OA without confirmatory objective testing.

Material safety data sheets (MSDSs) are an essential component of the occupational history.[43] They provide invaluable information regarding generic chemical names and specific constituents of raw materials being used in the workplace. They also provide standard information about threshold limit values (TLV) and permissible exposure levels (PEL) of potentially toxic and/or sensitizing agents.[43] When available,

---

TABLE 24.2

Criteria for Defining OA Proposed by the American College of Chest Physicians

  A. Diagnosis of asthma

  B. Onset of symptoms after entering the workplace

  C. Association between symptoms of asthma and work

  D. One or more of the following criteria:

    1. Workplace exposure to an agent or process known to give rise to OA

    2. Significant work-related changes in FEV_1 or PEF rate

    3. Significant-work related changes in nonspecific airway responsiveness

    4. Positive response to specific inhalation challenge tests with an agent to which the patient is exposed at work

    5. Onset of asthma with a clear association with a symptomatic exposure to an irritant agent in the workplace RADS

Requirements

  OA:

  Surveillance case definition: A + B+C + D1 or D2 or D3 or D4 or D5

  Medical case definition: A + B + C + D2 or D3 or D4 or D5

  Likely OA: A + B + C + D1

  Work-aggravated asthma: A + C (i.e., the subject was symptomatic or required medication before and had an increase in symptoms or medication requirement after entering a new occupational exposure setting)

Source: Tarlo, S.M., Balmes, J., Balkissoon, R., Beach, J., Beckett, W., Bernstein, D. et al., *Chest.*, 134, 1S–41S, 2008.

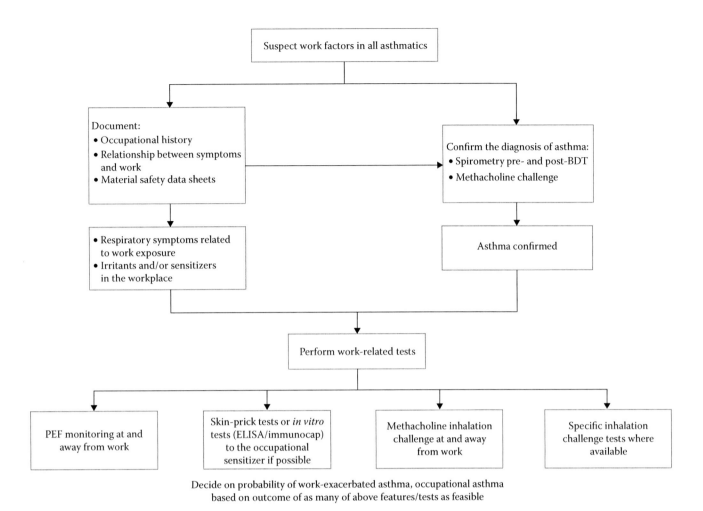

FIGURE 24.1   Algorithmic approach to the diagnosis of occupational asthma. BDT, bronchodilator therapy. (From Tarlo, S.M., Liss, G.M., Blanc, P.D., *Polskie Archiwum Medycyny Wewnetrznej.*, 119, 660–666, 2009.)

assistance from industrial hygienists or safety officers familiar with the workplace and the worker's exposure history should be sought. On occasion, these documents have proprietary agents not specifically listed that could cause OA. Therefore, it may be necessary for the clinician to contact the company to obtain additional exposure information.[43]

DIFFERENTIAL DIAGNOSIS

Diagnosis of OA can be incorrectly made in individuals with preexisting asthma due to nonworkplace allergens. In these cases, symptoms are aggravated by exposure to irritants, physical factors (e.g., cold air), or common indoor allergens (e.g., dust mites) in the workplace.[40] However, it should be emphasized that preexisting asthma does not preclude the development of OA. In these cases, workers may be experiencing work-exacerbated asthma or asthma due to a new workplace allergen or chemical exposure. At times, OA must also be distinguished from other diseases, such as vocal cord dysfunction, chronic obstructive lung disease, pneumoconiosis, bronchiolitis obliterans, and endotoxin-induced asthma-like syndromes such as grain fever or byssinosis.[40] These disorders are differentiated from OA by history, chest radiograph,

chest computerized tomography (CT) scan, lung volumes with diffusion capacity, and, if necessary, open lung biopsy. Chest radiographs and diffusing capacity of lung for carbon monoxide (DLCO) are normal in workers with OA.[40]

IMMUNOLOGIC ASSESSMENT

Immunologic mechanisms have been confirmed for many causes of OA. Therefore, it is important to investigate whether specific immune responses to suspected agents with allergenic potential are involved. Although identification of an immunologic response to a specific agent helps phenotype different forms of OA, it is usually not diagnostic. Such a response may only reflect exposure and the immunogenic nature of the inciting agent.[40] Cutaneous sensitization to an offending agent indicates a high risk for OA but lacks the specificity needed to diagnose OA. Several types of immune responses are associated with HMW and LMW agents that cause OA. Type I IgE-mediated immune responses have been identified for the majority of HMW proteins derived from a variety of plant and animal sources known to cause OA. IgE-mediated immune responses have also been identified as the underlying mechanism for several LMW chemical

TABLE 24.3

Key Elements of the Occupational History in the Evaluation of OA

I. Demographic Information

A. Identification and address

B. Personal data including sex, race, and age

C. Educational background with quantitation of the number of school years completed

II. Employment History

A. Current department and job description including dates begun, interrupted, and ended

B. List all other work processes and substances used in the employee's work environment. A schematic diagram of the workplace is helpful to identify indirect exposure to substances emanating from adjacent work stations

C. List prior jobs at current workplace with description of job, duration, and identification of material used

D. Work history describing employment preceding current workplace. Job descriptions and exposure history must be included

III. Symptoms

A. Categories:

1. Chest tightness, wheezing, cough, shortness of breath

2. Nasal rhinorrhea, sneezing, lacrimation, ocular itching

3. Systemic symptoms such as fever, arthralgias, and myalgias

B. Duration should be quantitated

C. Duration of employment at current job prior to onset of symptoms

D. Identify temporal pattern of symptoms in relationship to work

1. Immediate onset beginning at work with resolution soon after coming home

2. Delayed onset beginning 4–12 h after starting work or after coming home

3. Immediate onset followed by recovery with symptoms recurring 4–12 h after initial exposure to suspect agent at work

E. Improvement away from work

IV. Identify Potential Risk Factors

A. Obtain a smoking history along with current smoking status and quantitate number of pack years

B. Asthmatic symptoms preceding current work exposure

C. Atopic status

1. Identify consistent history of seasonal nasal or ocular symptoms

2. Family history of atopic disease

3. Confirmation by epicutaneous testing to a panel of common aeroallergens

D. History of accidental exposures to substances such as heated fumes or chemical spills

Source: Tarlo, S.M., Balmes, J., Balkissoon, R., Beach, J., Beckett, W., Bernstein, D. et al., *Chest.*, 134, 1S–41S, 2008.

agents, such as acid anhydrides and platinum salts. Although type II cytotoxic, type III immune-complex, and type IV cell-mediated immune responses have been linked to certain causes of OA, measures of specific IgE are usually the simplest and most readily available tests for diagnosing OA.[40]

HMW antigens are considered complete allergens because they do not require structural modification to elicit a specific immune response. *In vivo* skin testing and *in vitro* immunoassays have been used to identify sensitized individuals to these specific allergens. Examples of HMW allergens include proteins from animal dander, insect scales, food products, and enzymes used in the food manufacturing and pharmaceutical industries. LMW chemical agents in most instances require structural modification to act as complete antigens. Exceptions to this rule are platinum salts and sulfonechloramide. To investigate specific immune responses

of these chemicals, typically they are coupled to a carrier molecule such as an autologous human protein (e.g., human serum albumin [HSA]). The chemical hapten protein conjugate forms new antigenic determinants, which are capable of inducing an IgE-mediated response.[40]

Skin test or *in vitro* reagents used in the diagnosis of OA must be characterized and standardized as well as possible. Standardization should include identification of the allergen source, the extraction procedure, and its biochemical composition. Proper characterization should include total protein content, molecular weight range of proteins, isoelectric points of each protein, and identification of immunologic and allergenic components. The latter can be determined by a variety of techniques, such as enzyme-linked immunoabsorbent assay (ELISA), Western blotting, leukocyte histamine release assays, and endpoint skin test titration techniques.[40]

A limitation of skin or serologic testing to HMW and LMW agents is the lack of standardized skin test reagents and immunoassays. Studies comparing IgE serum-specific assays with skin prick testing have found fairly good correlations for some LMW agents like TMA.[44] Similarly, specific IgE assays and skin test reagents for natural rubber latex and cat and dog allergens have been found to have high positive and negative predictive values for occupational sensitization.[40]

Measurement of specific IgG antibodies by ELISA is often performed as part of immunosurveillance programs in industries where workers are exposed to agents known to cause OA. The significance of elevated specific IgG antibodies to a workplace allergen is less clear but for some agents such as isocyanates and acid anhydrides there is evidence to suggest it could represent a biologic marker of exposure.[44,45]

The proper interpretation of an immunologic test used in the diagnosis of OA requires validation against an accepted benchmark, such as the specific bronchoprovocation test (SBPT). In addition, proper standardization of an immunoassay always requires the use of well-established positive and negative control sera.[40] Other *in vitro* assays that have been proposed as biomarkers for OA include monocyte chemoattractant protein-1 (MCP-1), lymphocyte proliferation, and leukocyte histamine release, which have been used primarily as research tools in the investigation of workers with OA induced by various agents.[40,46] Skin test responses and *in vitro* specific antibody responses may decline within months or years after removal from exposure to the causative agent, which may limit their clinical utility in the evaluation of workers remotely exposed to an incriminated agent. Table 24.4 summarizes a representative number of HMW and LMW causes of OA and immunologic tests used for diagnosis.[13,40]

PHYSIOLOGIC ASSESSMENT

Many approaches have been used in measuring lung function in workers suspected of OA. It is recommended that lung function be monitored in the workplace during a known exposure to a suspected causative agent. However, this is not always logistically possible. Personnel experienced in proper performance of pulmonary function testing may not be readily available to conduct serial testing of lung function and employers may not be cooperative. Spirometry should include the forced expiratory volume in 1 s (FEV$_1$), forced vital capacity (FVC), and the maximum mid-expiratory flow rate (FEF25–75).[40] Assessment of cross-shift lung function (i.e., pre- and post-shift FEV$_1$) has been used to correlate asthma symptoms to workplace exposure, but this approach lacks sensitivity for confirming OA.[40] Multiple assessments of PEF at work (4–5 times per day) often capture enough data to diagnose or exclude OA.[40] Furthermore, cross-shift changes in a worker's lung function have been found to be directly proportional to their level of exposure to the sensitizing agent. Serial measurements of PEF, when performed properly, correlate moderately well with results of the SBPT used in the diagnosis of OA.[40] Serial PEF measurements

should be interpreted with caution due to patient noncompliance and the potential for falsification of measurements. Using computerized peak flow meters that record effort associated with each measurement, reproducibility, and the exact time of the reading may circumvent these problems.[40] Although not diagnostic, nonspecific bronchial hyperresponsiveness (NSBH) testing with agonists such as methacholine, histamine, and mannitol is essential for confirming the presence or absence of AHR, a central feature of asthma. Subjects with a positive methacholine test and evidence of specific IgE to a HMW are more likely to exhibit a positive SBPT to that agent. Negative tests of NSBH are most useful in excluding a current diagnosis of OA in a currently symptomatic exposed worker.[40]

The SBPT is considered the gold standard for diagnosis of OA. This test should only be administered in specially equipped centers under the supervision of physicians experienced in conducting this procedure.[40] Specific provocation testing is very time consuming and expensive to perform and therefore not readily available. However, if performed properly, the SBPT can be performed with minimal risk. Several airway response patterns may be elicited that are characteristic for workers presenting with OA.[40] An isolated EAR is characterized by the immediate onset of asthma symptoms after exposure to an agent that is more commonly associated with IgE-mediated OA. An isolated LAR, which occurs until 4–12 h after exposure to the challenge agent, is more characteristic of nonimmunologic OA induced by LMW chemical agents.[40] Finally, workers with OA may exhibit a DAR characterized by an EAR followed by a recovery period and then an LAR. Multiple physiologic patterns have been observed in OA caused by chemicals. For example, workers with diisocyanate-induced OA present 30%–50% of the time with DARs, 40% of the time with an isolated LAR, and <10% of the time with an isolated EAR.[24,40]

Asthma occurring in the workplace in the absence of a latency period is characteristic of RADS, also referred to as irritant-induced OA.[4] RADS typically occurs after one or more repetitive large inhalational exposure to a toxic chemical agent such as ammonia gas, acidic fumes, smoke, or spray paints.[4] RADS must be differentiated from the irritant symptoms that occur in patients with preexisting asthma. Irritant symptoms disappear promptly after cessation of exposure and are not associated with prolonged bronchoconstriction or bronchial hyperresponsiveness characteristic of RADS.[4] Workers with RADS typically do not manifest airway response patterns seen with OA induced by HMW and LMW agents.

CLINICAL ASSESSMENT OF A PATIENT WITH OCCUPATIONAL ASTHMA

As in the case summary presented in this chapter, the first step for assessing a suspected case of OA is to obtain a careful physician-administered history.[40,42] This can be greatly enhanced by using a validated occupational questionnaire to capture the necessary clinical and exposure information

TABLE 24.4

Etiologic Agents of HMW and LMW OA and Reported Immunologic Tests

Agent	In Vivo	In Vitro
Azodicarbonamide	Prick tests with 0.1%, 1%, and 5% azodicarbonamide	Not done
Baby's breath	Intradermal titration testing	RAST/histamine release
Bacillus subtilis enzymes	Prick tests with 0.05, 0.5, 5, and 10 mg/mL	RAST/radial immunodiffusion
Buckwheat flour	Prick test with 10 mg/mL	Reverse enzyme immunoassay/histamine release
Carmine dye	Skin test with Coccus cactus	RAST to dyes
Castor bean	Prick test with 1:100 extract	Not done
Chloramine-T, halazone	Scratch test at 10^{-5} dilution	Not done
Chromate	Prick test at 10, 5, 1, and 0.1 mg/mL $Cr_2(SO_4)_3$	RAST to HSA-chromium sulfate
Cobalt	Patch tests	RAST to HSA-cobalt sulfate
Coffee bean	Intradermal titration to coffee bean extract	RAST to coffee bean extract
Diazonium tetrafluoroborate (DTFB)	Not done	RAST to HSA-DTFB
Dimethylethanolamine	Prick tests to dimethylethanolamine undiluted at 1:10, 1:100, and 1:1000	Not done
Douglas fir tussock moth	Cutaneous tests with 1:25 extract	Histamine release
Dyes, textiles	Prick or scratch tests to dyes at 10 mg/mL in 50% glycerine	HSA-dye
Egg proteins	Prick tests with 1:10 w/v egg white, egg yolk, whole egg; prick tests to 10 mg/ml egg white fractions	RAST to egg proteins
Ethylenediamine	Intracutaneous test to 1:100 ethylenediamine	Not done
Furan binder	Not done	RAST to catalyst, sand, and furfuryl alcohol
Garlic	Prick test titrations beginning at 10^{-5} garlic extract	PTRIA for IgE against garlic extract
Grain dust, grain dust mite	Prick and intracutaneous tests with grain dust and grain mite	Not done
Grain weevil	Skin test to weevil extract	Not done
Gum acacia	Skin tests with gum arabic	Not done
Guar gum	Prick tests with 1 mg/mL guar gum	RAST with guar gum
Hexamethylene-diisocyanate (HDI)	Prick tests to HSA-HDI	ELISA to HSA-HDI
Hexahydrophthalic anhydride (HHPA)	Not done	RAST to HSA-HHPA
Hog trypsin	Skin test to trypsin	Histamine release
Laboratory animals	Skin tests with serum and urine extracts from animals	ELISA
Latex	Prick test using low ammonia latex solution	Not done
Locusts	Prick tests with locust extract at 0.1, 1, and 10 mg/mL	ELISA
Mealworm	Prick test titration beginning at 1:20 w/v *Tenebrio molitor* (TM) extract	RAST to TM extract
Diphenol methane diisocyanate (MDI)	Prick test with 5 mg/mL HSA-MDI; intradermal test with 1 and 10 μg/mL	ELISA to HSA-MDI
Mushroom	Prick test with mushroom extract	Not done
Nickel	Prick tests with $NiSO_4$ at 100, 10, 5, 1, and 0.1 mg/mL	RAST to HSA-$NiSO_4$
Papain	Skin test with papain at 1.25–20 mg/mL	RAST to papain
Pancreatic extract	Prick tests with 1:100 and 1:1000 extracts	Not done
Penicillin	Prick tests to ampicillin at 10^{-3}–10^{-2} mol/L, benzyl penicilloyl polylysine at 10^{-6} mol/L, and minor determinants at 10^{-2} mol/L	Not done
Penicillamine	Prick tests with penicillamine, major and minor penicillin determinants at 0.01, 0.1, and 1 mg/ml	Not done
Phthalic anhydride (PA) and tetrachlorophthalic anhydride (TCPA)	Prick and intradermal tests to HSA-PA and HSA-TCPA	ELISA; PTRIA to HSA-PA only
Platinum	Prick tests with complex platinum salts from 10^{-3} to 10^{-11} g/mL	RAST to $(NH_4)_2PtCl_2$, RAST to HSA-platinum and histamine release
Poultry mites	Skin tests with 1:10 w/v Northern fowl mite (NFM)	RAST to NFM
Protease bromelain	Prick test with bromelain at 10 mg/mL	RAST to bromelain
Redwood	Prick test to redwood sawdust extract	Not done
Spiramycin	Prick tests with 10 and 100 mg/mL spiramycin	Not done
Tobacco	Skin tests with green tobacco extract 10 mg/mL	RAST with green tobacco extract
Toluene diisocyanate (TDI)	Prick test to 5 mg/mL HSA-TDI	RAST and ELISA to HSA-TDI, histamine release
Trimellitic anhydride (TMA)	Prick tests to 3.4 mg/mL HSA-TMA and TMA in acetone	PTRIA with HSA-TMA
Western red cedar (WRC)	Prick tests with 25 mg/mL WRC extract; intracutaneous testing with 2.5 mg/mL WRC	Not done
Wheat flour	Prick tests with 10% w/v extract	RAST to wheat flour and wheat flour components

Source: Quirce, S., Bernstein, J.A., *Immunol. Allergy Clin. North Am.*, 31, 677–698, 2011.

and to help validate information obtained by the physician-administered history.[40] Workers with OA may present with dyspnea, chest tightness, wheezing, and cough in or out of the workplace. Upper airway symptoms such as rhinorrhea, nasal congestion, and ocular pruritus preceding the onset of asthmatic symptoms are especially characteristic of IgE-mediated sensitization to HMW agents.[47] Symptoms may begin after immediately starting a work shift (within 1–2 h) or several hours after starting work. Review of MSDSs is often very helpful for identifying agents known to cause OA.[43] If the history is positive for OA, a test of NSBH (i.e., methacholine or histamine provocation) should be performed. A negative methacholine test (PC20 >10 mg/mL) excludes AHR and is a good negative predictor for asthma. A positive methacholine test indicates the presence of AHR suggestive of asthma but is nonspecific and does not confirm a diagnosis of OA. In this case, assessment of lung function performed at and away from the workplace to demonstrate AHR around the suspected agent is very useful for supporting a diagnosis of OA.[42] When possible, a workplace challenge, which consists of supervised measurements of lung function (i.e., FEV_1) in the actual work site before and during work shifts for at least 1 week of work exposure, should be conducted. Improvement of symptoms and lung function after removal from the workplace with subsequent deterioration after reintroduction into the workplace further supports a diagnosis of OA, except in the case of RADS.[42] If a workplace challenge cannot be performed, PEF monitoring should be conducted over 2–3 weeks at work.[42] The worker should measure and record his or her PEF every 2 h at work and every 3–4 h while awake at home or at least four times a day. Work exposure, symptoms, and medication usage should be recorded in a diary during this time. Diurnal variability of >20% at work as compared with normal variability at home is consistent with OA.[40,42] The gold standard for the diagnosis of OA is the SBPT.[40,42] If a specific substance in the workplace is suspected of causing OA and the workplace challenge is equivocal, a SBPT may be necessary.[40,42] The PC20 ascertained by methacholine or histamine testing may be helpful for estimating the initial dose of an occupational agent prior to the specific inhalation challenge test. An SBPT should not be performed in workers with severe cardiac or pulmonary disease (FEV_1 <60%).[40,42] Specific inhalation challenge tests have also been used to document causation of OA by new substances in index cases and for medical/legal purposes in proving or excluding a worker's eligibility for workers' compensation. Although specific challenge tests confirm a diagnosis of OA if positive, negative tests do not always exclude the diagnosis in workers who have been removed from the workplace for a period of time, during which bronchial AHR to the suspected agent may have resolved. It is therefore important to perform a SBPT either before or shortly after removing the worker from his or her workplace. Other potential problems with specific inhalation challenge testing are poor standardization of methods used among different centers and inability to reproduce workplace exposure conditions in the laboratory including temperature, atmospheric pressure, and concentration.[40,42] As with any specific inhalation challenge, false positive and false negative tests can occur and therefore results must be interpreted with caution.[42] In addition to lung function assessment, it is important to identify the worker's allergic status by skin testing to common seasonal and perennial aeroallergens, especially for workers exposed to HMW agents. Skin prick testing to the suspected causative agent and/or specific IgE *in vitro* assays can also be performed when appropriate.[40,42]

TREATMENT

Once the diagnosis of OA has been confirmed, the treatment of choice is to remove the worker from further exposure.[42] Studies evaluating the clinical course of workers after removal from the workplace have found that persistence of their asthma was correlated with the duration of exposure and symptoms prior to diagnosis. Individuals with OA caused by diisocyanates or western red cedar wood dust had a better prognosis if they were diagnosed early, had relatively well-preserved lung function, and less AHR compared with symptomatic workers who remained in the workplace for longer periods of time and had greater deterioration of lung function, leading to chronic persistent asthma requiring increased medication use even after being removed from exposure. Use of respirators and other personal protective equipment (PPE) should be enforced for workers exposed to known causes of OA such as enzymes, isocyanates, and acid anhydrides. However, once OA has been established, use of PPE does not always prevent or reduce exposure or prevent clinical deterioration.[48] Some studies have suggested that certain types of respirators such as airstream helmets may offer adequate protection for the worker from the offending agent; however, they are generally not considered adequate substitutes for absolute avoidance measures.[49] Pharmacologic treatment of acute or chronic OA is similar to that of non-OA, which involves inhaled corticosteroids, with or without long acting beta$_2$-adrenergic agonists, leukotriene-modifying agents, xanthine oxidase inhibitors like theophylline, and, for severe asthma exacerbations, oral corticosteroids.[48,49] Medications can be used in various combinations depending on the severity of the worker's symptoms. Immunotherapy may play a role in the treatment of some forms of OA caused by HMW protein allergens such as laboratory animal proteins.[49]

PREVENTION AND IMMUNOSURVEILLANCE

The primary categories of prevention include reducing exposure to known occupational inciting agents, identifying susceptible workers and removing them from exposure, and administering workplace controls to reduce the number of workers exposed and the duration of their exposure.

It is important to educate at-risk atopic individuals about avoidance of occupations where the likelihood for developing OA is increased (e.g., laboratory handlers).[40,42,48,49] Effective prevention of OA requires cooperation between management and workers in the implementation of good industrial measures aimed at preventing exposure to agents known to cause OA. Every attempt should be made to minimize a worker's exposure to potentially problematic agent(s) through the institution of strict handling procedures. Workers should be continually educated about the importance of adhering to those procedures to avoid inadvertent exposures such as chemical spills.[40,42,48,49] Prescreening of already hired workers for atopy should be considered before assigning employees to jobs where they would have inhalational exposure to sensitizing proteins (e.g., latex, laboratory animals, and enzyme proteins). Comprehensive immuno-surveillance programs for detecting and monitoring workers at increased risk for exposure to known inducers of OA have been successfully implemented in industries that utilize enzymes and acid anhydrides in their manufacturing processes.[40]

REFERENCES

1. Bernstein IL, Chan-Yeung M, Malo J-L, Bernstein DI, (eds). *Asthma in the Workplace*, 3rd edn. New York: Taylor & Francis, 2006.
2. Bernstein DI. Allergic reactions to workplace allergens. *JAMA*. 1997;278(22):1907–1913.
3. Malo JL, Vandenplas O. Definitions and classification of work-related asthma. *Immunol Allergy Clin North Am*. 2011;31(4):645–662.
4. Brooks SM, Bernstein IL. Irritant-induced airway disorders. *Immunol Allergy Clin North Am*. 2011;31(4):747–768.
5. Szema AM. Work-exacerbated asthma. *Clin Chest Med*. 2012;33(4):617–624.
6. Smith AM. The epidemiology of work-related asthma. *Immunol Allergy Clin North Am*. 2011;31(4):663–675.
7. Reilly MJ, Rosenman KD, Watt FC, Schill D, Stanbury M, Trimbath LS, et al. Surveillance for occupational asthma: Michigan and New Jersey, 1988–1992. *MMWR CDC Surveill Summ*. 1994;43(1):9–17.
8. Oksa P. [Occupational asthma in Finland]. *Duodecim; laaketieteellinen aikakauskirja*. 2011;127(20):2225–2230.
9. To T, Tarlo SM, McLimont S, Haines T, Holness DL, Lougheed MD, et al. Feasibility of a provincial voluntary reporting system for work-related asthma in Ontario. *Can Respir J*. 2011;18(5):275–277.
10. Latza U, Baur X. Occupational obstructive airway diseases in Germany: Frequency and causes in an international comparison. *Am J Ind Med*. 2005;48(2):144–152.
11. Popin E, Kopferschmitt-Kubler MC, Gonzalez M, Brom M, Flesch F, Pauli G. [The incidence of occupational asthma in Alsace from 2001 to 2002. Results of intensification of the ONAP project in Alsace (2001–2002). Regional specificities]. *Rev Mal Respir*. 2008;25(7):806–813.
12. Bonneterre V, Faisandier L, Bicout D, Bernardet C, Piollat J, Ameille J, et al. Programmed health surveillance and detection of emerging diseases in occupational health: Contribution of the French national occupational disease surveillance and prevention network (RNV3P). *Occup Environ Med*. 2010;67(3):178–186.
13. Quirce S, Bernstein JA. Old and new causes of occupational asthma. *Immunol Allergy Clin North Am*. 2011;31(4):677–698.
14. Bush RK, Stave GM. Laboratory animal allergy: An update. *ILAR J/Natl Res Counc Inst Lab Anim Resour*. 2003;44(1):28–51.
15. Bakerly ND, Moore VC, Vellore AD, Jaakkola MS, Robertson AS, Burge PS. Fifteen-year trends in occupational asthma: Data from the Shield surveillance scheme. *Occup Med*. 2008;58(3):169–174.
16. Hur GY, Koh DH, Kim HA, Park HJ, Ye YM, Kim KS, et al. Prevalence of work-related symptoms and serum-specific antibodies to wheat flour in exposed workers in the bakery industry. *Respir Med*. 2008;102(4):548–555.
17. Le Moual N, Kauffmann F, Eisen EA, Kennedy SM. The healthy worker effect in asthma: Work may cause asthma, but asthma may also influence work. *Am J Respir Crit Care Med*. 2008;177(1):4–10.
18. Meyer JD, Holt DL, Chen Y, Cherry NM, McDonald JC. SWORD '99: Surveillance of work-related and occupational respiratory disease in the UK. *Occup Med*. 2001;51(3):204–208.
19. Lummus ZL, Wisnewski AV, Bernstein DI. Pathogenesis and disease mechanisms of occupational asthma. *Immunol Allergy Clin North Am*. 2011;31(4):699–716.
20. Gautrin D, Boulet LP, Boutet M, Dugas M, Bherer L, L'Archeveque J, et al. Is reactive airways dysfunction syndrome a variant of occupational asthma? *J Allergy Clin Immunol*. 1994;93(1 Pt 1):12–22.
21. Quirce S. Eosinophilic bronchitis in the workplace. *Curr Opin Allergy Clin Immunol*. 2004;4(2):87–91.
22. Lemiere C, Romeo P, Chaboillez S, Tremblay C, Malo JL. Airway inflammation and functional changes after exposure to different concentrations of isocyanates. *J Allergy Clin Immunol*. 2002;110(4):641–646.
23. Douwes J, Gibson P, Pekkanen J, Pearce N. Non-eosinophilic asthma: Importance and possible mechanisms. *Thorax*. 2002;57(7):643–648.
24. Bernstein JA. Overview of diisocyanate occupational asthma. *Toxicology*. 1996;111(1–3):181–189.
25. Zeiss CR, Mitchell JH, Van Peenen PF, Kavich D, Collins MJ, Grammer L, et al. A clinical and immunologic study of employees in a facility manufacturing trimellitic anhydride. *Allergy Proc*. 1992;13(4):193–198.
26. Zeiss CR, Patterson R, Pruzansky JJ, Miller MM, Rosenberg M, Levitz D. Trimellitic anhydride-induced airway syndromes: Clinical and immunologic studies. *J Allergy Clin Immunol*. 1977;60(2):96–103.
27. Ban M, Langonne I, Goutet M, Huguet N, Pepin E. Simultaneous analysis of the local and systemic immune responses in mice to study the occupational asthma mechanisms induced by chromium and platinum. *Toxicology*. 2010;277(1–3):29–37.
28. Regal JF. Immunologic effector mechanisms in animal models of occupational asthma. *J Immunot*. 2004;1(1):25–37.
29. Ward MD, Selgrade MK. Animal models for protein respiratory sensitizers. *Methods*. 2007;41(1):80–90.
30. Taylor AN. Role of human leukocyte antigen phenotype and exposure in development of occupational asthma. *Curr Opin Allergy Clin Immunol*. 2001;1(2):157–161.
31. Mapp CE, Beghe B, Balboni A, Zamorani G, Padoan M, Jovine L, et al. Association between HLA genes and susceptibility to toluene diisocyanate-induced asthma. *Clin Exp Allergy*. 2000;30(5):651–656.
32. Jones MG, Nielsen J, Welch J, Harris J, Welinder H, Bensryd I, et al. Association of HLA-DQ5 and HLA-DR1 with sensitization to organic acid anhydrides. *Clin Exp Allergy*. 2004;34(5):812–816.
33. Jeal H, Draper A, Jones M, Harris J, Welsh K, Taylor AN, et al. HLA associations with occupational sensitization to rat lipocalin allergens: A model for other animal allergies? *J Allergy Clin Immunol*. 2003;111(4):795–799.

34. Mapp CE, Fryer AA, De Marzo N, Pozzato V, Padoan M, Boschetto P, et al. Glutathione S-transferase GSTP1 is a susceptibility gene for occupational asthma induced by isocyanates. *J Allergy Clin Immunol*. 2002;109(5):867–872.

35. Yucesay B, Johnson V, Lummus ZL, Kissling GE, Fluharty K, Gautrin D, et al. Genetic variants in anti-oxidant genes are associated with diisocyanate-induced asthma. *Toxicol Sci*. 2012;129:166–173.

36. Bernstein DI, Kashon M, Lummus ZL, Johnson VJ, Fluharty K, Gautrin D, et al. CTNNA3 (α-catenin) gene variants are associated with diisocyanate asthma: A replication study in a Caucasian worker population. *Toxicol Sci*. 2013;131:242–246.

37. Wikman H, Piirila P, Rosenberg C, Luukkonen R, Kaaria K, Nordman H, et al. N-Acetyltransferase genotypes as modifiers of diisocyanate exposure-associated asthma risk. *Pharmacogenetics*. 2002;12(3):227–233.

38. Bernstein DI. Genetics of occupational asthma. *Curr Opin Allergy Clin Immunol*. 2011;11(2):86–89.

39. Bernstein DI, Wang N, Campo P, Chakraborty R, Smith A, Cartier A, et al. Diisocyanate asthma and gene-environment interactions with IL4RA, CD-14, and IL-13 genes. *Ann Allergy Asthma Immunol*. 2006;97(6):800–806.

40. Tarlo SM, Balmes J, Balkissoon R, Beach J, Beckett W, Bernstein D, et al. Diagnosis and management of work-related asthma: American College of Chest Physicians Consensus Statement. *Chest*. 2008;134(Suppl 3):1S–41S.

41. Nicholson PJ, Cullinan P, Burge S; British Occupational Health Research Foundation. Concise guidance: Diagnosis, management and prevention of occupational asthma. *Clin Med*. 2012;12(2):156–159.

42. Tarlo SM, Liss GM, Blanc PD. How to diagnose and treat work-related asthma: Key messages for clinical practice from the American college of chest physicians consensus statement. *Polskie Archiwum Medycyny Wewnetrznej*. 2009;119(10):660–666.

43. Bernstein JA. Material safety data sheets: Are they reliable in identifying human hazards? *J Allergy Clin Immunol*. 2002;110(1):35–38.

44. Bernstein JA, Ghosh D, Sublett WJ, Wells H, Levin L. Is trimellitic anhydride skin testing a sufficient screening tool for selectively identifying TMA-exposed workers with TMA-specific serum IgE antibodies? *J Occup Environ Med/Am Coll Occup Environ Med*. 2011;53(10):1122–1127.

45. Pronk A, Preller L, Raulf-Heimsoth M, Jonkers IC, Lammers JW, Wouters IM, et al. Respiratory symptoms, sensitization, and exposure response relationships in spray painters exposed to isocyanates. *Am J Respir Crit Care Med*. 2007;176(11):1090–1097.

46. Lummus ZL, Alam R, Bernstein JA, Bernstein DI. Diisocyanate antigen-enhanced production of monocyte chemoattractant protein-1, IL-8, and tumor necrosis factor-alpha by peripheral mononuclear cells of workers with occupational asthma. *J Allergy Clin Immunol*. 1998;102(2):265–274.

47. Sublett JW, Bernstein DI. Occupational rhinitis. *Immunol Allergy Clin North Am*. 2011;31(4):787–796.

48. Fishwick D, Barber CM, Bradshaw LM, Ayres JG, Barraclough R, Burge S, et al. Standards of care for occupational asthma: An update. *Thorax*. 2012;67(3):278–280.

49. Peden DB, Bush RK. Advances in environmental and occupational respiratory disease in 2010. *J Allergy Clin Immunol*. 2011;127(3):696–700.

25 Asthma in Pregnancy

Paul A. Greenberger

CONTENTS

CASE PRESENTATION

A 36-year-old woman (G 6, P4, A 1) with persistent moderate asthma, chronic rhinosinusitis with nasal polyps, allergic rhinitis (receiving allergen immunotherapy for over a year with dust mites, molds, and ragweed), and gastroesophageal reflux (GERD) presents for a routine follow-up visit and reports that she is 14 weeks pregnant. Her asthma is controlled. She is asymptomatic; albuterol rescue occurred just twice in the last 4 weeks and she has no nocturnal respiratory symptoms. She has pressure in her face over the maxillary sinuses and uses daily lansoprazole 30 mg to suppress heartburn. Her other medications include fluticasone/salmeterol (250/50 one inhalation twice a day), budesonide nasal spray (two each nostril), and cetirizine–pseudoephedrine (about 4 days/week). Previous pregnancies have aggravated her asthma, and she required short courses of prednisone to reestablish control. She experienced one stillbirth with a coiled umbilical cord resulting in fetal loss. She is not experiencing any systemic reactions to allergen immunotherapy and has received injections for 18 months. She avoids nonselective NSAIDS because of experiencing acute severe dyspnea after ingesting naproxen 400 mg.

INTRODUCTION

When a 36-year-old woman with asthma presents for an office visit and either reports that she is 14 weeks pregnant or is thinking of trying to become pregnant, she often will ask questions regarding (1) the potential severity of her asthma during pregnancy, (2) the safety of or actual indication for pharmacotherapy, (3) the possibility of preventing asthma in her baby by

a specific diet during gestation or during breast-feeding, and if the baby is born in fall or winter, and (4) whether she should receive influenza immunization. If she is receiving allergen immunotherapy, she will inquire (5) whether the injections should be discontinued and (6) whether the "shots" will prevent asthma or allergies in her baby.

Inadequately controlled asthma has been associated with many adverse outcomes including preterm births, small for gestational age infants, intrauterine growth restriction, low-birth-weight (term) infants, miscarriage, fetal demise, perinatal deaths, hypoxia-related or ischemic damage to the fetus resulting in cerebral palsy, and even congenital malformations.[1–10] The mother may develop preeclampsia or gestational diabetes and be more likely to require a cesarean delivery. Uncontrolled asthma can result in nocturnal asthma, unscheduled office visits, emergency department treatment and hospitalizations, and even fatalities in the mother. Alternatively, expert consensus reports (National Heart, Lung, and Blood Institute: National Asthma Education and Prevention Program [NAEPP] Expert Panel report 3 from 2004[11] and full report from 2007[12]), American College of Obstetrics and Gynecology guidelines,[13] the Global Initiative for Asthma (GINA),[14] and various studies and reviews[1,8,15–17] provide evidence and guidance for favorable outcomes and normal or near-normal babies with a basis for pharmacotherapy that is similar to that recommended for nonpregnant patients. For example, as in Steps 2 or 3 of the NAEPP report[12] of the National Heart, Lung, and Blood Institute of the United States or GINA,[14] inhaled corticosteroids (ICSs) are first-line therapy for persistent asthma. The short-acting beta₂-adrenergic agonist (SABA) albuterol (salbutamol) is recommended for women with intermittent or persistent asthma who require rescue therapy. Perhaps, most importantly, using medications for prevention of serious exacerbations of asthma and ongoing inadequately controlled asthma are advocated as compared with minimizing pharmacotherapy.

PHYSIOLOGY DURING PREGNANCY AND EFFECTS OF AN ACUTE EXACERBATION OF ASTHMA

Pregnancy is associated with alterations in maternal physiology that are impacted by inadequate control of asthma. When there is poorly controlled or uncontrolled asthma that results in maternal hypoxemia or hypoxia, the fetus also can be stressed when the low-oxygen intrauterine environment becomes compromised. Oxygen delivery to the fetus is dependent on maternal cardiac output to generate adequate blood flow to the uterus, an effectively functioning placenta, and sufficient maternal arterial oxygen content.[18] Because of the increase in heart rate and stroke volume and decreased vascular resistance, maternal cardiac output increases some 25% over prepregnant levels by 6 weeks of gestation and increases by 30%–60% as pregnancy progresses.[19,20] These changes result in greater preload and less afterload. The uterine blood flow increases as much as eightfold from about 50 mL/min to 400 mL/min by 20 weeks and remains at that level to term.[21] A pregnant woman's blood volume expands by 1200–1600 mL,[20] and total body water increases by approximately 5 L.[22] There is an increase of red cell mass by 17%–40% without any change in red cell life.[20] The expansion of plasma volume is greater than the increase in red cell mass, which results in the "physiologic anemia of pregnancy." The maternal hemoglobin concentration may be 11–12 g/dL. However, the increase in red cell mass helps in delivery of oxygen to the fetus.

The fetus grows in a low oxygen tension environment. The fetal hemoglobin oxygen dissociation curve is shifted to the left, meaning that it is steeper when compared with that of a nonpregnant, adult woman. The fetal hemoglobin concentration is 16.5 g/L, and fetal hemoglobin is 50% saturated at a pO_2 of 22 mmHg compared with 26–28 mm/Hg for maternal hemoglobin. Any major reduction in maternal arterial oxygen tension has the potential for immediate harm (potentially within a few minutes). Alternatively, when there are increases in the maternal arterial oxygen tension, the leftward shift of the fetal hemoglobin oxygen dissociation curve results in sharper increases in fetal oxygen saturation than in the mother's arterial blood. There is an expected respiratory alkalosis during pregnancy resulting in a shift of the maternal hemoglobin oxygen dissociation curve to the left, which does not favor unloading of oxygen from hemoglobin at the time of need. When the pregnant woman experiences an exacerbation of asthma resulting in hyperventilation, the maternal respiratory alkalosis could worsen the oxygen delivery to the fetus combined with ventilation–perfusion abnormalities that reduce the maternal oxygen tension. Thus, during the acute exacerbation of asthma producing hyperventilation (and reduced venous return) with the expected respiratory alkalosis in

pregnancy, maternal oxygen tension can decrease, and there is a shift in the maternal hemoglobin oxygen dissociation curve to the left. When the pregnant woman inspires higher concentrations of oxygen, the increase in her arterial oxygen tension can be expected (in most cases depending on severity of attack and any concurrent conditions such as pneumonia), but the increase in oxygen tension in the uterine veins is modest, consistent with a large maternal-uterine shunt. Should the acute exacerbation of asthma result in "normal" range pCO_2 and pH, this stage of asthma is especially dangerous for the mother as she could be developing acute respiratory acidosis with a continued rise in pCO_2. Intubation and controlled ventilation may be indicated as a life-saving measure. There is the possibility of stillbirth or fetal demise.

LESSONS LEARNED FROM PREGNANCIES OCCURRING AT HIGH ALTITUDES

Women living at high altitudes in Colorado (>8000 ft, 2500 m) deliver lighter-weight babies; they are reported to be 121 g lighter for 1000 m of elevation. This is thought to be related to slower fetal growth and not a shortened period of gestation.[23,24] When women were studied in La Paz (elevation 11,880 ft, 3600 m) and El Alto, Bolivia (elevation 14,470 ft, 4082 m), comparisons were made between Andean women who were born and reared at high altitudes and European women who had lived in the mountains for an average of 4 years.[24] During pregnancy, there were increases in resting ventilation and arterial oxygen saturation (from 91% to 94%), helping to offset the reduction in hemoglobin concentration of pregnancy. In comparison, although pregnant women living at sea level also increase their resting ventilation during pregnancy and PaO$_2$, there is no significant increase in maternal oxygen saturation as the PaO$_2$ is already close to maximal tension. Indeed, some pregnant women at sea level have resting PaO$_2$ > 100 mmHg.[25] The maternal arterial oxygen content can decrease at sea level because of the physiologic anemia of pregnancy. In contrast, at high altitudes, the increase in oxygen saturation is thought to maintain and protect the maternal arterial oxygen content, and this occurred in women of both Andean and European backgrounds. The uteroplacental circulation of Andean women appears to have adapted over time to achieve higher flow rates and for various reasons Andean women delivered babies on average 209 g heavier than babies born to European women.[24] If a woman living at sea level has significant hypoxemia from poorly controlled asthma, the compensatory mechanisms may be insufficient to avoid hypoxic harm in the fetus. For example, this author has observed that repeated episodes of acute severe asthma during pregnancy have been associated with cerebral palsy emerging in 9-month-old infants.

CHANGES IN RESPIRATORY PARAMETERS

At baseline, the respiratory rate, vital capacity, and total lung capacity generally are unchanged.[18] The residual volume and functional residual capacity are reduced as the diaphragm is more cephalad and flattened. There is reduced intrathoracic pressure that could favor earlier airway closure during exacerbations of asthma in pregnancy. During acute smooth muscle contraction of the bronchi in asthma, the pregnant woman needs to generate increased intrathoracic pressure to apply radial traction on the bronchi as a compensatory process to support patency of the airways. Minute ventilation does increase as much as 50% by late pregnancy.[18] The increased concentrations of estrogen and especially progesterone favor the increased ventilation and respiratory alkalosis. At the same time, oxygen consumption increases. The carotid body becomes more sensitive to reductions in oxygen, and these respiratory changes occur well before significant enlargement of the uterus. Most studies have found no important changes in bronchial responsiveness to methacholine; in one study there was doubling of the PC20, but the changes were from 0.35 mg/mL at baseline to 0.72 mg/mL during pregnancy.[26]

"Dyspnea" of pregnancy is not from airway obstruction but rather from progesterone-induced hyperventilation causing increased tidal volume in the first and second trimesters.[27] In later pregnancy, "dyspnea" also can be from the enlarging uterus.[27]

DISCUSSION

The incidence of asthma during pregnancy ranges from 8.4% to 13.9%[7,11,13,16,28] and the trend has been increasing just as the prevalence of asthma in the general population has been increasing (now being 25 million in the United States or 8.3% of the population).[29] The questions raised focus on the impact that pregnancy has on the severity of asthma, the safety (and necessity) for pharmacotherapy, what dietary changes during pregnancy should be incorporated to prevent or reduce the likelihood of asthma developing in the baby (or over time), to what extent breast-feeding and/or allergen immunotherapy will prevent/delay asthma or allergic disorders such as eczema or allergic rhinitis, and whether influenza immunization is necessary.

Effect of Pregnancy on Course of Asthma

The patient presented has persistent asthma requiring combination therapy; thus, she is at risk of worsening asthma as compared with the "prototype" pregnant woman with persistent asthma who is managed with an ICS as controller therapy. From a case-control series where nurse-interviewers spoke with women at 12 and 18 weeks of gestation and by 6 months postpartum, who did not have pulmonary function data but did record medications, 53% of women reported no change in symptoms during the pregnancy.[16] This average ranged from 69% in "well-controlled" to 41% in "poorly controlled" patients.[16] Of the 47% of pregnant women who had changes in their symptoms, about half of this group (24.6%) improved and the other half (22.4%) reported worsening. It is useful to know that if a pregnant woman reported being "well

controlled," she was likely to remain so, because just 16.7% of "well-controlled" women reported improving. In the pregnant women who were "poorly controlled," some 34.9% reported improving.[16] A target for system-wide improvement is why this percent was not greater. The authors noted that 63.3% of pregnant women whose asthma was "poorly controlled" did not use a controller medication, implying failure to receive evidence-based recommended pharmacotherapy.[16] Worsening of asthma was divided evenly over the three trimesters, whereas in those pregnant women who reported improvement in their asthma this change occurred more likely in the first (11.8%) than in the second (8.3%) or third (4.5%) trimester.[16] Based on pregnancies occurring from 1998 to 2006 in Massachusetts, this study presents opportunities for improvement in care of pregnant women with asthma. In another prospective study, where pregnant women were enrolled by 24 weeks of gestation (mean 15 weeks) and in which they were interviewed by research assistants in person in their places of residence and then by phone at weeks 20, 28, and 36 weeks gestation and in the hospital postpartum, severity of asthma (intermittent, persistent mild, moderate, or severe) and medications were assessed according to the GINA guidelines.[30] More women had intermittent asthma (57.5%) than persistent mild asthma (20.1%) and persistent moderate or severe asthma (22.5%).[30] Women with persistent asthma (mild or moderate/severe) were more likely to develop severe asthma during pregnancy compared with women with intermittent asthma. When analyzing all three severity groups prospectively, there was "little evidence of a change in asthma severity over the course of pregnancy."[30] The authors then analyzed whether the women were receiving GINA-recommended medications according to the severity class. Importantly, for all three classes, the average GINA severity score was lower if the medications being used were in accordance with guidelines.[30]

The old adage that "asthma in pregnancy improves in one-third of women, is unchanged in one-third of women, and worsens in one-third of women" is not supported by evidence.[16,30–33] More severe asthma is more likely to remain severe or exacerbation prone during pregnancy.[9,10] Women with persistent mild, moderate, or severe asthma are not taking medications according to recommended evidence, in particular the use of ICSs.[2,30,31] Furthermore, quality of life is reduced in early pregnancy, which can be associated with subsequent exacerbations, independent of FEV_1.[34] Asthma is a complex condition and there is heterogeneity of responses to treatment.[35] Perhaps it is not surprising that many general practitioners reported a lack of confidence and knowledge in making decisions in pregnant women with asthma.[36]

Safety of Pharmacotherapy during Pregnancy

Although the term "appropriate" for use in pregnancy may be preferred to "safety," the benefits of current medications required to achieve effective control of asthma outweigh any potential risks.[1,8,11–14,17,18,32] The evidence supporting ICSs continues to grow.[9,37–39]

For rescue treatment, most of the data for SABAs are for albuterol (salbutamol) whereas for LABAs the safety data is based on salmeterol compared to formoterol.[40] Evidence supporting experience with the leukotriene D_4 receptor antagonist, montelukast, has been published.[41,42]

It has been speculated that oral corticosteroid administration for treatment of exacerbations of asthma may contribute to reduced birth weights (200 g) in infants.[43] Nevertheless, inadequately controlled asthma is associated with reduced birth weights. The woman presented in the case discussion has prednisone available at home to use as part of her action plan. Table 25.1 lists appropriate drug therapies during pregnancy.

RECOMMENDATIONS ABOUT DIET DURING PREGNANCY AND EFFECTS OF BREAST-FEEDING

Restrictive diets during pregnancy and lactation such as avoidance of any milk, egg, peanuts, and tree nuts are not recommended as such an approach does not have long-term preventive benefits up to the first 4 years of life.[44] Delaying introduction of solid foods for infants (including fish, eggs, and foods containing peanuts) beyond the normally advised 4–6 months of age also was not recommended as a preventive strategy. Therefore, pregnant women should be encouraged to breast-feed as long as they are able to, but restrictive diets during gestation or lactation will not provide the desired reductions of allergic diseases and asthma in their babies.

RECOMMENDATIONS ABOUT RECEIVING IMMUNIZATION WITH INFLUENZA VACCINE

Women should receive annual inactivated influenza immunization, and injections can be administered at any time during gestation.[45]

RECOMMENDATIONS REGARDING CONTINUING SUBCUTANEOUS ALLERGEN IMMUNOTHERAPY

Subcutaneous allergen immunotherapy can be continued during pregnancy[46] unless there are administrative problems that interfere with good care such as the woman not appearing as required for weekly or biweekly injections, not waiting 30 min for observation, or having anaphylaxis ("systemic" reactions). Typically, subcutaneous allergen immunotherapy is not initiated during pregnancy.[47] The Joint Task Force on Practice Parameters of the American Academy of Allergy Asthma and Immunology, the American College of Allergy Asthma and Immunology, and Joint Council of Allergy Asthma and Immunology did not recommends that the woman should remain at the current step of the schedule and injections should not be increased according to the schedule.[47] However, for some patients this approach may be too conservative and would delay pregnant women from reaching more therapeutic maintenance dosages. There are currently no data to suggest that allergen immunotherapy is more likely to induce anaphylaxis during

TABLE 25.1
Drug Therapies for Asthma and Its Comorbidities That Are Considered Appropriate for Administration during Pregnancy

Asthma
- Albuterol
- Levalbuterol
- Salmeterol[a]
- Formoterol[a]
- Budesonide
- Fluticasone
- Beclomethasone dipropionate
- Prednisone
- Methylprednisolone
- Hydrocortisone
- Montelukast
- Cromolyn
- Theophylline
- Ipratropium bromide
- Inactivated influenza vaccine (second and third trimester but can be administered in first trimester)

Allergic Rhinitis
- Budesonide
- Beclomethasone dipropionate
- Fluticasone
- Loratadine
- Cetirizine
- Levocetirizine
- Diphenhydramine
- Chlorpheniramine

Nonallergic Rhinitis
- Above nasal corticosteroids
- Ipratropium bromide

Antibiotics
- Azithromycin
- Penicillins
- Cephalosporins
- Clindamycin

Gastroesophageal Reflux
- Cimetidine
- Famotidine
- Ranitidine
- Lansoprazole
- Esomeprazole
- Rabeprazole

Source: Bealert, S., Greenberger, P.A., *Allergy Asthma Proc.*, 33, S55–S57, 2012; Greenberger, P.A., *Patterson's Allergic Diseases*, 7th edn., Wolters Kluwer, Lippincott, Williams & Wilkins, Philadelphia, PA, 2009.

[a] Not indicated as monotherapy; use with an ICS for persistent asthma not controlled with ICS or montelukast monotherapy. See references [11–14] for stepwise management of asthma. There are more published data and years of use with salmeterol than formoterol.

gestation than in nonpregnant times. Thus, some physicians may choose to advise their pregnant patients on allergen immunotherapy to continue their regular injection schedule, which in this patient happens to be the maintenance dose.

WILL ALLERGEN IMMUNOTHERAPY IN THE MOTHER CONFER BENEFIT ON THE BABY?

There is no evidence for protection of the baby from asthma and atopic conditions when the mother receives subcutaneous allergen immunotherapy.[46] There will be expected transplacental delivery of anti-allergen IgG antibodies, but this effect does not translate into protection of the baby from subsequent development of asthma and atopic conditions. Other maternal antibodies do provide essential protection against infectious diseases for several months as the infant receives immunizations beginning at 2 months of age.

CONCLUSIONS

The pregnant asthma patient provides many challenges for the physician. It is essential to ensure that these patients are on appropriate controller therapy, to reassure them that the asthma controller medications they are taking are safe for the fetus, and to continuously emphasize to them the importance of complying with controller medications throughout their pregnancy. There are many specific questions that may arise during pregnancy for which the primary care physician should consider referring to an allergist/immunologist with experience managing pregnant asthma patients.

REFERENCES

1. Schatz M, Dombrowski MP. Asthma in pregnancy. *N Engl J Med* 2009;360:1862–1869.
2. Enriquez R, Griffin MR, Carroll KN, et al. Effect of maternal asthma and asthma control on pregnancy and perinatal outcomes. *J Allergy Clin Immunol* 2007;120:625–630.
3. Breton MC, Beauchesne M-F, Lemiere C, et al. Risk of perinatal mortality associated with asthma during pregnancy. *Thorax* 2009;64:101–106.
4. Bahna SL, Bjerkedal T. The course and outcome of pregnancy in women with bronchial asthma. *Acta Allergol* 1972;27:397–406.
5. Demissie K, Breckenridge MB, Rhoads GG. Infant and maternal outcomes in the pregnancies of asthmatic women. *Am J Respir Crit Care Med* 1998;158:1091–1095.
6. Blais L, Forget A. Asthma exacerbations during the first trimester of pregnancy and the risk of congenital malformations among asthmatic women. *J Allergy Clin Immunol* 2008;121:1379–1384.
7. Clifton VL, Engel P, Smith R, et al. Maternal and neonatal outcomes of pregnancies complicated by asthma in an Australian population. *Aust N Z J Obstet Gynaecol* 2009;49:619–626.
8. Bealert S, Greenberger PA. Chapter 16: Asthma in pregnancy. *Allergy Asthma Proc* 2012;33(Supp. 1):S55–S57.
9. Firoozi F, Lemiere C, Ducharme FM. Effect of maternal moderate to severe asthma on perinatal outcomes. *Respir Med* 2010;104:1278–1287.
10. Firoozi R, Lemiere C, Beauchesne M-F, et al. Impact of maternal asthma on perinatal outcomes: A two-stage sampling cohort study. *Eur J Epidemiol* 2012;27:205–214.
11. National Heart, Lung, and Blood Institute; National Asthma Education and Prevention Program Asthma and Pregnancy Working Group. NAEPP expert panel report. Managing asthma during pregnancy: Recommendations for pharmacologic treatment—2004 update. *J Allergy Clin Immunol* 2005;115:34–46.
12. National Asthma Education and Prevention Program. Expert panel report 3: Guidelines for the diagnosis and management of asthma—full report 2007. http://www.nhlbi.nih.gov/guidelines/asthma/asthgdln.pdf. Accessed 7/6/2012.
13. Dombrowski MP, Schatz M; ACOG Committee on Practice Bulletins-Obstetrics. ACOG practice bulletin: Clinical management guidelines for obstetrician-gynecologists number 90, February 2008: Asthma in pregnancy. *Obstet Gynecol* 2008;111:457–464.
14. Global Initiative for Asthma. Global strategy for asthma management and prevention. Updated 2011. www.ginaasthma.org. Accessed 7/26/2012.
15. Pali-Scholl I, Motala C, Jensen-Jarolim E. Asthma and allergic diseases in pregnancy: A review. *World Allergy Organiz J* 2009;2:26–36.
16. Louik C, Schatz M, Hernandez-Diaz S, et al. Asthma in pregnancy and its pharmacologic treatment. *Ann Allergy Asthma Immunol* 2010;105:110–117.
17. Greenberger PA, Patterson R. The outcomes of pregnancy complicated by severe asthma. *Alllergy Proc* 1988;9:539–543.
18. Greenberger PA. Allergic disorders and pregnancy. In: Grammer LC, Greenberger PA (eds.), *Patterson's Allergic Diseases*, 7th edn., pp. 622–632, 2009. Philadelphia, PA: Wolters Kluwer, Lippincott, Williams & Wilkins.
19. Robson SC, Hunter S, Boys RJ, et al. Serial study of factors influencing changes in cardiac output during human pregnancy. *Am J Physiol* 1989;256:H1060–H1065.
20. Ouzounian JG, Elkayam U. Physiologic changes during normal pregnancy and delivery. *Cardiol Clin* 2010;30:317–319.
21. Julian CG, Wilson MJ, Lopez M, et al. Augmented uterine artery blood-flow and oxygen delivery protect Andeans from altitude-associated reductions in fetal growth. *Am J Physiol Regul Integ Comp Physiol* 2009;296:R1564–R1575.
22. Coen van Hasselt JG, Green B, Morrish GA. Leveraging physiological data from literature into a pharmacokinetic model to support informative clinical study design in pregnant women. *Pharm Res* 2012;29:1609–1617.
23. Jensen GM, Moore LG. The effect of high altitude and other risk factors on birthweight: Independent or interactive effects? *Am J Public Health* 1997;87:1003–1007.
24. Vargas M, Vargas E, Julian CG, et al. Determinants of blood oxygenation during pregnancy in Andean and European residents of high altitude. *Am J Physiol Regul Integr Comp Physiol* 2007;293:R1303–R1312.
25. Templeton A, Kelman GR. Maternal blood gases, $(PA_{O_2}-Pa_{O_2})$, physiologic shunt and VD/VT in normal pregnancy. *Br J Anaesth* 1976;48:1001–1004.
26. Juniper EF, Daniel EE, Roberts RS, et al. Improvement in airway responsiveness and asthma severity during pregnancy. A prospective study. *Am Rev Respir Dis* 1989;140:924–931.
27. Gardner MO, Doyle NM. Asthma in pregnancy. *Obstet Gynecol Clin N Am* 2004;31:385–413.
28. Kwon HL, Triche EW, Belanger K, et al. The epidemiology of asthma during pregnancy: Prevalence, diagnosis, and symptoms. *Immunol Allergy Clin N Am* 2006;26:29–62.

29. CDC Centers for Disease Control and Prevention: Morbidity and Mortality Weekly Report MMWR. Vital signs: Asthma prevalence, disease characteristics, and self-management education—United States, 2001–2009. May 3, 2011/60 (early release); 1–7.

30. Belanger K, Hellenbrane ME, Holford TR, et al. Effect of pregnancy on maternal asthma symptoms and medication use. *Obstet Gynecol* 2010;115:559–567.

31. Bracken MB, Triche EW, Belanger K, et al. Asthma symptoms, severity, and drug therapy: A prospective study of effects on 2205 pregnancies. *Obstet Gynecol* 2003;102:739–752.

32. Turner ES, Greenberger PA, Patterson R. Management of the pregnant asthmatic patient. *Ann Intern Med* 1980;93:905–918.

33. Schatz M, Dombrowski MP, Wise R, et al. Asthma morbidity during pregnancy can be predicted by severity classification. *J Allergy Clin Immunol* 2003;112:283–288.

34. Schatz M, Dombrowski MP, Wise R, et al. The relationship of asthma-specific quality of life during pregnancy to subsequent asthma and perinatal morbidity. *J Asthma* 2010;47:46–50.

35. Greenberger PA. Personalized medicine for patients with asthma. *J Allergy Clin Immunol* 2010;125:305–306.

36. Lim AS, Stewart K, Abramson MJ, et al. Management of asthma in pregnant women by general practitioners: A cross sectional study. *BMC Fam Pract* 2011;12:121.

37. Norjavaara E, Gerhardsson de Verdier M. Normal pregnancy outcomes in a population-based study including 2968 pregnant women exposed to budesonide. *J Allergy Clin Immunol* 2003;111:736–742.

38. Martel M-J, Rey E, Beauchesne M-F, et al. Use of inhaled corticosteroids during pregnancy and risk of pregnancy induced hypertension: Nested case-control study. *BMJ* 2005;330:230.

39. Hodyl NA, Stark MJ, Osei-Kumah A, et al. Fetal glucocorticoid-regulated pathways are not affected by inhaled corticosteroid use for asthma during pregnancy. *Am J Respir Crit Care Med.* 2011;183:716–722.

40. Lim A, Stewart K, Konig K, et al. Systematic review of the safety of regular preventive asthma medications during pregnancy. *Ann Pharmacother* 2011;45:931–945.

41. Bakhireva LN, Jones, KL, Schatz M, et al. Safety of leukotriene antagonists in pregnancy. *J Allergy Clin Immunol* 2007;119:618–625.

42. Nelson LM, Shields KE, Cunningham ML, et al. Congenital malformations among infants born to women receiving montelukast, inhaled corticosteroids, and other asthma medications. *J Allergy Clin Immunol* 2012;129:251–254.

43. Bakhireva LN, Jones KJ, Schatz M, et al. Asthma medication use in pregnancy and fetal growth. *J Allergy Clin Immunol* 2005;116:503–509.

44. Greer FA, Sicherer SH, Burks AW, et al. Effects of early nutritional interventions on the development of atopic disease in infants and children: The role of maternal dietary restriction, breastfeeding, timing of introduction of complementary foods, and hydrolyzed formulas. *Pediatrics* 2008;121:183–191.

45. Prevention and control of influenza with vaccines: Interim recommendations of the Advisory Committee on Immunization Practice (ACIP), 2013. *Morb Mortal Wkly Rep* 2013;62:356.

46. Metzger WJ, Turner E, Patterson R. The safety of immunotherapy during pregnancy. *J Allergy Clin Immunol* 1978;61:268–272.

47. Joint Task Force on Practice Parameters: American Academy of Allergy Asthma and Immunology; American College of Allergy Asthma and Immunology; Joint Council of Allergy Asthma and Immunology. Allergen immunotherapy: A practice parameter second update. *J Allergy Clin Immunol* 2007;120:S25–S85.

26 Anxiety and Depression and Asthma

Alison C. McLeish, Kimberly M. Avallone, and Kristen M. Kraemer

CONTENTS

CASE PRESENTATION

KB was a 42-year-old white male with a history of progressive worsening of lower respiratory symptoms consisting of shortness of breath, chest tightness, wheezing, and cough. These symptoms developed gradually and resulted in four hospitalizations in the past 6 years. He reported that his symptoms were triggered by exercise, cold air, viral infections, dust, smoke, cleaning agents, and weather changes. He had been corticosteroid dependent for over 5 years with a minimal effective prednisone dose of 20 mg/day. He had no history of allergies or asthma as a child, but did have a family history of asthma. He was diagnosed with nasal polyps 10 years ago and underwent sinus surgery for a polypectomy. After the surgery, however, he continued to experience nasal congestion, anosmia, and postnasal drainage. Previously, he worked as a diesel machinist, but was forced to quit work and apply for disability due to the fumes. He was married with two children and was the primary homecare provider as his wife traveled extensively for work.

At presentation, KB appeared very calm, but was hesitant to volunteer information beyond answering specific questions he was asked. His past medical history was remarkable for acid reflux and weight gain from the prednisone. He denied a history of anxiety or depression. Allergy testing

to seasonal and perennial aeroallergens was negative. His FEV1 was 41%, which improved by 20% after administration of a bronchodilator, and there were no environmental factors at home identified as triggering his symptoms. Extensive asthma education was provided, and KB demonstrated good compliance with medications and office visits. However, repeated attempts to taper him off prednisone were unsuccessful, despite using other disease-modifying agents.

Further questioning to determine why the patient was unable to taper prednisone revealed that he was experiencing high levels of anxiety about recent financial and marital problems. He had recently moved out of the family home, and he and his wife were seeing a marriage counselor in an attempt to resolve their problems. KB also acknowledged that the physical limitations of his disease and inability to financially support his family contributed to his increased anxiety. As he was not receptive to treatment with anxiolytic medication, it was recommended that he see a psychologist for cognitive behavior therapy to treat his anxiety. This therapy helped him identify and change maladaptive thoughts and behaviors that contributed to his anxiety. As his symptoms decreased, KB began to exercise more and lose weight, and ended up moving back home with his wife and children. With continued therapy, he has been able to taper his daily prednisone dose to 7.5 mg/day while his asthma and nasal polyps have remained well controlled.

INTRODUCTION

Despite the existence of numerous effective treatment options, appropriate control of asthma symptoms is often difficult to achieve. In a recent survey of patients in the Asthma Care Network, nearly 75% reported symptoms indicative of poorly controlled asthma.[1] As a result, health-care expenditures related to asthma are higher than the costs associated with HIV/AIDS and tuberculosis combined, due in large part to poor asthma control.[2] Thus, identifying factors that contribute to poor asthma control is particularly important. It has long been appreciated that co-occurring psychological symptoms and disorders are fairly common among asthma patients. Indeed, recent epidemiological work indicates that individuals with asthma are nearly 1.7 times more likely than those without to have a lifetime history of any mental disorder.[3] Moreover, the presence of co-occurring psychopathology is related to greater difficulties in achieving and maintaining asthma control as well as more frequent asthma exacerbations.[4]

The purpose of the current chapter is to examine the association between asthma and both anxiety and depressive symptoms and disorders. The chapter will begin with a brief case study to illustrate some of the clinical issues associated with co-occurring asthma and anxiety and/or depression. Then we will provide a description of anxiety and depressive symptoms and disorders as well as clarification of appropriate terminology. Next, the prevalence of anxiety and mood disorders among individuals with asthma will be reviewed, with a particular focus on the association between asthma and panic disorder. Then, the effect of anxiety and depression on asthma-related outcomes will be examined (i.e., severity, control, symptom perception, quality of life, health-care use), followed by an examination of psychological interventions to address comorbid asthma and panic disorder. Next, a potential mechanism that contributes to the asthma–anxiety association, anxiety sensitivity (fear of one's own anxiety symptoms), will be examined. Lastly, limitations of the current literature and directions for future research will be discussed.

DEPRESSION AND ANXIETY OVERVIEW

Approximately half of the U.S. population will suffer from one or more psychiatric disorders at some point in their lifetime.[5] Of these disorders, mood and anxiety disorders are the most common, with lifetime prevalence rates of 21% and 29%, respectively.[5] Aside from a high prevalence rate, mood and anxiety disorders generally maintain a chronic, fluctuating course, resulting in substantial impairment across the life span. In addition, anxiety and mood disorders place a large burden on the financial and social resources of society. It is estimated that anxiety and mood disorders result in approximately $86 billion in direct and indirect costs in the United States each year.[6,7]

MOOD DISORDERS

Mood disorders, also called affective disorders, represent a category of mental health problems in which the primary underlying problem is an individual's persistent emotional state or mood. There are three primary mood disorders that are relevant to the current literature review: major depressive disorder (MDD), dysthymia, and bipolar disorder (formerly called manic depression). The lifetime prevalence rate of any mood disorder is 20.8%, with MDD being the most common (16.6%), followed by bipolar disorder (3.9%), and dysthymia (2.5%).[5] Mood disorders affect individuals of all ages, but they typically manifest in the midtwenties and are more common in women than men.[8]

MDD is what is often thought of by the term "depression" and is characterized by the presence of one or more major depressive episodes that cause significant distress and impairment. A major depressive episode is a period of two or more weeks of a depressed or irritable mood and/or markedly diminished interest or pleasure in all or almost all activities. These primary symptoms are accompanied by a combination of the following additional symptoms: significant weight loss or gain, insomnia or hypersomnia, fatigue, psychomotor agitation or retardation, feelings of worthlessness, difficulty concentrating, and suicidal ideation.[8] Dysthymia is often thought of as a less severe form of MDD, because many of the symptoms of MDD are present, but to a lesser degree. It is characterized by a chronic, low-grade depressed or irritable mood that lasts for at least 1 year. Bipolar disorder, in its most classic form, can be thought of as alternating periods of major depressive and manic episodes or unusual shifts in mood, energy, activity levels, and the ability to carry out everyday tasks. A manic episode is a period of abnormally elevated or irritable mood that lasts for at least 1 week and is accompanied by symptoms of inflated self-esteem, decreased need for sleep, pressured speech, racing thoughts, and increased activity.[8]

ANXIETY DISORDERS

Anxiety is a future-oriented, negative mood state that results in feelings of helplessness due to a perceived inability to control or predict events. Anxiety consists of symptoms across physiological (e.g., sympathetic nervous system activation), cognitive (e.g., hypervigilance, worry), and behavioral domains (e.g., avoidance, exaggerated startle response). While anxiety is a normal response to stressful events or the anticipation of such events, anxiety becomes abnormal when it is pervasive, persistent, and accompanied by excessive avoidance and clinically significant impairment. While prevalence rates vary across the specific anxiety disorders, the lifetime prevalence rate for any anxiety disorder is 28.8%.[5] The most common anxiety disorder is specific phobia with a lifetime prevalence rate of 12.5%, followed by social phobia (12.1%), posttraumatic stress disorder (PTSD; 6.8%), generalized anxiety disorder (GAD; 5.7%), separation anxiety disorder (5.2%), panic disorder (4.7%), obsessive–compulsive disorder (OCD; 1.6%), and agoraphobia without panic disorder (1.4%).[5]

A specific phobia is an extreme or irrational fear of a specific object or situation (e.g., heights, snakes, flying). Social phobia is a marked or persistent fear of social or performance situations involving unfamiliar people or scrutiny by others. PTSD consists of symptoms of reexperiencing (e.g., flashbacks), avoidance, and physiological arousal (e.g., exaggerated startle response) following exposure to a traumatic event where an individual experienced extreme fear, helplessness, or horror.[8] Generalized anxiety disorder is typically what is thought of by the term "anxiety" and consists of periods of intense worry that are excessive, pervasive, and uncontrollable. Separation anxiety disorder is a disorder of childhood only, that is characterized by developmentally inappropriate and excessive anxiety regarding separation from home or from those to whom the individual is attached. Panic disorder consists of recurrent or unexpected panic attacks (discrete periods of fear in which physical symptoms develop abruptly and peak within 10 min) as well as worry about future panic attacks and avoidance of situations that might produce panic attacks. OCD consists of intrusive and recurring thoughts (obsessions) that often result in repetitive behaviors or rituals that are repeated excessively to reduce anxiety (compulsions). Agoraphobia, or anxiety about being in a place or situation where escape might be difficult in the event of a panic attack, can occur within the context of panic disorder or alone.[8]

TERMINOLOGY

In the literature reviewed in the remainder of the chapter, mental health terms are not always used consistently or accurately. Thus, there is a need to clarify terms that will be used throughout the chapter. The terms "anxiety" and "depression" will be used to refer to global levels of anxiety and depression *symptoms* and not to clinical levels of anxiety and depression (i.e., *disorders*). When referring to clinical levels of anxiety and depression, the terms "anxiety disorders" and "mood disorders" will be used, or the specific anxiety or mood disorder will be identified. Although not an officially recognized category of disorders, the term "depressive disorders" is often used to indicate mood disorders that only include depression (e.g., MDD, dysphoria) and not mania (e.g., bipolar disorder) by many researchers. This term will be utilized in this manner throughout the chapter as well.

CO-OCCURRENCE OF ASTHMA AND ANXIETY AND MOOD DISORDERS

In addition to being common in the general population, anxiety and mood disorders are even more common among individuals with asthma. The presence of asthma has been linked with anxiety and mood disorders across developmental periods, and clinical and nonclinical samples, and using a variety of methodologies (e.g., longitudinal, cross-sectional, epidemiological).

CHILDREN

Epidemiological data indicate that children with asthma, compared with those without, are more likely to have any anxiety disorder (OR = 1.6), specific phobia (OR = 1.70), separation anxiety (OR = 1.82), and GAD (OR = 1.89), while children with a chronic illness other than asthma are more likely to meet criteria for any depressive disorder.[9] Similarly, in a nonclinical sample, adolescents with asthma, compared with those without, were nearly twice as likely to have an anxiety or depressive disorder.[10] Factors associated with the presence of comorbid depressive or anxiety disorders included female gender, more recent asthma diagnosis, living in a single-parent household, greater externalizing behaviors, and greater functional impairment.[10] However, at least one study has found that associations between asthma and depressive and anxiety disorders are no longer significant after controlling for confounding factors (e.g., exposure to childhood adversity).[11]

ADULTS

Findings from studies among adults generally mirror what is found in children and adolescents. On average, the prevalence rate of any anxiety disorder among adults with asthma is 34%.[12] The most common co-occurring anxiety diagnoses among adults with asthma are panic disorder (12%), agoraphobia (12%), and GAD (9%). Prevalence rates for these disorders are significantly higher than those found among individuals without asthma, while rates of specific phobia, social phobia, and PTSD are similar to, or lower than, rates among individuals without asthma.[12] Contrary to what has been found in children and adolescents with asthma, in a cross-national study of adults, early-onset MDD (OR = 1.91), panic disorder/agoraphobia (OR = 1.86), and any depressive/anxiety disorder (OR = 1.54) each predicted adult-onset asthma independent of the effects of childhood adversity.[13] In terms of differential associations based on asthma severity, current nonsevere asthma has been found to be associated with an increased likelihood of having any mood disorder (OR = 2.42), and current severe asthma has been associated with increased risk for any anxiety disorder (OR = 2.65), specific phobia (OR = 4.78), and panic disorder (OR = 4.61).[14] In this same study, lifetime severe asthma was associated with an increased risk for any anxiety disorder, panic disorder, specific phobia, social phobia, GAD, and bipolar disorder, while lifetime nonsevere asthma was associated with increased odds of any anxiety disorder, anxiety disorder not otherwise specified, and somatoform disorder.

ASTHMA AND PANIC PSYCHOPATHOLOGY

Although extant research has clearly documented an association between asthma and both depressive and anxiety disorders, there is evidence for a relatively specific association between asthma and panic psychopathology (i.e., panic attacks, panic disorder, and agoraphobia). Indeed, rates of panic attacks and panic disorder are consistently higher among individuals with asthma compared with the general population.[14,15] Moreover, there appears to be a dose–response relationship, such that with every additional panic symptom the likelihood of asthma increases.[15,16] A recent 20-year longitudinal study found a significant bidirectional relationship between the two; asthma was a significant predictor of future panic disorder (OR = 4.5), and panic disorder predicted later asthma activity (OR = 6.3).[16]

IMPACT OF CO-OCCURRING ANXIETY AND DEPRESSION

ASTHMA SEVERITY

Due to the high rates of co-occurrence between asthma and both anxiety and depression, researchers have begun to examine the effects of these comorbid mental health conditions on asthma severity, including asthma symptoms and pulmonary function. Among youth, the presence of one or more anxiety or depressive disorders has been found to be associated with greater asthma symptoms, with a linear increase in asthma symptoms as severity of anxiety and depressive disorders increases.[17] Similarly, depression has been found to be associated with greater asthma severity and a greater risk for future hospitalization due to asthma.[18]

In terms of pulmonary function, one study found that the presence of depression, but not anxiety, was associated with decreased FEV_1 and FEV_1/FVC values, independent of asthma severity.[19] The nonsignificant findings for anxiety, however, may be due to the small sample size in this study ($n = 38$). When looking at diagnoses, current or lifetime MDD, but not GAD, panic disorder, or PTSD, are predictive of slightly lower FEV_1 and FEV25%–75%, but only among males.[20] The results, however, have not always been consistent. Indeed, Lavoie and colleagues found no differences between those with and without a mood or anxiety disorder in terms of pulmonary function, asthma duration, asthma severity, presence of atopy, and number of emergency department visits (ED) or hospitalizations in the past year.[21]

There are a few studies examining associations between anxiety and depression and asthma-related death, with conflicting results. In one historical cohort and nested case control study, there was an increased mortality rate among asthma patients with comorbid depression[22] (OR = 1.87); however, the authors caution that the cause of this association has yet to be examined. On the other hand, other work has found similar or even lower mortality rates among asthma patients reporting depression or anxiety symptoms.[23,24] There is also a small but growing body of literature examining increased risk of suicidal ideation (OR = 2.3), suicide attempts (OR = 3.5), and death by suicide among individuals with asthma.[25-27] There are, however, a number of methodological limitations to many of the studies in this area; thus, further research is needed before any definitive conclusions about the impact of depression or anxiety on asthma-related death as well as the impact of asthma on suicidal ideation and behavior can be made.

ASTHMA CONTROL

The results for asthma control, on the other hand, are more consistent. The majority of studies in this domain have found that anxiety and depression (both symptoms and disorders) are associated with poorer asthma control.[21,28,29] Compared with individuals without psychiatric disorders, individuals with comorbid anxiety and depressive disorders report greater bronchodilator use, more nocturnal waking, and worse symptoms in the morning, shortness of breath, and wheezing, despite no differences in measures of lung function.[29] In an epidemiological survey, individuals with an anxiety or depressive disorder were more likely to have had an asthma attack in the past 30 days and more than three ED or doctor's office visits in the past year.[30] Further, individuals with a lifetime history of an anxiety disorder were nearly twice as likely to have used an inhaler more than 30 times in the past 30 days compared with those without such a history.

There is some question as to whether the effects of depression on asthma are stronger or more severe than the effects of anxiety. Although the body of literature is small, a few studies have found that only those with depressive, but not anxiety, disorders reported poorer asthma control.[21,31] However, there are also studies that have found that both anxiety and depression are independent predictors of asthma control.[28] Similar contradictory findings can be seen when looking at the interaction of anxiety and depression. Lavoie and colleagues found no significant increase in risk for poorer asthma control associated with the presence of both anxiety and depressive disorders.[21] However, another study found that only a combination of anxiety and depression was a significant predictor of poor asthma control.[32]

SYMPTOM PERCEPTION

One potential explanation for the association between anxiety and depression and poor asthma control is that these conditions affect symptom perception, a key component in asthma management. Previous research indicates that anxiety and depression are associated with greater frequency of self-reported hyperventilation and airway obstruction symptoms.[33] However, it is unclear whether individuals with comorbid asthma and anxiety or depression perceive, report, or recall their asthma symptoms differently, or whether they are truly experiencing more symptoms. One study examined symptom perception in childhood asthma and found that, after controlling for pulmonary function, trait anxiety was associated with heightened symptom perception at baseline, but not during a methacholine challenge.[34] Such findings lend support to the idea that individuals with high anxiety tend to pay more attention to (i.e., overperceive) ambiguous (i.e., mild) symptoms, but are able to accurately perceive symptoms of changes in bronchoconstriction. However, patients with comorbid asthma and panic disorder have been found to report greater levels of dyspnea, compared with those with asthma only, when experiencing the same reduction of lung function during a histamine challenge.[35]

QUALITY OF LIFE

Given these reports of poorer asthma control, it is not surprising that anxiety and depression are associated with poorer asthma-related and overall quality of life as well as increased functional limitations.[4,18,21,29,36–38] Indeed, individuals with asthma and a lifetime diagnosis of an anxiety or depressive disorder are more likely to report frequent physical distress, mental distress, and activity limitations as well as fair/poor general health, greater life dissatisfaction, and lack of social support.[30] The findings are less clear when trying to discern the unique effects of symptoms of depression and anxiety on quality of life. Some studies have found that when controlling for the effects of anxiety, depression is no longer a significant predictor of quality of life.[32] On the other hand, in a study of patients with poorly controlled asthma, when controlling for the effects of anxiety, only depression was found to be a significant predictor of poorer quality of life.[33] The substantial overlap between depression and anxiety symptoms may partly explain these inconsistent findings. Similar inconsistencies have been found when trying to determine whether the presence of both anxiety and depression is worse than either alone. One study found an additive negative effect of having depression in addition to anxiety in terms of quality of life;[32] however, no such additive effect was found in a study of patients with poorly controlled asthma.[33]

HEALTH-CARE USE

Depression and anxiety have also been associated with greater asthma-related health-care use.[28] Higher levels of anxiety are associated with higher rates of ED visits, more frequent routine and unscheduled medical visits and overnight hospitalizations, greater use of short-acting beta-agonists, and more frequent need for oral corticosteroid treatment.[28] Independent of objective pulmonary functioning, individuals with anxiety tend to overuse short-acting beta-agonist medication, receive more intensive corticosteroid regimens, and have longer and more frequent hospitalizations.[39–41] Comorbid asthma and panic disorder seem to be particularly problematic. These patients are over six times as likely to visit their primary care provider and report greater use of short-acting beta-agonists compared with those with asthma only.[4,42]

At least two studies have found that depression, but not anxiety, is associated with greater health-care use. In one, depression, but not anxiety, was found to be associated with more frequent unscheduled doctor's visits.[33] Another found that depression was associated with more hospital visits and greater number of days on oral corticosteroids in the past year, even after controlling for anxiety.[36] While the majority of studies have focused on asthma-related health-care use, it should be noted that at least one study found that the increase in health-care costs among individuals with asthma and comorbid anxiety and depression was related to treatment of the mental health condition and not to asthma.[38]

INTERVENTIONS FOR CO-OCCURRING ANXIETY AND DEPRESSION

With the high rates of depression and anxiety found among individuals with asthma and the resulting increases in morbidity and functional impairment, there is a clear need for interventions to treat these comorbid problems. Thus, it is surprising that, despite the existence of well-validated and highly efficacious cognitive behavioral treatments for anxiety and depressive disorders, there has been little attempt to apply cognitive behavioral principles to develop efficacious treatments for asthma patients with comorbid anxiety or depression. Cognitive behavioral therapy (CBT) in this context would focus on understanding and changing dysfunctional behaviors and beliefs about bodily symptoms and the asthma diagnosis itself (e.g., perceived burden associated with asthma management).

Due to their high rates of co-occurrence, the majority of work in this area has focused on developing interventions to treat comorbid asthma and panic disorder. To date, there have been two different CBT interventions developed to treat comorbid asthma and panic disorder. The first intervention was a nurse-administered 8-week group treatment program that combined CBT for panic disorder with asthma education.[43] The CBT portion of the treatment program consisted of four major components: (1) psychoeducation regarding the nature of anxiety and panic; (2) cognitive therapy techniques to identify, monitor, and modify cognitive misappraisals that contribute to and maintain panic symptoms; (3) training on diaphragmatic breathing to reduce physical symptoms that may elicit panic attacks; and (4) interoceptive exposure exercises designed to reduce fear of the bodily sensations associated with anxiety and panic attack symptoms.

The asthma education portion of the treatment consisted of six components: (1) information regarding airway inflammation and bronchoconstriction; (2) information about the correct use and side effects of short- and long-acting asthma medications; (3) inhaler techniques; (4) instruction about self-monitoring of symptoms; (5) asthma triggers and control strategies; and (6) action plans. Each treatment session contained a CBT component and an asthma education component. For the first 4 weeks, participants met twice weekly in small groups for 90-min sessions. For the last 4 weeks, sessions were held weekly, for a total of 12 treatment sessions. Results in a study of women only indicated that, compared with a wait-list control, the treatment program resulted in significant reduction of frequency of panic symptoms, general anxiety, and anxiety sensitivity (fear of anxiety-related sensations), and improvements in asthma-related quality of life and morning PEF ratings. The improvements in all outcomes except quality of life were maintained throughout the 6-month follow-up period.

The second intervention was similar to the first and was a pilot test of the efficacy of a 14-session and 8-session protocol that combined components of CBT for panic disorder with asthma self-management programs.[44] The 14-session protocol consisted of education about asthma, proper medication use, and differentiating between asthma and panic symptoms (Sessions 1–2); progressive muscle relaxation and breathing retraining (Sessions 3–5); cognitive restructuring and asthma problem solving (Sessions 6–7); exposure (Sessions 8–10); asthma and medication, effective communication with doctors (Session 11); smoking reduction and treatment of agoraphobic symptoms (Session 12); assertiveness training (Session 13); and relapse prevention (Session 14). The 8-session protocol was a condensed version of the 14-session version. Both protocols resulted in a more than 50% decrease in panic symptoms, significant decreases in asthma symptoms, and improved asthma-related quality of life. The 14-session protocol also resulted in decreased short-acting beta-agonist use; however, there was significantly greater dropout rate in the 14-session (50%) compared with the 8-session protocol (18%).

There has been one examination of a CBT-based prevention program to treat individuals with asthma and high levels of anxiety and asthma-related panic fear, which would place these individuals at higher risk for developing a comorbid anxiety disorder.[45] As with the previous two studies, this intervention combined education about asthma and anxiety, CBT, and asthma self-management. Treatment was tailored to each individual based on a functional analysis of the relationship between his or her specific situational triggers, asthma-related beliefs, maladaptive cognitions, attention focus, and physiological factors. Based on this analysis, the intervention could contain the following components: (1) education about asthma and how to differentiate between asthma and anxiety symptoms; (2) self-monitoring of anxiety-related cognitions, particularly those involving catastrophic misinterpretation of bodily sensations; (3) attention retraining; (4) exposure; (5) education about methods to control hyperventilation; (6) identifying panic fear triggers; (7) improving problem-solving skills; and (8) exploration of dysfunctional asthma-related beliefs. After an introductory 1.5-h session, sessions were 1 h in length and occurred weekly for 4–6 weeks. Results indicated that the intervention resulted in a significant reduction of asthma-related panic fear, but not general anxiety, by the end of treatment, and this reduction was maintained at the 6-month follow-up. There were also significant improvements in asthma-related quality of life and depression at the end of treatment, but these gains were not maintained at the 6-month follow-up.

ANXIETY SENSITIVITY: A POTENTIAL PSYCHOLOGICAL MECHANISM

Research has clearly documented substantial negative health effects as well as personal and economic costs associated with co-occurring asthma and depression and/or anxiety, particularly for co-occurring panic disorder. However, little is known about the etiology of these associations and what factors may serve to maintain them. Efforts to understand these underlying mechanisms would not only fill an

important gap within the empirical literature, but would also provide specific targets for intervention efforts that could improve asthma control and ultimately reduce health-care costs. One way in which to accomplish this task is to identify malleable psychological risk factors for not only mood and anxiety symptoms and disorders, but also for poor asthma control. Given the particularly strong relationship between asthma and panic disorder, we focus here on one panic-related risk factor that has been receiving increased research attention in terms of its association with asthma, namely anxiety sensitivity.

Anxiety sensitivity is a modifiable cognitive predisposition defined as the fear of anxiety-related physical and psychological sensations that is theoretically and empirically distinct from the tendency to experience negative affect.[46] Anxiety sensitivity encompasses three lower-order dimensions: physical, cognitive, and social concerns that load onto a single higher-order factor.[47] When anxious, individuals with high anxiety sensitivity become acutely fearful due to beliefs that these anxiety-related interoceptive sensations have harmful physical, psychological, or social consequences. In line with this theory, anxiety sensitivity is concurrently and prospectively associated with an increased risk of anxiety symptoms and with the onset of certain anxiety disorders, most notably panic disorder and PTSD.[48,49]

Although not yet empirically tested, a cognitive behavioral model may help explain how anxiety sensitivity impacts asthma. Individuals with asthma tend to be fearful of pulmonary-based and other bodily sensations and may react with greater levels of anxiety or related negative affect when confronted with such stressors. Since anxiety sensitivity results in the amplification of negative emotional experiences, an individual with asthma who is high in anxiety sensitivity would perceive bodily sensations associated with autonomic arousal as a sign of imminent harm, resulting in greater distress about these physical sensations and an increased tendency to catastrophize about them, resulting in avoidance of situations that may elicit such sensations. As a result, this asthma patient with high anxiety sensitivity would likely experience elevated levels of anxiety and be at risk for developing panic disorder as well as increased asthma symptoms and exacerbations.

Research examining anxiety sensitivity and asthma, although limited, is promising. For example, anxiety sensitivity has been shown to significantly predict panic in response to symptoms of asthma (i.e., panic fear) independently of asthma severity.[50] Other work has found that patients with atopic asthma have higher levels of anxiety sensitivity than those with nonatopic asthma.[51] In terms of asthma-related outcomes, anxiety sensitivity, particularly the physical concerns facet, has been found to significantly predict asthma control and asthma-related quality of life among individuals with self-reported and physician-verified asthma diagnoses.[52,53] These effects were significant even after controlling for relevant demographic variables and negative affect. These findings suggest that individuals with asthma who are fearful of physiological arousal are a particularly "at risk" population for poor asthma control and that there may be utility in reducing anxiety sensitivity levels to improve asthma control.

SUMMARY

Overall, extant research indicates a significant association between asthma and depression and anxiety in terms of both global symptoms and specific disorders, most notably panic disorder. The presence of co-occurring anxiety and depression negatively impacts asthma, particularly in terms of asthma control, quality of life, and health-care usage. Although the findings are not consistent, co-occurring anxiety and depression do appear to be associated with greater asthma severity in terms of more severe and frequent symptoms, more frequent hospitalizations, and greater medication use. However, the majority of studies also found that there was no effect of co-occurring anxiety and depression on objective measures of lung function. Indeed, it appears as if one of the primary ways in which anxiety, in particular, exerts its influence on asthma is through increased symptom perception, particularly for ambiguous symptoms. Such overperception of symptoms is problematic as individuals with asthma rely on their subjective experience of asthma symptoms to guide the management of their asthma and physicians tend to rely more heavily on patients' subjective reports of asthma symptoms than on objective assessments of lung function to inform treatment decisions (e.g., medication class or dosage).[54] As a result, co-occurring anxiety and depression appear to result in poorer asthma outcomes in the absence of actual physical causes. Thus, interventions to treat anxiety and depression are needed to reduce this overperception. Although there are psychological treatments for comorbid asthma and panic disorder, little attention has been given to developing preventive interventions for asthma patients that would target risk factors for developing comorbid anxiety or mood disorders. One potential target that has been identified is anxiety sensitivity. Exposure-based techniques to reduce anxiety sensitivity have been used to improve outcomes in other health problems (e.g., smoking cessation),[55] but have yet to be applied among asthma patients. Such interventions are shorter than existing CBT interventions for comorbid anxiety and asthma and can easily be implemented in a clinic setting.

LIMITATIONS AND FUTURE DIRECTIONS

Although a great deal of research attention has been paid to co-occurring asthma and depression and anxiety, a number of directions for research in this area remain relatively unexplored. Much of this research has focused on documenting this co-occurrence and its effects, and less research attention has been paid to developing and testing theoretical models to explain the etiology and maintenance of this co-occurrence. Such a theory would not only guide research, but also provide a framework for understanding how data from various studies fit together. Furthermore, it is difficult to draw definitive conclusions about the associations between anxiety and depression and asthma based on the numerous discrepancies found in extant research. These discrepancies are due, in part, to the types of samples used (e.g., community vs. clinical), but also to what specifically is being examined (e.g., anxiety or depression or both) and how variables are defined. In terms of anxiety and depression, both have been looked at as symptoms as well as clinical disorders. No studies, to our knowledge, have examined the differential effects on asthma outcomes of subclinical levels of anxiety and depression symptoms compared with actual clinical anxiety and depressive disorders. Such work would provide important information about which levels of anxiety and depression are particularly problematic, and what specific effects these differing levels have on asthma. Further, it may be useful to clarify the definition of the constructs used as well as the method of their assessment to increase consistency across studies.

Along these same lines, researchers often combine a wide range of anxiety or mood disorders into one group, rather than examining each disorder individually. This strategy is understandable, as relatively large sample sizes are needed to have sufficient representation of each disorder. However, it is then difficult to ascertain associations between specific anxiety or mood disorders and asthma. Moreover, studies looking at classes of disorders do not necessarily include all disorders within a certain class. That is, when researchers examine anxiety disorders, they typically do not include every anxiety disorder. Thus, even the conclusions about anxiety disorders as a class can be somewhat misleading since they do not cover all anxiety disorders. Similarly, researchers have focused primarily on the depression end of the spectrum of mood disorders, and little research has been done on the effects of disorders involving mania (e.g., bipolar disorder). This lack of attention is unfortunate as at least one study found that bipolar disorder is associated with lifetime severe asthma.[14]

More research is needed to examine the differential effects of depression and anxiety on asthma. Several studies attempted to determine whether anxiety or depression, or both, exerted a stronger negative effect on asthma, with conflicting results.[21,28,31–33] There is substantial symptom overlap between anxiety and depression, and most self-report measures of depression and anxiety do not take this overlap into consideration. The tripartite model is one attempt to differentiate between anxiety and depression. This model posits that negative affectivity serves as a general distress factor, lack of positive affect is specific to depression, and autonomic arousal is specific to anxiety.[56] Measures based on this conceptualization (e.g., Inventory of Depression and Anxiety Symptoms) contain scales that assess symptoms specific to anxiety and specific to depression.[56] Use of such measures in future research may help clarify the differential effects of depression and anxiety. In addition, there is a need to more clearly differentiate between subjective and objective measures of asthma outcomes. Research has shown that asthma patients with co-occurring anxiety, in particular, tend to perceive more symptoms than would be expected based on objective measures of lung function.[35] Unfortunately, various measures of asthma control and asthma severity are largely based on patients' subjective reports of symptoms. Thus, it is unclear to what extent anxiety and depression actually exert a negative influence on asthma outcome measures as the effects of depression and anxiety on symptom perception could confound significant findings.

The majority of studies have compared individuals with asthma to those without; however, anxiety and depression are commonly found among most chronic medical conditions. Thus, it is important to understand how much of the link between anxiety and depression and asthma is specific to asthma, rather than related to having a chronic medical condition in general. Sixth, future research would benefit from examining the role of so-called "third variables" in the co-occurrence of anxiety and depression and asthma. For example, there appear to be certain differential effects based on age[11,13] and gender[20] that need further examination. Moreover, recent research examining the role of anxiety-related risk factors (e.g., anxiety sensitivity) in this association highlights the importance of examining malleable psychological risk factors as well.

Lastly, this body of literature would benefit from greater use of laboratory-based studies. Such studies could examine "on-line" responding to symptoms of depression and anxiety among individuals with asthma. For example, laboratory-based emotion elicitation procedures could be used to examine how experiencing anxiety or depression symptoms impact physiological responding, perceptions of asthma control, and medication use. This information would not only inform theoretical models of co-occurring asthma and anxiety and depression, but also facilitate the examination of the individual and interactive effects of depression and anxiety. Ultimately, such knowledge could be used to develop targeted interventions for individuals with co-occurring asthma and depression or anxiety that would improve asthma management and reduce asthma-related health-care costs.

REFERENCES

1. Carlton BG, Lucas DO, Ellis EF, et al. The status of asthma control and asthma prescribing practices in the United States: Results of a large prospective asthma control survey of primary care practices. *J Asthma* 2005;42:529–535.
2. World Health Organization. Bronchial Asthma Fact Sheet no. 206. January 2000. Available: https://apps.who.int/inf-fs/en/fact206.html.
3. Goodwin RD, Pagura J, Cox B, et al. Asthma and mental disorders in Canada: Impact on functional and mental health service use. *J Psychosom Res* 2010;68:165–173.
4. Feldman JM, Lehrer PM, Borson S, et al. Health care use and quality of life among patients with asthma and panic disorder. *J Asthma* 2005;42:179–184.
5. Kessler RC, Berglund P, Demler O, et al. Lifetime prevalence and age-of-onset distributions of DSM-IV disorders in the National Comorbidity Survey Replication. *Arch Gen Psychiat* 2005;62:593–602.
6. Greenberg PE, Sisitsky T, Kessler RC, et al. The economic burden of anxiety disorders in the 1990s. *J Clin Psychiat* 1999;60:427–435.
7. Hall RC, Wise MG. The clinical and financial burden of mood disorders. Cost and outcome. *Psychosomatics* 1995;36:11–18.

8. American Psychological Association. *Diagnostic and Statistical Manual of Mental Disorders* (4th edn., text revision). Washington, DC: APA, 2000.
9. Ortega AN, Huertas SE, Canino G, et al. Childhood asthma, chronic illness, and psychiatric disorders. *J Nerv Ment Dis* 2002;190:275–281.
10. Katon W, Lozano P, Russo J, et al. The prevalence of DSM-IV anxiety and depressive disorders in youth with asthma compared with controls. *J Adolesc Health* 2007;41:455–463.
11. Goodwin RD, Fergusson DM, Horwood LJ. Asthma and depressive and anxiety disorders among young persons in the community. *Psychol Med* 2004;34:1465–1474.
12. Weiser EB. The prevalence of anxiety disorders among adults with asthma: A meta-analytic review. *J Clin Psychol Med Settings* 2007;14:297–307.
13. Patten SB, Williams JV, Lavorato DH, et al. Major depression as a risk factor for chronic disease incidence: Longitudinal analyses in a general population cohort. *Gen Hosp Psychiat* 2008;30:407–413.
14. Goodwin RD, Jacobi F, Thefeld W. Mental disorders and asthma in the community. *Arch Gen Psychiat* 2003;60:1125–1130.
15. Goodwin RD, Pine DS, Hoven CW. Asthma and panic attacks among youth in the community. *J Asthma* 2003;40:139–145.
16. Hasler G, Gergen PJ, Kleinbaum DG, et al. Asthma and panic in young adults: A 20-year prospective community study. *Am J Respir Crit Care Med* 2005;171:1224–1230.
17. Richardson LP, Lozano P, Russo J, et al. Asthma symptom burden: Relationship to asthma severity and anxiety and depression symptoms. *Pediatrics* 2006;118:1042–1051.
18. Eisner MD, Katz PP, Lactao G, et al. Impact of depressive symptoms on adult asthma outcomes. *Ann Allergy Asthma Immunol* 2005;94:566–574.
19. Krommydas GC, Gourgoulianis KI, Angelopoulos NV, et al. Depression and pulmonary function in outpatients with asthma. *Respir Med* 2004;98:220–224.
20. Hayatbakhsh MR, Najman JM, Clavarino A, et al. Association of psychiatric disorders, asthma and lung function in early adulthood. *J Asthma* 2010;47:786–791.
21. Lavoie KL, Bacon SL, Barone S, et al. What is worse for asthma control and quality of life: Depressive disorders, anxiety disorders, or both? *Chest* 2006;130:1039–1047.
22. Walters P, Schofield P, Howard L, et al. The relationship between asthma and depression in primary care patients: A historical cohort and nested case control study. *PLoS ONE* 2011;6:e20750.
23. Kolbe J, Fergusson W, Vamos M, et al. Case-control study of severe life threatening asthma (SLTA) in adults: Psychological factors. *Thorax* 2002;57:317–322.
24. Sturdy PM, Victor CR, Anderson HR, et al. Psychological, social and health behaviour risk factors for deaths certified as asthma: A national case-control study. *Thorax* 2002;57:1034–1039.
25. Goodwin RD, Eaton WW. Asthma, suicidal ideation, and suicide attempts: Findings from the Baltimore epidemiologic catchment area follow-up. *Am J Public Health* 2005;95(4):717–722.
26. Kuo CJ, Chen VC, Lee WC, et al. Asthma and suicide mortality in young people: A 12-year follow-up study. *Am J Psychiat* 2010;167(9):1092–1099.
27. Goodwin R. Asthma and suicide: Current knowledge and future directions. *Curr Psychiat Rep* 2012;14:30–35.
28. Di Marco F, Verga M, Santus P, et al. Close correlation between anxiety, depression, and asthma control. *Respir Med* 2010;104:22–28.

29. Lavoie KL, Cartier A, Labrecque M, et al. Are psychiatric disorders associated with worse asthma control and quality of life in asthma patients? *Respir Med* 2005;99:1249–1257.

30. Strine TW, Mokdad AH, Balluz LS, et al. Impact of depression and anxiety on quality of life, health behaviors, and asthma control among adults in the United States with asthma, 2006. *J Asthma* 2008;45:123–133.

31. Trzcińska H, Przybylski G, Kozłowski B, et al. Analysis of the relation between level of asthma control and depression and anxiety. *Med Sci Monit* 2012;18:190–194.

32. Urrutia I, Aguirre U, Pascual S, et al. Impact of anxiety and depression on disease control and quality of life in asthma patients. *J Asthma* 2012;49:201–208.

33. Deshmukh VM, Toelle BG, Usherwood T, et al. The association of comorbid anxiety and depression with asthma-related quality of life and symptom perception in adults. *Respirology* 2008;13:695–702.

34. Chen E, Hermann C, Rodgers D, et al. Symptom perception in childhood asthma: The role of anxiety and asthma severity. *Health Psychol* 2006;25:389–395.

35. Van Peski-Oosterbaan AS, Spinhoven P, Van der Does AJ, et al. Is there a specific relationship between asthma and panic disorder? *Behav Res Ther* 1996;34:333–340.

36. Kullowatz A, Kanniess F, Dahme B, et al. Association of depression and anxiety with health care use and quality of life in asthma patients. *Respir Med* 2007;101:638–644.

37. Mancuso CA, Peterson MG, Charlson ME. Effects of depressive symptoms on health-related quality of life in asthma patients. *J Gen Intern Med* 2000;15:301–310.

38. McCauley E, Katon W, Russo J, et al. Impact of anxiety and depression on functional impairment in adolescents with asthma. *Gen Hosp Psychiat* 2007;29:214–222.

39. Dahlem NW, Kinsman RA, Horton DJ. Panic-fear in asthma: Requests for as-needed medications in relation to pulmonary function measurements. *J Allergy Clin Immunol* 1977;60:295–300.

40. Dirks JF, Kinsman RA, Horton DJ, et al. Panic-fear in asthma: Rehospitalization following intensive long-term treatment. *Psychosom Med* 1978;40:5–13.

41. Dirks JF, Kinsman RA, Jones NF, et al. Panic-fear: A personality dimension related to length of hospitalization in respiratory illness. *J Asthma Res* 1977;14:61–71.

42. Feldman JM, Siddique MI, Thompson NS, et al. The role of panic-fear in comorbid asthma and panic disorder. *J Anxiety Disord* 2009;23:178–184.

43. Ross CJ, Davis TM, MacDonald GF. Cognitive-behavioral treatment combined with asthma education for adults with asthma and coexisting panic disorder. *Clin Nurs Res* 2005;14:131–157.

44. Lehrer PM, Karavidas MK, Lu SE, et al. Psychological treatment of comorbid asthma and panic disorder: A pilot study. *J Anxiety Disord* 2008;22:671–683.

45. Parry GD, Cooper CL, Moore JM, et al. Cognitive behavioural intervention for adults with anxiety complications of asthma: Prospective randomised trial. *Respir Med* 2012;106(6):802–810.

46. McNally RJ. Anxiety sensitivity and panic disorder. *Biol Psychiat* 2002;52:938–946.

47. Zinbarg RE, Barlow DH, Brown TA. Hierarchical structure and general factor saturation of the Anxiety Sensitivity Index: Evidence and implications. *Psychol Assess* 1997;9:277–284.

48. Feldner MT, Zvolensky MJ, Schmidt NB, et al. A prospective test of anxiety sensitivity as a moderator of the relation between gender and posttraumatic symptom maintenance among high anxiety sensitive young adults. *Depress Anxiety* 2008;25:190–199.

49. Schmidt NB, Lerew DR, Jackson RJ. The role of anxiety sensitivity in the pathogenesis of panic: Prospective evaluation of spontaneous panic attacks during acute stress. *J Abnorm Psychol* 1997;106:355–364.

50. Carr RE, Lehrer PM, Hochron SM. Predictors of panic-fear in asthma. *Health Psychol* 1995;14:421–426.

51. Barone S, Bacon SL, Campbell TS, et al. The association between anxiety sensitivity and atopy in adult asthmatics. *J Behav Med* 2008;31:331–339.

52. McLeish AC, Zvolensky MJ, Luberto CM. The role of anxiety sensitivity in terms of asthma control: A pilot test among young adult asthmatics. *J Health Psychol* 2011;16:439–444.

53. Avallone KM, McLeish AC, Luberto CM, Bernstein JA. Anxiety sensitivity, asthma control, and quality of life in adults with asthma. *J Asthma* 2012;49:57–62.

54. Apter AJ, Affleck G, Reisine ST, et al. Perception of airway obstruction in asthma: Sequential daily analyses of symptoms, peak expiratory flow rate, and mood. *J Allergy Clin Immunol* 1997;99:605–612.

55. Zvolensky MJ, Yartz AR, Gregor K, et al. Interoceptive exposure-based cessation intervention for smokers high in anxiety sensitivity: A case series. *J Cogn Psychother* 2008;22:346–365.

56. Watson D, O'Hara MW, Simms LJ, et al. Development and validation of the Inventory of Depression and Anxiety Symptoms (IDAS). *Psychol Assess* 2007;19:253–268.

Section VII

Approach to Asthma Worldwide
and in the Primary Care Setting

27 Managing Asthma and Allergy
A Countrywide Approach to Integrating Care

Tari Haahtela

CONTENTS

SUMMARY

In Finland, a comprehensive and nationwide *Asthma Programme 1994–2004* was undertaken to improve asthma care and prevent the predicted increase in costs. The main goal was to lessen the burden of asthma on individuals and society. The program has been a success, which is attributed to early diagnosis, active anti-inflammatory treatment from the outset of disease, guided self-management, and effective networking with general practitioners, nurses, pharmacists, and nongovernmental organization (NGO) patient advocates (i.e., patient associations). The Finnish experience demonstrated that careful planning and simple interventions (i.e., defined goals and systematic follow-up), over a relatively short period of time, significantly reduced patient morbidity and the economic burden associated with asthma on society. The proper management of asthma involves all stakeholders, not just the patient. Most of the suffering due to asthma is unnecessary and considerable cost savings can be obtained if the best clinical practices are implemented in a systematic way. However, reducing the incidence of asthma remains a challenge. In the footsteps of the *Asthma Programme*, a new *Allergy Programme 2008–2018* is being implemented in Finland to extend the benefits of the Asthma Programme to other allergic conditions. The preliminary outcomes of this program, the purpose of which is to increase immunological tolerance by promoting both primary and secondary prevention, appear promising.

ASTHMA BURDEN

Asthma is an important public health issue and causes significant suffering and disability resulting in increased healthcare costs.

The scale of the asthma and allergy epidemic around the world is tremendous. The number of patients suffering from asthma has doubled over the past 10 years. The World Health Organization (WHO) estimates that 300 million people around the world are affected by this disease and its incidence is still rising; it is projected to afflict 100 million patients by 2025.

Approximately 250,000 people are estimated to die prematurely each year as a result of asthma,[1,2] although overall mortality rates have fallen since the 1980s.[1] Although asthma deaths represent only the tip of the asthma burden pyramid (Figure 27.1), they reflect the overall lack of efficacy and organization of treating patients. It is the author's conservative estimate that in the European Union at least 2 million hospital days have been allocated for acute asthma treatment. No estimate exists for emergency room visit numbers.

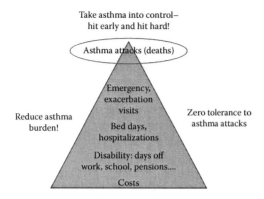

FIGURE 27.1 Asthma deaths comprise only the very top of the asthma burden pyramid.

Not surprisingly, asthma is associated with enormous health-care expenditures. Almost 10 years ago the annual asthma-related costs in the EU amounted to €18 billion, while the estimated loss of productivity was approximately €10 billion per year. A systematic review showed that despite the availability of effective therapies, the costs of treating asthma are increasing.[3]

FAILURES AND PITFALLS OF TREATMENT

Asthma usually responds well to appropriate medication. The treatment of choice for asthma is inhaled corticosteroids (ICSs), which control airway inflammation and relieve bronchoconstriction. If optimally utilized, mortality in asthma could be almost abolished and hospital days reduced significantly.

Why treatment still fails far too often is still unclear. From the public health perspective, the key issue is to implement the best standards of care in everyday practice. Effective implementation requires networking with general practitioners (GPs), nurses, pharmacists, and patient advocacy organizations. Family doctors, primary care physicians, and pediatricians are usually the patient's first contact with health care and therefore play a vital role in the early diagnosis and introduction of appropriate treatment.[4] All health-care professionals should be aware of the excellent possibilities of significantly improving asthma outcomes.

There are numerous national and international guidelines for the evaluation, management, and treatment of asthma. However, the critical charge is to effectively implement these recommendations into practice. While evidence-based medicine (EBM) is an important tool, it is used retrospectively; what is needed is an approach that allows the doctor to currently treat a patient and plan for future treatment. A system is needed to adapt EBM guidelines sensibly to individual patient care. They are not army rules that can be applied to everyone!

Individual patients should be educated to understand their disease and provided with tools for self-management. *Guided self-management* is the key to proactively prevent attacks and exacerbations, which cause the most trouble and costs (Figure 27.2). A concept of mini-attacks could be adapted:

every time the patient needs a short (rapid)-acting beta$_2$-adrenergic agonist (SABA) for breathlessness, it is a *mini-attack*! The patient should know what to do when the need for treatment is increasing.

Patients only take 30%–40% of their prescribed doses of inhaled medication.[5] For tablets the adherence is 60%–70%.[5] Inhalation technique is inadequate in at least 50% of patients, and should be taught properly at the first opportunity and checked regularly.

At the population level, most asthma (70%–80%) is intermittent or mild, and the treatment is relatively simple [reference needed]. More clinical studies should be done at the mild end of the asthma spectrum to guide for proper treatment strategies. Intermittent asthma could be treated intermittently; persistent disease needs regular maintenance medication.

In creating clinically relevant treatment strategies, we should realize that most asthma drug studies have been performed in patients with moderately persistent asthma in order to show differences between drugs. The results have often been carelessly generalized to the asthmatic population in general; when strictly speaking they are applicable only to those fulfilling the study-specific inclusion and exclusion criteria. We need better evidence for different treatment approaches in *real-life* situations, especially for patients at the mild end of the severity spectrum.[6]

Patients with moderate to severe asthma should be carefully monitored, because they are most at risk of the need for future emergency treatment, long-term lung function decline, and increased health-care utilization costs. The problem is often that insufficient anti-inflammatory treatment is prescribed, and that patients rely too much on symptomatic beta$_2$-agonist use. The global guidelines (GINA) had the foresight to focus on and emphasize the need for *asthma control* in 2006. If control is inadequate, the anti-inflammatory treatment needs optimization, and the clinician needs to ask some questions such as: Is the patient really taking it? Is the inhalation technique correct? Does the patient need more effective anti-inflammatory medication or higher doses? Is there something in the medication that, in fact, worsens asthma control (such as regular use of high doses of beta$_2$-agonists, or nonselective beta-blockers for cardiovascular problems).

First-line, early, and effective use of ICSs has revolutionized asthma treatment. However it is unknown whether ICSs prevent lung function decline (measured by FEV_1), which may take place over the years in moderate to severe asthma and is caused by permanent structural changes of the airway wall (remodeling). In other words, do ICSs have the potential to change the natural course of asthma? The first study that suggested this may be the case was Haahtela et al.,[7] and 10-year observational data from Denmark seem to confirm this.[8] Busse et al.[9] and O'Byrne et al.[10] also showed that severe asthma exacerbations are associated with a more rapid decline in lung function, and maintenance treatment with low doses of ICSs prevents severe asthma-related events and attenuates lung function decline. The question, however, remains open.

Adult asthma control

Card/stamp + net/mobile-version

Doctor-nurse-pharmacist   Patient-guided self-management

Ask patient-is he/she doing   OK?   Notice symptom increase   YES

1. Reliever max 2 dose/wk   ☐   1. Needing more reliever?   ☐

2. Symptoms max 2 day/wk   ☐   2. Feeling cold, flu?   ☐

3. Symptoms max 1 night/wk   ☐   3. Coughing ▲Wheezing▲   ☐

4. No activity restrictions   ☐   4. Exercise tolerance▼   ☐

5. PEF-var.max 50 l/min/wk   ☐   5. Morning-PEF▼   ☐

                                              ▶ PEF-decreases from ___ to ___

Ask yourself-is the treatment   OK?   Stop attack (exacerbation)

1. Reliever need minimal   ☐   1. Increase controller 2–4 fold (2–4 wk),
                                                 or start a course of controller (4 wk)   ☐

2. Controller dose adequate   ☐   2. Start to use reliever regularily (2–4 wk) ☐

3. Adherent to treatment   ☐   3. If on Combi, double the dose (2 wk)   ☐

4. Correct inhalation   ☐   4. Prednisolon tabl. 20 mg/day (1–2 wk)   ☐

5. Exacerbation plan exists   ☐   5. Go to emergency, if no help   ☐

▶ Good morning PEF_____   6. Later, check controller treatment ☐

Doctor/nurse uses the check-list to assure asthma control, and guide the patient to self-management.

Zero tolerance to asthma attacks

FIGURE 27.2 Example of guided self-management in adult asthma. Key questions for family doctors and nurses to find out disease control (*left*). Key points for the patient to notice symptom increase and stop exacerbation proactively (*right*). (From Haahtela, T., Tuomisto, L.E., Pietinalho, A., Klaukka, T., Erhola, M., Kaila, M., Nieminen, M.M., Kontula, E., Laitinen, L.A., *Thorax*, 61, 663–670, 2006.)

At the population level, most asthma is intermittent or mild and relatively easy to control. These patients do not face any clinically significant lung function loss over time, whatever the treatment. Nevertheless, the ICS-responsive inflammatory changes seem to be present even in the mildest forms of asthma, or even in patients with asthma-like symptoms (or pre-asthma).[6] Therefore, these patients should be prescribed anti-inflammatory or controller treatment rather than beta$_2$-agonists alone.[11] It is also evident that many adults and children with mild forms of disease can cope with intermittent rather than continuous treatment.[12,13] In these patients, the effect of ICSs on lung function is difficult or even impossible to verify.

It is increasingly clear that genetic polymorphism affects individual patients' responses to drugs. While many patients respond to low doses of ICSs, there are patients who need high doses and do not demonstrate the expected clinical result. True corticosteroid resistance is very rare; however, if the patient has comorbidities like chronic obstructive pulmonary disease (COPD), the ICS effect may only be modest. About 80% of patients do benefit from leukotriene antagonists (LTRAs), but 20% do not. After an initial trial of therapy (1–3 months), the drug should be dropped if no obvious improvement is observed. LTRAs are anti-inflammatory and may control mild asthma alone and more severe disease combined with ICSs. LTRAs are quite free from side effects.

Beta$_2$-receptor tolerance develops early, during the first few weeks of treatment, in a marked proportion of asthmatics. Often this is relatively harmless, if ICSs are used at the same time. However, some of these patients may deteriorate with regular high-dose long-acting beta$_2$-adrenergic agonists (LABAs). Rapid-acting beta$_2$-agonists are essential for rescue use, but fixed combinations of ICSs and LABAs are increasingly used in maintenance treatment of all asthma whether mild or severe. The combination preparations have, indeed, decreased exacerbations in specified patient groups.[14,15] LABAs do not, however, tackle the inflammation, and regular administration causes tachyphylaxis,[16] which means a reduced preventive effect on exercise-induced bronchoconstriction as well as reduced bronchodilator effect.[17] LABAs should be introduced for long-term maintenance only after some thought, and always concomitantly with ICSs in patients who are not controlled with anti-inflammatory treatment alone. While patients should not be undertreated, which is still commonplace, there is an emerging problem due to overtreatment.[18]

It is conceivable that in the not-too-distant future, pharmacogenomics will provide clinicians with affordable genetic tests that may predict drug response and especially explain failures. (See Chapter 3 to read further on this exciting concept.)

THE FINNISH INITIATIVE

A national asthma implementation program was undertaken in Finland in 1994–2004 (population 5.4 million).[19–21] Of particular importance for the development of asthma care in Finland was the new knowledge starting to evolve from the mid-1980s onward that asthma was primarily an inflammatory disease.[22] Early and precise diagnosis of patients with respiratory symptoms suggestive of asthma was emphasized, and anti-inflammatory medication with ICSs was introduced as first-line treatment.[23] The program focused on early diagnosis, active anti-inflammatory treatment from the outset, guided self-management, and effective networking with GPs and pharmacists.

The new knowledge about asthma was rapidly and consistently implemented in general clinical practice through a nationwide program initiated by the Ministry of Health and Social Welfare.[19] Strategic information, education, and effective networking with different stakeholders were key to the successful implementation of this project (Figure 27.3).

Cooperation between primary care physicians, nurses, physiotherapists, pharmacists, and the pharmaceutical industry, the latter being involved mainly in the production of approved educational information material, resulted in a rapid breakthrough, which was achieved at a relatively low cost.

A major contributing factor was that many of the studies resulting in the new understanding of asthma had been performed "at home" by Finnish investigators.

GOALS: SIMPLE AND MEASURABLE

Five specific goals were set. For example, two goals were decreasing the number of hospital days caused by asthma by 50% and reducing the annual cost related to treating asthma per patient by 50% (see Box 27.1). The program comprised both evidence-based management guidelines, available to GPs and nurses via the Internet since 2000, and an action plan with defined tools to achieve the goals.

The action plan focused on implementation of new diagnostic and treatment strategies, especially for primary care. At that time the new medical knowledge was, "Asthma is an inflammatory disease and should be treated as such from the very beginning." The key to implementation was the presence

---

BOX 27.1   ASTHMA PROGRAM 1994–2004 GOALS

1. Patients with early asthma recover.
2. Patients feel well (QoL), and lung function and capacity for work correspond to age.
3. Percentage of patients with severe and moderate asthma falls from 40% to 20% (asthma barometer).
4. Number of bed days of asthma decreases by 50%, to 50,000 a year.
5. Annual costs per patient fall by 50% with more effective preventive treatment.

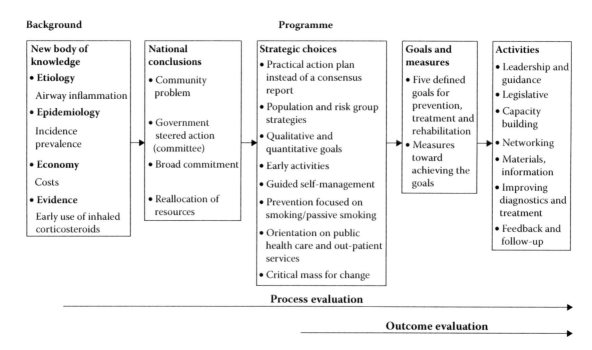

FIGURE 27.3   Finnish Asthma Program 1994–2004. Flowchart of strategic planning. (From Haahtela, T., Laitinen, L.A., *Clin. Exp. Allergy*, 26, 1–24, 1996.)

of an effective network of asthma-responsible professionals and development of an evaluation strategy. In 1997, Finnish pharmacies were included in the *Pharmacy Program*, and in 2002 a *Childhood Asthma Mini-Program* was launched to address the special needs of small children.

RESULTS: THE BURDEN OF ASTHMA HAS DECREASED

As a result of this comprehensive program, the burden of asthma in Finland has decreased considerably.[20,21] Key indicators have fallen significantly: the number of hospital days reduced by 86% from around 110,000 (1993) to 15,000 (2010) and disability pensions reduced by 76% from 1993 to 2003. In recent years, only a few asthma deaths per year under the age of 65 have been recorded. In young age groups there is virtually no asthma mortality. Medicine use, especially early use of ICSs to deal with the airway inflammatory process, had increased by 75% during the early years of the Program (1994–1999).

COSTS ARE DOWN FOR PATIENTS AND SOCIETY

In spite of the still slightly increasing prevalence of asthma, the overall costs related to asthma (compensation for disability, medicines, hospital care, and outpatient doctor visits) have leveled off and started to decrease.[21,24] This has been in stark contrast to what was predicted. The overall cost of treating asthma in 1993 was approximately $US446 million, including loss of productivity. By 2010, this figure had dropped to $US360 million. The total asthma costs in 2010 (health-care, drugs, disability and production loss) were predicted to vary from $US783 million (minimum scenario) to $US1253 million (maximum scenario). The cost prediction is a theoretical model, but shows the enormous potential of cost savings by improving treatment. The estimate of the potential savings for the year 2010 alone was $US423–893 million, depending on the scenario used.

Annual costs per patient attributable to asthma have been reduced by more than 50%. The extra costs of planning and implementing the program have been relatively small, primarily because most of the activities were carried out as part of the routine work of the clinicians and administrators.

PATIENT BENEFITS: EARLY DETECTION, TIMELY TREATMENT

For the patient, the main improvement has been early detection of the disease and its timely treatment: "Hit early and hit hard!" Patients with chronic asthma have been educated to employ *guided self-management*, an approach that encourages them to be proactive in stopping asthma attacks (Figure 27.2). Effective *networking* of specialists with asthma-responsible GPs (n = 200), asthma nurses (n = 700), and asthma-responsible pharmacists (n = 700) has also considerably improved overall asthma awareness and care in Finland. Patients are definitely doing better; for example, there has been a reduction of almost 80% over the past 10 years in the number of asthma patients receiving disability pensions.

OTHER COUNTRIES: SAME SUCCESS

In other countries, similarly defined asthma programs have been shown to be cost-effective, have been associated with a gain in quality-adjusted life years (QALY),[25,26] and have resulted in improvements in quality of life, asthma symptoms, and lung function at lower costs compared with usual care.[27,28]

The results from Finland and other countries do not leave much room for argument. The programs have not been able to halt the continuing rise in asthma incidence, but have markedly reduced mortality, hospital days, and disability. Asthma programs or campaigns in Australia,[29] Poland,[30,31] Japan,[32] Brazil,[33,34] Canada,[35] Singapore,[36] and Tonga,[37] just to mention a few, have considerably reduced the burden of asthma over the last 10 years.

EXPANDING TO ALL ALLERGIC CONDITIONS

Following in the footsteps of the Asthma Program, the *Finnish Allergy Program 2008–2018* was recently launched to combat the allergy epidemic.[38,39] This new initiative, which included asthma, was developed to expand the excellent asthma results to all other allergic conditions, with emphasis on changing the management approach to focus on prevention as well as treatment. The long-term aim of this extended program was to decrease the incidence of asthma and allergies.

The Finnish initiative is a comprehensive plan designed to change the course of allergy in society. This was launched to increase both immunological and psychological tolerance and to change attitudes to support health, not just allergy. Allergy health emphasizes that those with allergic symptoms should not be prevented from living a normal life. For severe allergies, *early and effective treatment* is strongly emphasized. *Guided self-management* is again the key to stopping attacks proactively.

NEW KNOWLEDGE: A PREREQUISITE TO MOTIVATION

The prevalence of allergic diseases has grown in Finland during the past 50 years, similarly to what has been observed for many other industrialized and urbanized countries. Although the origin of allergy remains unresolved, an increasing body of evidence indicates that modern man living in an urban built environment is deprived of environmental protective factors (e.g., soil microorganisms) that are fundamental for normal tolerance development. Reduced contact with natural, biodiverse environments may adversely affect the human commensal microbiota and its immunomodulatory capacity. Recent results from North Karelian teenagers have prompted the so-called *biodiversity hypothesis*, which expands the well known "hygiene and microbial deprivation" hypotheses by taking into account the interrelationships of three DNA compartments: human cells, skin-mucosal microbiomes, and environmental microbiomes.[40–42]

The current dogma of allergen avoidance has not proved effective in halting the "allergy epidemic," although allergen avoidance is, and will remain, a cornerstone in the treatment armamentarium of allergic patients. It is the Finnish consensus that restoring and strengthening *tolerance* is the key to a balanced immune system and should be a focus of research in the future (Box 27.2). Understanding the mechanisms of tolerance will serve to pave the way from the central emphasis on treatment to prevention and improved public health.

BOX 27.2 PRACTICAL ADVICE FOR PROFESSIONALS TO HELP PATIENTS BUILD UP AND IMPROVE IMMUNE TOLERANCE AND PREVENT AND TREAT INFLAMMATION

Primary prevention

- Support breastfeeding. Solid foods from 4–6 months.
- Do not avoid environmental exposure unnecessarily (e.g., foods, pets).
- Strengthen immunity by increasing connection to natural environments.
- Strengthen immunity by regular physical exercise.
- Strengthen immunity by healthy diet (e.g., traditional Mediterranean or Baltic type).
- Use antibiotics with care. Majority of microbes are useful and support health.
- Probiotic bacteria in fermented food or other preparations may strengthen immunity.
- Do not smoke.

Secondary (tertiary) prevention

- Regular physical exercise is anti-inflammatory.
- Healthy diet is anti-inflammatory (Mediterranean- or Baltic-type diet improves asthma control).
- Fermented food or other preparations, including probiotic bacteria, are anti-inflammatory.
- Allergen-specific immunotherapy:
  - Allergens as is (foods)
  - Sublingual tablets or drops (e.g., timothy, birch pollen, mites?)
  - Subcutaneous injections.
- Hit early and hit hard respiratory/skin inflammation with anti-inflammatory medication. Find maintenance treatment for long-term control.
- Do not smoke.

(From Haahtela, T., von Hertzen, L., Mäkelä, M.J., and Hannuksela, N., *Allergy*, 63, 634–645, 2008).

INSPIRING GOALS

The 10-year implementation program aims to reduce the burden of allergies at both the individual and societal levels.

Allergy Program goals:

1. Prevent the development of allergic symptoms
2. Increase tolerance against allergens
3. Improve diagnostic quality
4. Decrease work-related allergies
5. Allocate resources to manage and prevent asthma and allergy attacks
6. Decrease costs due to allergic diseases

The goals are also numeric if the program is successful, for example, asthma emergency visits should drop 40% in 10 years.

DEFINED METHODS

For each goal, specific tasks, tools, and evaluation methods have been defined. We have developed tools for practical implementation for *childhood allergies*.[43,44] Mild allergic symptoms are common and should not be treated unnecessarily. Mild allergy is not predestined to become more severe in time and outcomes are generally favorable.[45]

Severe forms of allergy require specific focus. To help patients proactively stop allergic reactions and exacerbations, simple self-management plans have been launched for allergic rhinitis, anaphylaxis, asthma, asthma in small children, atopic eczema, food allergy, and urticaria. Patients are trained in self-management. Disease control is strongly emphasized and education is provided for both health-care personnel and patients. Allergic inflammation in asthma, atopic dermatitis, and rhinitis are treated most effectively very early on in the course of illness.[46] The importance of patient follow-up and long-term maintenance therapy is stressed. For children with mild persistent asthma (the majority!), a strategy of intermittent (periodic) treatment has been developed.[47]

Immunotherapy and especially sublingual immunotherapy (SLIT) are advocated where feasible. Food allergy diets are critically reevaluated and stopped if possible. Specific oral tolerance induction (SOTI) for milk, wheat, and peanuts has been studied intensively and employed increasingly in clinical practice.[48] Long avoidance lists of allergens or irritants have been eliminated. Avoidance must be based on proper diagnostic work-up and recommendations must be precise regarding what should be avoided and for how long. In patients with troublesome food allergies, a clear shift from passive avoidance to active treatment has been taken.

Nationwide implementation acts through the network of local public health coordinators (GPs, nurses, pharmacists). In addition, three NGOs started a 5-year project in 2011 to implement these new recommendations among allergic people and the general public.

All 21 central hospital districts are currently carrying out a three-step educational process:

- Two-hour program launch sessions for opinion leaders, coordinators, and educators of NGOs
- Educational sessions in large health center
- One-day courses in central hospitals for local health-care personnel

During 2008–2013, the Finnish Lung Health Association (Filha) organized 200 educational events with 12,000 participants (25% physicians, 50% nurses, 10% pharmacists, 15% others). The main themes were the allergy–healthy child, anaphylaxis, food allergy, improving tolerance, and asthma. Fifteen allergy-testing centers have been audited for good diagnostic practice and, if approved, are given a certificate.

Outcomes and Preliminary Results

For outcome evaluation, repeated surveys are performed and health-care registers employed at the beginning, at 5 years, and at the end of the program. The messages of the program have been well received by health-care personnel, and attitudes are changing. For example, GPs scored the message of improving tolerance 9.1 on a scale 4–10. In an Internet-based Gallup survey, allergic people gave the best score to the message "support health, not allergy," and only 12% agreed with the claim "avoidance is the best strategy to combat allergy."

The preliminary results are promising. Emergency visits and hospital days caused by asthma are in steady decline (54% during the last 10 years), but to reduce them further perhaps requires an approach that targets at-risk groups.[49] For example, small children and women over 60 years of age could be our focus for further intervention.

Anaphylaxis emergency visits have increased, which may have resulted from improved education and awareness. Asthma and anaphylaxis visits vary considerably between different regions of the country, which is probably a reflection of variable health-care practices rather than true differences in occurrence. Asthma seems to have become a milder disease, or better controlled, according to a pharmacy barometer survey: 10% of asthmatics evaluated their disease as severe in 2001, while the corresponding figure was 4% in 2010.[50]

Several health-care indicators are demonstrating that the allergy burden is leveling off in Finland and even decreasing.

Cooperation Both Nationally and Internationally

The Finnish program, or parts of it, is associated with the World Allergy Organization (WAO),[51] Global Initiative for Asthma (GINA),[52] and WHO/GARD (Global Alliance against Chronic Respiratory Diseases). The program has been developed further and enlarged along with a European Union-funded project: Mechanisms of Development of Allergy (MeDALL).[53] A Norwegian Allergy Program is being developed and, together with the Finnish one, will provide a model for others to modify and improve their programs to meet their special needs.

The key messages

- Endorse health, not allergy.
- Strengthen tolerance.
- Adopt a new attitude to allergy. Avoid allergens, only if mandatory.
- Recognize and treat severe allergies early. Prevent attacks.
- Improve air quality. Stop smoking.

STOP ASTHMA DEATHS

It is time to halt asthma attacks and stop deaths. In Finland (population 5.4 million), only a few asthma deaths are registered annually in the population under the age of 65 years. However every asthma death is an accident and potentially preventable. Overall asthma severity determines the attack risk, and a new classification for severity has been published.[54] Simple tools for clinical work are needed. WHO has a performance score from 0 to 5 for cancer patients.[55] This idea could be modified for asthma based on symptoms, disability, and medication (Table 27.1). The suggested classification is tentative and calls for validation.

GINA has put forward a 5-year challenge to reduce hospitalizations for asthma attacks by 50%.[56] GARD provides an ideal framework to work toward this goal.[57]

WHAT HAVE WE LEARNED?

Reduction of the asthma burden is relatively simple, if the best clinical practices are employed. Effective medication exists, especially ICSs and combination products of ICSs and LABAs. Recently, asthma projects and programs in Argentina, Australia, Brazil, China, Japan, Mexico, the Philippines, Russia, South Africa, and Turkey were discussed by a group of asthma care experts who are part of

---

TABLE 27.1

Asthma Performance (AP) Score for Health-Care Providers

0—*No symptoms.* No medication. Fully active and able to carry on predisease activities without restriction.

1—*Symptoms but not disabled.* Occasional symptoms and medication. Not restricted in normal activities (e.g., housework, office work, play).

2—*Symptoms and mildly disabled.* Symptoms every week and more regular medication. Occasionally restricted in normal activities.

3—*Symptoms and moderately disabled.* Symptoms on most days and regular medication. Restricted in normal activities.

4—*Symptoms and severely disabled.* Continuous symptoms. Regular medication with several drugs. Difficult to carry on self-care.

5—*Symptoms life-threatening.* Immediate emergency treatment needed.

Notes: Scale from no symptoms = 0 to life-threatening symptoms = 5. The AP score can help to transfer information between health-care providers and patients and improve communication of asthma severity. The performance scores have not been validated as such.

the Advancing Asthma Care Network.[58] The expert group concluded that the major barriers for a successful program are low rates of dissemination and implementation of treatment guidelines; low levels of continuing medical education and training of primary health-care professionals; and poor access to and distribution of ICSs. In countries with less well developed asthma programs, underdiagnosis and undertreatment further limit the success.

For all allergic conditions, where prevalence of allergic individuals is rising in the rapidly urbanizing populations, it is time to reevaluate the paradigm and implement new types of interventions.[51] National and local action plans that have been demonstrated to work, with clear targets and defined tools, are needed to meet the challenge.[59] Allergy is a community problem requiring community actions. Interesting examples are the Finnish and Korean[60] initiatives, where multisector cooperation is taking place (government, academic institutions, private organizations, local communities, media) to tackle the asthma and allergy burden.

REFERENCES

1. Bousquet J, Khaltaev N. *Global Surveillance, Prevention and Control of Chronic Respiratory Diseases: A Comprehensive Approach*. World Health Organization, Geneva, 2007.
2. Bousquet J, Burney PG, Zuberbier T, Cauwenberge PV, Akdis CA, Bindslev-Jensen C, Bonini S, et al. GA2LEN (Global Allergy and Asthma European Network) addresses the allergy and asthma "epidemic." *Allergy* 2009;64:969–977.
3. Bahadori K, Doyle-Waters MM, Marra C, Lynd L, Alasaly K, Swiston J, FitzGerald JM. Economic burden of asthma: A systematic review. *BMC Pulm Med* 2009;9:24.
4. van Weel C, Bateman ED, Bousquet J, Reid J, Grouse L, Schermer T, Valovirta E, Zhong N. Asthma management pocket reference 2008. *Allergy* 2008;63:997–1004.
5. Jones C, Santanello NC, Boccuzzi SJ, Wogen J, Strub P, Nelsen LM. Adherence to prescribed treatment for asthma: Evidence from pharmacy benefits data. J Asthma 2003;40:93–101.
6. Rytilä P, Metso T, Heikkinen K, Saarelainen P, Helenius IJ, Haahtela T. Airway inflammation in patients with symptoms suggesting asthma but with normal lung function. *Eur Respir J* 2000;16:824–830.
7. Haahtela T, Järvinen M, Kava T, Kiviranta K, Koskinen S, Lehtonen K, Nikander K, et al. Effects of reducing or discontinuing inhaled budesonide in patients with mild asthma. *N Engl J Med* 1994;331:700–705.
8. Lange P, Scharling H, Ulrik CS, Vestbo J. Inhaled corticosteroids and decline of lung function in community residents with asthma. *Thorax* 2006;61(2):100–104.
9. Busse WW, Pedersen S, Pauwels RA, Tan WC, Chen YZ, Lamm CJ, O'Byrne PM; START Investigators Group. The Inhaled Steroid Treatment As Regular Therapy in Early Asthma (START) study 5-year follow-up: Effectiveness of early intervention with budesonide in mild persistent asthma. *J Allergy Clin Immunol* 2008;121:1167–1174.
10. O'Byrne PM, Pedersen S, Lamm CJ, Tan WC, Busse WW; START Investigators Group. Severe exacerbations and decline in lung function in asthma. *Am J Respir Crit Care Med* 2009;179(1):19–24.
11. Haahtela T, Tamminen K, Malmberg LP, Zetterström O, Karjalainen J, Ylä-Outinen H, Svahn T, Ekström T, Selroos O. Formoterol as needed with or without budesonide in patients with intermittent asthma and raised NO levels in exhaled air: A SOMA study. *Eur Respir J* 2006;28:748–755.
12. Boushey HA, Sorkness CA, King TS, Sullivan SD, Fahy JV, Lazarus SC, Chinchilli VM, et al. Daily versus as-needed corticosteroids for mild persistent asthma. *N Engl J Med* 2005;352(15):1519–1528.
13. Turpeinen M, Nikander K, Pelkonen A, Syvänen P, Sorva R, Raitio H, Malmberg P, Juntunen-Backman K, Haahtela T. Daily versus as-needed inhaled corticosteroid for mild persistent asthma. The Helsinki early intervention childhood asthma study. *Arch Dis Child* 2008;93:654–659.
14. Pauwels RA, Löfdahl CG, Postma DS, Tattersfield AE, O'Byrne P, Barnes PJ, Ullman A. Effect of inhaled formoterol and budesonide on exacerbations of asthma. Formoterol and Corticosteroids Establishing Therapy (FACET) International Study Group. *N Engl J Med* 1997;337:1405–1411.
15. Bateman ED, Boushey HA, Bousquet J, Busse WW, Clark TJ, Pauwels RA, Pedersen SE; GOAL Investigators Group. Can guideline-defined asthma control be achieved? The Gaining Optimal Asthma ControL study. *Am J Respir Crit Care Med* 2004;170(8):836–844.
16. Hancox RJ, Anderson SD. Current issues with beta-2-adrenoceptor agonists. *Clin Rev Allergy Immunol* 2006;31:1–295.
17. van der Woude HJ, Winter TH, Aalbers R. Decreased bronchodilating effect of salbutamol in relieving methacholine induced moderate to severe bronchoconstriction during high dose treatment with long acting beta2 agonists. *Thorax* 2001;56(7):529–535.
18. Caudri D, Wijga AH, Smit HA, Koppelman GH, Kerkhof M, Hoekstra MO, Brunekreef B, de Jongste JC. Asthma symptoms and medication in the PIAMA birth cohort: Evidence for under and overtreatment. *Pediatr Allergy Immunol* 2011;22:652–659.
19. Haahtela T, Laitinen LA. Asthma Programme in Finland 1994–2004. *Clin Exp Allergy* 1996;26(Suppl. 1):1–24.
20. Haahtela T, Klaukka T, Koskela K, Erhola M, Laitinen L. Asthma programme in Finland: A community problems needs community solutions. *Thorax* 2001;56:806–814.
21. Haahtela T, Tuomisto LE, Pietinalho A, Klaukka T, Erhola M, Kaila M, Nieminen MM, Kontula E, Laitinen LA. A 10 year asthma programme in Finland: Major change for the better. *Thorax* 2006;61:663–670.
22. Laitinen LA, Heino M, Laitinen A, Kava T, Haahtela T. Damage of the airway epithelium and bronchial reactivity in patients with asthma. *Am Rev Respir Dis* 1985;131:599–606.
23. Haahtela T, Järvinen M, Kava T, Kiviranta K, Koskinen S, Lehtonen K, Nikander K, et al. Comparison of a B2-agonist, terbutaline, with an inhaled corticosteroid, budesonide in newly detected asthma. *N Engl J Med* 1991;325:388–392.
24. Reissell E, Herse F, Väänänen J, Karjalainen J, Klaukka T, Haahtela T. Asthma costs in Finland. A public health model to indicate cost effectiveness during 20 years. *Finn Med J* 2010;9:811–816 (in Finnish with English summary).
25. Schermer TR, Thoonen BP, van den Boom G, Akkermans RP, Grol RP, Folgering HT, van Weel C, van Schayck CP. Randomized controlled economic evaluation of asthma self-management in primary health care. *Am J Respir Crit Care Med* 2002;166:1062–1072.
26. Steuten L, Palmer S, Vrijhoef B, van Merode F, Spreeuwenberg C, Severens H. Cost-utility of a disease management program for patients with asthma. *Int J Technol Assess Health Care* 2007;23:184–191.

27. Petro W, Schulenburg JM, Greiner W, Weithase J, Schülke A, Metzdorf N. Efficacy of a disease management programme in asthma. *Pneumologie* 2005;59:101–107.

28. Plaza V, Cobos A, Ignacio-García JM, Molina J, Bergoñón S, García-Alonso F, Espinosa C; Grupo Investigador AsmaCare. Cost-effectiveness of an intervention based on the Global Initiative for Asthma (GINA) recommendations using a computerized clinical decision support system: A physicians randomized trial. *Med Clin (Barc)* 2005;124:201–206.

29. McCaul KA, Wakefield MA, Roder DM, Ruffin RE, Heard AR, Alpers JH, Staugas RE. Trends in hospital readmission for asthma: Has the Australian National Asthma Campaign had an effect? *Med J Aust* 2000;172:62–66.

30. Stelmach W, Majak P, Jerzynska J, Stelmach I. Early effects of Asthma Prevention Program on asthma diagnosis and hospitalization in urban population of Poland. *Allergy* 2005;60:606–610.

31. Kuna P, Kupczyk M, Kupryś-Lipińska I. POLASTMA: National Programme of Elary Diagnostics and Treatment of Asthma. ISBN 978-83-929380-1-9, 2009, http://www.mojaastma.org.pl/files/polastma_en.pdf.

32. Adachi M, Ohta K, Morikawa A, Nishima S, Tokunaga S, Disantostefano RL. Changes in asthma insights and reality in Japan (AIRJ) in 2005 since 2000. *Arerugi* 2008;57:107–120.

33. Franco R, Santos AC, Nascimento HF, Souza-Machado C, Ponte E, Souza-Machado A, Loureiro S, Barreto ML, Rodrigues LC, Cruz AA. Cost-effectiveness analysis of a state funded programme for control of severe asthma. *BMC Public Health* 2007; 7:82–89.

34. Souza-Machado C, Souza-Machado A, Franco R, Ponte EV, Barreto ML, Rodrigues LC, Bousquet J, Cruz AA. Rapid reduction in hospitalizations after an intervention to manage severe asthma. *Eur Respir J* 2010;35:515–521.

35. Boulet LP, Dorval E, Labrecque M, Turgeon M, Montague T, Thivierge RL. Towards Excellence in Asthma Management: Final report of an eight-year program aimed at reducing care gaps in asthma management in Quebec. *Can Respir J* 2008;15(6):302–310. Review.

36. Chong PN, Tan NC, Lim TK. Impact of the Singapore National Asthma Program (SNAP) on preventor-reliever prescription ratio in polyclinics. *Ann Acad Med Singap* 2008;37:114–117.

37. Foliaki S, Fakakovikaetau T, D'Souza W, Latu S, Tutone V, Cheng S, Pearce N. Reduction in asthma morbidity following a community-based asthma self-management programme in Tonga. *Int J Tuberc Lung Dis* 2009;13:142–147.

38. Haahtela T, von Hertzen L, Mäkelä MJ, Hannuksela N, Allergy Programme Working Group. Finnish Allergy Programme 2008–2018: Time to act and change the course. *Allergy* 2008;63:634–645.

39. von Hertzen L, Savolainen J, Hannuksela M, Klaukka T, Lauerma A, Klaukka T, Pekkanen J, et al. Scientific rational for the Finnish Allergy Programme 2008–2018: Emphasis on prevention and endorsing tolerance. *Allergy* 2009;64:678–701.

40. Laatikainen T, von Hertzen L, Koskinen JP, Mäkelä MJ, Jousilahti P, Kosunen TU, Vlasoff T, Ahlström M, Vartiainen E, Haahtela T. Allergy gap between Finnish and Russian Karelia on increase. *Allergy* 2011;66:886–892.

41. von Hertzen L, Hanski I, Haahtela T. Natural immunity. Biodiversity loss and inflammatory diseases are two global megatrends that might be related. *EMBO Rep* 2011;12:1089–1093.

42. Hanski I, von Hertzen L, Fyhrqvist N, Koskinen K, Torppa K, Laatikainen T, Karisola P, et al. Environmental biodiversity, human microbiota and allergy are interrelated. *Proc Natl Acad Sci U S A* 2012;109:8334–8339.

43. Pelkonen AS, Kuitunen M, Dunder T, Reijonen T, Valovirta E, Mäkelä MJ, Finnish Allergy Programme. Allergy in children: Practical recommendations of the Finnish Allergy Programme 2008–2018 for prevention, diagnosis, and treatment. *Pediatr Allergy Immunol* 2012;23:103–116.

44. Mäkelä MJ, Pelkonen A, Valovirta E, Haahtela T. The challenge of relaying the right public health message in allergy. *Pediatr Allergy Immunol* 2012;23:102.

45. Teppo H, Revonta M, Haahtela T. Allergic rhinitis and asthma have generally good outcome and little effect on quality of life: A 10-year follow-up. *Allergy* 2011;66:1123–1125.

46. Reitamo S, Remitz A, Haahtela T. Hit early and hit hard in atopic dermatitis and not only in asthma. *Allergy* 2009;64:503–504.

47. Turpeinen M, Pelkonen A, Selroos O, Nikander K, Haahtela T. Continuous versus intermittent inhaled corticosteroid (budesonide) for mild persistent asthma in children—Not too much, not too little. *Thorax* 2012;67:100–102.

48. Mäkelä M, Kulmala P, Pelkonen AS, Remes S, Kuitunen M. Food hyposensitization: New approach and treatment for food allergies. *Duodecim* 2011;127:1263–1271 (in Finnish).

49. Kauppi P, Linna M, Martikainen J, Mäkelä MJ, Haahtela T. Follow-up of the Finnish Asthma Programme 2000–2010: Reduction of hospital burden needs risk group rethinking. *Thorax* 2012;68(3):292–293.

50. Kauppi P, et al. Pharmacy allergy barometer survey, 2013, personal communication.

51. Pawankar R, Canonica GW, Holgate ST, Lockey RF (eds.). *World Allergy Organization (WAO) White Book on Allergy.* WAO, 2011.

52. Boulet LP, FitzGerald JM, Levy ML, Cruz ASA, Pedersen S, Haahtela T, Bateman ED. A guide to the translation of the Global Initiative for Asthma (GINA) strategy into improved care. *Eur Respir J* 2012;39:1220–1229.

53. Bousquet J, Anto J, Auffray C, Akdis M, Cambon-Thomsen A, Keil T, Haahtela T, et al. MeDALL (Mechanisms of the Development of ALLergy): An integrated approach from phenotypes to systems medicine. *Allergy* 2011;66:596–604.

54. Bousquet J, Bachert C, Canonica GW, Casale TB, Cruz AA, Lockey RJ, Zuberbier T; Extended Global Allergy and Asthma European Network, World Allergy Organization and Allergic Rhinitis and its Impact on Asthma Study Group. Unmet needs in severe chronic upper airway disease (SCUAD). *J Allergy Clin Immunol* 2009;124:428–433.

55. Oken MM, Creech RH, Tormey DC, Horton J, Davis TE, McFadden ET, Carbone PP. Toxicity and response criteria of the Eastern Cooperative Oncology Group. *Am J Clin Oncol* 1982;5:649–655.

56. Fitzgerald JM, Bateman E, Hurd S, Boulet LP, Haahtela T, Cruz AA, Levy ML. The GINA Asthma Challenge: Reducing asthma hospitalisations. *Eur Respir J* 2011;38:997–998.

57. Bousquet J, Dahl R, Khaltaev N. Global Alliance against chronic respiratory diseases. *Eur Respir J* 2007; 29:233–239.

58. Lalloo UG, Walters RD, Adachi M, deGuia T, Emelyanov A, Fritscher CC, Hong J, et al. Asthma programmes in diverse regions of the world: Challenges, successes and lessons learnt. *Int J Tuberc Lung Dis* 2011;15:1574–1587.

59. Kupczyk M, Haahtela T, Cruz A, Kuna P. Reduction of asthma burden is possible through National Asthma Plans. *Allergy* 2010;65:415–419.

60. Chung EH, Seo SH, Seo HJ, Jou HM, Kim YA, Kim YT. *Prevention and Control of Asthma and Allergic Diseases in Korea*; WAO XXII World Allergy Congress; 2011 December 4–8; Mexico, Cancun. WAO, Milwaukee, 2011. Abstract 4114.

28 Primary Care Setting and Integrating Care across Primary/Secondary Care Interface

Barbara P. Yawn

CONTENTS

CASE PRESENTATION

CASES

Mary and John are 12-year-old twins whose asthma was diagnosed at ages 10 and 6 years, respectively. Both were diagnosed with persistent asthma and both began therapy with moderate-dose inhaled corticosteroid (ICS). After this, the courses of their diseases differed.

John is an athlete whose asthma was adequately controlled until about 2 years ago. Now he consistently has problems during soccer and basketball practice. In addition, he awakes several nights a month. While his spirometry is within normal limits, he continues to remain poorly controlled. Over the past 2 years, he has progressed from his moderate-dose ICS to a high-dose combination of ICS and long-acting beta-adrenoceptor agonist (LABA) but continues to use his short-acting beta$_2$-adrenoceptor agonist (SABA) almost daily with limited results. He is waking up

to 2–3 nights a month coughing and had to sit out the last soccer practice. His family physician has assessed potential allergens with in vitro assays with positive results for grasses and trees. John does not appear to have seasonal symptoms but with the constant problems, seasonal assessment is difficult. John's mother is ready for a specialty consultation and his family physician wonders if it is time to consider omalizumab.

On the other hand, Mary's asthma was well controlled immediately with moderate-dose ICS and remains controlled most of the time. However, in the spring and fall for the past 2 years, Mary has had severe exacerbations even requiring hospitalization this March. After the hospitalization, Mary finished a 21-day course of oral steroids and her asthma has been under good control on moderate-dose ICS plus LABA for May, June, and July. Mary, her mother, and the family physician welcome a second opinion and she will see the allergist on the same day as her brother.

John's visit reveals a common but often unrecognized problem. John's inhaler technique is very poor for both his dry powder inhaler and his metered-dose inhaler. Thinking back, it becomes clear that John's problems began when he started using his medications in his room rather than with parental supervision. Since then his inhaler technique has apparently deteriorated. With an appropriate technique and improved adherence, John's asthma is again well controlled on moderate-dose ICS and preexercise use of SABA. The allergist dismissed John with an updated asthma action plan and a suggestion to the family physician to assess inhaler technique at each visit.

Mary's visit takes longer and includes a detailed allergy history and targeted allergy skin testing. The allergist recommends consideration of either allergy desensitization or anti-IgE therapy. Mary and her mother want to talk with their family physician as well as Mary's father and return to the allergist in 2 weeks to make a decision. The allergist provides a detailed consultation summary to the family and Mary's family physician. All agree that Mary's asthma care will be a collaboration between her personal family physician and the allergist.

COMMENT

John's consultation probably could have been avoided if the primary care physician had a systematic approach to not only assessing control but also assessing the common causes of asthma being out of control. Mary's posthospital referral is recommended in all current asthma guidelines and provided options that are seldom available in primary care.

INTRODUCTION

Asthma is one of the most common chronic conditions for both adults and children. Rates vary by country and are high in the most developed countries: 14%–15% in the United Kingdom, New Zealand, Canada, Australia, and Ireland and 11% in the United States. Developing countries report wider variations: 13% in Peru, 12% in Costa Rica, 8% in Africa, and only 2% in China, with many cases likely to be unreported or undiagnosed. Rates in schoolchildren are always higher than those in adults[1] (see ref. 2 for the United States and ref. 3 for the world). The estimated percentage of those with asthma who have persistent asthma varies widely but is seldom estimated as less than 50% of all asthma.[4–6] Because asthma is such a common condition and associated with exacerbations or "attacks" requiring immediate care and intervention, it is not surprising that the vast majority of people with asthma and asthma exacerbations are cared for by primary care physicians. The reliance on primary care is true even in places like the United States where specialists are common.[1,7,8]

Data from many countries demonstrate the vast opportunities to improve asthma care and patient outcomes.[4,6,9–15]

Some allergists, especially in the United States, continue to provide data that people with asthma have better outcomes when cared for by an asthma specialist.[4,16] Whether this is due entirely to the additional training and expertise of the allergist or to the allergists' care system is not clear.[10,16] Based on information from management of other chronic conditions, improving the primary care systems of care is very likely to improve asthma outcomes as it has improved outcomes for people with diabetes.[17,18] Asthma specialist care systems can be adapted and transferred to primary care sites and for many that is what is happening in quality-improvement (QI) programs for asthma management.[19] Not all attempts at improvement have been successful, but some specific tasks appear to be universally helpful. The next section of this chapter will address asthma care in primary care practices. Many of the issues discussed are addressed in greater depth in other chapters in this book. When possible, reference is made to other chapters to guide you to tools and information that can facilitate implementation of suggestions in this chapter.

ASTHMA GUIDELINES IN PRACTICE

Several national and international guidelines have been produced to direct asthma management—Global Initiative for Asthma (GINA), Scottish Intercollegiate Guidelines Network (SIGN), National Heart, Lung, and Blood Institute (NHLBI), International Primary Care Respiratory Group (IPCRG), Dutch GP guidelines, and Australian guidelines (see Chapter 5, this volume). Unfortunately, few of the guidelines can be transferred directly to daily practice activities.[20–23] For example, asthma control tools have been developed to facilitate assessment of asthma response to therapy and the adequacy of asthma management.[24–29] These tools were developed in response to identified gaps in practice, specifically, the failure of most medical encounter notes to include the information required to quantify asthma signs and symptoms.[23,30] The control tools are used to calculate a score that suggests the patient's asthma is "in control," "poorly controlled," or somewhere between, for example, Asthma Control Test (ACT), Asthma Therapy Assessment Questionnaire (ATTAQ), Asthma Control Questionnaire (ACQ), and Asthma Apgar.[24–26,29] The ACT and ACQ both have separate tools for children while the Asthma Apgar is designed to be used by parents of very young children, adolescents, and adults. After quickly assessing control, it is then the responsibility of the physician or other clinician to determine next steps. Limited data are available on the impact of incorporation of these tools into routine practice.[26] Most of the literature on the tools addresses their validation and translation to other languages, as well as cross-comparisons among the tools.[24,25,27,31,32] The Asthma APGAR goes beyond assessing control to assess potential causes for inadequate control and is linked to a care algorithm based on the 2007 US asthma guidelines to guide next steps[26] (Figure 28.1).

A = Activities
P = Persistent
G = triGGers
A = Asthma medications
R = Response to therapy

Asthma APGAR

P = Asthma Plan
L = Lung function
U = Use of inhaler
S = Steroids

Please circle your answers:

A 1. In the past 2 weeks, how many times did any breathing problems (such as asthma) interfere with your **ACTIVITIES** or activities you wanted to do?

    Never   1 – 2 times   3 or more times

P 2. How many **DAYS** in the past 2 weeks did you have shortness of breath, wheezing, chest tightness, cough or felt you should use your rescue inhaler?

    None   1 – 2 DAYS   3 or more DAYS

3. How many **NIGHTS** in the past 2 weeks did you wake up or have trouble sleeping due to coughing, shortness of breath, wheezing, chest tightness or get up to use your rescue medication?

    None   1 – 2 NIGHTS   3 or more NIGHTS

G 4. Do you know what makes your breathing problems or asthma worse?

    Yes   No   Unsure

   • **Please circle things that make your breathing problems or asthma worse:**

   Cigarettes   Smoke   Cold Air   Colds   Exercise   Dust   Dust Mites

   Trees   Flowers   Cats   Dogs   Mold   Other: _____

   • **Can you avoid the things that make your breathing problems or asthma wores?**

    Seldom   Sometimes   Most of the times

A 5. List or describe medications you've taken for breathing problems or asthma in the past 2 weeks: Remember you may use Nasal, Oral, or Inhaler medications.

Breathing or Asthma Medication	When taken?		Reasons for taking medication:	Reasons for not taking medication:
	☐ Daily	☐ As needed		
	☐ Daily	☐ As needed		
	☐ Daily	☐ As needed		
	☐ Daily	☐ As needed		

R 6. When I use my breathing or asthma medicines I feel:

    Worse   No Different   A Little Better   A Lot Better

FIGURE 28.1 Asthma Apgar patient survey.

All of the asthma guidelines suggest management steps in response to asthma control problems. For example, in the 2007 NHLBI guidelines, an often ignored box to the right of the steps of therapy says, "assess adherence, triggers and inhaler techniques before stepping it up."[33,34]

The British Thoracic Society guidelines also specifically state, "Before initiating a new drug therapy practitioners should check compliance with existing therapies, inhaler technique, and eliminate trigger factors."[35] Despite these statements, in most primary patient care settings, poor control results in an increase in medication without further assessment of why the current therapy is not effective.[23,26,30] Common causes of poor or inadequate control include lack of adherence to current management program due to too many medications and cost, poor inhaler technique, and triggers that are unrecognized or not avoided.[34] Physicians and other clinicians cite time constraints, discomfort in "confronting" patients about adherence, and limited knowledge of inhaler techniques as reasons to skip these steps and move forward with step-ups of therapy.[36,37] Failing to assess the common causes of poor or inadequate asthma control can result in a perception of a person having "difficult-to-control asthma" with resultant over-medication.[15,26] Stepping up may not result in improved outcomes.

For example, patients who are unable to adhere to their current medication regimen or unable to get medications to the target organ due to poor inhaler technique or incorrect prescribed inhaler type are unlikely to have better control after adding yet another drug.[15] For all of these reasons, the system changes to improve asthma care need to go beyond simply adding a control test assessment during asthma visits.

ASSESSING ASTHMA CONTROL

Tools such as the ACT, the ATTAQ, and the ACQ have proven to be valid and reliable at quantifying asthma control, some in many languages[24,25,30] (see Chapter 16, this volume). But as noted above, most national and primary care asthma guidelines require more than a simple control score to guide asthma care.[33–35,38–44] The Asthma Apgar goes beyond control questions and asks patients about triggers, and medications taken and not taken and why, as well as solicits a patient judgment of the effect of therapy on the asthma symptoms. Linked to an algorithm for next steps, the Asthma Apgar guides next steps through assessment of steps of care beyond simply increasing medications[26] (Figure 28.2). The use of exhaled nitric oxide may also help.[45] While usually considered a test to identify out-of-control asthma, it may also be used to demonstrate to patients the impact of actually using their medications. In busy primary care practices where physicians address multiple conditions in any single visit, having a system and tools to guide next steps may improve outcomes to a greater degree than a simple assessment of control status.

ASSESSING INHALER TECHNIQUE

Every primary care site should have the ability to teach and assess inhaler technique. Simply asking if the patient is able to use the inhaler regularly, how often, why, and why not is a good start but insufficient. Consider this part of the adherence or compliance assessment and intervention. If the person's inhaler technique is poor, they may not be getting the medication into the lungs effectively, making them nonadherent even if they never "miss a dose." Most practices with systems of asthma care assign this task to a nonphysician such as a clinical nurse specialist in the United Kingdom, the Netherlands, and Australia, or an asthma educator in the United States. In observational studies, neither the health-care professional nor the patient demonstrated adequate inhaler technique more than 50% of the time.[46–48] If the health professional has a poor grasp of inhaler technique, who is competent to teach the patient?[49] (See Chapters 14 and 15, this volume.)

IDENTIFICATION OF AND EDUCATION ABOUT ASTHMA TRIGGERS

Trigger assessment is an essential part of every primary care evaluation of asthma. Even if the patient is well controlled, identifying and confirming methods to avoid triggers may prevent future exacerbations. While the Asthma Apgar addresses patient-suspected triggers and can be used to start the discussion of triggers, some patients will require a more extensive assessment of allergies, which can be facilitated using a list of potential allergens and a discussion of seasonal symptoms. Many patients are aware of triggers including tobacco, wood-fire smoke, animals, and plants but have just never been asked what they believe are their allergies. The primary care office can be the site of blood tests to screen for allergies or "in some countries" skin testing.[50] In other countries or regions, in-depth allergy assessment and initiation of anti-IgE or immune therapy is best considered part of shared care with an allergist (see Chapter 10, this volume). Shared care will be the focus of the later part of this chapter.

COMORBID CONDITIONS

Often overlooked but an important part of asthma and allergy evaluation is assessment for allergic rhinitis. Allergic rhinitis can be a substantial barrier to good asthma control. Allergic Rhinitis and Its Impact on Asthma (ARIA) provides guidelines for allergic rhinitis in asthma.[41,51] Few practical tools have been developed to translate these guidelines into everyday practice. However, a few simple questions may begin this process and many patients are aware of allergies[26,34] (see Chapter 8, this volume).

ASSESSING ADHERENCE

Adherence is a known barrier to management of all chronic diseases and asthma is no exception.[18,37] Comments about

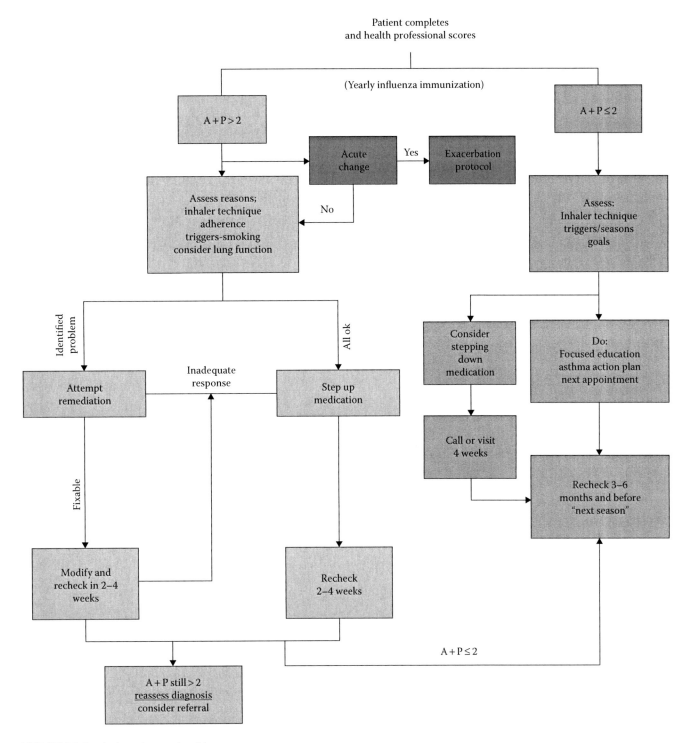

FIGURE 28.2   Asthma Apgar algorithm.

medication adherence should be prefaced with comments such as "Many people find it difficult to take all of their medications all of time. How often have you been able to take your medications?" When using the Asthma Apgar, the list of medications written by patients, as well as answers about why they take the medications and why not, can lead to a nonconfrontational review of adherence. Qualitative studies report that patients are willing to address the issue of nonadherence. In addition, asking them why they take their

medications may highlight the fact that patients do or do not understand the concept of daily "controller" medications and those to be used for acute symptoms. (See Chapter 14, this volume.)

UNINTENTIONAL NONADHERENCE

Deciding how to address adherence may be easier if it is possible to categorize the type of nonadherence.[18,37]

Unintentional nonadherence includes forgetting medications or taking them incorrectly, for example, or poor inhaler technique. Reminders, medication placement near site of a common activity, or simplifying a complex therapy regimen can improve unintentional nonadherence. Knowing that failure to take the medication is unintentional saves the primary care office personnel the time that might be spent trying to convince the patient that they need the medication and allows them to move directly to problem solving with the patient.

INTENTIONAL NONADHERENCE

Intentional nonadherence may vary from inability to afford the medications to fear of side effects, concerns about medication dependency, failure to accept the diagnosis, and failure to accept the chronic nature of asthma. One of the most common types of nonadherence is discontinuing medications when control is good—because symptoms are in abeyance.[52] Intentional nonadherence can be more time consuming to address and may require collaboration with a social worker to identify financial resources or an asthma educator or pharmacist to help affirm the risk and benefit of asthma medication usage.

ASSESSING LUNG FUNCTION

Spirometry use in asthma has limited evidence on which to base recommendations but is recommended for the confirmation of reversible airflow obstruction and, therefore, diagnosis in suspected asthma in adults and children over ages 5–7 years by the U.S. and the Australian national asthma guidelines.[34,53] The British guidelines are more permissive, suggesting that spirometry is important for patients with less than a high probability of asthma. For patients with a high probability risk of asthma, spirometry is ideal, but not required, to confirm the diagnosis unless a trial of therapy does not result in improvement.[35,39] Quality-assured spirometry is an important tool for primary care practices and should be available for assessment of asthma diagnosis, especially in those with less clear clinical assessment for asthma, when trying to differentiate COPD from asthma and for patients whose asthma is difficult to control, requiring multiple therapies.[9] The data to support the use of spirometry for monitoring asthma care are less sound.[54,55] The SIGN guidelines suggest spirometry for monitoring difficult-to-control asthma and for people with occupational exposures in order to assess possible reversible lung function when exposed.[35]

Many primary care practices do not have easily accessible spirometry testing onsite to facilitate patient access. When spirometry is available on site, problems often still arise related to the quality of tests performed[56–58] and the accuracy of interpretation of the results. Sharing spirometry care with a respiratory therapist, a respiratory nurse specialist, another primary care physician with expertise

TABLE 28.1
Systematizing Care

- Consider carrying out routine reviews by telephone for people with asthma.
- In primary care, people with asthma should be reviewed regularly by a nurse or doctor with appropriate training in asthma management.
- The review should incorporate a written action plan.
- Primary care practices should maintain and use a register of people with asthma.
- Clinical review should be structured and utilize a standard recording system.
- Feedback of audit data to clinicians should link guidelines recommendations to management of individual patients.

in performing quality assured spirometry, or a specialist in this field may improve both the quality of the tests performed and the interpretation and use of the results for clinical practice.[59] In fact, working together to make high-quality-assured spirometry available to primary care patients may be a first simple step to implementing shared care (Table 28.1).

Some patients require more care or more intensive care than is feasible in the primary care office. While guidelines often define when patients with asthma should be referred for specialty care, that decision is best made by the physician and the patient and family. Some primary care teams are quite comfortable caring for patients with moderate to moderately severe asthma and do so. Other primary care teams have trouble caring for even mild or intermittent asthma, usually due to the lack of an asthma care system.

PRIMARY CARE TEAMS

Developing primary care teams and delegating responsibilities to appropriately trained individuals, rather than relying on physicians alone, is a major advance when developing care systems and implementing the medical home concept.[60] In several countries that have a national health system, other groups of health professionals have been developed to provide asthma care both for those with stable asthma and for those with more difficult-to-control asthma. Practice nurses have been trained to provide routine asthma care and support the primary care physicians' practices.[34,35,53] Some sites define "specialty respiratory nurses" who see complicated patients and help monitor their asthma.[28,29] The final level of referral remains the specialist physician—an allergist or a respirologist. All of these levels and layers can work together to provide shared care but only if that shared care is intentional rather than happenstance.[7] Shared care assures that the patient has access to the specialty services they need while retaining the whole person care that all children and adults require, including care for other acute or chronic conditions and preventive services. This is also the basic premise of the medical home and family medicine.

SPECIALIST REFERRAL

The timing for referral of a person with asthma to additional services will vary based on many factors (Table 28.2). While guidelines have suggested benchmarks for referral, each guideline is a little different and not easily translated to a global set of recommendations. The primary care physician/ team and the patient/parents are the final arbiters of this decision. A request for additional care and support from either group should result in discussion of the referral, including what is desired from the referral and whether asthma care will also continue at the primary care site.

COMMUNICATION

Communication is the biggest issue in shared care. Before communicating, the primary care physician or team must consider three things: (1) Why is a referral being made? (2) To whom should communication be made? and (3) What information do you want back following the referral?[7] The purpose of the communication is to prevent some of the potential adverse outcomes of shared care, such as fragmented care, patient/family confusion due to multiple and differing health care messages, patient and provider uncertainty of the role(s) of each of the individuals involved in the patient's care, and failure to address the whole person and potential comorbidities. Each of these concerns can be addressed briefly in the referral communication. For example, in your referral letter or even on the asthma action plan, list the terms that you and the patient use to talk about asthma—reactive airway disease, recurrent wheezing, and so on. If a doctor uses general terms to identify medications, these should be included in the letter and on the asthma action plan; for example, rescue medications or acute medications, e.g., short-acting bronchodilators; controller, maintenance, or anti-inflammatory medications, e.g., ICSs; and combination medications or leukotriene modifiers. Of

---

TABLE 28.2

Reasons for Referral for Additional Asthma Care

- Level of asthma problems
- Age of the person with asthma
- Ability of the primary care practice to help the patient/family obtain and maintain adequate asthma control
- Number and type of asthma-related staff and expertise available in the local office
- Local availability and accessibility of other asthma support health-care professionals and services
- Primary care physician comfort and expertise in caring for people with asthma
- Financial issues

---

course, include the generic names of each type used so the consultant has both the medical information and a communication strategy for talking with the patient. In addition, the referrer should detail those medications prescribed for allergic rhinitis such as intranasal steroids or antihistamines, as well as any comorbidity such as depression, anxiety, or the possibility of coexisting asthma and COPD so these can be considered in the consultant's care and recommendations and are not reevaluated with the tests you have already completed.

REFERRAL TEMPLATE LETTERS

While each referral can result in a one-off letter, it is easier and more efficient to develop a template or list of topics to be included in the referral letter. That template should be incorporated into the electronic medical record and require only a couple of keystrokes to access. Boxes 28.1 and 28.2 are examples of templates for use in such letters or communication. This template is a combination of published templates and the experience of the author. It is not, to date, evidence based.

Deciding to send a letter to the specialist is an obvious choice when referring a patient. However, determining who else might be appropriate for formal communication depends on the stability of the asthma, the ease of obtaining and maintaining control, who is available in your region, and what usual referral patterns have been established. For example, Dr. Smith in the United Kingdom, the Netherlands, or Australia may ask the asthma practice nurse or a specialty nurse to spend extra time with a patient who needs further assessment of triggers and an allergy history. In the United States help may be required by the generalist for identification of the type of trigger, an allergy assessment, or spirometry, prompting referral to an allergist's or pulmonologist's office.

While some large health-care systems and organizations do have disease management nurses, to date few U.S. sites have office-based asthma practice nurses or regional asthma practice nurses that can support asthma patients from several practices. Asthma educators are able to support patients and families with longer and repeated episodes of asthma education and even spirometry in some cases, but they are not able to provide asthma care and pharmaceutical therapy oversight. So while shared care may appear quite different in various countries, actually it is very similar with just a broad range of different people fulfilling the roles of educator, support person, spirometry technician, prescriber, and expert. In all situations, people with asthma should have their health care anchored in a setting that not only provides and coordinates care of asthma, but also helps integrate asthma care into the care for the whole person. In the United States, this is called the "medical home," with similar concepts for primary care around the world. For patients who are frequent attendees of the emergency department (ED), urgent care, or hospital casualty units for their asthma, the referring doctor could consider sending communication to those sites. Often

BOX 28.1   EXAMPLE OF REFERRAL LETTER TOPICS

Summary of asthma to date

- Date of diagnosis: be specific about what the condition has been called with patient (reactive airway disease, asthma, recurrent wheezing, etc.)
- Current medications and duration
- Previous medications and, if not successful, why (inadequate control, patient unable to use, lack of compliance, adverse effects, patient concerns, other reasons)

Why is the referral being made now?

- Recent hospitalization, severe exacerbations, frequent exacerbations
- Assessment of triggers/allergies
- Patient request

What do you want from the referral?

- Help assessing next steps in therapy
- Additional education
- Help confirming diagnosis
- Patient/family reassurance

What do you want for future care of this individual?

- Transfer of asthma care to others
- Shared care with specialist visits once a year and interaction with referring physician as needed
- One-time assessment
- Treatment for allergies such as immunotherapy
- Management of therapy that primary care physician is uncomfortable monitoring, e.g., anti-IgE or daily oral steroids or other

What do you want back?

- Care plan, including asthma action plan for home and school or work
- Results of any assessments
- Suggested time for next visit
- A call or e-mail immediately if asthma is the wrong diagnosis

01/01/2013
Dr. Airway
Family Care Facility
1010 Asthma Lane
Triggers, USA
Phone 222-333-4444
Fax 222-333-4445

Mary Teenager
05/05/1998
9394 Wheeze Avenue
Nebulize, USA

Dear Dr. Bronchi,

I am referring Mary Teenager to you for a second opinion regarding her asthma care. Mary is 14, with a 4-year history of persistent asthma. She is well controlled most of the time on moderate-dose ICS (fluticasone 100 mg used BID). However, she has had moderate to severe exacerbations spring and fall for the past 2 years requiring a hospitalization this spring. Please see attached hospital discharge summary. She did respond to oral steroids, antibiotics, and regular nebulized bronchodilator. Following her March admission she has been adequately controlled (Asthma Apgar score of less than 2) in May, June, and July. She does clearly have seasonal triggers but is unsure what they are. No one in her family smokes and she does not appear to have seasonal allergic rhinitis.

Both she and her family would like you to help assess the cause of the exacerbations and suggest an approach to prevent future exacerbations, including possible allergy testing and consideration of immunotherapy or anti-IgE therapy. I hope to remain Mary's primary asthma contact since your office is over 90 miles from where she lives.

I look forward to your assessment and recommendations for her future care. (Please see my attached questions.)

Sincerely,
Dr. Airway

BOX 28.2 ATTACHMENT TO REFERRAL LETTER

Mary Teenager
05/05/1998

1. Do you agree that she has uncontrolled asthma?
2. Do you see reasons other than inability to avoid allergens?
3. Is she a candidate for allergy testing and if so can you provide please?
4. Is she a candidate for anti-IgE?
5. Is she a candidate for desensitization or immunotherapy?

I would like to continue to be the primary contact for Mary since she is so far from your office site.

I would certainly anticipate that she may need to be seen multiple times for regulation of anti-IgE therapy or beginning of immunotherapy.

I am comfortable managing stable anti-IgE therapy. I am also comfortable overseeing immunotherapy once a regular dose is established. My nursing staff and I have done this for more than 25 patients in the past 3 years.

---

the ED physicians have only what the patient reports and perhaps past notes from other ED visits. Providing the ED with the list of current medications, current asthma action plan, and your e-mail or postal address or telephone number could facilitate those follow-up visits we all wish would happen whenever our patient visits the ED or hospital. Initiating communication not only models communication but provides the ED personnel with added support in caring for patients in a potential crisis. Simply putting a well-written asthma action plan on an inexpensive flash drive that you can provide to your patients with multiple ED or hospital visits will allow you to maximize the effort spent on developing that action plan without requiring you to write numerous types of notes and letters to other providers. (See Chapters 14 and 16, this volume.)

IMPROVING QUALITY OF REFERRAL OUTCOME

The referring doctor could include an outline detailing his or her expectation concerning the consultation with the specialist, and a request for the consultant to respond in a timely manner, before the patient returns for a primary care consultation. This will help the referring doctor reaffirm recommendations made during the consultant visit.

SHARING CARE WITH OTHERS BEYOND SPECIALIZED SERVICES

For children, shared care will go beyond the patient, family, practice team, respiratory nurses, and specialists. Children spend a good portion of their day in school and often experience asthma problems during school. Adults most commonly work outside the home and many preschoolers attend day care. Therefore, care will be shared with the school, work, or day care. In schools and in some work places, nurses are on-site all or part of each day. But those nurses may not be trained to deal with asthma specifically, as respiratory practice nurses are.[28,61] Many school and worksite nurses have limited asthma care knowledge or experience. They require clear and thorough guidance in the assessment and treatment of asthma problems. This guidance is often provided in an asthma action plan that can be provided to both the person (family) with asthma and their school, day care or work site. (See Chapters 13, 14, and 16, this volume.)

Sharing care with schools has been expanded beyond care of those with identified asthma to an attempt to include those who have apparent or potential asthma but remain unrecognized and undiagnosed.[62,63] In less developed countries, the International Study of Asthma and Allergies in Childhood (ISAAC) was successful in identifying those with potential asthma, but providing the required follow-up evaluation and care was often beyond the ability and resources of the county's health-care system.[64] In the United States, school-based asthma screening has not been found to be successful in identifying new cases; however, it was able to identify children whose asthma was out of control. Therefore, working with schools may facilitate the broad-based care anchored in the community that is likely to be most effective in improving asthma control, especially in children.

SUMMARY

Primary care physicians (and nurses in some countries) continue to have many opportunities to improve asthma diagnosis and chronic care and to reduce emergency and hospital-based utilization for asthma.[15] This requires a willingness and ability to share care within the office team and with patients and their families, as well as to extend the shared management to include appropriate others from school, work, or day care personnel to respiratory nurses or asthma specialists. Asthma management is a team exercise. Teams are more likely to succeed when they have an integrated management plan with a designated role for each member and systems in place to ensure effective communication to reassess the process of care provision and patient outcomes so adjustments can be made when necessary.

ACKNOWLEDGMENTS

The author appreciates the assistance of Dawn Elfstrand in the preparation of this chapter.

REFERENCES

1. Braman SS. The global burden of asthma. *Chest* 2006;130:4s–12s.
2. Mannino DM, Homa DM, Pertowski CA, Ashizawa A, Nixon LL, Johnson CA, Ball LB, Jack E, Kang DS. Surveillance for Asthma: United States, 1960–1995. *MMWR Morb Mortal Wkly Rep* 1998;47(SS-1):1–28.
3. WHO (World Health Organization). Bronchial asthma. Fact sheet no. 206. WHO, Geneva, www.who.int/mediacentre/factsheets/fs206/en. (Accessed 23 October 2011).
4. Bandiola C, Badiella L, Plaza V, Prieto L, Molina J, Villa JR, Cimas E. Women, patients with severe asthma and patients attended by primary care physicians are at higher risk of suffering from poorly controlled asthma. *Prim Care Respir J* 2009;18:294–299.
5. Shah S, Sawyer S, Mellis CM, et al. Improving paediatric asthma outcomes in primary health care: A randomised trial. *Med J Aust* 2011;195:405–409.
6. Barton C, Proudfoot J, Amoroso C, et al. Management of asthma in Australian general practice: Care is still not in line with clinical practice guidelines. *Prim Care Respir J* 2009;18(2):100–105.
7. Levy M, Couriel J, Clark R, Holgate S, Chauhan A. *Share Care for Asthma*. ISIS Medical Media, Oxford, 1997.
8. PHF (Public Health Foundation). We can do better: Improving asthma outcomes in America. PHF, Washington, DC, January, 2009.
9. Yawn BP, Enright PL, Lemanske RF, Israel E, Pace W, Wollan P, Boushey H. Spirometry can be done in family physicians' offices and alters clinical decisions in management of asthma and COPD. *Chest* 2007;132(4):1162–1168.
10. Yawn BP. The role of the primary care physician in helping adolescent and adult patient improve asthma control. *Mayo Clin Proc* 2011;86:894–902.
11. Rank MA, Wollan P, Li JT, Yawn BP. Trigger recognition and management in poorly controlled asthmatics. *Allergy Asthma Proc* 2010;31(6):99–105.
12. Stanford RH, Yancey SW, Stempel DA. Asthma control differences between inhaled corticosteroids likely related to differences in patient severity. *J Allergy Clin Immunol* 2011;127(3):835; author reply 835–836.
13. Sullivan PW, Ghushchyan VH, Slejko JF, Belozeroff V, Globe DR, Lin SL. The burden of adult asthma in the United States: Evidence from the Medical Expenditure Panel Survey. *J Allergy Clin Immunol* 2011;127(2):363–369; e1–e3.
14. Campbell SM, Reeves D, Kontopantelis E, Sibbald B, Roland M. Effects of pay for performance on the quality of primary care in England. *N Engl J Med* 2009;361:368–378.
15. Hancox RJ, Le Souef PN, Anderson GP, Reddel HK, Change AB, Beasley R. Asthma: Time to confront some inconvenient truths. *Respirology* 2010;15:194–201.
16. Vollmer WM, O'Hollaren M, Ettinger KM, et al. Specialty difference in the management of asthma: A cross-sectional assessment of allergists' patients and generalists' patients in a large HMO. *Arch Intern Med* 1997;137:1201–1208.
17. Grimshaw JM, Shirran L, Thomas R, et al. Changing provider behavior: An overview of systematic reviews of interventions. *Med Care* 2001;39:112–145.
18. Haynes RB, Ackloo E, Sahota N, et al. Interventions for enhancing medication adherence. *Cochrane Database Syst Rev* 2009;3:CD00011.
19. National Asthma Council Australia, http://www.national-asthma.org.au/.
20. Burgers JS, Grol RP, Zaat JO, et al. Characteristics of effective clinical guidelines for general practice. *Br J Gen Pract* 2003;53:15–19.
21. Weinberger M. Seventeen years of asthma guidelines: Why hasn't the outcome improved for children? *J Pediatr* 2009;154:786–788.
22. Cabana MD, Rand CS, Powe NR, et al. Why don't physicians follow clinical practice guidelines. A framework for improvement. *JAMA* 1999;282:1458–1465.
23. Yawn BP, van der Molen T, Humbert M. Asthma management: Are GINA guidelines appropriate for daily clinical practice? *Prim Care Respir J* 2005;14(6):294–302.
24. Nathan RA, Sorkness CA, Kosinski M, et al. Development of the asthma control test: A survey for assessing asthma control. *J Allergy Clin Immunol* 2004;113(1):59–65.
25. Juniper EF, Bousquet J, Abetz L, Bateman ED. Identifying 'well-controlled' and 'not well-controlled' asthma using the Asthma Control Questionnaire. *Respir Med* 2006;100(4):616–621.
26. Yawn BP, Bertram S, Wollan P. Introduction of Asthma APGAR tools improve asthma management in primary care practices. *J Asthma Allergy* 2008;1:1–10.
27. Liu AH, Zeiger R, Sorkness C, et al. Development and cross-sectional validation of Childhood Asthma Control Test. *J Allergy Clin Immunol* 2007;119(4):817–825.
28. Pinnock H. Asthma: BMJ Masterclass for GPs. *BMJ* 2007;334(7598):847–850.
29. Vollmer WM, Markson LE, O'Connor E, et al. Association of asthma control with health care untilization: A prospective evaluation. *Am J Respir Crit Care Med* 2002;165(2):195–199.
30. Vollmer WM. Assessment of asthma control and severity. *Ann Allergy Asthma Immunol* 2004;93(5):409–413; quiz 414–416, 492.
31. Zhou X, Ding FM, Lin JT, et al. Validity of Asthma Control Test in Chinese patients. *Chin Med J* 2007;120(12):1037–1041.
32. Vega JM, Badia X, Badiola C, et al. Validation of the Spanish version of the Asthma Control Test. *J Asthma* 2007;44(10):867–872.
33. Levy ML, Fletcher M, Price DB, Hausen T, Halbert RJ, Yawn BP. International Primary Care Respiratory Group (IPCRG) Guidelines: Diagnosis of respiratory diseases in primary care. *Prim Care Respir J* 2006;15(1):20–34.

34. National, Heart, Lung and Blood Institute. Guidelines for the diagnosis and management of asthma (EPR-3). National Institutes of Health, Bethesda, MD, 2007, http://www.nhlbi.nih.gov/guidelines/asthma/.

35. British Thoracic Society. British guideline on the management of asthma: Quick reference guide. British Thoracic Society, London, 2011, http://www.sign.ac.uk/pdf/qrg101.pdf.

36. Williams LK, Pladevall M, Hi H, et al. Relationship between adherence to inhaled corticosteroids and poor outcomes among adults with asthma. *J Allergy Clin Immunol* 2004;114:1288–1293.

37. Bender B. Physician-patient communication as a tool that can change adherence. *Ann Allergy Asthma Immunol* 2009;103(1):1–2.

38. Reid PP, Compton WD, Grossman JH, Fanjiang, G (eds). *Building a Better Delivery System: A New Engineering/Health Care Partnership.* National Academies Press, Washington, DC, 2005.

39. Hagmolen of Ten Have W, van den Berg N, van der Palen J, van Aalderen WMC, Bindela PJE. Implementation of an asthma guideline for the management of childhood asthma in general practice: A randomised controlled trial. *Prim Care Respir J* 2008;17(2):90–96.

40. Global Initiative for Asthma. Global strategy for asthma management and prevention. National Institutes of Health, NIH publication no. 06–3659, www.ginasthma.org, 2006.

41. Bousquet J, Schünemann HJ, Zuberbier T, et al. Development and implementation of guidelines in allergic rhinitis: An ARIA-GA2LEN paper. *Allergy* 2010;65(10):1212–1221.

42. Smith AD, Cowan JO, Brassett KP, Herbison GP, Taylor DR. Use of exhaled nitric oxide measurements to guide treat in chronic asthma. *N Engl J Med* 2005;352(21):2163–2173.

43. van Beerendonk I, Mesters I, Muddle AN, et al. Assessment of the inhalation technique in outpatients with asthma or chronic obstructive pulmonary disease using a metered-dose inhaler or dry powder device. *J Asthma* 1998;35:273–279.

44. National Asthma Council Australia. Understanding asthma, http://www.nationalasthma.org.au/understanding-asthma.

45. Fink JB, Rubin BK. Problems with inhaler use: A call for improved clinician and patient education. *Respir Care* 2005;50:1360–1374.

46. Jensen JK, Jakobsen MK. Allergiudredning i almen praksis i Arhus Amt. Kvalitetsvurdering af diagnostik, behandling og patientinstruktion. III. Allergidiagnostik. *Ugeskr Laeger* 2006;168(13):1336–1340.

47. Yawn BP, Wollan PC, Bertram SL, Lowe D, Butterfield JH, Bonde D, Li JT. Asthma treatment in a population-based cohort: Putting step-up and step-down treatment changes in context. *Mayo Clin Proc* 2007;82(4):414–421.

48. Hesselink AE, Penninx BW, van der Windt DA, et al. Effectiveness of an education programme by a general practice assistant for asthma and COPD patients: Results from a randomised controlled trial. *Patient Educ Couns* 2004;55(1):121–128.

49. National Asthma Council Australia. How-to videos: Standard MDI, http://www.nationalasthma.org.au/how-to-videos/using-your-inhaler/standard-mdi.

50. Holton C, Crockett A, Nelson M, Ryan P, Wood-Baker R, Stocks N, Briggs N, Beilby J. Does spirometry training in general practice improve quality and outcomes of asthma care? *Int J Qual Health Care* 2011;23(5):545–553.

51. Guidry GG, Roche N. Incorrect use of metered-dose inhalers by medical personnel. *Chest* 1992;101:31–33.

52. D'Urzo AD. Must family physicians use spirometry in managing asthma patients? NO. *Can Fam Phys* 2010;56:127–128.

53. National Asthma Council Australia. *Asthma Management Handbook*, 6th edn. National Asthma Council Australia, Melbourne, 2006, http://www.nationalasthma.org.au/uploads/handbook/370-amh2006_web_5.pdf.

54. Dombkowski KJ, Hassan F, Wasilevich EA, Clark SJ. Spirometry use among pediatric primary care physicians. *Pediatrics* 2010;126(4):682–687.

55. Poels PJ, Schermer TR, Thoonen BP, Jacobs JE, Akkermans RP, de Vries Robbe PF, Quanjer PH, Bottema BJ, van Weel C. Spirometry expert support in family practice: A cluster-randomised trial. *Prim Care Respir J* 2009;18(3):189–197.

56. Gillette C, Loughlin CE, Sleath BL, Williams DM, Davis SD. Quality of pulmonary function testing in 3 large primary care pediatric clinics in rural North Carolina. *N C Med J* 2011;72(2):105–110.

57. Lindberg M, Ahlner J, Ekstrom T. Asthma nurse practice improves outcomes and reduces costs in primary health care. *Scand J Caring Sci* 2002;16:73–78.

58. Yawn BP, Wollan P, Scanlon PD, Kurland M. Outcome results of a school-based screening program for undertreated asthma. *Ann Allergy Asthma Immunol* 2003;90(5):508–515.

59. Anderson HR, Gupta R, Kapetanakis V, Asher MI, Clayton T, Robertson CF, Strachan DP, and the ISAAC Steering Committee. International correlations between indicators of prevalence, hospital admissions and mortality for asthma in children. *Int J Epidemiol* 2008;37(3):573–582.

60. Mitchell D. Asthma home care cuts kids' hospital visits. Emax Health 5 May, 2010, http://www.emaxhealth.com/1275/asthma-home-care-cuts-kids-hospital-visits.html.

61. Wilson KD, Moonie S, Sterling DA, Gillespie KN, Kurz RS. Examining the consulting physician model to enhance the school nurse role of children with asthma. *J Sch Health* 2009;79(1):1–7.

62. Yawn BP. Asthma screening, case identification and treatment in school-based programs. *Curr Opin Pulm Med* 2006;12(1):23–27.

63. Moricca ML, Grasska MA, BMarthaler M, Morphew T, Wiesmuller PC, Galant SP. School asthma screening and case management: Attendance and learning outcomes. *J Sch Nurs* 2013;29(2):104–112.

64. Ellwood P, Asher MI, Beasley R, Clayton TO, Stewart AW; ISAAC Steering Committee. The international study of asthma and allergies in childhood (ISAAC): Phase three rationale and methods. *Int J Tuberc Lung Dis* 2005;9(1):10–16.

29 Preventing Asthma Death
Primary Care Setting

Mark L. Levy

CONTENTS

CASE PRESENTATION

MR died due to an acute asthma attack at the age of 12 years. He had suffered from asthma since the age of 3 months. He had eczema, peanut allergy, and a strong family history of asthma. He had been prescribed inhaled topical corticosteroids, a reliever inhaler, an oral leukotriene receptor antagonist (LTRA), and an injectable adrenaline device. He had been taught to use a spacer device with his pressurized metered-dose inhalers, but had not been using the corticosteroid inhaler regularly in his last few years of life. His repeat prescription record showed that he had been issued prescriptions for nine salbutamol inhalers and three beclometasone inhalers in the 12 months before he died. He had not regularly attended planned routine checks at the general practitioner; he had, however, been seen in the local emergency department (ED) on two occasions in the 2 months preceding his death. The notes from these attendances indicated he had presented with upper respiratory tract infections associated with wheezing. He had been treated with antibiotics and nebulized salbutamol on the second occasion. He was not seen by a doctor or nurse in follow-up after these episodes and there was no evidence in the record of follow-up arrangements made by either the hospital or his general practitioner after these episodes. His final, fatal attack occurred when the family was away on a camping holiday. He had been coughing and wheezing for two nights. For these last few days, he had needed to use his salbutamol inhaler every 3–4 h, and when he finally became very distressed and short of breath his parents called for an emergency ambulance, which responded within 8 min. By this time he had collapsed and was cyanosed. Despite resuscitation attempts both en route to and in the hospital ED, he failed to recover consciousness.

COMMENT ON THE CASE

This child's medical history illustrates a number of problems associated with the management of people with asthma in a general practice. While this was an extreme and tragic case, similar problems and themes are evident in many patients dying from asthma. The child was diagnosed at an early age and had features associated with a high risk of dying from asthma, but his adherence to advice was poor, and the delay in calling for help in his fatal attack indicated a possible lack of personal or parental awareness of action to be taken during an attack. This could be because the family was not provided with an action plan, or if one was provided it was not adhered to. The failure of his parents to bring him for routine follow-up consultations may also be due to their lack of awareness of his risk status and the risks associated with asthma or alternatively poor awareness of asthma guidelines on the part of his general practitioner. There were a number of missed opportunities where health professionals may have intervened. These include failure to detect and act on the child's poor adherence to medication, failure to attend routine follow-ups and to use his preventer medication regularly, and most importantly failure to recognize that excess prescriptions for short-acting beta-agonist inhalers had been issued. The failure of health professionals to review this child after ED admissions was another missed opportunity.

INTRODUCTION

There are not many published examples of high-quality, practical implementation of research findings or guidelines in the management of asthma.[1,2] Management of patients who die or nearly die from acute asthma is no exception; repeated studies demonstrate aspects in their management, on the part of the patients themselves or their health professionals, that could have prevented many of these deaths.[3–11] Sadly, potentially preventable factors identified in early studies on asthma deaths[3,7] have again been found in subsequent research.[8,10,12] This chapter will summarize and discuss the findings and recommendations of these studies and provide practical recommendations for their implementation. As diagnosis and management of asthma is well covered in other chapters of the book, the reader is directed to those for more detail. This chapter should assist primary health care professionals (general practitioners and nurses) in reducing the incidence of severe and fatal episodes of acute asthma. Furthermore, Chapter 14 provides a number of practical examples for improving both health-care delivery and adherence to medical advice, and complements many of the messages in this chapter.

LESSONS FROM CONFIDENTIAL INQUIRIES AND ASTHMA DEATH REVIEWS

A number of themes emerge from the confidential inquiries on asthma death. These include issues related to assessment, chronic and acute management, and patient education.

ASSESSMENT

Failure to assess asthma control routinely and to assess the severity of asthma exacerbations has been recognized for over 50 years.[3,11] In the British Thoracic Association's confidential inquiry into 92 asthma deaths in 1979, the authors concluded that a possible explanation for the perception that many of the 92 cases they studied were precipitous or sudden occurrences was that patients, clinicians, and families had underestimated the underlying severity of asthma in these people.[3] In fact, only 20% of deaths were sudden in the recent East of England Confidential Inquiry.[10] That the severity of fatal attacks was not recognized by the majority of individuals concerned[3] indicates that patients and families may not have been taught to recognize danger signs, health professional may not have sought or recognized these factors, or maybe objective measurements were not performed.[8] The ongoing confidential enquiries in eastern England in the United Kingdom have reported improvements in the use of objective assessment of

asthma control, particularly lung function[10,13,14]; however, in their latest report, nearly 20% of those who died had not had a recent peak flow assessment either in the primary or secondary care setting. Sturdy et al.,[9] in their large case control study, noted that among those who died from asthma there were fewer general practice contacts in the previous year and fewer peak expiratory flow recordings in the 3 months preceding their index attacks.

Follow-up and assessment of patients after an acute attack are recommended by national and international guidelines and yet failure to do this has been noted as a problem in past and recent studies on asthma deaths.[3,9,10]

CHRONIC MANAGEMENT

Following the early asthma death confidential inquiries[3,11] and an international task force meeting[7] to discuss lessons learned from these studies, both national and international guidelines and strategy documents were published in the early 1990s. Despite these developments, recent studies have demonstrated that implementation of asthma guidelines by health professionals varies considerably.[1] Inadequate prescribing of preventer medication, particularly inhaled corticosteroids, as well as underuse of systemic corticosteroids in acute attacks has been a common observation in confidential inquiries as well as in case control studies of severe asthma attacks. The association between excess use of short-acting beta$_2$-adrenergic agonists (SABAs) and increased risk of asthma death has been identified in a number of studies, one of the earliest being in 1994.[15] Yet, excessive reliance on SABAs by both patients and health professionals persists.[8,10] In addition, studies demonstrate that health professionals seem to underprescribe inhaled corticosteroids for prevention and systemic corticosteroids for acute asthma, and fail to implement routine management and follow-up.[3,10,16,17] Surprisingly, incorrect drug treatment was noted in one study where nearly 40% of the 20 children who died from asthma attacks were prescribed long-acting beta-agonists (LABAs) without concurrent inhaled corticosteroids.[12] One pediatric study found that 18 out of 35 (51%) children under 16 who died from asthma had been chronically undertreated,[16] while another reported inadequate assessment or therapy of asthma in 68% of 51 people under 20 years who died from asthma.[17]

Furthermore, studies have concluded that in many cases overall care of people before their asthma deaths was below expected standards,[10] and that specialist care was not sought, or was delayed, in both primary and secondary care (the latter while people were inpatients in hospital).[10]

Organization of care provision has been implicated in poor outcomes for people with asthma. Delayed access to care is one factor: a case control study comparing near-fatal and fatal cases due to asthma concluded there was a delay in access to acute treatment in 28% of the 80 fatalities studied.[18] Second, not having systems in place for follow-up of nonattenders and failure to recognize poor prognostic risk factors have also been cited as causes for concern.[10]

Failure to recognize poor prognostic risk factors of dying from asthma and subsequently taking appropriate action to gain and maintain control of the disease has been frequently noted in studies on asthma death.[3,7,10,11]

PATIENT EDUCATION

While a number of studies report cases of nonadherence to medical advice by patients, a number also report delays in seeking help during fatal attacks.[3,8,18] This is possibly due to poor adherence to treatment advice, but is more likely to be related to lack of provision by health professionals or underuse of personal asthma action plans by patients (see Chapters 13 and 14). While primary care consultations are relatively brief, people are exposed to their health-care professional for a considerable period of time overall and each of these episodes presents an opportunity for education.

ACUTE ASTHMA MANAGEMENT AND FOLLOW-UP IN GENERAL PRACTICE

Failure to identify asthma exacerbations, to recognize the severity of uncontrolled or acute asthma, and to treat these patients appropriately has been documented in studies on asthma deaths. In particular, a lack of formal assessment including medical history, symptoms and signs, and objective measurements of asthma control and lung function has been noted. Furthermore, confidential inquiries as well as case control studies have concluded there were undue delays in receiving treatment for fatal attacks of asthma.[9,18] Over the last few decades, health professionals in primary care, for example in the United Kingdom, have seen a dramatic increase of workload in terms of patient demand. Furthermore, largely due to changes in funding structure, many sessional or part-time doctors are employed in primary care. As a result, patients experience significant delays in obtaining appointments with their usual doctors, as well as a consequent loss in continuity of care. Finally, undertreatment of acute asthma attacks, especially the failure to use systemic corticosteroids, has been a recurrent theme underlying the conclusions of asthma death studies.[3,7,10,11] Either these drugs are not used at all or they are not used in adequate doses for a long enough duration.

PREVENTING ASTHMA DEATHS IN PRIMARY CARE

Although the nature of general practice varies from country to country, a number of opportunities for identifying asthma patients at risk are evident in most settings. These arise during routine consultations, for conditions other than asthma, where a few carefully planned questions can determine whether someone's asthma is poorly controlled. For example, asking a few questions about the presence of respiratory symptoms in the day or night, and about limitation of activity, can lead to conclusions about the level of asthma control. Similarly, a quick perusal of medical records can assist in determining whether the patient is adhering to medical advice by collecting preventer prescriptions, attending at appropriate intervals for routine review, or being prescribed excess reliever medication. Evidence of consultations with other colleagues in the same practice, attendance of EDs, or admissions to the hospital for asthma will also appear in the record. Accepting that they have an extremely difficult task, with limited time, to deal with all sorts of medical and social problems, health professionals in primary care need to try to move away from an approach that deals only with the patient's presenting symptoms. By identifying patients at risk, in a dynamic ongoing manner, patients' well-being can be improved while decreasing workload through reduction of acute crises in the future.

OPPORTUNITIES FOR INTERVENTION

The advent of computerized record systems in primary care has been extremely positive in some respects, but, as is often the case, the value of the system depends entirely on the quality of information entered by the human operator. Prescribing has certainly been made safer, with alerts on past allergies and potential drug interactions, and also through maintenance of a clear legible record of prescriptions issued. However, medical record entries are often in the form of short coded items without much information describing the underlying rationale for clinical decisions. In essence, many primary care computerized record systems are simply used as a repository for a sometimes very brief record, and the power of using the data dynamically and interactively has not yet been systematically harnessed in routine clinical practice.

Primary care and pharmacy prescription records have been used for years by funders, researchers, and advisers to management, although there is little evidence in the literature that these records are integrated with those in primary care and used dynamically in assessing risk and identifying patients in need of optimization of care. With modern computer systems it should be possible for software to flag certain issues during the consultation. For example, when an asthmatic patient consults, a flag could alert the practitioner to the number of beta$_2$-agonist bronchodilator prescriptions issued in the last year. The system could also display the proportion of inhaled corticosteroid prescriptions to SABAs and LABAs. In the absence of a computer system, a manual record could be organized to provide the same sort of information. For example, a page in the record could be dedicated to each repeat drug prescribed, perhaps a page for each SABA, and one for each inhaled corticosteroid prescribed, numbered and dated so a quick glance will reveal those under- or overusing their drugs. These types of systems could alert the clinician, at the time the patient consults, that further intervention may be needed. Suissa and colleagues[15] noted many years ago that a pattern of increased use of beta$_2$-agonist inhalers was associated with an increased risk of having a life-threatening asthma attack, yet a high proportion of children who died in the last decade from asthma had been prescribed excess SABAs.[10] Ideally, there should be systems for integrating pharmacy records—for example, on dispensing or actual "pick-up rates" by patients collecting medication—with those in primary care (see Chapter 14). Therefore, by implementing systems for recognizing this pattern, general practitioners and pharmacists are uniquely placed to identify people in need of an urgent asthma evaluation. Another example from general practice is that many patients are able to obtain refill prescriptions without seeing a doctor or nurse. A quick perusal of the prescribing history by the doctor, before signing one of these refills, could help identify those who are receiving an excess of SABAs or too few controller medications. These patients could be instructed to make an office appointment when coming to pick up their prescription. Furthermore, in keeping with prescribing advice, those taking LABAs as monotherapy without inhaled corticosteroids could also be identified and told to make an office appointment immediately.

FOCUSED ASTHMA REVIEWS: ACHIEVING AND MAINTAINING CONTROL

Asthma reviews are usually done either as a planned routine assessment or opportunistically when a patient consults for some other reason. The principles of these reviews have been well described in international and national guidelines and should include confirmation of the diagnosis, assessment of asthma control, identification of risk factors particular to that patient, checking of adherence, inhaler technique, optimization of medication, and provision or updating of a personal asthma action plan. All of these subjects are covered in detail throughout this book and some of the practical issues related to primary care are discussed in this chapter.

One of the major criticisms of primary care management of asthma relates to delay and accuracy of diagnosis. Considering that family doctors deal with a multitude of medical and social problems, it is not surprising that these issues exist. The nature of general practice where patients may consult a number of different health professionals from different disciplines at various times results in delayed diagnosis and lack of continuity of care, resulting in variable consistency of advice or treatment. This is further compounded by ever-changing demands on these health professionals by governments and local funding bodies, coupled with an ever-increasing paper mountain of guidelines and cost-cutting directives covering the vast range of disease areas dealt with by these doctors and nurses. Nonetheless, efficient systems do need to be in place to ensure high-quality, safe care of patients, which begins with establishing an accurate diagnosis. Previously, we demonstrated the extraordinary delays that can occur in diagnosing asthma in general practice[19,20] and recommended a few possible solutions.[21] These included searching through past records for clues to the patient's atopic status such as allergic rhinitis and asthma, as well as a record of prescriptions for inhalers whenever an undiagnosed patient consulted with respiratory symptoms. In this way, the "reflex" prescription issue of an antibiotic for presumed acute infection rather than a chronic underlying disease may be resisted. By accurately recording the medical history as well as the rationale for a final diagnosis in the office notes, in the form of a summary or problem-orientated system, future management should improve. If this is done well, health professionals can utilize the records as a valuable resource in deciding on management when patients consult. Furthermore, as many research studies recruit patients from primary care on the basis of "physician-diagnosed asthma," it is important to accurately record the subjective and objective criteria in support of this diagnosis.

Some have suggested setting up asthma "at-risk registers" in primary care. The justification for this would be to prioritize those patients at risk for severe asthma and to reduce workload. This would result in a list of patients that should be more closely monitored and more aggressively treated in the outpatient setting. However, this argument is flawed in a number of ways, particularly since asthma control is a dynamic process and therefore a classification of an asthma sufferer as "at risk" is only valid on the day of assessment. Since asthma may change status from day to day, it is possible for someone to be well controlled one day, and admitted to an intensive care unit for an acute severe attack on another. Therefore, unless there is a dynamic system for updating patients' risk status it may be very dangerous to put some on a register. While it would be a good idea to know about those people with brittle asthma and those that are under the care of specialists for true severe asthma, it is another matter to create a general asthma at-risk register. There is obviously concern that those not on the "at-risk" registers may get substandard care.[10,22] It could be said that all asthmatic people are potentially at risk, given that up to 50% of people who die from asthma and a high proportion of those who have severe attacks are deemed to have had "mild asthma".[12,23,24] In addition to recalling and assessing those patients after they have been treated for acute attacks, systems should be in place to opportunistically identify poorly controlled asthmatics.

Therefore, a dynamic process of assessment is needed when determining the risks to individuals with asthma. The GINA Strategy document[25] was one of the first to focus on assessment of asthma control and risks, with the aim of achieving and maintaining control to prevent asthma attacks. This hypothesis was confirmed in a number of studies. Bateman et al.[26] demonstrated a six-fold increased risk of future asthma exacerbations in people with poorly controlled asthma using the GINA Control Tool. Wei et al. showed that both partly and poorly controlled patients (using the Asthma Control Test) were at risk of having future asthma exacerbations as well as unplanned and emergency visits.[27] Therefore it seems sensible to assess asthma control at every opportunity in the primary care setting.

There is some confusion between the terms "control" and "severity" when classifying asthma patients, which may result in inconsistent care provided for those with this disease, including their current need for treatment and frequency of routine office visit follow-ups. Essentially, chronic severity of asthma relates to the amount of treatment required to achieve symptom control, whereas acute severity is determined by the presence of symptoms, signs, and physiological indices.[25,28,29] Humbert et al.[30] described very clearly the rationale against using "chronic severity" of asthma as a basis for clinical decisions; this is not a static phenomenon and there was limited evidence that severity was of value in predicting the effects of long-term outcomes from treatment. In fact, they recommended periodic assessment of asthma control as more relevant and useful.

There are a number of methods available for assessment of asthma control that include evaluation of symptoms, the effect of the person's asthma on their lifestyle, their use of rescue medication, and lung function measurement. Despite the existence of a number of instruments and tools, including the Asthma Control Test,[31] the GINA Control Tool,[25] the Royal College of Physicians "3 Questions",[32] and the Asthma Control Questionnaire (ACQ),[33] this assessment is not often done routinely in primary care.

It is not enough to assess asthma control. Having determined that a person's asthma is poorly controlled, it is clearly incumbent upon the clinician to then ascertain the possible reason(s) for this and to take appropriate action to gain control. This would include an assessment of adherence to medication and inhaler technique. As described above, the former is fairly straightforward to establish in primary care by simply counting the number of prescriptions issued for SABAs and preventer medication. Thus, providing some information on asthma control (prescription of more than four to six SABA inhalers a year indicates possible poor control) and the proportion of inhaled corticosteroid to SABA prescriptions acts as a surrogate measure for both the clinician's and the patient's adherence to asthma guidelines. Clearly, patients using excess SABAs should be prescribed a preventer medication. Similarly, someone who has had prescriptions for short courses of systemic corticosteroids is possibly at risk for further exacerbations. Of course, while this will establish the number of prescriptions issued, it will not determine whether the medication has been dispensed by a pharmacist or has actually been taken by the person.

Patients unable to use their inhalers (particularly pressurized metered-dose inhalers) should be either taught to do so or prescribed an alternative device.[34,35] This could be in the form of a completely different device or the addition of a spacer inhaler. There is mounting evidence that asthma control is adversely affected by poor inhaler technique and therefore it is vital to ensure that patients can take their medication properly.[36]

RECOGNIZING AND MANAGING ASTHMA ATTACKS IN PRIMARY CARE

Diagnosis of asthma in general practice requires initial recognition and confirmation of the disease, recognition and diagnosis of uncontrolled episodes of asthma, and assessment of the severity of these exacerbations. General practitioners

manage a large variety of conditions in patients presenting to their offices, and it can be sometimes very challenging to identify those developing an asthma exacerbation. While the management of acute asthma exacerbations is detailed elsewhere in this book, the key challenge for the health professional in primary care is to diagnose an asthma attack or exacerbation in a very busy general clinic where most ailments are relatively minor. Therefore, maintaining a high index of suspicion for an impending asthma attack in any patient presenting with respiratory symptoms, regardless of whether or not they had been previously diagnosed with asthma, is essential. While the symptoms may be sudden and associated with overt wheezing, an asthma exacerbation in many patients may be insidious without overt clues to an impending attack. For example, a child who presents with a history from the mother of severe wheezing and coughing during the night may look perfectly well with a clear chest examination. However, the current situation may simply be due to the effect of a high-dose bronchodilator or oral corticosteroids administered during the night if the mother has followed the asthma action plan previously provided. It would be a mistake to send that child home without appropriate advice or management. Similarly it would be a mistake not to take seriously a patient's history of using an excessive amount of short-acting bronchodilator prior to their office visit for respiratory symptoms. A primary care physician, therefore, needs to be very familiar with the natural history and management of asthma exacerbations in order to prevent the development of severe attacks. Clues to developing asthma attacks in primary care need to be detected through a very careful history including a history of reduced effectiveness of reliever drugs; ongoing nighttime symptoms; ongoing respiratory symptoms following a virus infection; and increased variability of peak flow measurements. In those patients with allergic rhinitis, increased symptoms on exposure to indoor or outdoor allergic and nonallergic triggers could herald an asthma exacerbation. Furthermore, an exacerbation could be precipitated on exposure to a variety of environmental triggers in poorly controlled asthma. Therefore, someone with poorly controlled asthma consulting with respiratory symptoms should be treated fairly rigorously. Depending on their reported triggers, consideration should be given for allergy consultation.

The severity of the attack can be determined using the suggested tables from international[25] or local guidelines based on history, examination, oxygen saturation, and vital signs. It is helpful to have a reference copy of these tables in each consulting room. Establishing asthma severity helps the determination whether it is necessary to transfer the patient to secondary care. Clearly someone with an acute severe or life-threatening attack should be transferred to an appropriate facility as soon as possible. In other cases, a system for ongoing assessment during treatment is helpful, to facilitate decisions on management as the situation progresses. The author uses a timed chart detailing vital signs, peak expiratory flow, oxygen saturation, and oxygen flow rates (http://www.consultmarklevy.com/academic_services/other.php).

This information is recorded and can be used to supplement notes sent to the hospital if that decision is taken. This is helpful because many general practitioners have had the experience of sending a patient with acute asthma attack to the hospital after initial treatment, only to find the patient has been discharged home after a short 4 h time span while the acute drugs are still exhibiting an effect. These patients often need to be readmitted. Treatment would include high-dose bronchodilators, systemic corticosteroids, and oxygen. In those patients not admitted to hospital, in addition to a home supply of oral corticosteroids, optimization of treatment, and checking inhaler technique, providing a peak flow meter and diary to enable the patient to monitor progress until the episode has resolved is very beneficial. In this way an informed decision can be made as to when it may be safe to discontinue oral corticosteroids. Follow-up appointments to ensure that the patient is adhering to agreed medical management plans are essential. It is important to communicate the need for more frequent office visits until asthma control can be established.

Follow-Up after Attacks Treated in Primary or Secondary Care

Every patient should be seen by their physician within a few days after an asthma exacerbation. This applies to all exacerbations whether they occur in a primary or secondary care setting, or even where patients have self-treated an attack according to a previously agreed self-management action plan. This is often not done, as evidenced by the numerous studies on near-fatal attacks and in confidential inquiries on asthma deaths where the individuals had suffered a previous attack. The review is an opportunity not only to monitor the person's progress toward satisfactory recovery to optimize treatment, but also to try to identify barriers to adherence and where things may have gone wrong. Asking for and reviewing a peak flow chart helps to reinforce adherent behavior in future. Questions to consider asking include: When did the symptoms start? How bad were they? Was there any response to self-treatment? Did the person have and follow an action plan? Did they try and get an appointment to see the general practitioner or asthma nurse? What happened? Were they seen in an ED or urgent care center? (See Chapter 14 for examples of improving both understanding and improvement of adherence through mutual agreement between the patient and health professional, to reduce future asthma attacks.)

Essentially, by conducting a thorough review after initial treatment, both the health professional and the patient can learn from this experience how to prevent future attacks.

CONCLUSION

Lessons learned from the circumstances surrounding the tragic avoidable deaths due directly or indirectly to poorly controlled asthma provide an extremely rich source of educational information to guide health professionals as well as patients and their families through proper asthma management. Case reviews, medical audit,[37] and participation in confidential inquiries following an acute attack or asthma death provide a method for learning from our patients and improving asthma care overall.

REFERENCES

1. Boulet LP, FitzGerald JM, Levy ML, Cruz AA, Pedersen S, Haahtela T, et al. A guide to the translation of the Global Initiative for Asthma (GINA) strategy into improved care. *Eur Respir J*. 2012;39(5):1220–1229.
2. Bayes HK, Oyeniran O, Shepherd M, Walters M. Clinical audit: Management of acute severe asthma in west Glasgow. *Scot Med J*. 2010;55(1):6–9.
3. British Thoracic A. Death from asthma in two regions. *Br Med J*. 1982;285:1251–1255.
4. Benatar SR, Ainslie GM. Deaths from asthma in Cape Town, 1980–1982. *S Afr Med J*. 1986;69(11):669–671.
5. MacDonald JB, MacDonald ET, Seaton A, Williams DA. Asthma deaths in Cardiff 1963–1974: 53 deaths in hospital. *Br Med J*. 1976;2(6038):721–723.
6. MacDonald JB, Seaton A, Williams DA. Asthma deaths in Cardiff 1963–1974: 90 deaths outside hospital. *Br Med J*. 1976;1(6024):1493–1495.
7. Proceedings of the Asthma Mortality Task Force. November 13–16, 1986, Bethesda, Maryland. *J Allergy Clin Immunol*. 1987;80:361–514.
8. Bucknall CE, Slack R, Godley CC, Mackay TW, Wright SC. Scottish Confidential Inquiry into Asthma Deaths (SCIAD), 1994–1996. *Thorax*. 1999;54(11):978–984.
9. Sturdy PM, Butland BK, Anderson HR, Ayres JG, Bland JM, Harrison BDW, et al. Deaths certified as asthma and use of medical services: A national case-control study. *Thorax*. 2005;60(11):909–915.
10. Harrison B, Stephenson P, Mohan G, Nasser S. An ongoing confidential enquiry into asthma deaths in the Eastern Region of the UK, 2001–2003. *Primary Care Respir J*. 2005;14(6):303–313.
11. Fraser PM, Speizer FE, Waters SDM, Doll R, Mann NM. The circumstances preceding death from asthma in young people in 1968–1969. *Br J Dis Chest*. 1971;65(2):71–84.
12. Anagnostou K, Harrison B, Iles R, Nasser S. Risk factors for childhood asthma deaths from the UK Eastern Region Confidential Enquiry 2001–2006. *Prim Care Respir J*. 2012;21(1):71–77.
13. Wareham NJ, Harrison BDW, Jenkins PF, Nicholls J, Stableforth DE. A district confidential enquiry into deaths due to asthma. *Thorax*. 1993;48(11):1117–1120.
14. Mohan G, Harrison BDW, Badminton RM, Mildenhall S, Wareham NJ. A confidential enquiry into deaths caused by asthma in an English health region: Implications for general practice. *Br J Gen Pract*. 1996;46(410):529–532.
15. Suissa S, Blais L, Ernst P. Patterns of increasing beta-2-agonist use and the risk of fatal or near-fatal asthma. *Eur Respir J*. 1994;7(9):1602–1609.
16. Fletcher HJ, Ibrahim SA, Speight N. Survey of asthma deaths in the Northern region, 1970–85. *Arch Dis Child*. 1990;65(2):163–167.
17. Robertson CF, Rubinfeld AR, Bowes G. Pediatric asthma deaths in Victoria: The mild are at risk. *Pediatr Pulmonol*. 1992;13(2):95–100.

18. Campbell DA, McLennan G, Coates JR, Frith PA, Gluyas PA, Latimer KM, et al. A comparison of asthma deaths and near-fatal asthma attacks in South Australia. *Eur Respir J.* 1994;7(3):490–497.

19. Levy M, Bell L. General practice audit of asthma in childhood. *Br Med J.* 1984;289(6452):1115–1158.

20. Levy M, Parmar M, Coetzee D, Duffy SW. Respiratory consultations in asthmatic compared with non-asthmatic children in general practice. *Br Med J.* 1985;291(6487):29–30.

21. Levy M. Delay in diagnosing asthma: Is the nature of general practice to blame? *J R Coll Gen Pract.* 1986;36(283):52–53.

22. Levy ML. Obtaining outcome data on asthma management: The UK national review of asthma deaths. *Prim Care Respir J.* 2012;21(1):18.

23. Fabbri LM, Stoloff S. Is mild asthma really 'mild'? *Int J Clin Pract.* 2005;59(6):692–703.

24. Robertson CF, Bishop J, Dalton M, Caust J, Nolan TM, Olinsky A, et al. Prevalence of asthma in regional victorian schoolchildren [see comments]. *Med J Aust.* 1992;156(12):831–833.

25. The Global Strategy for Asthma Management and Prevention, Global Initiative for Asthma (GINA). Updated 2011. Available from: http://www.ginasthma.org. Last accessed 2011.

26. Bateman ED, Reddel HK, Eriksson G, Peterson S, Ostlund O, Sears MR, et al. Overall asthma control: The relationship between current control and future risk. *J Allergy Clin Immunol.* 2010;125(3):600–608.e6.

27. Wei H, Zhou T, Wang L, Zhang H, Fu J, Ji Y, et al. Current asthma control predicts future risk of asthma exacerbation: A 12-month prospective cohort study. *Chinese Med J.* 2012;125(17):2986–2993.

28. Reddel HK, Taylor DR, Bateman ED, Boulet LP, Boushey HA, Busse WW, et al. An official American Thoracic Society/European Respiratory Society statement: Asthma control and exacerbations: Standardizing endpoints for clinical asthma trials and clinical practice. *Am J Respir Crit Care Med.* 2009;180(1):59–99.

29. Taylor DR, Bateman ED, Boulet LP, Boushey HA, Busse WW, Casale TB, et al. A new perspective on concepts of asthma severity and control. *Eur Respir J.* 2008;32(3):545–554.

30. Humbert M, Holgate S, Boulet LP, Bousquet J. Asthma control or severity: That is the question. *Allergy: Eur J Allergy Clin Immunol.* 2007;62(2):95–101.

31. Nathan RA, Sorkness CA, Kosinski M, Schatz M, Li JT, Marcus P, et al. Development of the Asthma Control Test: A survey for assessing asthma control. *J Allergy Clin Immunol.* 2004;113(1):59–65.

32. Pearson MG, Bucknall CE (eds.). *Measuring Clinical Outcome in Asthma: A Patient Focused Approach.* London: Royal College of Physicians, 1999.

33. Juniper EF, O'Byrne PM, Guyatt GH, Ferrie PJ, King DR. Development and validation of a questionnaire to measure asthma control. *Eur Respir J.* 1999;14(4):902–907.

34. Crompton GK. Problems patients have using pressurized aerosol inhalers. *Eur J Respir Dis.* 1982;63(Suppl. 119):101–104.

35. Lavorini F, Levy ML, Corrigan C, Crompton G, on behalf of the AWG. The ADMIT series: Issues in inhalation therapy. (6) Training tools for inhalation devices. *Primary Care Respir J.* 2010;19(4):335–341.

36. Levy ML, Hardwell A, McKnight E, Holmes J. Asthma patients' inability to use a pressurised metered-dose inhaler (pMDI) correctly correlates with poor asthma control as defined by the Global Initiative for Asthma (GINA) strategy: A retrospective analysis. *Prim Care Respir J.* 2013. Available from http://dx.doi.org/10.4104/pcrj.2013.00084.

37. A system for doing medical audit. www.guideline-audit.com (in particular the one on acute asthma exacerbation management based on the GINA Strategy document, www.ginasthma.org). Accessed 21 September 2013.

Index